Ghazanfar Khadim, MD
FACC, FSCAI
8/13/2010

Ghazanfar Khadim, MD
FACC, FSCAI
8/13/2010

Transcatheter Closure of ASDs and PFOs

A Comprehensive Assessment

Transcatheter Closure of ASDs and PFOs

A Comprehensive Assessment

Ziyad M. Hijazi, MD, MPH, FSCAI, FACC, FAAP
Director of the Rush Center for Congenital and Structural Heart Disease, Pediatric Cardiology Section Chief, and Professor of Pediatrics and Internal Medicine, Rush University Medical Center, Chicago, Illinois

Ted Feldman, MD, FSCAI, FACC, FESC
Director of the Cardiac Catheterization Laboratory, NorthShore University HealthSystem–Evanston Hospital, Evanston, Illinois

Mustafa H. Abdullah Al-Qbandi, MD, DCH, FAAP, FRCPC, FAAC, FSCAI
Consultant Pediatrician, Pediatric Cardiologist, and Head of Pediatric Cardiology Unit, Chest Diseases Hospital, Kuwait Cardiac Centre, Kuwait

Horst Sievert, MD, FSCAI, FACC, FESC, FICA
Director of the CardioVascular Center Frankfurt, Sankt Katharinen Hospital, Frankfurt; Director of the Department of Internal Medicine, Cardiology and Vascular Medicine, Sankt Katharinen Hospital, Frankfurt; Professor of Medicine, Johann Wolfgang Goethe University, Frankfurt, Germany

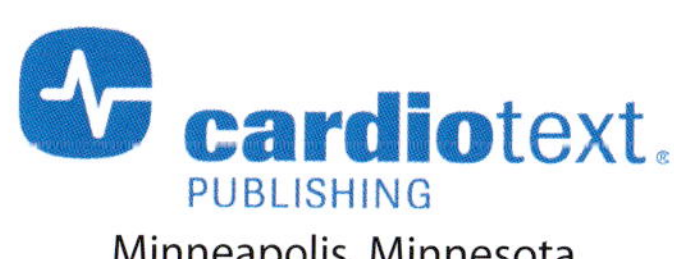

cardiotext PUBLISHING
Minneapolis, Minnesota

Cardiotext Publishing, LLC
3405 W. 44th Street
Minneapolis, MN 55410
USA

www.cardiotextpublishing.com

Any updates to this book may be found at: www.cardiotextpublishing.com/titles/detail/9780979016493

Supplemental video content for this book may be found at: www.cardiotextpublishing.com/sites/transcatheter-closure/

Devices on the front cover (left to right): AMPLATZER Septal Occluder, AGA Medical Corporation; BioSTAR Septal Occluder, NMT Medical, Inc.; GORE HELEX Septal Occluder, W.L. Gore & Associates; Figulla Flex, Occlutech; Coherex FlatStent EF, Coherex Medical, Inc. All devices are reprinted with permission. All rights reserved.

Comments, inquiries, and requests for bulk sales can be directed to the publisher at: info@cardiotextpublishing.com.

Unless otherwise stated, all figures and tables in this book are used courtesy of the authors.

♾ Printed on acid-free paper.

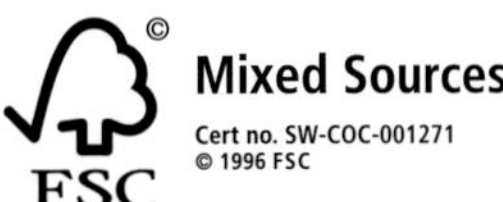

This book is printed on 100% FSC-certified paper from well-managed forests, where people, wildlife, and the environment benefit from the forestry practices. Forest Stewardship Council certification is globally recognized for ensuring well-managed forests.

Cover and book design by Zan Ceeley, Trio Bookworks

Library of Congress Control Number: 2010924349

ISBN-13: 978-0-9790164-9-3

Printed in Canada

15   14   13   12   11   10   1   2   3   4   5   6   7   8   9   10

Contents

■ Part I: Anatomy, Pathophysiology, and Natural History

■ Part IV: Devices

EDITORS

Ziyad M. Hijazi MD, MPH, FSCAI, FACC, FAAP
Director of the Rush Center for Congenital and Structural Heart Disease, Pediatric Cardiology Section Chief, and Professor of Pediatrics and Internal Medicine, Rush University Medical Center, Chicago, Illinois

Ted Feldman MD, FSCAI, FACC, FESC
Director of the Cardiac Catheterization Laboratory, NorthShore University HealthSystem–Evanston Hospital, Evanston, Illinois

Mustafa H. Abdullah Al-Qbandi MD, DCH, FAAP, FRCPC, FAAC, FSCAI
Consultant Pediatrician, Pediatric Cardiologist, and Head of Pediatric Cardiology Unit, Chest Diseases Hospital, Kuwait Cardiac Centre, Kuwait

Horst Sievert MD, FSCAI, FACC, FESC, FICA
Director of the CardioVascular Center Frankfurt, Sankt Katharinen Hospital, Frankfurt; Director of the Department of Internal Medicine, Cardiology and Vascular Medicine, Sankt Katharinen Hospital, Frankfurt; Professor of Medicine, Johann Wolfgang Goethe University, Frankfurt, Germany

CONTRIBUTORS

Wail Alkashkari MD
Rush Center for Congenital and Structural Heart Disease, Rush University Medical Center, Chicago, Illinois

Zahid Amin MD

Professor of Pediatrics, and Director of Cardiac Catheterization and Hybrid Suites, Rush Center for Congenital and Structural Heart Disease, Rush University Medical Center, Chicago, Illinois

Stephan Baldus MD

Department of Cardiology, University Heart Center, University Medical Center Hamburg-Eppendorf, Hamburg, Germany

Prof. Felix Berger MD

Director of the Department of Congenital Heart Disease/Pediatric Cardiology, German Heart Institute Berlin and Charité–Medical University Berlin, Germany

Stefan Bertog MD

CardioVascular Center Frankfurt, Germany

Qi-Ling Cao MD

Associate Professor, and Director of Echocardiography Research Laboratory, Rush Center for Congenital and Structural Heart Disease, Section of Cardiology, Department of Pediatrics, Rush University Medical Center, Chicago, Illinois

John D. Carroll MD

Professor of Medicine, University of Colorado, Denver; Director of Interventional Cardiology and Medical Director of Cardiac and Vascular Center, University of Colorado Hospital, Denver, Colorado

Mehmet Cilingiroglu MD, FESC, FACC, FSCAI

NorthShore University HealthSystem–Evanston Hospital, Evanston, Illinois

John D. Coulson MD

Clinical Associate, Division of Pediatric Cardiology, Department of Pediatrics, Johns Hopkins University, Baltimore, Maryland

Lisa C. A. D'Alessandro MD

Division of Cardiology, The Children's Hospital of Philadelphia, Philadelphia, Pennsylvania

Pedro J. del Nido MD

William E. Ladd Professor and Chairman of the Department of Cardiac Surgery, Children's Hospital–Boston, Harvard Medical School, Boston, Massachusetts

Carol A. Devellian BS

Vice President, Research and Development, NMT Medical, Inc., Boston, Massachusetts

Thomas Doyle MD

Ann and Monroe Carell Jr. Family Associate Professor of Pediatrics, Vanderbilt University; Clinical Director of the Division of Pediatric Cardiology; Monroe Carell Jr. Children's Hospital at Vanderbilt, Nashville, Tennessee

Matthew Egan MD

Heart Center, Nationwide Children's Hospital, Columbus, Ohio

Peter Ewert MD, PhD

Deputy Director of the Department of Congenital Heart Disease/Pediatric Cardiology, and Head of the Catheterization Laboratory, German Heart Institute Berlin; Department of Pediatric Cardiology, Pediatric Intensive Care, Congenital Heart Diseases in Adults, Senior Lecturer, Department of Pediatrics, Otto Heubner Center for Pediatric and Adolescent Medicine, Charité–Medical University Berlin, Germany

Gregory A. Fleming MD, MSCI
Clinical Instructor, Division of Pediatric Cardiology, Monroe Carell Jr. Children's Hospital at Vanderbilt, Nashville, Tennessee

Mark A. Fogel MD, FACC, FAHA, FAAP
Associate Professor of Cardiology and Radiology; Director of Cardiac Magnetic Resonance, Division of Cardiology, The Children's Hospital of Philadelphia, University of Pennsylvania School of Medicine, Philadelphia, Pennsylvania

Thomas J. Forbes MD, FSCAI, FACC
Associate Professor, Carman and Ann Adams Department of Pediatrics, and Director of the Cardiac Catheterization Laboratory, Wayne State University School of Medicine, Children's Hospital of Michigan, Detroit, Michigan

Jennifer Franke MD
CardioVascular Center Frankfurt, Germany

Olaf Franzen MD
Department of Cardiology, University Heart Center, University Medical Center Hamburg-Eppendorf, Hamburg, Germany

Franz Freudenthal MD
Department of Pediatric Cardiology, Kardiozentrum, La Paz, Bolivia

Thomas P. Graham Jr. MD
Emeritus Professsor, Pediatric Heart Institute, Thomas P. Graham Jr. Division of Pediatric Cardiology, Monroe Carell Jr. Children's Hospital at Vanderbilt, Nashville, Tennessee

Miguel Granja MD
Chief of the Interventional Cardiology Laboratory at the Pedro de Elizalde Children's Hospital of Buenos Aires; Chief of Interventional Cardiology in Congenital Heart Disease Laboratories, Heart Institute of the Italian Hospital of Buenos Aires; Associate Professor, University of Buenos Aires, Argentina.

William E. Hellenbrand MD
Director of the Division of Pediatric Cardiology, Columbia College of Physicians and Surgeons, Morgan Stanley Children's Hospital of New York–Presbyterian, New York

Ralf J. Holzer MD, MSc, FSCAI
Assistant Director of the Cardiac Catheterization & Interventional Therapy, The Heart Center, Nationwide Children's Hospital, Columbus, Ohio; Associate Professor of Pediatrics, The Ohio State University School of Medicine, Columbus, Ohio

Sonya Joy
CardioVascular Center Frankfurt, Germany

Terry Dean King MD
Director of Pediatrics, St. Francis Medical Center, Monroe, Louisiana; Clinical Professor of Pediatrics, LSU School of Medicine; Clinical Professor of Pediatrics, Tulane School of Medicine, New Orleans, Louisiana

Stephanie M. Kladakis PhD
Program Manager, NMT Medical, Inc., Boston, Massachusetts

Ryan Ko MBBS, MPCP
Adult Congenital Heart Disease Unit, Royal Brompton Hospital, London, United Kingdom

Paul Kramer MD, FACC, FSCAI
Director of the Cardiac Catheterization Laboratory, Liberty Regional Cardiac and Vascular Center, Liberty Hospital, Liberty, Missouri

Larry A. Latson MD
Center for Pediatric and Congenital Heart Diseases, Children's Hospital, Cleveland Clinic, Cleveland, Ohio

Trong-Phi Lê MD
Head of Pediatric Catheterization Laboratory, Vice Director of the Department of Pediatric Cardiology, Heart Center, University of Hamburg, Germany

Tina Lehr
CardioVascular Center Frankfurt, Germany

Nicolas Majunke MD
CardioVascular Center Frankfurt, Germany; Heart Center, Department of Internal Medicine/Cardiology, University of Leipzig, Leipzig, Germany

Noel L. Mills MD
Clinical Professor of Surgery, Tulane School of Medicine, New Orleans, Louisiana

Tarek S. Momenah MBBS, DCH, FAAP, FRCPC, FACC
Senior Consultant and Director of Pediatric Cardiology Department, Prince Sultan Cardiac Center, Riyadh, Kingdom of Saudi Arabia

John W. Moore MD, MPH
Professor of Pediatrics, Pediatric Cardiology Section Chief, Department of Pediatrics, University of California–San Diego School of Medicine; Director of the Division of Cardiology, Rady Children's Hospital, San Diego, California

Michael J. Mullen MD, FRCP
Lead for Structural Heart Intervention, Consultant Cardiologist, The Heart Hospital, University College Hospital, NHS Foundation Trust, London, United Kingdom

Steven W. Opolski MS
Senior Technical Consultant, NMT Medical, Inc., Boston, Massachusetts

Akash R. Patel MD
Division of Cardiology, The Children's Hospital of Philadelphia, Philadelphia, Pennsylvania

Robert A. Quaife MD
Director of Advanced Cardiac Imaging; Associate Professor of Medicine and Radiology, Cardiac and Vascular Center, University of Colorado, Denver, Colorado

Kristina Renkhoff
CardioVascular Center Frankfurt, Germany

Anas Salkini MD
Senior Interventional Pediatric Cardiology Fellow, Section of Cardiology, Department of Pediatrics, University of California–San Diego School of Medicine, Rady Children's Hospital, San Diego, California

Girish S. Shirali MBBS, FACC, FASE
Professor, Departments of Pediatrics and Obstetrics/Gynecology; Vice-Chairman for Fellowship Education, Department of Pediatrics; Director of Pediatric Echocardiography; Director of Pediatric Cardiology Fellowship Training, Medical University of South Carolina, Charleston, South Carolina

Basilios E. Sideris BS (Biomedical Engineering)
Athenian Institute of Pediatric Cardiology, Athens, Greece

Eleftherios B. Sideris MD
Director of the Athenian Institute of Pediatric Cardiology, Athens, Greece

Jonathan Tobis MD
Director of Interventional Cardiology, UCLA Medical Center; Professor of Medicine, David Geffen School of Medicine at the University of California, Los Angeles (UCLA), California

Sara M. Trucco MD
Pediatric Interventional Catheterization Fellow, Columbia College of Physicians and Surgeons, Morgan Stanley Children's Hospital of New York–Presbyterian, New York

Daniel R. Turner MD, FAAP, FACC
Associate Professor, Carman and Ann Adams Department of Pediatrics, Wayne State University School of Medicine; Interventional Cardiologist, Children's Hospital of Michigan, Detroit, Michigan

Nikolay V. Vasilyev MD
Staff Scientist, Department of Cardiac Surgery, Children's Hospital–Boston; Instructor in Surgery, Division of Surgery, Harvard Medical School, Boston, Massachusetts

Swarnendra Verma MD
Division of Interventional Cardiology, UCLA Medical Center, David Geffen School of Medicine at the University of California, Los Angeles

Paul M. Weinberg MD, FAAP, FACC
Director of the Fellowship Training Program in Pediatric Cardiology, Senior Cardiologist, and Professor of Pediatrics and Pediatric Pathology and Laboratory Medicine, The Children's Hospital of Philadelphia, University of Pennsylvania School of Medicine, Philadelphia, Pennsylvania

John A. Wright Jr. MS
Director of Research and Development, NMT Medical, Inc., Boston, Massachusetts

Nina Wunderlich MD
CardioVascular Center Frankfurt, Germany

Sinai C. Zyblewski MD
Assistant Professor, Pediatric Cardiology, Medical University of South Carolina, Charleston, South Carolina

Charles E. Mullins, MD

Professor Emeritus of Pediatrics, Baylor College of Medicine, Houston, Texas

REFLECTING ON MY OWN 49-YEAR CAREER as a pediatric cardiologist, it is hard to comprehend what has been achieved in the repair of atrial septal defects (ASDs) during that period of time. While still in medical school, I had the privilege of witnessing a very new and exciting "open heart" surgical closure of an ASD. This was accomplished using the new technique of hypothermic cardiac arrest (ice in a bathtub). At the time, this intracardiac repair was undoubtedly revolutionary, but the actual procedure seemed barbaric, too. Even as a medical student, I knew there had to be a better way. By the time I began my cardiology residency a few years later, cardiopulmonary bypass had become almost routine. With that, the surgical repair of ASDs already was being considered a simple and low-risk procedure. But, in addition to the risks of the early bypass procedures, it still required opening the chest and the heart, which, at the very least, was quite uncomfortable for the patient, the parents, and the physicians caring for them.

In 1966, Dr. William J. Rashkind published his paper on the improbable procedure of using a catheter with a balloon at its tip for the *creation* of ASDs in very sick infants *in the catheterization laboratory*. This procedure was to replace the high-risk, "closed" surgical procedure that was used for the same palliation. The Rashkind septostomy procedure saved thousands of infants' lives, but of probably equal importance, it stimulated the creative imagination of many pediatric cardiologists. If we could create defects in the septum with a catheter, why couldn't we close cardiac defects with a catheter delivered device? Early and fairly crude devices for closure of the patent ductus appeared almost immediately. But the dream for a catheter-delivered device for atrial septal defects was not realized, even in its most rudimentary form, for almost another decade. Once demonstrated to be feasible, the procedures and devices for catheter-delivered device closure of ASDs evolved into the standard of care over the next three decades.

Transcatheter Closure of ASDs and PFOs: A Comprehensive Assessment provides a comprehensive view of the long and arduous course taken in order to progress from the surgical repair of secundum ASDs, to the early devices, and finally to the more sophisticated catheter devices and procedures, which we now take for granted. It also extensively covers the technical aspect of the earlier as well as the very latest devices along with the details of the procedures for implanting them and the particular advantages and problems of each device.

Considering the progress that has occurred in catheter closure of ASDs since the 1970s, it is hard to imagine that, in the ensuing three or four decades, there could possibly be comparable advances in the management of ASDs. But, although we now have effective and safe catheter-delivered devices applicable for almost 80% of atrial defects, the goal of the perfect device/procedure still leaves much to be accomplished in the future. The ultimate catheter-delivered atrial septal occlusion device will have to be simple to implant, delivered through an even smaller catheter system, preferably leave no residual or permanent foreign material in the body, and have no real or potential risks to the patient.

For the practitioner today, this book presents a wealth of practical material that is invaluable for the current management of ASDs and provides a glimpse into the future of treating them.

INTEREST IN THE ATRIAL SEPTAL DEFECT (ASD) and patent foramen ovales (PFOs) was sparked in the mid-1970s when Terry D. King, MD, an interventional cardiologist, and Noel Mills, MD, a cardiac surgeon, performed the first transcatheter closure of an ASD on a 17-year-old female. Since that time, interventional congenital cardiologists have been on a mission: to create devices and procedures that enable physicians to close defects in the atrial septum as effectively as our colleagues in surgery do, and of course without the morbidity of open surgery.

When Steven Korn from Cardiotext Publishing approached us to write a book, we were not sure what to write about. We have edited a few books in the past related to different topics in congenital and structural heart disease intervention. But while we were discussing the project, we were surprised to realize that there is no book dedicated to the atrial septum at all. Therefore, the idea of writing such a book was born.

We have assembled the best of the best to contribute to this exciting project, organizing their work in four sections that comprehensively present the most important areas of knowledge for today's practitioners.

Part I discusses anatomy, pathophysiology, and natural history. We believe that every physician treating patients with ASDs and PFOs should have full knowledge of the anatomy, pathophysiology, and natural history of the disease process. Part II addresses imaging of the septum and the assessment of the defects, reviewing all of the imaging modalities, from transthoracic and transesophageal echocardiography to computed tomography and magnetic resonance imaging of the septum. Part III focuses on the technical aspects of closure of ASDs and PFOs. Each chapter discusses in detail specific technical details encountered in clinical practice. And part IV examines the devices available to interventional cardiologists. We made every attempt to include all available devices. If a device was not mentioned, this was not intentional. Also, we were as careful as possible to be fair when providing details about the most commonly used devices.

We hope that you will enjoy reading this book, and we know that you will glean information that will help you take care of your patients.

We would like to thank all of our patients. It is from them that we collect images for teaching ourselves to be better doctors.

Finally, we would like to give a big thank you to Steven Korn, Mike Crouchet, and Caitlin Crouchet with Cardiotext Publishing and to Zan Ceeley with Trio Bookworks for keeping us on time and providing us with the best support to achieve this project.

—Ziyad M. Hijazi,
Ted Feldman,
Mustafa H. Abdullah al-Qbandi,
and Horst Sievert

I want to thank Steve Korn, Mike Crouchet, and Caitlin Crouchet from Cardiotext Publishing for their efforts in pushing hard for this book. I would like to thank and dedicate this book to all my patients all over the world with ASDs and PFOs who I treated over the years—you have taught me what I know today. I want to thank my family for their support during the writing of this book and throughout my professional career, which would have been impossible without their help, dedication, and understanding. Finally, I want to thank Dr. Charles "Chuck" Mullins for agreeing to write the foreword. Dr. Mullins has been a great friend for many years and his contributions to our field are seen every day in our catheterization laboratories.

ZH

Special thanks to our patients, who have formed the basis of our experience. A great cath lab axiom says, "Good judgment comes from experience, and experience comes from bad judgment." One of the best outcomes from this book that we can hope for is the sharing of experience and a contribution to procedure decision making for many of our colleagues that comes without the expense of too many difficult procedures. Shared learning in the interventional community is transmitted in many forms, and we hope this book and the collected knowledge and experience it contains will be among them.

TF

I would like to express my gratitude to the staff at Hospital for Sick Children in Toronto, who taught me the essentials of pediatric cardiology. It was my great fortune to have a chance to work with Dr. Robert M. Freedom and Dr. Jeff Smallhorn, who played a key role in upgrading my academic career as a pediatric cardiologist, from resident to staff position, during the period of 1995–2001. During my career in Kuwait, I came to know Professor Ziyad M. Hijazi, who used to help us in some difficult interventional cases during his many visits to Kuwait. I would like to very much thank Professor Hijazi for his continuous teaching and giving me a chance in being one of the editors of this book. Finally, I would like to thank my wife and children, for their patience and consideration, and to dedicate this book to my mother and father. My family's love and support during this endeavor has been of the utmost importance.

MHAQ

Dr. Ziyad M. Hijazi suggested that we all should write a paragraph of acknowledgment. My initial thought was that it would not be appropriate to thank our families in this kind of book. However, Ziyad replied "of course you can thank your family! I did!"

So I take this opportunity to thank my family, my children Niko, Inga, Eiko, and Kolja, and especially my lovely wife, Nicola, not only for their help regarding this book but for their patience and continuous support over the years.

HS

PART I

Anatomy, Pathophysiology, and Natural History

Anatomy of the Atrial Septum

Akash R. Patel, Lisa C. A. D'Alessandro, and Paul M. Weinberg

Normal Atrial Septal Embryology and Anatomy

The atrial septum is composed largely of the septum primum and septum secundum. The septum primum has its embryological origin from the atrial roof and migrates anteriorly and somewhat inferiorly toward the endocardial cushions. The space between the crescent-like septum primum and the atrioventricular endocardial cushions is the embryonic ostium primum. The most superior aspect of the septum primum forms a half-moon shape with the two ends typically attaching to the left side of the septum secundum. During the growth of the septum, the space between the two septa constitutes the ostium secundum. Once the septum primum attaches to the septum secundum, this space becomes the foramen ovale. The inferior portion of the septum primum is contiguous with the vestibular spine, a structure that originates from the right pulmonary ridge and provides for the joining of the septum primum with the endocardial cushions and the closure of ostium primum. This region becomes muscularized and transitions to the gossamer valve of the fossa ovalis, viz., septum primum.

Septum secundum forms as an infolding of the roof of the atria at the point of indentation by the embryonic truncus, to the right of the septum primum.[1] As will be discussed later, in certain cases the septum secundum may be very shallow or nonexistent and may not be adjacent to the septum primum. The leading edge of the septum secundum becomes the superior limbus of the fossa ovalis and normally allows apposition of the valve of fossa ovalis and therefore

Transcatheter Closure of ASDs and PFOs: A Comprehensive Assessment. © 2010 Ziyad M. Hijazi, Ted Feldman, Mustafa H. Abdullah Al-Qbandi, and Horst Sievert, editors. Cardiotext Publishing, ISBN: 978-0-9790164-9-3.

functional closure of the ostium secundum (foramen ovale). Thus the foramen ovale (or fossa ovalis), between these structures, is not a true deficiency in the atrial septum but rather an interatrial communication, which is vital in prenatal circulation. The atrial septation nears completion by 3 months gestation; although in most cases the septum primum is cellophane-like until the end of gestation or even after birth, with muscularization continuing postnatally (Fig 1.1).

Anatomically, the atrial septum is composed of an interatrial portion, dividing the left and right atrium, and an atrioventricular portion, dividing the right atrium and left ventricle.[1,2] The interatrial portion is composed of septum primum, septum secundum, and part of the atrioventricular canal septum. The interatrial portion measures 4- to 8-mm thick in adolescents and adults except for the valve of the fossa ovalis, which measures 1 mm in thickness.[3] The atrioventricular portion is composed of the atrioventricular canal septum. The muscular portion of the atrioventricular septum measures approximately 10 mm in thickness, and the membranous portion measures 1 mm.[3] With age, the atrial septum thickens and anatomic sealing of the patent foramen ovale occurs in two-thirds of patients[4,5] (Fig 1.2).

Structures adjacent to the septum are important when considering atrial septal anatomy.[1,3,4] Anterosuperiorly, septum secundum abuts the right aortic sinus of Valsalva. The atrioventricular portion of the atrial septum lies anteroinferiorly and adjacent to the septal leaflet of the tricuspid valve and the right coronary–noncoronary aortic commissure. This region contains the atrioventricular node. Consideration should also be given to the systemic venous connections, right pulmonary veins, coronary sinus, and eustachian valve when determining atrial septal interventions.

Patent Foramen Ovale

As mentioned before, the patent foramen ovale is a gap between the septum secundum, which forms the limbus of the fossa ovalis, and septum primum, which forms the flap valve that covers the fossa ovalis.[1,6,7] Based on autopsy studies, the patent foramen ovale is circular to elliptical in shape and located in the anterosuperior portion of the atrial septum. The patent foramen ovale diameter ranges from 1 to 19 mm with a mean of 4.9 mm.[8] The patent foramen ovale length, also referred to as the tunnel length, ranges from 3 to 18 mm with a mean of 8 mm.[7] Both the diameter and length increase with age but not

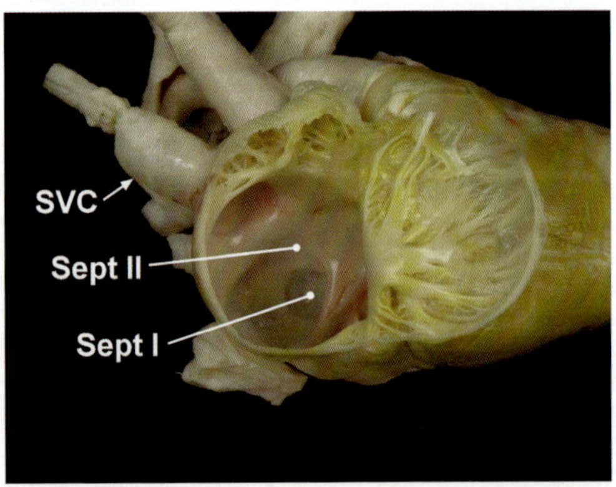

Fig 1.1A—Right atrial view of atrial septum in an infant. Septum primum (Sept I) is the thin flap valve of the foramen ovale, which closes against the thick muscular septum secundum (Sept II). Sept II is medial to the entrance of the superior vena cava (SVC).

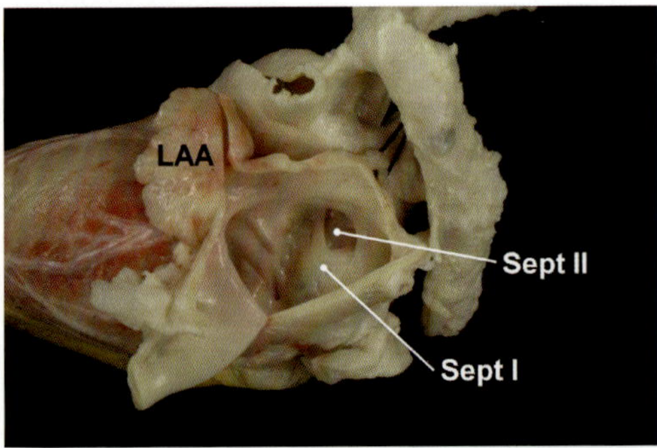

Fig 1.1B—Left atrial view of atrial septum in an infant. Note the half-moon shape of the superior margin of Sept I as it attaches to Sept II. This is the location of the foramen ovale. Abbreviation: LAA, left atrial appendage.

body surface area. The mean diameter is 3.4 mm in the first decade of life and 5.8 mm in the 10th decade of life.[8] It is important to note that there are limited evaluations on size correlation between those based on pathologic specimens and those obtained by echocardiography and balloon sizing.

The effective size of the foramen ovale is not only dependent on the size of the space between the two septal components but also the degree of valvar competency.[9] Valvar competency occurs when there is appropriate apposition of the valve of the fossa ovalis and septum secundum to completely cover the foramen ovale. There can be valvar incompetency in three scenarios. First, stretching of the superior limbus of the fossa ovalis seen in atrial dilation leads to a lack of apposition with the valve of fossa ovalis. Second, aneurysmal formation of the septum primum prevents complete closure of the interatrial communication. Third, the patent foramen ovale can be associated with deficiencies of septum primum, resulting in a true secundum ASD.

When choosing the correct closure device, consider the mechanism of the interatrial communication and the relationship of the patent foramen ovale to its surrounding structures. The patent foramen is located in the superior portion of the atrial septum.[8] The crescentic superior boundary of the foramen is the superior limbus of the fossa ovalis—the muscular septum secundum.[6] There is no true inferior boundary as mentioned because this defect is a flap-valve communication that creates a tunneled interatrial communication.[10] However, the superior margin of the septum primum has a rather consistent half-moon shape that forms the lower boundary of the foramen ovale. Based on an autopsy study, the average distance from the patent foramen ovale to the superior vena cava is 12.2 mm and 8.1 mm to the aortic annulus.[7] These measurements did not increase with age but rather with increasing body surface area.[7]

Ostium Secundum ASD

Ostium secundum atrial septal defects (ASDs) are the most common ASDs. The defects are due to deficiency in septum primum or, rarely, an "unguarded" foramen ovale from deficiency in septum secundum.

The vast majority of these defects are a complete absence (Fig 1.3), deficiency (Figs 1.4 and 1.5), or multiple fenestrations of septum primum (Figs 1.6 and 1.7).[11–13] When the fossa ovalis valve is absent, the defect is typically circular. The superior limbus forms the superior and posterosuperior boundaries of the defect. The absence of the fossa ovalis valve may result

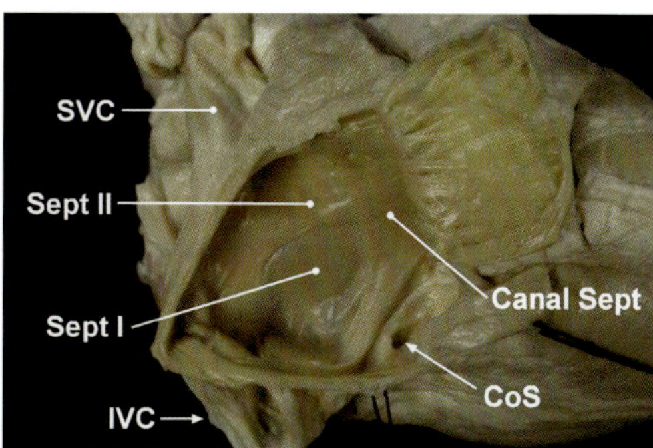

Fig 1.2A—Right atrial view of mature atrial septum. Sept I is thick and muscularized. The superior margin as seen from the right atrial side is the fossa ovalis. Sept II covers Sept I. Between Sept I and the atrioventricular valve is the canal septum (Canal Sept). Abbreviations: CoS, coronary sinus ostium; IVC, inferior vena cava.

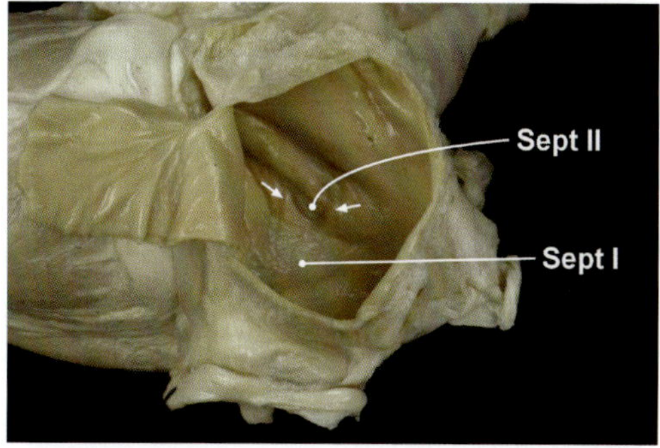

Fig 1.2B—Left atrial view of mature atrial septum. Even though the foramen ovale is sealed, the two attachments of Sept I to Sept II (arrows) with the intervening half-moon shape of the superior margin of Sept I are easily visible.

in shallow posteroinferior and inferior rims. The atrial floor between the superior limbus and the atrioventricular septum does however form an anterior ridge. With deficiency of the valve of the fossa ovalis, the ASD is typically elliptical in shape and centrally located but can assume almost any shape or location within septum primum. The rims include the remaining septum primum plus septum secundum superiorly and posteriorly, the canal septum anteriorly, and septum primum plus left venous valve of the inferior vena cava inferiorly. Similarly, fenestrations can be variable and located anywhere in the contiguous septum primum, which can result in variable amounts of rim. In situations in which either atrium is dilated, septum primum may become stretched, while the two main attachments on either side of the half-moon shaped superior edge remain fixed. This stretching of septum primum results in incompetence of the fossa ovalis valve, and may be considered the "foramen ovale" type of ostium secundum ASD without there being frank deficiency of septum primum.

A rare cause of an ostium secundum ASD is complete absence or incomplete development of the superior limbus of septum secundum, typically in association with left-sided juxtaposition of the atrial appendages.[11-13] The superior limbus from posterosuperior to anterosuperior is underdeveloped or absent because of the marked rightward position of the great arteries (which normally indent the roof of the atria and initiate the infolding, which results in septum secundum). Not only does the absence or shallow nature of septum secundum result in the inability to form the flap-valve mechanism of the fossa ovalis, but in many cases, septum primum is deviated markedly to the left with its superior portion positioned horizontally with attachment to the left lateral atrial wall between the two juxtaposed appendages. This results in an ASD located in the half-moon–shaped septum primum between the right atrium, superiorly, and the left atrium, inferiorly. What would have been the superior rim is insufficient and formed by the lateral atrial wall. The posteroinferior, inferior, and anteroinferior rims are sufficient and formed by the valve of the fossa ovalis.

The secundum ASD type, size, and shape can vary greatly. It is important to note that all these defects involve the fossa ovalis and do not include the vena cava, right pulmonary veins, coronary sinus, or atrioventricular valves. However, relationships to these structures remain important when considering device closure.[3,5] Identification of the enface anatomic rims viewed from the right atrial surface are defined as follows[14]: the posterosuperior rim is the distance to the superior vena cava, the anterosuperior rim is the distance to the aorta, the posteroinferior rim is the distance to the inferior vena cava, the anteroinferior rim is the distance to the tricuspid valve. Other

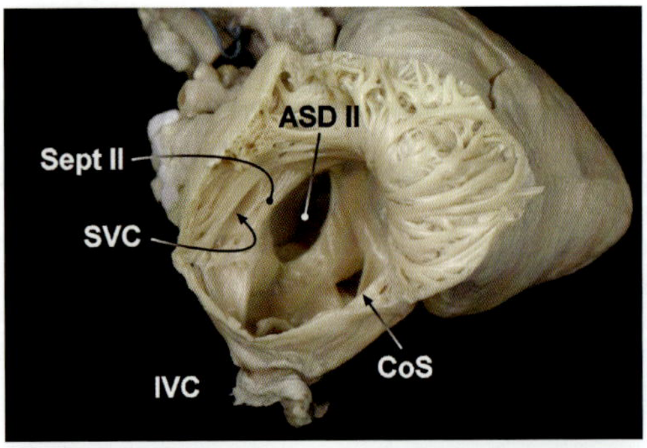

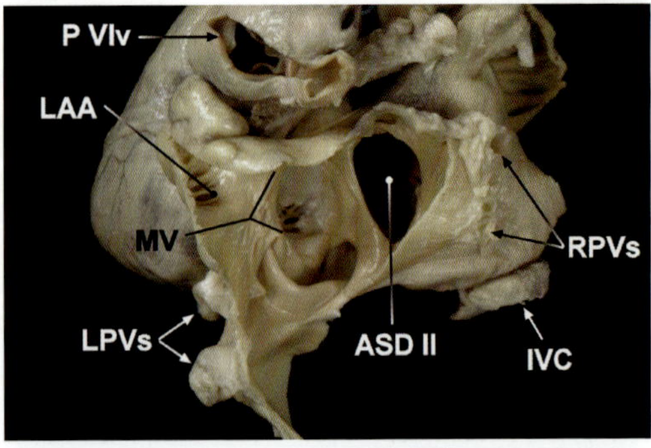

Fig 1.3A—Right atrial view of large ostium secundum atrial septal defect (ASD II). Sept II forms the superior margin of the defect and the canal septum the anterior margin. Variable amounts of inferior and posterior rims are present.

Fig 1.3B—Left atrial view of same defect. Note the relationship of the defect to the right (RPVs) and left pulmonary veins (LPVs) and to the mitral valve (MV).
Abbreviation: P Vlv, pulmonary valve.

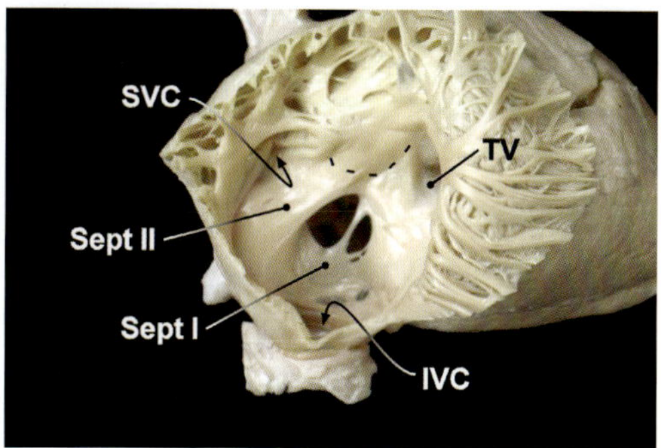

Fig 1.4A—Right atrial view of ASD II with persistent remnants of Sept I. Note the location of the right sinus of Valsalva (dotted line) within the anterosuperior rim of the ASD. Abbreviation: TV, tricuspid valve.

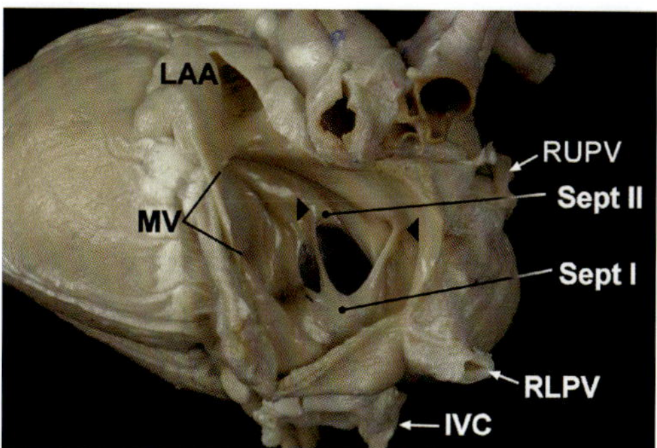

Fig 1.4B—Left atrial view of same defect. Note the persistent attachments of Sept I to Sept II (black arrows). Abbreviations: RLPV, right lower pulmonary vein; RUPV, right upper pulmonary vein.

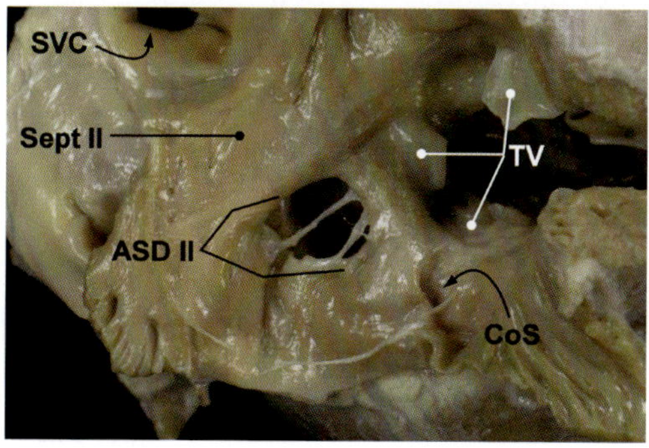

Fig 1.5A—Right atrial view of ASD II with strands of persistent Sept I. Note relationship to tricuspid valve (TV) and coronary sinus ostium (CoS).

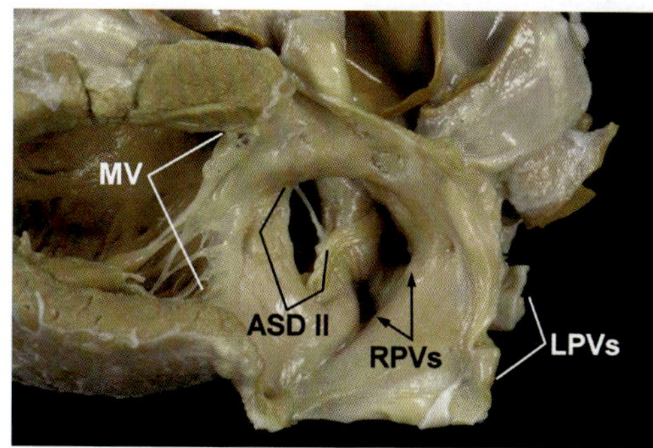

Fig 1.5B—Left atrial view of same defect. Note proximity to mitral valve (MV).

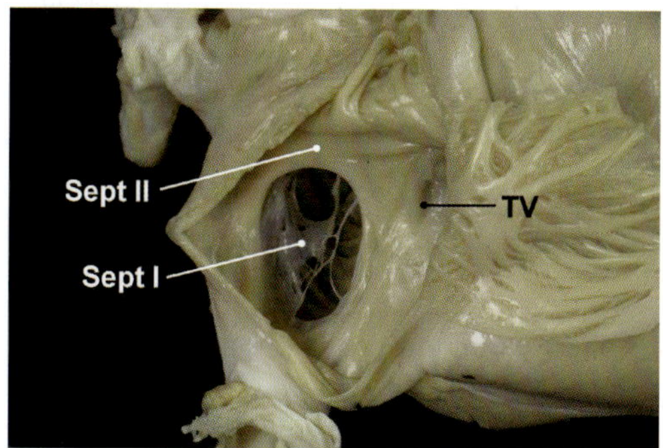

Fig 1.6A—Right atrial view of fenestrated Sept I.

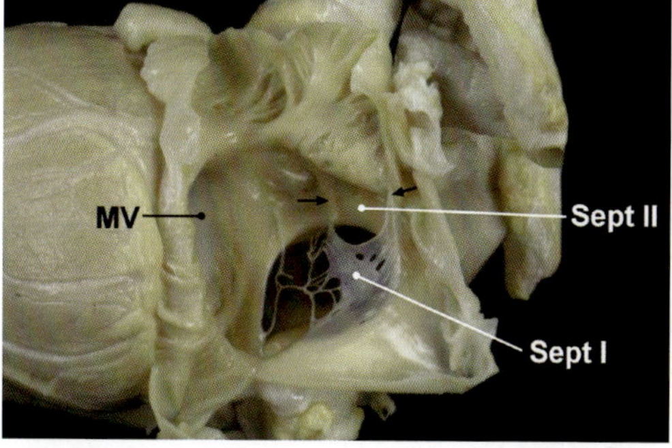

Fig 1.6B—Left atrial view of same defect. Note the normal attachments of Sept I to Sept II (black arrows).

nearby structures to avoid with device closure include the coronary sinus and the right pulmonary veins. Also the left venous valve of the inferior vena cava, which is normally adherent to the atrial septum, may be separated from it by several millimeters. In that situation it can be confused with the posteroinferior rim, but is not capable of anchoring a device. Furthermore, the eustachian valve can also be mistaken for the inferior rim of an ASD.

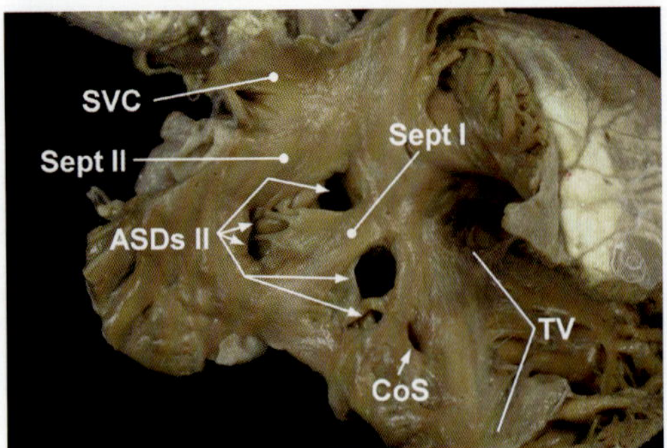

Fig 1.7A—Right atrial view of multiple ASDs II within muscular Sept I.

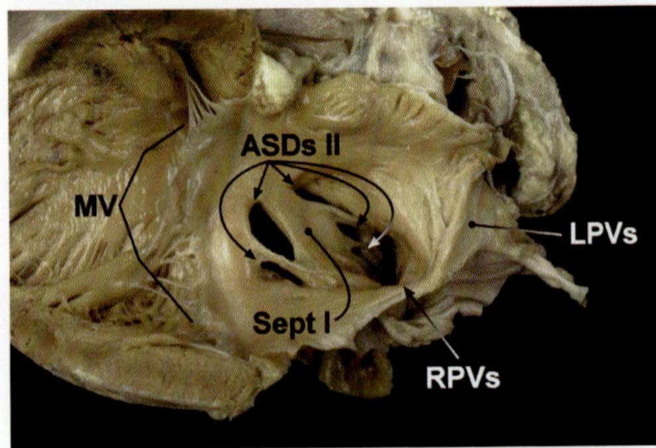

Fig 1.7B—Left atrial view of same defects.

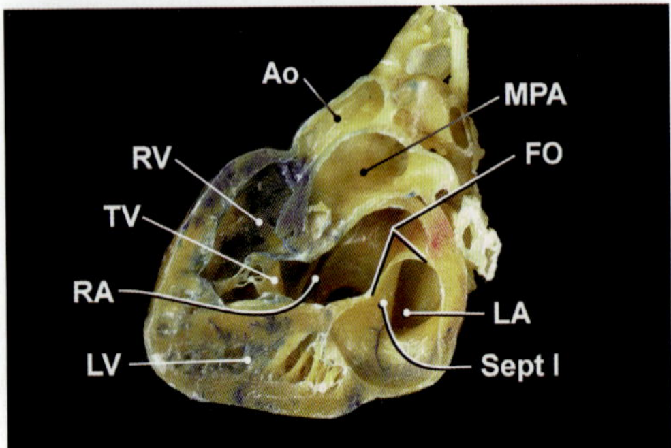

Fig 1.8A—Left-sided juxtaposition of atrial appendages, sagittal section, right side. Note horizontal Sept I with unguarded foramen ovale (FO) permitting blood flow between superiorly located right atrium (RA) and inferiorly located left atrium (LA). Abbreviations: Ao, aorta; LV, left ventricle; RV, right ventricle.

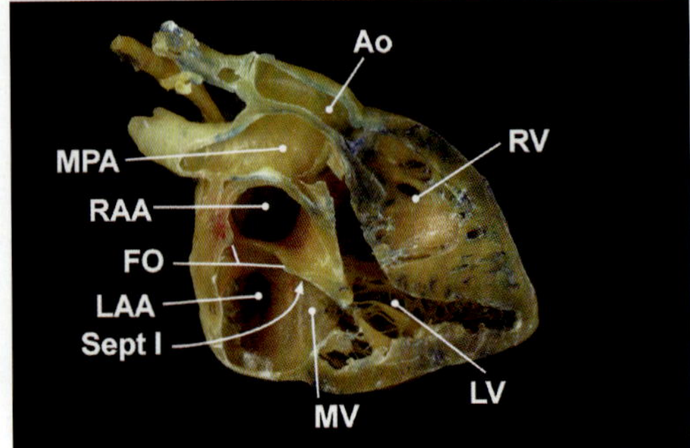

Fig 1.8B—Left side of same specimen demonstrates the horizontal Sept I extending to the lateral atrial wall between left atrial appendage (LAA) and right atrial appendage (RAA).

Deviation of Septum Primum

Leftward and/or posterior deviation of the atrial septum is another mechanism of inter-atrial communication. There are four different types of deviation of septum primum: (1) that seen with left-sided juxtaposition of the atrial septum (described earlier); (2) deviation of the anterosuperior portion of septum primum relative to septum secundum associated with hypoplasia or atresia of the left-sided atrioventricular valve, usually as part of hypoplastic left heart syndrome; (3) deviation of the anterior portion of septum primum in the setting of unbalanced atrioventricular canal at atrial level, also known as double outlet right atrium; and (4) deviation of the posterior aspect of the atrial septum to the left of some or all pulmonary vein orifices.

In juxtaposition of the atrial appendages, the atrial septum may have a horizontal orientation at its superior aspect when there is little or no septum secundum (Fig 1.8). The half-moon–shaped opening at the upper end of septum primum, being "unguarded" by septum secundum, is effectively an ostium secundum ASD. The margins of the defect are septum primum anteriorly, rightward, and posteriorly, and atrial wall leftward.

Leftward and posterior deviation of the anterosuperior portion of septum primum is the second most common atrial septal configuration in hypoplastic left heart syndrome. Most of these cases have mitral and aortic atresia. In one series of 129 patients with left atrioventricular valve hypoplasia (129 patients with normally aligned great arteries and two ventricles, 29 with double outlet right ventricle [DORV], and 8 with single ventricle), 62 patients had deviation of the atrial septum primum.[15] Although casual inspection appears to show a large ostium secundum ASD from apparent absence of septum primum at its expected location immediately to the left of septum secundum; in fact, septum primum is present but, being

deviated to the left, leaves a gap between the two septa (Fig 1.9). Furthermore, the superior aspect of septum primum is attached to the roof of the left atrium near the mouth of the atrial appendage rather than to the left side of septum secundum. Once again there is an "unguarded" foramen ovale far to the left of septum secundum making it more difficult to pass a catheter across the foramen ovale. In addition, the left atrium is usually quite small making balloon septostomy challenging if one can enter the left atrium. Unlike the normally attached septum primum where increased pulmonary venous return after birth stretches the foramen ovale, some cases of this form of displaced septum primum can actually lead to postnatal obstruction of the foramen ovale as septum primum is forced against the roof of the atrium.

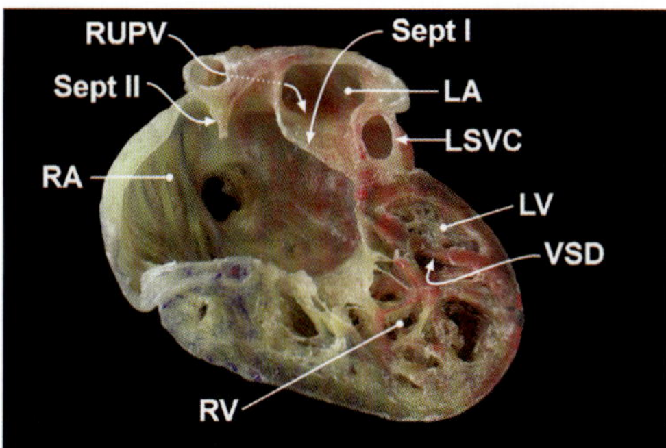

Fig 1.9A—Lower section of four-chamber view of hypoplastic left heart with leftward displacement of Sept I relative to Sept II. Note how Sept I forms a hood over right upper pulmonary vein (RUPV). These patients typically have mitral atresia (ie, no connection between left atrium [LA] and left ventricle [LV]). This case has a small LV with a ventricular septal defect (VSD). There is also a persistent left superior vena cava (LSVC).

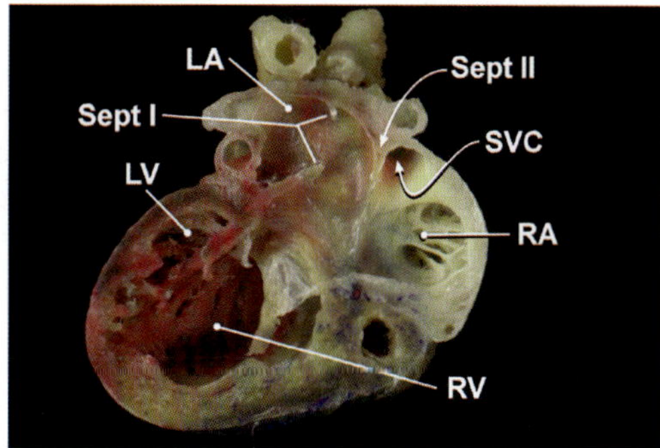

Fig 1.9B—Upper section of same specimen. Note the large gap between the two attachments of Sept I to the roof of left atrium (LA) and Sept II, in its normal location, medial to superior vena cava (SVC).

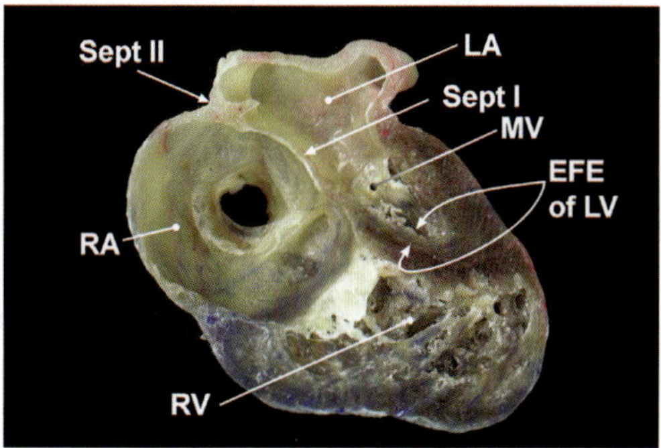

Fig 1.9C—Comparison view of specimen with hypoplastic left heart but normal atrial septum, that is, Sept I attached to Sept II. These patients typically have a patent MV and often have endocardial fibroelastosis (EFE) of the left ventricle (LV).

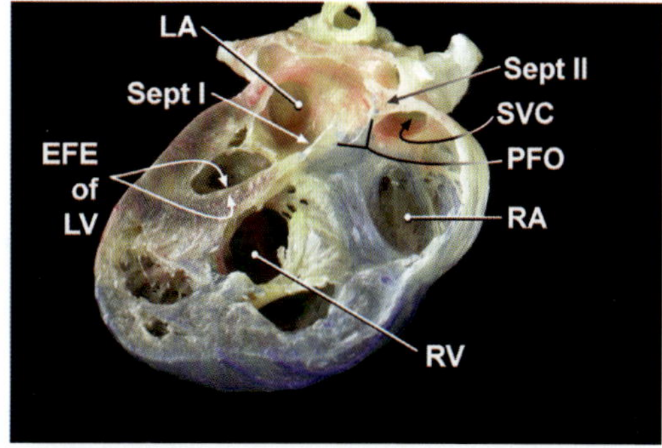

Fig 1.9D—Upper section of same specimen as in part C. Note that there is no gap between attachments of Sept I and Sept II.

Fig 1.9 continues on following page

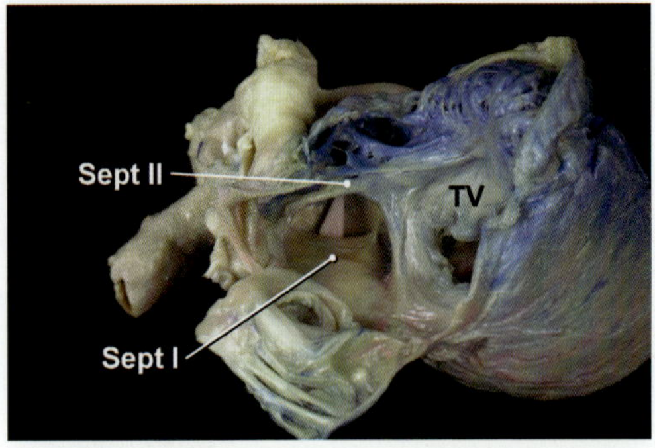

Fig 1.9E—Right atrial view of case similar to parts A and B with marked displacement of Sept I away from Sept II. Arrow-shaped probe in foramen ovale.

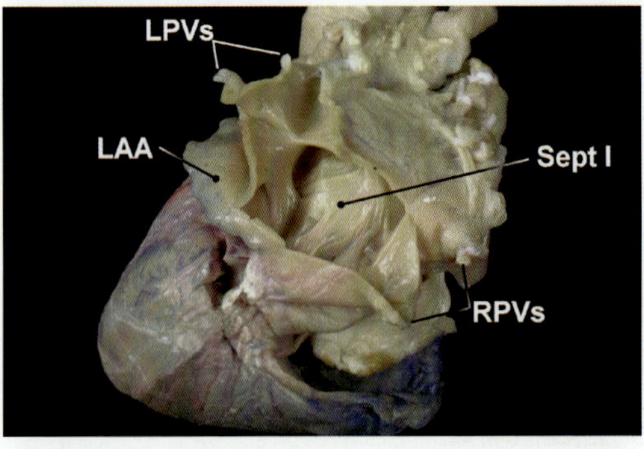

Fig 1.9F—Left atrial view of same specimen as in part E. Note small volume of left atrium with Sept I attached closer to pulmonary vein entrances than normal. However, pulmonary veins are still to the left of Sept I.

Deviation of the anterior portion of septum primum in cases of common atrioventricular canal is a rare form of unbalanced canal at the atrial rather than ventricular level.[16] Similar to the previous type, the surgeon's view from the right atrium can be mistaken for a common atrium with absence of the atrial septum, when, in fact, the atrial septum is deviated far to the left of its expected location. As such, the deviated septum can be mistaken for the left atrial free wall with associated common atrium. Thus if the apparent ASD is closed with a patch, significant pulmonary venous obstruction can result from the persistent deviated atrial septum. In this form the left atrium "sees" only a small fraction of the left side of the common AV valve, while the right atrium "sees" both sides of the valve—so-called double outlet right atrium.

Leftward deviation of the posterior aspect of septum primum is a rare but important etiology of intracardiac partial or total anomalous pulmonary venous return but with normal pulmonary venous connection.[17] In other words, the pulmonary veins enter the left atrium normally, but the septum primum is attached to the left of some or all of the pulmonary veins. In this situation, there is a large left-to-right shunt at the atrial level (anomalous pulmonary venous *return*) despite normal pulmonary venous *connection*. The degree of displacement can be described relative to the entrance of the pulmo-

nary veins: between the right and left pulmonary veins, or lateral to the entrance of the left pulmonary veins. When the septum is to the left of all pulmonary veins, systemic output is from that portion of pulmonary venous return that passes through the foramen ovale. Unlike total anomalous pulmonary venous connection, the streaming of pulmonary venous blood through the foramen ovale yields normal systemic saturation; whereas in total anomalous pulmonary venous connection the systemic flow is mildly desaturated because of total mixing at right atrial level.

Interatrial Communications Not Amenable to Device Closure

Coronary sinus defects, sinus venosus defects, and ostium primum ASDs are interatrial communications that are not amenable to catheter-based device closure because of the anatomic nature of the lesions.

Coronary sinus defects are quite rare, occurring in < 1%, and are not true defects in the atrial septum.[18] Rather there is an interatrial communication that exists due to a defect in the wall between the coronary sinus and the left atrium—the sinus septum (Fig 1.10). The defect

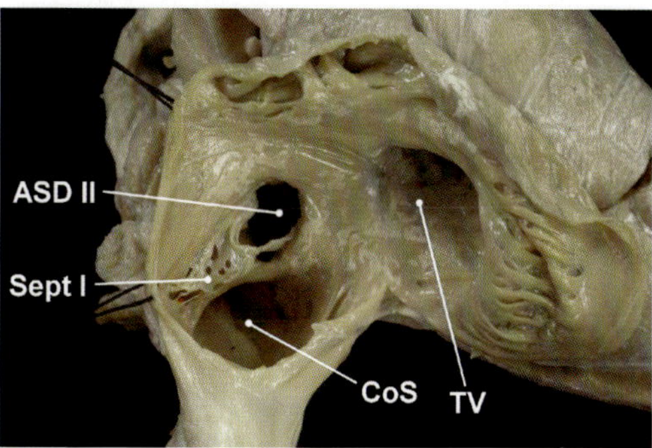

Fig 1.10A—Right atrial view of enlarged coronary sinus ostium (CoS) and ASD II in a patient with a partially unroofed coronary sinus (shown in part B). Note the fenestrations in Sept I. Although there appears to be a lower rim to the ASD II, the sinus septum (shown in part B) would, most likely, preclude proper seating of a device. The CoS is effectively an ASD because of the ability for left atrial blood to pass from left atrium (LA) through the sinus septal defect to the CoS to the right atrium (RA).

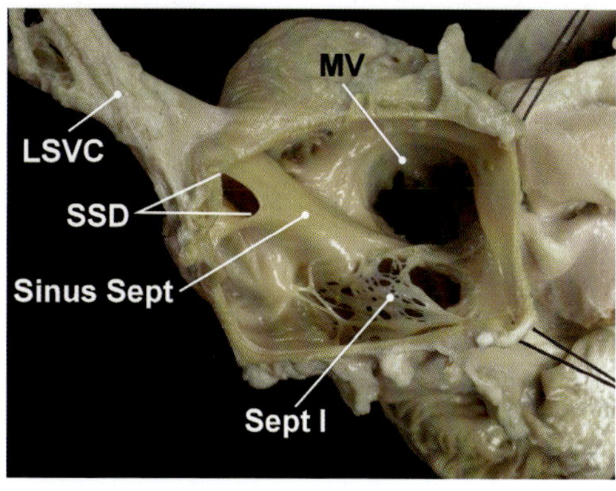

Fig 1.10B—Left atrial view of same specimen as in part A. Note left superior vena cava (LSVC) to coronary sinus ostium (CoS) with the sinus septum (Sinus Sept) indicated. There is a sinus septal defect (SSD) in this wall between the dilated CoS and the left atrium (LA). There are two sites of left-to-right shunt: through the fenestrated Sept I and through the SSD to CoS.

is often located at the site of the coronary sinus ostium with a dilated coronary sinus. It is inferior and anterior to the fossa ovalis and superior and anterior to the inferior vena cava-right atrial junction. The coronary sinus is either partially or completely unroofed.[18] In the partially unroofed coronary sinus, the boundaries of the defect are the remnants of the coronary sinus septum.[19-22] In the completely and incompletely unroofed coronary sinus, the perceived defect viewed from the right atrium is actually the coronary sinus ostium.[18,23] The coronary sinus defect is usually associated with a persistent left superior vena cava and in the completely unroofed defect, the left superior vena cava attaches to the roof of the left atrium.[23,24] Surgery is required to close the sinus septal defect or reroute the left superior vena cava, so that device closure of the coronary sinus ostium defect is not advisable. These defects are often associated with a variety of other congenital cardiac malformations.

Sinus venosus defects account for 4% to 11% of atrial level communications and are also not true defects in the atrial septum.[18] Rather there is an interatrial communication created by an abnormal connection of the right pulmo-

nary vein or veins, the superior vena cava, or the inferior vena cava to both atria such that the mouth of the vein(s) or cava straddle the atrial septum.[25-28] The most common variant is the sinus venosus defect of the superior vena cava type.[25,29,30] In this instance, the right upper and/or middle pulmonary vein insertions straddle the atrial septum at the superior vena cava-to-right atrial junction (Fig 1.11). This results in the creation of an interatrial communication from the left atrium to the right atrium. The anterior and inferior boundary of the defect is the posterosuperior portion of the septum secundum. The remaining boundaries are the ostia of the pulmonary veins and superior vena cava. Rarely one can see a superior vena cava alone straddling the septum—so-called right superior vena cava to left atrium[31]—with essentially normal pulmonary venous connection (Fig 1.12). This too is a form of sinus venosus defect of the superior vena caval type. The other major sinus venosus defect is that of the inferior vena cava type.[25,30] In this instance, the inferior vena cava straddles the atrial septum, usually without pulmonary venous abnormality (Fig 1.13), but occasionally with involvement of the right lower pulmonary vein. This creates an interatrial communication

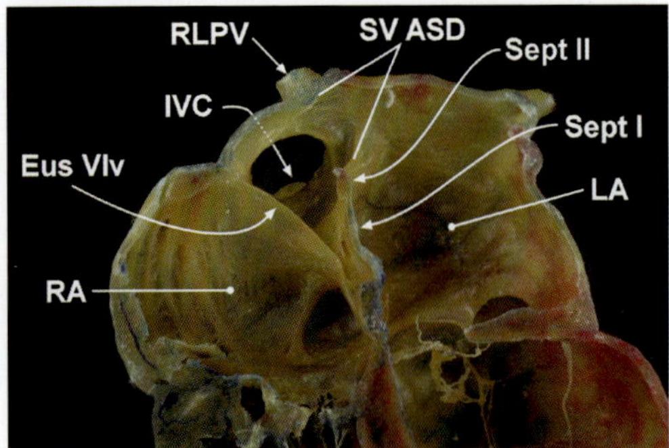

Fig 1.11A—Four-chamber view, inferior half showing a sinus venosus atrial septal defect (SV ASD). Note the entrance of the right lower pulmonary vein (RLPV) behind the atrial septum—both Sept II and Sept I. Even though this part of the defect is close to the inferior vena cava (IVC), the IVC is entirely to the right of the septum indicating that it is the mouth of the RLPV that *is* the SV ASD. Abbreviation: Eus VIV, Eustachian valve.

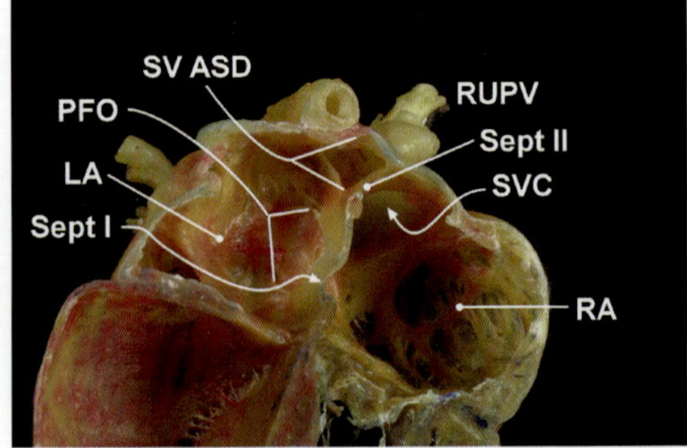

Fig 1.11B—Superior half of specimen shown in part A. Right upper pulmonary vein (RUPV) straddles the atrial septum behind Sept II and Sept I, both of which are well formed (ie, not defective). Note that the SV ASD is relatively remote from the patent foramen ovale (PFO) and from the entrance of the superior vena cava (SVC).

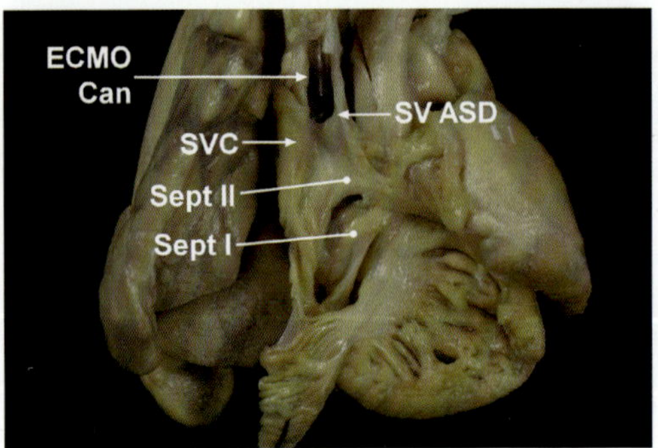

Fig 1.12—Right atrial and opened superior vena cava (SVC) view of SV ASD demonstrating an ECMO cannula (ECMO Can) passing through the defect to the left atrium. The atrial septum itself—Sept I and Sept II—looks normal.

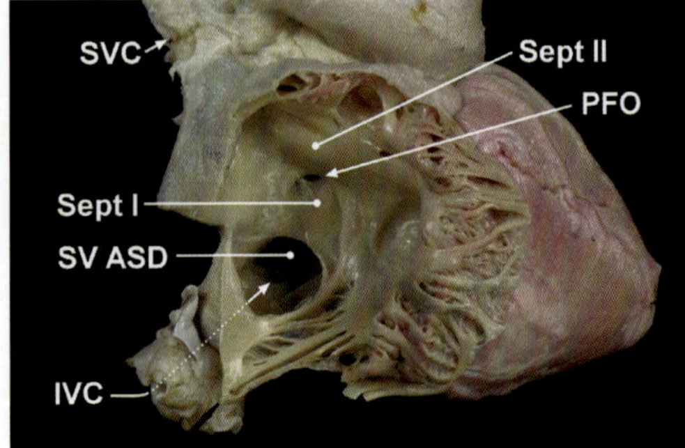

Fig 1.13A—Right atrial view of SV ASD of the inferior vena cava (IVC) type. Note the entrance of the IVC below Sept I so that the mouth of the IVC *is* the SV ASD. Note the normal superior aspect of Sept I with a patent foramen ovale (PFO).

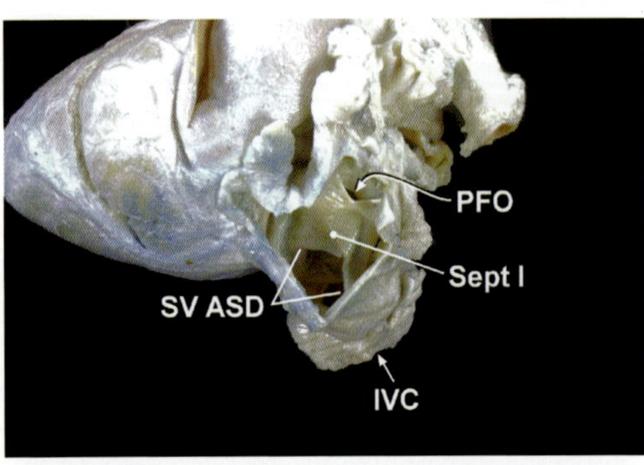

Fig 1.13B—Left atrial view of same specimen as in part A. Normal Sept I and patent foramen ovale (PFO) are noted.

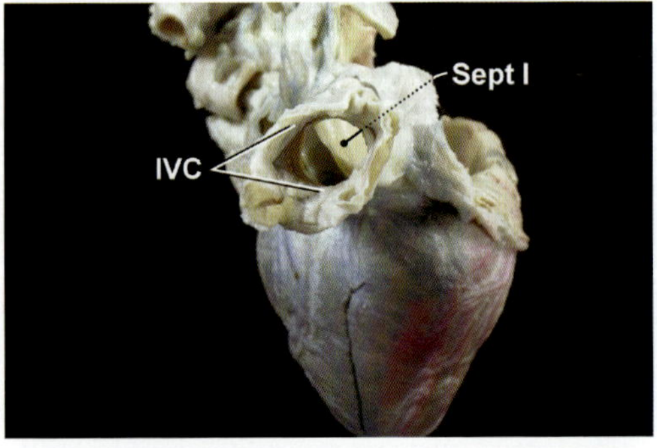

Fig 1.13C—Inferior view through the inferior vena cava (IVC) shows that it straddles Sept I thus entering both right atrium (RA) and left atrium (LA).

with the superior and anterior boundary of the defect being the inferior portion of septum primum. The remaining boundaries are the ostia of the inferior vena cava and possibly a pulmonary vein. The atrial septum has no defect in either condition but rather a "defect" that allows for blood to cross from the left atrium to the right atrium through the mouth of one or more venous structures as they straddle the atrial septum. Because a large portion of the boundary of these defects is straddling vein, device closure is not feasible.

Ostium primum ASDs are defects in the canal septum.[32–35] The defect is due to failure of division of the embryonic atrioventricular canal and specifically to failure of fusion of septum primum with the endocardial cushions. The defect is in the portion of the septum located between the septum primum and the common atrioventricular valve (Fig 1.14). The boundaries of the defect include septum primum posteriorly and superiorly and the atrioventricular valves anterior and inferiorly. Because the anterior and inferior border is the atrioventricular valve, device closure is not feasible.

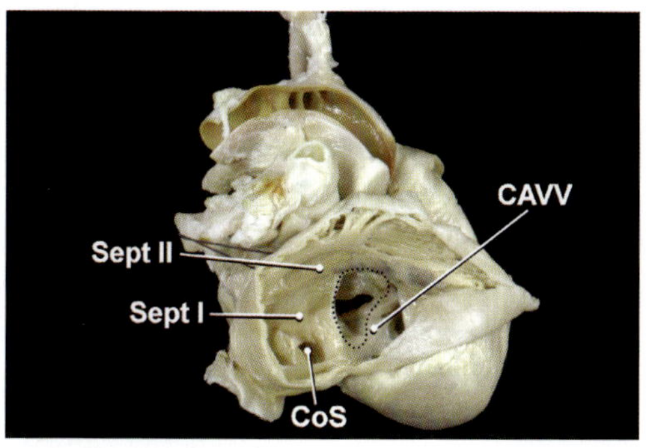

Fig 1.14A—Right atrial view of ostium primum atrial septal defect (dotted line) seen in common atrioventricular canal. The posterior border of the defect is the normal appearing Sept I, the superior border is Sept II, but the anterior and inferior border is the common atrioventricular valve (CAVV). In this case of so-called incomplete or partial atrioventricular canal, there is a strip of valve tissue that divides the valve into one with two orifices (seen on either side of the dotted line).

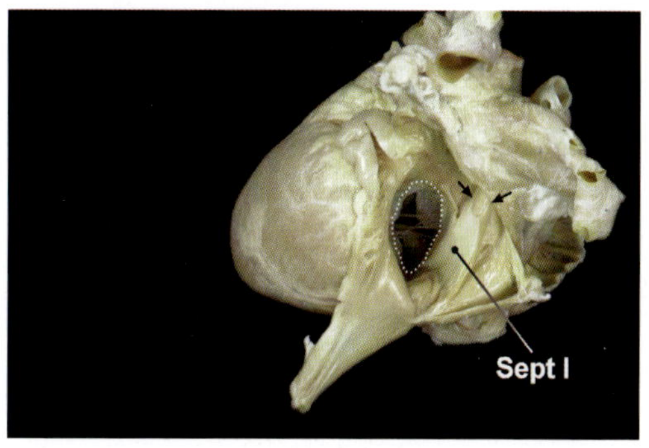

Fig 1.14B—Left atrial view of same specimen as in part A showing the ostium primum atrial septal defect (dotted line). Note the normal Sept I posterior to the defect with the two normal attachments (black arrows) of Sept I to Sept II on either side of the half-moon shaped edge of the foramen ovale.

References

1. Anderson RH, Brown NA, Webb S. Development and structure of the atrial septum. *Heart.* 2002:88(1);104–110,

2. Sweeney LJ, Rosenquist GC. The normal anatomy of the atrial septum in the human heart. *Am Heart J.* 1979;98:51–54.

3. Edwards W. Cardiac anatomy and examination of cardiac specimens. Atrial Septum. In: Allen HD, Driscoll DJ, Shaddy RE, Feltes TF, eds. *Moss and Adams' Heart Disease in Infants, Children,* *and Adolescents: Including the Fetus and Young Adult.* 7th ed. Philadelphia: Wolters Kluwer, 2007;(vol 1):10–11.

4. Hutchins GM, Moore GW, Jones JF, et al. Postnatal endocardial fibroelastosis of the valve of the foramen ovale. *Am J Cardiol.* 1981;47:90–94.

5. Porter CJ, Edwards W. Atrial septal defects. Anatomy, embryology, and pathology. In: Allen HD, Driscoll DJ, Shaddy RE, Feltes TF, eds. *Moss and Adams' Heart Disease in Infants, Children, and Adolescents: Including the Fetus and Young*

Adult. 7th ed. Philadelphia: Wolters Kluwer, 2007;(vol 1): 632–645.

6. McKenzie JA, Edwards WD, Hagler DJ. Anatomy of the patent foramen ovale for the interventionalist. *Cathet Cardiovasc Intervent*. 2009; 73(6):821–826.

7. Hagen P, Scholz D, Edwards W. Incidence and size of patent foramen ovale during the first 10 decades of life: An autopsy study of 965 normal hearts. *Mayo Clin Proc*. 1984;59:17–20.

8. Ho SY, McCarthy KP, Rigby ML. Morphological features pertinent to interventional closure of patent oval foramen. *J Interv Cardiol*. 2003;16:33–38.

9. Marshall AC, Lock JE. Structural and compliant anatomy of the patent foramen ovale in patients undergoing transcatheter closure. *Am Heart J*. 2000;140:303–307.

10. Spence MS, Khan AA, Mullen MJ. Balloon assessment of patent foramen ovale morphology and the modification of tunnels using a balloon detunnelisation technique. *Cathet Cardiovasc Intervent*. 2008;71:222–228.

11. Blom NA, Ottenkamp J, Jongeneel TH, DeRuiter MC, Gittenberger-de Groot AC. Morphogenetic differences of secundum atrial septal defects. *Pediatr Cardiol*. 2005;25(4):338–343.

12. Chan KC, Godman MJ. Morphological variations of fossa ovalis atrial septal defects (secundum): feasibility for transcutaneous closure with the clam-shell device. *Br Heart J*. 1993; 69(1):52–55.

13. Ferreira SM, Ho SY, Anderson RH. Morphological study of defects of the atrial septum within the oval fossa: implications for transcatheter closure of left-to-right shunt. *Br Heart J*. 1992;67(4):316–320.

14. Marx GR, Sherwood MG, Fleishman C, Van Praagh R. Three-dimensional echocardiography of the atrial septum. *Echocardiography*. 2001;18(5):433–443.

15 Chin AJ, Weinberg PM, Barber G. Subcostal two-dimensional echocardiographic identification of anomalous attachment of septum primum in patients with left atrioventricular valve underdevelopment. *J Am Coll Cardiol*. 1990;15:678–681.

16. Cohen MS, Weinberg PM, Coon PD, Gaynor JW, Rychik J. Deviation of atrial septum primum in association with normal left atrioventricular valve size. *J Am Soc Echocardiogr*. 2001;14:732–737.

17. Van Praagh S, Carrera ME, Sanders S, Mayer JE Jr, Van Praagh R. Partial or total direct pulmonary venous drainage to right atrium due to malposition of septum primum. *Chest*. 1995;107(6):1488–1498.

18. Geva T. Anomalies of the atrial septum. In: Lai W, Mertens K, Cohen M, Geva T, eds. *Echocardiography in Pediatric and Congenital Heart Disease: From Fetus to Adult*. Hoboken: NJ: Wiley-Blackwell, 2009;15.

19. Rose AG, Beckman CB, Edwards JE. Communication between coronary sinus and left atrium. *Br Heart J*. 1974;36:182–185.

20. Freedom RM, Culham JA, Rowe RD. Left atrial to coronary sinus fenestration (partially unroofed coronary sinus): morphological and angiocardiographic observations. *Br Heart J*. 1981;46:63–68.

21. Knauth A, McCarthy KP, Webb S, et al. Interatrial communication through the mouth of the coronary sinus. *Cardiol Young*. 2002;12: 364–372.

22. Adatia I, Gittenberger-De Groot AC. Unroofed coronary sinus and coronary sinus orifice atresia: Implications for management of complex congenital heart disease. *JACC*. 1995; 25(4):948–953.

23. Raghib G, Ruttenberg HD, Anderson RC, Amplatz K, Adams Jr P, Edwards JE. Termination of left superior vena cava in left atrium, atrial septal defect, and absence of coronary sinus: a developmental complex. *Circulation*. 1965;31:906–918.

24. Ootaki Y, Yamaguchi M, Yoshimura N, Oka S, Yoshida M, Hasegawa T. Unroofed coronary sinus syndrome: diagnosis, classification, and surgical treatment. *J Thorac Cardiovasc Surg*. 2003;126:1655–1656.

25. Van Praagh S, Carrera ME, Sanders SP, et al. Sinus venosus defects: unroofing of the right pulmonary veins-anatomic and echocardiographic findings and surgical treatment. *Am Heart J*. 1994;128:365–379.

26. Anderson RH, Ettedgui JA, Devine WA. Sinus venous defect. *Am Heart J.* 1995;129:1229–1230.

27. Van Praagh S, Carrera ME, Sanders SP, et al. Sinus venosus defect [reply]. *Am Heart J.* 1995;129:1231–1232.

28. Blom NA, Gittenberger-de Groot AC, Jongeneel TH, et al. Normal development of the pulmonary veins in human embryos and formulation of a morphogenetic concept for sinus venosus defects. *Am J Cardiol.* 2001;87:305–309.

29. Li J, Al Zaghal AM, Anderson RH. The nature of the superior sinus venosus defect. *Clin Anat.* 1998;11:349–352.

30. Al Zaghal AM, Ahmed M, Li J, et al. Anatomical criteria for diagnosis of sinus venosus syndrome. *Heart.* 1997;78:298–304.

31. Van Praagh S, Geva T, Lock JE, Nido PJ, Vance MS, Van Praagh R. Biatrial or left atrial drainage of the right superior vena cava: anatomic, morphogenetic, and surgical considerations—report of three new cases and literature review. *Pediatr Cardiol.* 2003;24(4):350–363,

32. Cohen MS. Common atrioventricular canal defects anomalies of the atrial septum. In: Lai W, Mertens K, Cohen M, Geva T, eds. *Echocardiography in Pediatric and Congenital Heart Disease: From Fetus to Adult.* Hoboken: NJ: Wiley-Blackwell, 2009;230–248.

33. Pillai R, Ho SY, Anderson RH, Lincoln C. Ostium primum atrioventricular septal defect: an anatomical and surgical review. *Ann Thorac Surg.* 1986;41(4):458–461.

34. Penkoske PA, Neches WH, Anderson RH, Zuberuhler JR. Further observations on the morphology of atrioventricular septal defects. *J Thorac Cardiovasc Surg.* 1985;90:611–622.

35. Piero GP, Leon MG, Wilkinson JG, Lozsadi K, Macartney FJ, Anderson RH. Morphology and classification of atrioventricular defects. *Am Heart J.* 1979;42:621–632.

2

Natural and Unnatural History of a Secundum ASD

Gregory A. Fleming, Thomas Doyle, and Thomas P. Graham Jr.

Introduction

Secundum atrial septal defect (ASD) is one of the most common forms of congenital heart defect, with an estimated incidence of 0.2 to 0.5 per 1000 live births.[1-3] ASD accounts for 6% to 10% of all defects at birth, and excluding bicuspid aortic valves, is the most common congenital heart defect presenting in adults.[1,2,4] It affects approximately twice as many females as males.[5] Although the majority of defects are sporadic, they can be associated with other complex cardiac defects and genetic syndromes, such as Holt-Oram Syndrome and Ellis van Creveld syndrome.[6]

An ASD creates a source for intracardiac shunting at the atrial level. The direction of shunting across the ASD is determined by the diastolic properties of the right and left ventricles. In a small ASD, the left atrial pressure is typically slightly higher than the right atrial pressure and left to right shunting occurs mainly in diastole. With large defects, the right and left atrial pressures are equal and left to right shunting occurs due to the increased distensibility and compliance of the right ventricle compared to the left ventricle. The degree of shunting is determined by the size of the defect and the compliance of the two ventricles.[7] Chronic volume overload to the right-sided structures leads to dilation of the right atrium and right ventricle and dilation of the entire pulmonary bed. Over time, microscopic changes can occur in the lungs with medial hypertrophy of the muscular pulmonary arteries and veins and muscularization of the pulmonary arterioles, ultimately leading to pulmonary vascular disease and pulmonary hypertension.[8]

Transcatheter Closure of ASDs and PFOs: A Comprehensive Assessment. © 2010 Ziyad M. Hijazi, Ted Feldman, Mustafa H. Abdullah Al-Qbandi, and Horst Sievert, editors. Cardiotext Publishing, ISBN: 978-0-9790164-9-3.

The natural history of children and adults with an isolated ASD as well as the natural history following surgical or percutaneous closure of an ASD in children and adults are reviewed in this chapter. Currently, most hemodynamically significant ASDs are diagnosed and closed at an early age, making the natural history somewhat difficult to assess. Several observational studies describing the natural history of ASDs were published before the age of enhanced diagnosis by echocardiography.[9–11] Selection bias is a common error in these early observational studies because many of them focused on patients who were brought to medical attention after the onset of symptoms. It is clear from these studies that an unrepaired, hemodynamically significant ASD leads to significant morbidity in adulthood and reduces life expectancy.[9,10,12]

Natural History of an Atrial Septal Defect Diagnosed in Childhood

The right ventricle is relatively stiff in early infancy, and there is little left to right shunting. As the pulmonary vascular resistance drops in the first month of life, the diastolic properties of the right ventricle change allowing more left to right shunt.[13] Infants with an ASD are usually asymptomatic, however, there are rare reports of infants who develop heart failure, and it is not clear what the etiology is, as their hemodynamic features are no different from infants who remain asymptomatic.[14]

When a family is presented with the diagnosis of a secundum ASD in their child, the discussion often turns to the question of what will happen to the ASD over time. A number of studies have addressed this issue.[5,15–18] Results of studies have varied depending on a number of variables such as method of diagnosis, exclusion criteria, age of patients at diagnosis, and length of follow-up. In 1973, Mody published a series of 40 patients with clinical evidence of cardiac enlargement and pulmonary overcirculation who were diagnosed with an ASD at cardiac catheterization.[18] In this study, 11 of 20 patients diagnosed prior to 1 year of age had spontaneous closure of their ASD during follow-up, whereas spontaneous closure did not occur in any patients diagnosed after 1 year of age.[18] Although this study could not quantify the anatomic size of each ASD, it did suggest that the age at diagnosis could help determine the likelihood of spontaneous closure of an ASD over time.

The development of two-dimensional (2D) echocardiography provided the ability to detect atrial septal defects of all sizes, as well as the ability to follow their size over time. Radzik et al[17] followed 101 consecutive infants who were referred at < 3 months of age for a murmur and subsequently diagnosed with an interatrial communication. The study did not exclude infants felt to have a patent foramen ovale. Infants were divided into groups based on the size of their ASD. In this study, all defects < 3 mm in diameter and 87% of defects < 5 mm in diameter closed spontaneously, whereas spontaneous closure did not occur in any infant with defects > 8mm in diameter.[17] Similar findings were noted by Helgason and Jonsdottir,[5] who followed all children in Iceland diagnosed with a secundum ASD of at least 4 mm in diameter by echocardiogram during a 10-year period. In their study, the age of patients at diagnosis ranged from 1 week to 10 years of age. They found that 62% of defects 4 mm in diameter closed spontaneously, whereas 16 of 17 patients with defects 5 to 6 mm in diameter had either a reduction in size (5 patients) or complete closure (11 patients). Only one of eight patients with a defect 7 to 8 mm in diameter had spontaneous closure with four other defects becoming smaller over time. Similar to the report by Radzik,[17] there was no spontaneous closure in defects > 8 mm in diameter with 24 of 26 such defects requiring surgical closure. Interestingly, the median age at diagnosis of patients with defects > 8 mm was 14 months compared to 1 month for those with 4 mm defects. Of note, one patient in the 4-mm group and one in the 5- to 6-mm group actually had significant increase in the size of the defect during follow-up.[5]

In 2002, Texas Children's Hospital published their experience with isolated ASDs > 3 mm in diameter between the years 1991 and 1998 and found a significant increase in size over time with all ASD sizes. In 34 patients with an ASD between 3 and 6 mm in diameter, they surprisingly found that 17 defects increased in size during follow-up, with 7 defects enlarging to between 8 and 12 mm in diameter, and 3 defects increasing in size to > 12 mm in diameter. Similarly, 8 of 40 moderate-sized defects increased to > 12 mm in diameter. Overall, 66% of their patients had an increase in defect size during follow-up. The mean age at diagnosis in this group of patients was older than other studies at 4.5 years, and this may account for the large percentage of defects that enlarged overtime.[16]

In a study from Austria published in 2006, 200 consecutive patients with ASDs ≥ 4 mm in diameter were followed for > 6 months. Similar to the study by Helgason and Jonsdottir, they found smaller defects in the younger children and larger defects in those diagnosed at a later age. They hypothesized that this finding was either because many ASDs may be an incidental finding on echocardiograms in younger children or that there may be growth of an ASD over time. In their series, 77% of defects decreased in size over time whereas only 18% increased in size. In addition, there was a strong association between defect size at diagnosis and spontaneous closure. Of the defects measuring 4 to 5 mm in diameter, 56% closed spontaneously during follow-up, whereas none of the defects > 10 mm in diameter closed spontaneously. Surgical or device closure was required in 77% of patients with defects > 10 mm. They also found a strong correlation between age at diagnosis and the incidence of spontaneous closure with spontaneous closure occurring in 39% of patients diagnosed at < 1 year of age compared to only 19% of patients diagnosed at > 1 year of age. Using a multivariate analysis, smaller ASD diameter and younger age at diagnosis were both independent predictors of spontaneous

closure or regression in ASD size to < 3 mm in diameter.[15]

In summary, the two most important predictors of spontaneous closure of a secundum ASD appear to be the age at diagnosis and the size of the defect. Defects that measure < 3 mm in diameter diagnosed in the first few months of life will most likely close spontaneously. Children diagnosed at < 1 year of age with defects < 6 mm in diameter are likely to undergo complete spontaneous closure or regression of their ASD to < 3 mm. Defects > 8 mm are much less likely to become smaller over time and have a significant chance of requiring surgical or percutaneous closure in the future, regardless of age at diagnosis. Defects > 3 mm in diameter have the potential to increase in size over time, however this seems more likely in children diagnosed after 1 year of age and in those with larger defects at the time of diagnosis.

Natural History
of an Unrepaired ASD

An ASD usually has a benign clinical course in children.[19] Complications of an unrepaired ASD occur in adulthood and can include right ventricular failure, atrial arrhythmias, paradoxical embolization, pulmonary hypertension, and cyanosis secondary to reversal of shunt from pulmonary vascular disease (Eisenmenger syndrome).[10,20–22]

Chronic volume overload to the lungs from an ASD may lead to progressive dyspnea and recurrent respiratory infections. As pulmonary vascular disease develops, symptoms of right ventricular heart failure develop. Symptoms are rare in childhood but are progressive with age.[19] Commonly cited early observational studies reported a very low prevalence of symptoms before the age of 30 with about half of the patients becoming symptomatic by 45 years of age and the most common symptoms being exertional dyspnea and fatigue.[9,10] Konstantinides et al reported the presence of exertional dyspnea in 75% and peripheral edema in 24% of patients with an ASD evaluated at a mean age of 56 years, and 29% of these patients were classified as New York Heart Association (NYHA) class III or IV.[23] Craig and Selzer found that congestive heart failure developed after the age of 40 in their study of patients who were > 18 years of age at diagnosis.[10] Adults with an unrepaired ASD were found to have moderately reduced ventilatory function and markedly reduced exercise capacity by pulmonary function and cardiopulmonary exercise testing.[24,25] Cyanosis is also a late symptom seen in patients with an ASD and is usually secondary to pulmonary vascular disease causing right to left shunt at the atrial level.[20] Although rare before 20 years of age, the incidence of cyanosis increases with age, and in Dexter's early hemodynamic studies of patients with an ASD, 37% had a measurable decrease in oxygen saturation at cardiac catheterization.[7] Konstantinides et al reported cyanosis in 27% of patients studied at a mean age of 56 years and Attie et al reported a mean oxygen saturation of 89% in patients studied at a mean age of 50.8 years.[23,26]

Atrial arrhythmias, primarily atrial flutter and atrial fibrillation, are well-documented complications of an unrepaired ASD and, like other complications, are rare during childhood.[22] Although, the risk of atrial arrhythmias is extremely low in patients before the age of 40, the risk increases with older age and higher mean pulmonary artery pressure.[22,27] The prevalence of atrial arrhythmias in the fifth decade has been reported at 19% to 22%, and patients with atrial arrhythmias are more likely to be classified as NYHA classes III or IV.[27,28]

Pulmonary hypertension and pulmonary vascular disease is one of the most important complications of an ASD. Determining the true incidence of pulmonary hypertension in patients with an unrepaired ASD is complicated because studies have used differing criteria to define significant pulmonary hypertension. Pulmonary hypertension rarely develops before 18 years of age in an uncomplicated, unrepaired ASD.[10,11,29] The incidence of pulmonary hypertension between 20 and 40 years of age in

early natural history studies ranged from 14% to 18%.[9,10] Pulmonary hypertension has been shown to be more common in females, and the prevalence increases with age.[10,11,29] Once pulmonary vascular disease develops, it may be progressive and may significantly alter the clinical course and prognosis of a patient with an ASD, including their outcome after surgical repair.[29]

The presence of an ASD allows for systemic embolism of thrombus or air in the presence of transient increases in right atrial pressure that create a right to left shunt. Paradoxical embolism can lead to significant complications including cryptogenic stroke as well as ischemic damage to other major organs.[21,30] Pregnancy is associated with an increased risk of stroke from various etiologies, and the risk of paradoxical embolism due to the presence of a patent foramen ovale or ASD may be increased during pregnancy.[31,32] Transcatheter closure of atrial septal defects has been performed during pregnancy in these situations.[33] Additionally, the presence of an unrepaired ASD during pregnancy is associated with increased risk of maternal pre-eclampsia and fetal mortality.[34]

Early natural history studies of patients with an ASD indicate reduced survival, with an average age at death of 37 to 49 years.[9–11,35] Causes of death in earlier reports were most frequently due to congestive heart failure, pulmonary arterial thrombosis, and bronchopulmonary infections.[10] As mentioned earlier, the selection bias present in these early studies likely overestimates the mortality figures. More recent studies suggest a better prognosis, and survival to 90 years of age has been reported in patients with an unrepaired ASD.[28,35,36] Campbell calculated survival rates for each decade in patients with an ASD based on both necropsy reports and longitudinal studies, and his calculations show < 1% per year mortality rate in the first two decades; increasing in successive decades to 7.5% per year in the sixth decade.[12]

In summary, an ASD is well tolerated during childhood with symptoms developing during early adulthood. Although early natural history studies may have overestimated the true mortality and morbidity of patients with an ASD, it is clear that patients with an ASD are prone to developing significant complications such as heart failure, atrial arrhythmias, and pulmonary vascular disease during early adulthood, ultimately leading to reduced life expectancy.

Unnatural history of an ASD: surgical closure

It is generally accepted that children and young adults with evidence of a hemodynamically significant ASD resulting in right atrial and/or right ventricular volume overload should have their ASD closed either surgically or percutaneously. Guidelines from the American Heart Association (AHA) recommend closure of a secundum ASD in the presence of symptoms or evidence of a large shunt; defined as the presence of a diastolic flow rumble, electrocardiographic evidence of right ventricular hypertrophy, chest radiographic evidence of cardiomegaly or increased pulmonary vascular markings, echocardiographic evidence of right ventricular enlargement or paradoxical septal motion, or a pulmonary to systemic flow ratio (Qp:Qs) ≥ 1.5.[37] Surgical closure of a secundum ASD is both safe and effective. The long-term survival of patients who have surgical closure of an ASD during childhood is similar to age and sex matched controls with no heart disease.[38,39] Roos-Hesslink et al demonstrated this point in a longitudinal study of 135 patients who underwent surgical ASD closure during childhood, reporting no cardiovascular mortality and no evidence of stroke, heart failure, or pulmonary hypertension in any patients at 15- and 26-year follow-up evaluations.[38] In addition, the prevalence of atrial arrhythmias was only 6% at 15-year follow-up with an additional 2% at 26-year follow-up, which is much lower than that seen after surgical ASD closure in adults as well as in adults with an unrepaired ASD.[27,38,39] Despite excellent clinical outcomes following surgical ASD repair, right ventricular enlargement and abnormal ventricular septal wall motion

may persist.[40] In long-term follow-up of 104 patients repaired prior to the age of 15 years, Meijboon et al found persistent right ventricular enlargement in 26%.[41]

Younger patients appear to have better long-term prognosis than older patients following surgical ASD closure. A comparison between patients with surgical closure of an ASD during childhood to patients with surgical closure as adults demonstrated more frequent development of late heart failure, stroke, and atrial arrhythmias in the older group, and age at operation was an independent predictor of long-term survival.[39] There has been some controversy as to whether older adults truly benefit from surgical closure of an ASD. A historical, prospective, nonrandomized study published in 1994 evaluated patients over the age of 45 who had previously been diagnosed with an ASD, and compared patients who underwent surgical closure to those who had medical management. The study reported no significant difference in survival, symptoms, or other morbidities between the two groups.[28] However, several studies show that patients older than the age of 40 do well after surgical ASD closure, with improvement in symptoms and overall mortality compared to medical treatment alone.[23,26,42] In 2001, Attie et al reported the results of their prospective, randomized controlled trial, in which patients more than 40 years old with an ASD were assigned to either surgical or medical management. Their study showed surgery improved both the composite of major cardiovascular events as well as overall mortality compared to medical management.[26] In addition, exercise capacity as measured by cardiopulmonary exercise testing, significantly improves following either surgical or transcatheter closure of an ASD in older patients, even in those who reported no symptoms prior to closure.[24,25] Unfortunately, the risk of late atrial arrhythmias does not seem to change significantly following surgical repair at an older age compared to patients with an unrepaired ASD.[27] Older age at the time of surgery (> 40 years), the presence of preoperative atrial fibrillation or flutter, and the presence of early postoperative atrial fibrillation or flutter were all found to be independent predictors of late atrial arrhythmias.[27] The fact that little improvement is seen in atrial arrhythmias following closure in adults is likely due to structural changes having already occurred in the atrial tissue. The addition of the Cox maze procedure at the time of surgical ASD closure has been associated with a decreased incidence of atrial arrhythmias postoperatively at short and intermediate follow-up.[43,44]

Pulmonary vascular disease and fixed pulmonary hypertension in patients with an unrepaired ASD is associated with high mortality postoperatively, and maintaining an atrial septal communication may be necessary in these patients to allow for right to left shunting at the atrial level to maintain an adequate cardiac output at the expense of cyanosis. Steel et al reported low postoperative mortality and regression of symptoms in patients with total pulmonary resistance < 15 Wood units/M^2, however total pulmonary resistance > 15 Wood units/M^2 was associated with poor long-term survival. In addition, preoperative oxygen saturation was predictive of outcome in patients with borderline total pulmonary resistance.[29]

Unnatural history of an ASD: transcatheter closure

Transcatheter closure of a secundum ASD was first performed by King and Mills in 1976 using a double umbrella device, and the procedure has evolved significantly since that time with the development of several different devices.[45,46] Transcatheter closure of a secundum ASD has been shown to be safe and efficacious in both children and adults, having similar short-term success rate and mortality as surgery.[47–50] In addition, Du et al reported decreased morbidity and length of hospital stay with transcatheter closure compared to surgery.[47]

The CardioSEAL/STARFlex and AMPLATZER Septal Occluder (ASO) devices account for the majority of follow-up data regarding transcatheter closure of atrial septal defects. Histologic analysis of piglets who underwent ASD closure with an ASO device demonstrate complete neoendocardium coverage of both the right and left atrial discs by 1–3 months after device placement.[51] The success rate of closure with the ASO device has been very high in multiple studies, and residual shunting is rarely more than trivial to mild following device placement.[47,48,52–54] An early study published by Chan et al in 1999 reported complete closure in 85% of patients at 24 hours from closure with an ASO device, and complete closure in 99% at 3 months after the procedure.[54] In 2002, Du et al reported results on 423 patients who had defects closed with an ASO device, demonstrating complete closure of the defect in 73% of patients at 24 hours and in 98% of patients at 6-months follow-up.[47] Although residual shunting more than a month after closure is rare with the ASO device, it has been shown to be more frequent following closure with the CardioSEAL or STARFlex device. In a study published in 2004, Butera et al compared 153 patients who had defects closed with an ASO device to 121 patients with defects that were closed with either the CardioSEAL or STARFlex device. Their study showed residual shunting at discharge in only 3% of patients closed with an ASO device compared to 21% of patients whose defect was closed with either the CardioSEAL or STARFlex device, and there was no significant difference in closure rates between the CardioSEAL and STARFlex devices.[55]

Periprocedural complications with transcatheter closure are uncommon, the most common and significant short-term complication being device embolization or malposition that requires percutaneous or surgical removal of the device.[56] A review of the Manufacturer and User Facility Device Experience (MAUDE) database for ASO devices reported an overall mortality of < 0.1%, with 0.83% of cases requiring a rescue operation for adverse events related to device placement.[57] Cardiac perforation due to erosion of the device through cardiac structures has been a rare but serious and life-threatening complication following ASD closure with the

ASO device, resulting in a change in the device sizing guidelines.[58,59] Cardiac perforations typically occur within 3 days of the procedure, however, they have been reported as long as 3 years after the procedure.[58]

Transcatheter closure of a secundum ASD has only recently gained wide acceptance, and therefore surveillance and collection of data for long-term results and complications is ongoing. Masura et al reported no residual shunt, no significant complications, and no death at a median follow up of 78 months in 151 patients who underwent closure of a secundum ASD with an ASO device.[49] This and other studies show that midterm outcomes following transcatheter closure of a secundum ASD are very good in both children and adults, and late complications related to the device are uncommon.[49,50,56]

Following device closure of an ASD, there is evidence of regression of the right atrial and right ventricular enlargement.[60,61] In a study of 38 patients undergoing transcatheter ASD closure, Kort et al demonstrated normalization of right ventricular size 24 months after transcatheter ASD closure. Although there was also significant reduction in right atrial size, the right atrial size remained large compared to controls at 24 months. The authors also noted greater reduction in right atrial size in patients closed at a younger age, suggesting that younger patients may have a greater potential for remodeling. In contrast, no relationship between the age at closure and the change in the right ventricular volume was evident.[60]

In summary, a secundum ASD is a common congenital heart defect with good prognosis during childhood and the development of significant morbidity and mortality during early adulthood. Surgical and transcatheter closure of an ASD are both safe and effective, decreasing the morbidity and mortality associated with an unrepaired ASD. Although long-term results regarding transcatheter closure are still being evaluated; with appropriate patient selection, it is associated with similar safety and efficacy as surgical closure.

References

1. Carlgren LE. The incidence of congenital heart disease in children born in Gothenburg 1941–1950. *Br Heart J.* 1959;21(1):40–50.

2. Dickinson DF, Arnold R, Wilkinson JL. Congenital heart disease among 160 480 liveborn children in Liverpool 1960 to 1969. Implications for surgical treatment. *Br Heart J.* 1981;46(1):55–62.

3. Ferencz C, Rubin JD, McCarter RJ, et al. Congenital heart disease: prevalence at livebirth. The Baltimore-Washington Infant Study. *Am J Epidemiol.* 1985;121(1):31–36.

4. Fuster V, Brandenburg RO, McGoon DC, Giuliani ER. Clinical approach and management of congenital heart disease in the adolescent and adult. *Cardiovasc Clin.* 1980;10(3): 161–197.

5. Helgason H, Jonsdottir G. Spontaneous closure of atrial septal defects. *Pediatr Cardiol.* 1999;20(3):195–199.

6. Vaughan CJ, Basson CT. Molecular determinants of atrial and ventricular septal defects and patent ductus arteriosus. *Am J Med Genet.* 2000;97(4):304–309.

7. Dexter L. Atrial septal defect. *Br Heart J.* 1956;18(2):209–225.

8. Haworth SG, Hislop AA. Pulmonary vascular development: normal values of peripheral vascular structure. *Am J Cardiol.* 1983;52(5): 578–583.

9. Campbell M, Neill C, Suzman S. The prognosis of atrial septal defect. *Br Med J.* 1957;1 (5032):1375–1383.

10. Craig RJ, Selzer A. Natural history and prognosis of atrial septal defect. *Circulation.* 1968; 37(5):805–815.

11. Markman P, Howitt G, Wade EG. Atrial septal defect in the middle-aged and elderly. *Q J Med.* 1965;34(136):409–426.

12. Campbell M. Natural history of atrial septal defect. *Br Heart J.* 1970;32(6):820–826.

13. Mathew R, Thilenius OG, Arcilla RA. Comparative response of right and left ventricles to volume overload. *Am J Cardiol.* 1976;38(2):209–217.

14. Mainwaring RD, Mirali-Akbar H, Lamberti JJ, Moore JW. Secundum-type atrial septal defects

with failure to thrive in the first year of life. *J Cardiol Surg.* 1996;11(2):116–120.

15. Hanslik A, Pospisil U, Salzer-Muhar U, Greber-Platzer S, Male C. Predictors of spontaneous closure of isolated secundum atrial septal defect in children: a longitudinal study. *Pediatrics.* 2006;118(4):1560–1565.

16. McMahon CJ, Feltes TF, Fraley JK, et al. Natural history of growth of secundum atrial septal defects and implications for transcatheter closure. *Heart.* 2002;87(3):256–259.

17. Radzik D, Davignon A, van Doesburg N, Fournier A, Marchand T, Ducharme G. Predictive factors for spontaneous closure of atrial septal defects diagnosed in the first 3 months of life. *J Am Coll Cardiol.* 1993;22(3):851–853.

18. Mody MR. Serial hemodynamic observations in secundum atrial septal defect with special reference to spontaneous closure. *Am J Cardiol.* 1973;32(7):978–981.

19. Rostad H, Sorland S. Atrial septal defect of secundum type in patients under 40 years of age. A review of 481 operated cases. Symptoms, signs, treatment and early results. *Scand J Thorac Cardiovasc Surg.* 1979;13(2):123–127.

20. Beghetti M, Galie N. Eisenmenger syndrome a clinical perspective in a new therapeutic era of pulmonary arterial hypertension. *J Am Coll Cardiol.* 2009;53(9):733–740.

21. Bartz PJ, Cetta F, Cabalka AK, et al. Paradoxical emboli in children and young adults: role of atrial septal defect and patent foramen ovale device closure. *Mayo Clin Proc.* 2006;81(5):615–618.

22. Berger F, Vogel M, Kramer A, et al. Incidence of atrial flutter/fibrillation in adults with atrial septal defect before and after surgery. *Ann Thorac Surg.* 1999;68(1):75–78.

23. Konstantinides S, Geibel A, Olschewski M, et al. A comparison of surgical and medical therapy for atrial septal defect in adults. *N Engl J Med.* 1995;333(8):469–473.

24. Helber U, Baumann R, Seboldt H, Reinhard U, Hoffmeister HM. Atrial septal defect in adults: cardiopulmonary exercise capacity before and 4 months and 10 years after defect closure. *J Am Coll Cardiol.* 1997;29(6):1345–1350.

25. Brochu MC, Baril JF, Dore A, Juneau M, De Guise P, Mercier LA. Improvement in exercise capacity in asymptomatic and mildly symptomatic adults after atrial septal defect percutaneous closure. *Circulation.* 2002;106(14):1821–1826.

26. Attie F, Rosas M, Granados N, Zabal C, Buendia A, Calderon J. Surgical treatment for secundum atrial septal defects in patients >40 years old. A randomized clinical trial. *J Am Coll Cardiol.* 2001;38(7):2035–2042.

27. Gatzoulis MA, Freeman MA, Siu SC, Webb GD, Harris L. Atrial arrhythmia after surgical closure of atrial septal defects in adults. *N Engl J Med.* 1999;340(11):839–846.

28. Shah D, Azhar M, Oakley CM, Cleland JG, Nihoyannopoulos P. Natural history of secundum atrial septal defect in adults after medical or surgical treatment: a historical prospective study. *Br Heart J.* 1994;71(3):224–227; discussion 228.

29. Steele PM, Fuster V, Cohen M, Ritter DG, McGoon DC. Isolated atrial septal defect with pulmonary vascular obstructive disease–long-term follow-up and prediction of outcome after surgical correction. *Circulation.* 1987;76(5):1037–1042.

30. Loscalzo J. Paradoxical embolism: clinical presentation, diagnostic strategies, and therapeutic options. *Am Heart J.* 1986;112(1):141–145.

31. Treadwell SD, Thanvi B, Robinson TG. Stroke in pregnancy and the puerperium. *Postgrad Med J.* 2008;84(991):238–245.

32. Kozelj M, Novak-Antolic Z, Grad A, Peternel P. Patent foramen ovale as a potential cause of paradoxical embolism in the postpartum period. *Eur J Obstet Gynecol Reprod Biol.* 1999;84(1):55–57.

33. Schrale RG, Ormerod J, Ormerod OJ. Percutaneous device closure of the patent foramen ovale during pregnancy. *Cathet Cardiovasc Interv.* 2007;69(4):579–583.

34. Yap SC, Drenthen W, Meijboom FJ, et al. Comparison of pregnancy outcomes in women with repaired versus unrepaired atrial septal defect. *BJOG.* 2009;116(12):1593-601.

35. Perloff JK. Ostium secundum atrial septal defect–survival for 87 and 94 years. *Am J Cardiol.* 1984;53(2):388–389.

36. Nomura M, Nakaya Y, Kishi F, et al. A 90-year old patient with atrial septal defect and sinus rhythm. *Acta Cardiol.* 1996;51(4):377–380.

37. Driscoll D, Allen HD, Atkins DL, et al. Guidelines for evaluation and management of common congenital cardiac problems in infants, children, and adolescents. A statement for healthcare professionals from the Committee on Congenital Cardiac Defects of the Council on Cardiovascular Disease in the Young, American Heart Association. *Circulation.* 1994;90(4):2180–2188.

38. Roos-Hesselink JW, Meijboom FJ, Spitaels SE, et al. Excellent survival and low incidence of arrhythmias, stroke and heart failure long-term after surgical ASD closure at young age. A prospective follow-up study of 21–33 years. *Eur Heart J.* 2003;24(2):190–197.

39. Murphy JG, Gersh BJ, McGoon MD, et al. Long-term outcome after surgical repair of isolated atrial septal defect. Follow-up at 27 to 32 years. *N Engl J Med.* 1990;323(24):1645–1650.

40. Pearlman AS, Borer JS, Clark CE, et al. Abnormal right ventricular size and ventricular septal motion after atrial septal defect closure: etiology and functional significance. *Am J Cardiol.* 1978;41(2):295–301.

41. Meijboom F, Hess J, Szatmari A, et al. Long-term follow-up (9 to 20 years) after surgical closure of atrial septal defect at a young age. *Am J Cardiol.* 1993;72(18):1431–1434.

42. John Sutton MG, Tajik AJ, McGoon DC. Atrial septal defect in patients ages 60 years or older: operative results and long-term postoperative follow-up. *Circulation.* 1981;64(2):402–409.

43. Sandoval N, Velasco VM, Orjuela H, et al. Concomitant mitral valve or atrial septal defect surgery and the modified Cox-maze procedure. *Am J Cardiol.* 1996;77(8):591–596.

44. Bonchek LI, Burlingame MW, Worley SJ, Vazales BE, Lundy EF. Cox/maze procedure for atrial septal defect with atrial fibrillation: management strategies. *Ann Thorac Surg.* 1993;55(3):607–610.

45. King TD, Thompson SL, Steiner C, Mills NL. Secundum atrial septal defect. Nonoperative closure during cardiac catheterization. *JAMA.* 1976;235(23):2506–2509.

46. Majunke N, Sievert H. ASD/PFO devices: what is in the pipeline? *J Interv Cardiol.* 2007;20(6):517–523.

47. Du ZD, Hijazi ZM, Kleinman CS, Silverman NH, Larntz K. Comparison between transcatheter and surgical closure of secundum atrial septal defect in children and adults: results of a multicenter nonrandomized trial. *J Am Coll Cardiol.* 2002;39(11):1836–1844.

48. Masura J, Gavora P, Formanek A, Hijazi ZM. Transcatheter closure of secundum atrial septal defects using the new self-centering AMPLATZER septal occluder: initial human experience. *Cathet Cardiovasc Diagn.* 1997;42(4):388–393.

49. Masura J, Gavora P, Podnar T. Long-term outcome of transcatheter secundum-type atrial septal defect closure using AMPLATZER septal occluders. *J Am Coll Cardiol.* 2005;45(4):505–507.

50. Butera G, De Rosa G, Chessa M, et al. Transcatheter closure of atrial septal defect in young children: results and follow-up. *J Am Coll Cardiol.* 2003;42(2):241–245.

51. Sharafuddin MJ, Gu X, Titus JL, Urness M, Cervera-Ceballos JJ, Amplatz K. Transvenous closure of secundum atrial septal defects: preliminary results with a new self-expanding nitinol prosthesis in a swine model. *Circulation.* 1997;95(8):2162–2168.

52. Thanopoulos BD, Laskari CV, Tsaousis GS, Zarayelyan A, Vekiou A, Papadopoulos GS. Closure of atrial septal defects with the AMPLATZER occlusion device: preliminary results. *J Am Coll Cardiol.* 1998;31(5):1110–1116.

53. Hijazi ZM, Cao Q-L, Patel HT, Rhodes J, Hanlon KM. Transesophageal echocardiographic results of catheter closure of atrial septal defect in children and adults using the AMPLATZER device. *Am J Cardiol.* 2000;85(11):1387–1390.

54. Chan KC, Godman MJ, Walsh K, Wilson N, Redington A, Gibbs JL. Transcatheter closure of atrial septal defect and interatrial communications with a new self expanding nitinol double disc device (AMPLATZER septal occluder): multicentre UK experience. *Heart.* 1999;82(3):300–306.

55. Butera G, Carminati M, Chessa M, et al. CardioSEAL/STARFlex versus AMPLATZER devices for percutaneous closure of small to moderate (up to 18 mm) atrial septal defects. *Am Heart J.* 2004,148(3).507–510.

56. Chessa M, Carminati M, Butera G, et al. Early and late complications associated with transcatheter occlusion of secundum atrial septal defect. *J Am Coll Cardiol.* 2002;39(6):1061–1065.

57. DiBardino DJ, McElhinney DB, Kaza AK, Mayer JE, Jr. Analysis of the US Food and Drug Administration Manufacturer and User Facility Device Experience database for adverse events involving AMPLATZER septal occluder devices and comparison with the Society of Thoracic Surgery congenital cardiac surgery database. *J Thorac Cardiovasc Surg.* 2009;137(6):1334–1341.

58. Divekar A, Gaamangwe T, Shaikh N, Raabe M, Ducas J. Cardiac perforation after device closure of atrial septal defects with the AMPLATZER septal occluder. *J Am Coll Cardiol.* 2005;45(8):1213–1218.

59. Amin Z, Hijazi ZM, Bass JL, Cheatham JP, Hellenbrand WE, Kleinman CS. Erosion of AMPLATZER septal occluder device after closure of secundum atrial septal defects: review of registry of complications and recommendations to minimize future risk. *Cathet Cardiovasc Interv.* 2004;63(4):496–502.

60. Kort HW, Balzer DT, Johnson MC. Resolution of right heart enlargement after closure of secundum atrial septal defect with transcatheter technique. *J Am Coll Cardiol.* 2001;38(5):1528–1532.

61. Teo KS, Carbone A, Piantadosi C, et al. Cardiac MRI assessment of left and right ventricular parameters in healthy Australian normal volunteers. *Heart Lung Circ.* 2008;17(4):313–317.

3

ASDs:

Clinical Perspectives

Wail Alkashkari and Ziyad M. Hijazi

Atrial Septal Defect

Definition

Atrial septal defects (ASDs) are congenital cardiac defects that allow communication between the left and right atria and account for 10% of all congenital heart disease (CHD). There are several different types of ASDs. The most common is secundum, present in the region of the fossa ovalis and accounting for 75% of all ASDs. Secundum ASD is the most common CHD in adult patients after bicuspid aortic valve. It is more common in females with a female to male ratio of 2:1.

The primum ASD (15%–20% of ASD cases) is positioned in the inferior part of the atrial septum, near the crux of the heart. This defect is associated with atrioventricular septal defects. The sinus venosus type (5%–10% of ASD cases) is located in the superior or inferior part of the septum, near the superior or inferior vena cava entry to the right atrium. The superior type is usually associated with partial anomalous pulmonary venous drainage.

The uncommon coronary sinus septal defect (< 1%), allows shunting through the ostium of the coronary sinus.

Patent foramen ovale (PFO) is a flaplike communication in which the septum primum covering the fossa ovalis overlaps with the superior limbic band of the septum secundum. In some patients, the septum primum or secundum is aneurysmal and may have multiple small fenestrations.

Transcatheter Closure of ASDs and PFOs: A Comprehensive Assessment. © 2010 Ziyad M. Hijazi, Ted Feldman, Mustafa H. Abdullah Al-Qbandi, and Horst Sievert, editors. Cardiotext Publishing, ISBN: 978-0-9790164-9-3.

Genetics

In the majority of the ASD cases there is no genetic predisposition, however, familial occurrence of secundum ASDs is well recognized, and in some kindreds, a defect has been localized to chromosome 5. Familial ASD associated with AV conduction defect is an autosomal dominant trait, with mutation in the cardiac homeobox transcription factor gene NKX2-5. Genetic syndromes with skeletal abnormalities associated with ASD include a variety of heart-hand syndromes, of which Holt-Oram syndrome is best known, which is due to mutation in TBX5. Both secundum and primum ASDs are associated with trisomy 21. The risk of transmission of CHD to offspring of women with sporadic ASD is estimated at 8% to 10%.

Associated lesions

When an ASD is the primary diagnosis, associated malformations occur in 30% of the cases. As part of the atrioventricular septal defect, the primum ASD is nearly always accompanied by a cleft in the anterior mitral valve leaflet. As mentioned, superior sinus venosus defect is frequently (in 80%–90%) associated with partial anomalous pulmonary veinous drainage. The secundum ASD is rarely associated with partial anomalous return of the right pulmonary veins. Mitral valve prolapse is frequently seen in patients with ASD. Valvular pulmonic stenosis is frequently seen in association with ASD and in some cases, mild RV outflow tract gradient caused by increased flow across the structurally normal valve is seen. Coronary sinus septal defect (unroofed coronary sinus) can be associated with partial or total anomalous pulmonary venous connection and/or a persistent left superior vena cava draining to the coronary sinus or left atrium.

Pathophysiology

An ASD allows shunting between the two atria. The magnitude and direction of shunt depends on defect size, the relative compliance of the ventricles, and the status of the atrioventricular valves. Generally the difference between pressures in either atrium is low, and the left-to-right direction of the shunt is due to the higher compliance (less stiffness) of the right ventricle compared to the left ventricle resulting in left-to-right shunt.

In infancy, the right ventricle is thick, stiff, and not very compliant. Therefore, a minimal amount of left-to-right shunting occurs. In the first few weeks of life, pulmonary vascular resistance (PVR) decreases, the right ventricle becomes more compliant, and the magnitude of left-to-right shunt increases.

In adults, the shunting is still mostly left to right. In conditions associated with a reduction in left ventricular compliance and an increase in left atrial pressure (systemic hypertension, ischemic heart disease, left heart failure, and mitral valve dysfunction), the magnitude of the left-to-right shunt increases. Simultaneous right-to-left shunt occurs in the presence of significant tricuspid regurgitation especially if directed into the defect, or when the right ventricular end-diastolic pressure is elevated (eg, RV failure, pulmonary valve disease, or pulmonary hypertension), or in cases in which the superior or inferior vena cavae are superimposed on the left atrium in sinus venosus defects.

A left-to-right shunt at the atrial level results in a volume overload and dilatation of the right atrium, right ventricle, and pulmonary artery; at a later stage, in the presence of tricuspid regurgitation, regurgitant volume through the tricuspid valve contributes further to right heart chambers dilatation. Eventually right ventricular systolic dysfunction will occur.

At younger ages, the increased pulmonary blood flow does not result in severe pulmonary hypertension, as the pulmonary vascular bed may dilate considerably. Therefore, the rise in pulmonary artery pressure in childhood and young age is limited and is due to a high pulmonary blood flow rate with normal PVR. However, a high pulmonary blood flow occurring for a number of years may result in endothelial injury of the pulmonary vessels, depletion of the vasodilator reserve, and pulmonary vascular bed remodeling. This may result in an increase in PVR and severe pulmonary hypertension. Factors contributing to the rise in pulmonary artery pressure include actual changes in the pulmonary vascular bed; left-heart disease; and hypoxic pulmonary hypertension in the presence of chronic lung disease or sleep apnea syndrome. A severely dilated pulmonary artery in older age may be associated with formation of mural thrombi and distal embolism into the pulmonary vascular bed. This may also worsen pulmonary hypertension. Further, underlying genetic factors can modify the phenotype and predispose the patient to the development of severe pulmonary vascular disease in the presence of a shunt at the atrial level.

During exercise, pulmonary artery pressure tends to rise in healthy individuals too, and is proportionate to cardiac output.[1] However, the rise in pulmonary artery pressure in individuals older than 50 years of age is steeper. Older adults with ASD have been shown to have an abnormal rise in pulmonary artery pressure compared with controls. Patients with ASD and pulmonary hypertension have significantly reduced oxygen consumption during exertion; in patients without significant pulmonary hypertension, peak oxygen consumption correlates inversely with the size of the left-to-right shunt.[2] Defect closure is followed by a fall in pulmonary artery pressure, even in older patients, unless there is irreversible, advanced disease in the pulmonary vascular bed (Eisenmenger syndrome). Eisenmenger syndrome is defined as an extreme form of pulmonary vascular disease with pulmonary artery pressures at or near systemic level, and reversed or bidirectional shunting at atrial, ventricular, or arterial levels. It is rarely associated with ASD (1%–6%), with higher incidence in females compared to male patients.

In ASD, the left ventricle is oppressed by a dilated right ventricle and left ventricular diastolic function is abnormal. However, left ventricular systolic function is usually normal and does not diminish until an appreciably paradoxical movement of the interventricular septum occurs. Diastolic function of the left ventricle is adversely affected by the volume-overloaded right ventricle (interventricular interaction). Inadequate filling and the oppression of the left ventricle over a prolonged period results in its hypoplasia with a risk of left heart failure following defect closure.

Clinical findings

Presentation

In childhood, ASD usually presents with a murmur and is asymptomatic. Occasionally, infants may present with breathlessness, recurrent chest infections, and even heart failure. Failure to thrive is an uncommon presentation. In the current era, many children are referred to a pediatric cardiologist for spurious reasons and found incidentally to have an ASD on echocardiographic evaluation.

A typical feature of ASD in adulthood is its prolonged asymptomatic course. In their youth, many patients with even a large ASD practiced sports experiencing no problems at all. Symptoms develop insidiously, most often after the age of 40 or 50. In women, the clinical status may deteriorate during pregnancy or after delivery. In adults with an ASD who are < 40 years of age, there is no correlation between symptoms (NYHA class) and the size of a shunt. But, the development of symptoms does correlate with age. Most patients with an ASD who are in their sixties experience problems; however, exertional dyspnea and reduced physical fitness are usually ascribed by these patients to physiological changes associated with aging, and lifestyle is modified accordingly. Major and limiting problems are often experienced after age 65 years. The clinical course of a nonoperated ASD in adulthood may be significantly affected by associated cardiovascular disease such as hypertension, coronary artery disease, and mitral regurgitation, as the compliance and the filling pressures of the ventricles change with subsequent impact on the size and direction of the shunt at the atrial level. Therefore, even patients with small (< 10 mm) defects can present with significant symptoms. Patients with unoperated ASD older than 60 years of age very often develop atrial fibrillation. Atrial fibrillation or atrial flutter is an age-related reflection of the atrial stretch, which seldom occurs in those younger than 40 years of age.

Occasionally ASDs in adulthood are diagnosed for the first time accidentally due to an abnormal clinical finding or abnormal electrocardiogram (ECG), chest x-ray (CXR), or echocardiography performed for other medical reasons.

Symptoms

Symptoms may include the following:

- Reduced exercise tolerance, tiredness
- Exertional dyspnea
- Palpitations (due to supraventricular arrhythmias, frequent atrial fibrillation/atrial flutter in older age), or syncope for sick sinus syndrome
- Atypical chest pain (right ventricular ischemia)
- Frequent respiratory tract infections
- Signs of right-heart failure
- Paradoxical embolism from peripheral venous or pelvic vein thrombosis, atrial arrhythmias, unfiltered intravenous infusion, or indwelling venous catheters

Clinical findings

- The patients are usually pink; cyanosis suggests severe pulmonary hypertension with reversed shunting in the presence of a secundum ASD or superior sinus venosus defect; cyanosis can also reflect associated pulmonary stenosis, a coronary sinus defect, or an inferior sinus venosus defect (with a prominent Eustachian valve directing the blood to the left atrium).
- Right ventricular heave, but the left ventricular impulse is usually normal
- Wide and fixed split of the second heart sound above the pulmonary artery (delayed pulmonary artery valve closure); a loud pulmonary component reflects severe pulmonary hypertension
- Ejection systolic murmur heard best at the left sternal border (increased blood flow through the pulmonary artery orifice

(relative pulmonary stenosis); sometimes, a pulmonary ejection click can be heard
- Diastolic murmur at the lower right sternal border due to increased blood flow through the tricuspid orifice specially if the Qp:Qs ratio is more than 2.5:1 (relative tricuspid stenosis)
- Examination should focus also on the status of the left heart pathology; an example of that is pansystolic murmur can be heard in the presence of mitral regurgitation on the apex. The clinical findings and auscultation may be completely discrete and *unremarkable*.

Electrocardiogram

In secundum ASD, the rhythm can be sinus, atrial flutter, or atrial fibrillation. Right atrial overload can be present (P-Pulmonale). Right axis deviation and right ventricular hypertrophy (tall R wave in V_1) reflects right ventricular volume overload/hypertrophy. Incomplete right bundle branch block (shape rSr' or rsR' in leads V_1–V_3) is a feature of delayed activation of the dilated right ventricle. First-degree atrioventricular block can be found in the presence of secundum ASD, and this is due to intra-atrial and sometimes H-V conduction delay but it can also be found in older patients with a secundum ASD and this is due to AV nodal delay.

Crochetage, a notch seen in the QRS in leads II and III, has also been reported in secundum ASD.

In primum ASD, left axis deviation (superior axis) and first-degree atrioventricular block can be found and this is due to the anatomic position of the conduction bundle and should not be confused with bifascicular block.

Junctional (coronary sinus) rhythm (negative P wave) reflects the absence of a sinus node and is frequently seen in the presence of a superior sinus venosus defect.

Complete heart block may be present in association with familial ASDs.

Chest x-ray

The cardiac silhouette is enlarged (right atrium and right ventricle). A prominent, dilated pulmonary artery and dilated hilar vessels can be present, and a lifted cardiac apex reflects the presence of right ventricular dilatation. Pulmonary plethora reflects increased pulmonary blood flow (left-to-right shunt). A small aortic knuckle reflects a chronic low systemic blood flow in the presence of an important left-to-right shunt.

Echocardiography

A TTE (transthoracic echocardiography) is the primary diagnostic imaging modality for ASD; in children most of the information can be obtained from TTE but in adults, TEE (transesophageal echocardiography) is important to complete the necessary information. The study should include two-dimensional (2D) imaging of the atrial septum from the parasternal short axis view at the base of the heart, apical, and subcostal view with color Doppler demonstration of shunting. The following parameters are assessed:

- Presence and type of defect
- Exact defect size determined in at least two planes, the biggest measured size is of importance
- Distance of defect rims from other structures by TEE (atrioventricular valves, coronary sinus, superior and inferior caval veins, aorta, and pulmonary veins)
- Quality of atrial septal margins (rims) around the defect (by TEE)
- Entry of pulmonary veins to rule out their anomalous return
- Right ventricular size, its function, and signs of volume overload (paradoxical movement of the interventricular septum)
- Magnitude of the left-to-right shunt using noninvasive calculation of the pulmonary to systemic blood flow ratio (Qp/Qs)—this is of little use
- Pulmonary artery pressure derived from noninvasive calculation of the right ventricular systolic pressure in the presence of tricuspid regurgitation (modified Bernoulli equation), provided there is no pulmonary stenosis. The degree of

the Tricuspid regurgitation is very important as this may influence the mode of repair

- Any other associated congenital anomalies, including another ASD, pulmonary stenosis, ventricular septal defect, etc.
- Size, systolic, and diastolic function of the left ventricle, which chronically fills inadequately
- Mitral valve prolapse and magnitude of mitral regurgitation, if present
- Width of the proximal segment of the main pulmonary artery with respect to the potential presence of pulmonary artery aneurysms and mural thrombi

In addition to the above-mentioned points, the following important points should be considered during evaluation of ASD:

- False-positive diagnosis of ASD can result from either apparent septal dropout on 2D echocardiography images or misinterpretation by color Doppler of vena caval inflow as shunt flow. The use of contrast echocardiography or TEE will prevent false-positive interpretations. Patients with partial anomalous pulmonary venous drainage without an ASD will have RV volume overload and may be erroneously presumed to have an ASD.
- False-negative diagnoses are relatively common in adults with poor-quality transthoracic images, especially in patients with sinus venosus ASD. Because of its superior location, the superior sinus venosus defect is most often missed by TTE. Patients with an unexplained RV volume overload by TTE should be studied by TEE or another imaging modality to fully evaluate the atrial septum and pulmonary veins and to rule out defects in the roof of the coronary sinus.
- A large coronary sinus orifice with evidence of atrial shunting may indicate a defect in the roof of the coronary sinus (eg, sinoseptal defects). Thus, the entire

coronary sinus roof should be imaged when this is suspected. When a coronary sinoseptal defect is associated with lesions that cause right-to-left shunting, the orifice of the coronary sinus may not be enlarged and the defect not recognized until after definitive surgery, at which time a left-to-right shunt may occur. With PAH (pulmonary arterial hypertension), the low velocity of the shunt flow across the coronary sinoseptal defect may be difficult to distinguish from other low-velocity flow within the atria.

- Contrast echocardiography with intravenous agitated saline injection is used to confirm the presence of a right-to-left atrial shunt if imaging and color Doppler are not conclusive. Additionally, the presence of negative contrast in the right atrium may be helpful in identifying a left-to-right shunt. If a left-to-right shunt or RV volume overload is recognized but unexplained, the patient should be referred to an ACHD (adult congenital heart disease) center for further imaging studies.

Magnetic resonance and computed tomography

Magnetic resonance imaging (MRI) provides an additional noninvasive imaging modality if findings by echocardiography are uncertain. Direct visualization of the defect and pulmonary veins is possible, RV volume and function can be quantified (gold standard), and estimates of shunt size can also be obtained. Contrast-enhanced cardiovascular computed tomography can also provide diagnostic information although the radiation exposure limits its utility in most cases; computerized tomography (CT) scanning is an alternative if the patient is claustrophobic or if there is a contraindication of a cardiac MRI (eg, a pacemaker).

Catheterization

Catheterization is not required to establish the diagnosis of ASD. It is indicated:

- When there is a need to determine PVR and pulmonary vascular reactivity in the presence of pulmonary hypertension
- In the presence of partial anomalous return of pulmonary veins, unless the course of all pulmonary veins is completely clear based on echocardiography, MRI or CT angiography
- To perform selective coronary angiography in patients older than 40 years of age, or in younger individuals with risk factors of coronary artery disease (CAD) or angina pain, or if there is suspicion of congenital coronary artery anomaly or perioperative injury
- Exceptionally to determine shunt size, only if the hemodynamic relevance of the defect is not clear from echocardiography

Of course, if the intention is to close the defect percutaneously, a hemodynamic study can be done at the same time.

Exercise testing

Exercise testing can be useful to document exercise capacity in patients with symptoms that are discrepant with clinical findings or to document changes in oxygen saturation in patients with PAH. Maximal exercise testing is not recommended in ASD with severe PAH, however.

Management

Indications for closure of ASDs

Large defects with evidence of RV volume overload on echocardiography usually only cause symptoms in the third decade of life or beyond, and closure is usually indicated to prevent long-term complications even if the patient is asymptomatic.

It is of great importance to understand the natural history of unoperated ASD to understand why we are keen to close the hemodynamically significant ASD even in asymptomatic patients. It is mainly to prevent long-term complications, which include premature death, atrial arrhythmias, reduced exercise tolerance, hemodynamically significant TR (tricuspid regurgitation), right-to-left shunting and embolism during pregnancy, overt congestive cardiac failure, or pulmonary vascular disease that may develop in up to 5% to 10% of affected (mainly female) individuals.

In patients undergoing ASD closure before 24 years of age, the long-term survival does not differ from the general population at large. Significantly shorter survival rates have been reported in patients with pulmonary hypertension (PAP ≥ 40 mm Hg) not having the ASD closed until after 24 years of age.[3] Closure in patients older than 40 years of age, while reducing mortality, improving symptoms, and reducing the incidence of functional deterioration and the incidence of heart failure compared with a conservatively managed control group, did not result in a reduced incidence of arrhythmia or stroke on long-term follow-up.[4] Independent mortality predictors were functional NYHA Class III–IV, PAP > 40 mm Hg and Qp:Qs ratio of > 3.5:1.

The development of symptoms or complications does not preclude the patients with ASD from closure regardless of age. Closure will prevent further deterioration and probably will reverse or normalize the complication especially RV dilatation, RV failure, and TR.[5] In patients with atrial flutter or fibrillation, defect closure may be complemented with radiofrequency ablation, ablation of cavo-tricuspid isthmus, or atrial surgery (Maze procedure).

If the patient developed PAH, complete assessment of reversibility of pulmonary vascular disease should be done before closure, and closure may be considered in the presence of net left-to-right shunting, pulmonary artery pressure less than two thirds systemic levels, PVR less than two thirds systemic vascular resistance, or when responsive to either pulmonary vasodilator therapy or test occlusion of the defect (patients should be treated in conjunction with providers who have expertise in the management of pulmonary hypertensive syndromes).

Closure of an ASD also is reasonable in the presence of paradoxical embolism and documented orthodeoxia-platypnea syndrome.

Closure of ASD should be considered and discussed with patients in some cases as prophylaxis even if the defect is small. An example of that is in professional divers and patients undergoing pacemaker implantation due to the risk of paradoxical embolism.

Pregnancy and delivery are generally well tolerated, even by patients with an unclosed ASD with a significant left-to-right shunt. However, clinical symptoms may emerge or deteriorate during pregnancy or after childbirth. During pregnancy and delivery there is an increased risk of paradoxical embolism, regardless of the defect size. It is more appropriate in our opinion to close the defect before planned pregnancy even if it is hemodynamically not significant. Sudden major loss of blood, leading to hypovolemia, systemic vasoconstriction, reduced venous return, increase in the left-to-right shunt, and a decrease in cardiac output, is poorly tolerated. Careful discussion about the need for antiplatelet therapy for several months after device closure is important for patients who intend to become pregnant after a device has been placed. Pregnancy is contraindicated in patients with Eisenmenger syndrome.

Contraindications for closure of ASDs
Small ASDs with a diameter of < 5 mm and no evidence of RV volume overload do not impact the natural history of the individual and thus may not require closure in male patients unless associated with paradoxical embolism.

Routine follow-up of the patient with a small ASD without evidence of RV enlargement or PAH should include assessment of symptoms, especially arrhythmias, and possible paradoxical embolic events. A repeat echocardiogram should be obtained every 2 to 3 years to assess RV size, function, and pulmonary pressure. Reductions in LV compliance related to hypertension, coronary artery disease, or acquired valvular disease increase the degree of left-to-right shunt across an existing ASD so some authors advocate biannual echocardiography in these populations.

Absolute contraindication for ASD closure is the development of severe irreversible PAH

(PVR > 8 Woods units) and no evidence of a left-to-right shunt.

Relative contraindication includes poor state of the patient with other serious conditions and comorbidities. Patients with elevated left atrial pressure due to left ventricular dysfunction pose a special problem and are discussed in the chapter on ASD closure in older patients.

Options for ASD closure

Surgical closure

Until recently, surgical closure has been the "gold standard" form of treatment, with excellent late outcome.

The surgical approach is via midline sternotomy or right thoracotomy. Minimally invasive technique through a right thoracotomy is used in some centers. Primary operation includes pericardial patch closure (autologous material, bovine pericardium, or artificial material) or direct suture closure depending on the type and defect size. The mortality for surgical closure of ASD is reported as 0.3% in the STS database for procedures performed between 1998 and 2002.[6] Complications include:

- Incomplete closure
- Obliteration of the inferior vena caval orifice
- Acute left-heart failure after surgical ASD closure, leading to death or reoperation with a need for partial shunt restoration reported in earlier series in about 2% of cases[7,8]
- Postpericardiotomy syndrome with pericardial and pleural effusions
- Arrhythmias common after surgical ASD closure, especially in elderly patients; supraventricular arrhythmia is most often involved
- Anomalous pulmonary vein orifice obstruction by patch in sinus venosus-type defect (redirection of the right pulmonary vein[s] through a baffle)
- Cyanosis, if the vena cava inferior has been inadvertently detoured to the left atrium

- Local and systemic complications related to cardiac surgical procedure

The development of percutaneous transcatheter closure techniques has provided an alternative method of closure for uncomplicated secundum ASDs with appropriate morphology. The majority of secundum ASDs can be closed with a percutaneous catheter technique. When this is not feasible or is not appropriate, surgical closure is recommended.

Surgical approach is indicated in the following conditions:

- Primum ASD
- Sinus venosus ASD
- Coronary sinus ASD
- Patients with associated anomalous pulmonary venous drainage
- Associated other cardiac indications for surgery (need for correction of other cardiac congenital anomalies, or valvular abnormalities or need for CABG)
- If the atrial septum morphology in secundum ASD is not appropriate for percutaneous closure (deficient rims)

Catheter-based closure of secundum ASDs

Because of the good outcome and low rates of complications, device closure has replaced surgical closure, and has become the method of choice to close morphologically suitable secundum ASD in the absence of any other associated defects.

There are several devices available for use. Percutaneous closure can be considered for defects up to 38 mm in stretched diameter. Adequate septal tissue rims must be present to anchor the device. Adequate rims indicate the presence of > 5-mm distance from the ASD to the superior and inferior vena cava; right upper and lower pulmonary veins; coronary sinus; and mitral or tricuspid valve (a deficient anterior rim toward aorta is not a contraindication for closure).

Relative contraindications for device closure include active infection and the presence of contraindication for antiplatelet therapy.

Any catheter-based arrhythmia procedure should be performed prior to device closure because access to the left atrium will be difficult afterwards.

In large series, using the AMPLATZER occluder or the HELEX device, the complication rates were < 10%, whereas serious complications occurred in the range of 0.3% to 1%.[12,14]

Complications of catheter-based ASD closure devices include:

- Arrhythmias, both during the procedure and within the first 3 months after the procedure; however, they are usually transient and their incidence is not high. They include atrial flutter or fibrillation; and there have been rare reports of complete atrioventricular block. The long-term risk of supraventricular arrhythmias is unknown.
- Transient pericardial effusion
- Thrombus on the left atrial disc, possibly with peripheral embolism
- Occluder malposition and its interference with surrounding structures, which may require surgical revision. If this complication is noted during the procedure, the AMPLATZER occluder or the HELEX device can be repositioned or removed.
- Occluder release and embolism (migration) is one of the most serious complications, which may potentially require cardiac surgical removal. In large series, occluder embolism has been reported to occur in 1.4% to 3.5% of cases, and more frequently with bigger occluder models. Embolism into the right ventricle and pulmonary artery is more frequent, whereas embolism to the left ventricle is rare.
- Perforation of the right or left atrial wall or aorta is a rare, but potentially lethal complication; it requires acute cardiosurgical revision. Patient monitoring during the first 24 to 48 hours after transcatheter closure is recommended.[9] See chapters 12–15 and chapter 22 for a more in-depth discussion of these complications.
- Occluder deformation has been reported

when using an oversize Amplatz occluder whose neck tends to bulge in smaller defects ("mushrooming") or Cobra head malformation, with disc twisting, a rare complication.

- A rise in left atrial pressure has been reported following catheter-based ASD closure in patients older than 60 years of age, in as many as 39% of cases.[10]
- Acute left-heart decompensation is a potential risk in elderly patients with a small left ventricle or in patients with left ventricular diastolic dysfunction (eg, a long history of hypertension). However, serious left-heart failure with pulmonary edema and the need for mechanical artificial ventilation after catheter-based ASD closure has only been described as a case report. Pretreatment with an ACE inhibitor/angiotensin II inhibitor/calcium antagonists with diuretics may be required to optimize hemodynamics/left ventricular filling pressures.
- Air embolism when using an improper technique of occluder insertion
- Occluder insertion may interfere with right atrial structures such as Eustachian valve and Chiari's network.
- Hemolysis has been reported very rarely.[11]
- Local complications in the groin after percutaneous puncture

However, the complication rate was lower and the length of hospital stay was shorter for the device closure than for surgical closure.[12] Kim et al reported that percutaneous ASD closure with the AMPLATZER Septal Occluder not only had equal effectiveness but also cost less compared to surgical closure.[13]

Conclusion

ASD is a common congenital cardiac defect. Full knowledge of the anatomy, physiology, and indications for closure is of paramount importance for the appropriate management of such patients.

References

1. Oelberg DA, Marcotte F, Kreisman H, et al. Evaluation of right ventricular systolic pressure during incremental exercise by Doppler echocardiography in adults with atrial septal defect. *Chest.* 1998;113(6):1459–1465.

2. Kobayashi Y, Nakanishi N, Kosakai Y. Pre- and postoperative exercise capacity associated with hemodynamics in adult patients with atrial septal defect: A retrospective study. *Eur J Cardiothorac Surg.* 1997;11(6):1062–1066.

3. Murphy JG, Gersh BJ, McGoon MD, et al. Long-term outcome after surgical repair of isolated atrial septa defect. *N Engl J Med.* 1990;323:1645–1650.

4. Gatzoulis MA, Freeman MA, Siu SC, Webb GD, Harris L. Atrial arrhythmias after surgical closure of atrial septal defects in adults. *N Engl J Med.* 1999;340:839–846.

5. Popelová J, Hlaváček K, Honěk T, Špatenka J, Kölbel F. Atrial septal defect in adults. *Can J Cardiol.* 1996;12(10):983–988.

6. STS congenital heart surgery data summary available at: http://www.sts.org.

7. Bayer J, Brunner L, Hugel W, et al. Acute left heart failure following repair of atrial septal defects. Its treatment by reopening. *Thoraachir Vask Chir.* 1975;23:346–349.

8. Beyer J. Atrial septal defect: acute left heart failure after surgical closure. *Ann Thorac Surg.* 1978;25:36–43.

9. Amin Z, Hijazi ZM, Bass JL, et al. Erosion of Amplatzer septal occluder device after closure of secundum atrial septal defects: Review of registry of complications and recommendations to minimize future risk. *Cathet Cardiovasc Interv.* 2004;63 (4):496-502

10. Ewert P, Berger F, Nagdyman N, et al. Masked left-ventricular restriction in elderly patients with atrial septal defects: A contraindication for closure? *Cathet Cardiovasc Interv.* 2001;52 (2):177–180.

11. Lambert V, Belli E, Piot JD, Planche C, Losay J. Hemolysis, a rare complication after percutaneous closure of an atrial septal defect. *Arch Mal Coeur Vaiss.* 2000;93(5):623–625.

12. Du ZD, Hijazi ZM, Kleinman CS, et al. for the AMPLATZER Investigators. Comparison between transcatheter and surgical closure of secundum atrial septal defect in children and adult: results of multicenter nonrandomized trial. *J Am Coll Cardiol.* 2002;39:1836–1844.

13. Kim JJ, Hijazi ZM. Clinical outcomes and costs of AMPLATZER transcatheter closure as compared to surgical closure of ostium secundum ASD. *Med Sci Monit.* 2002;8:CR 787–791.

14. Jones TK, Latson LA, Zahn E, et al. Results of the U.S. Multicenter Pivotal Study of the HELEX Septal Occluder for Percutaneous Closure of Secundum Atrial Septal Defects. *J Am Coll Cardiol.* 2007;49:2215–2221.

4

Historical Perspectives on ASD Device Closure

Terry Dean King and Noel L. Mills

*A hundred times every day, I remind myself
that my inner and outer life depend on the
labors of other men, living and dead, and
that I must exert myself in order to
give in same measure as I have received
and am still receiving.*
—Albert Einstein

Introduction

Over the past 40 years, tremendous advances have been made in the evolution of the field of pediatric interventional cardiology. Since the embryonic experimental device in the early 1970s, the field slowly progressed to a worldwide effort to master nonoperative closure of atrial septal defects (ASDs) and more. Beginning with stainless steel and Dacron, new met-als, materials, and technologies have made miniaturization and safety a reality. This chapter covers the initial efforts up to and including current technologies. The more recent devices and closure techniques are mentioned but will be covered in greater detail in later chapters.

It would be inappropriate not to acknowledge what our surgical colleagues have contributed to our foundations and continue to do even today. It has, and will always remain a collaborative effort across multiple disciplines, that enable us all to move forward.

Historical Surgical Background

The interatrial septum (IAS) has been of interest for more than 150 years. The first reported paradoxical embolus through a patent foramen ovale (PFO) is attributed to Julius Cohnheim (1839–1884).[1] Since that time, there have been many reports of paradoxical emboli through the IAS.

In 1939, Gross[2] reported patent ductus arteriosus (PDA) ligation (performed August 17, 1938) and Gross and Hufnagel[3] reported experimental coarctectomy in 1945. Also in 1945, Crafoord and Nylin[4] reported coarctectomy in two patients (12 and 27 years old) performed in October 1944. Surgical focus turned to repair of the IAS in the late 1940s. In 1947, Cohn[5] began experimental closure of ASDs in dogs and in 1948 Murray[6] reported extracardiac surgical closure of an ASD in a 12-year-old child; however, subsequent cardiac catheterization revealed the defect was only partially closed.[7]

The first reported attempt of ASD closure using cardiopulmonary bypass by Dennis et al[8] was in April of 1951; however, at surgery the patient was found to have primum ASD and ultimately expired. Device closure of an ASD using two nylon buttons (forerunner of catheter device closure) in an experimental model was described by Hufnagel and Gillespie[9] in 1951. The buttons were attached to an outer and inner rod that could be inserted through the right atrial appendage atriotomy to close surgically created ASDs in dogs.

In September 1952, Drs. John Lewis and Mansur Taufic are credited with repair of an ASD in a 5-year-old female under general anesthesia and general hypothermia with inflow occlusion.[10] That same year, Gross [11] reported the use of the "well technique" with direct suture closure of an ASD. In May 1953, John Gibbon[12] used cardiopulmonary bypass to repair an ASD in an 18-year-old female and is credited as the first to do so. In Germany, Derra et al[13] reported successful closure of an ASD using surface hypothermia with inflow occlusion in 1955.

Surgical closure of ASDs became increasingly more successful in the 1950s using cardiopulmonary bypass and would later become the gold standard of therapy. Surgical repair still enjoys a low morbidity and mortality status. However, other schools of thought regarding interventional techniques were evolving to repair the IAS and PDA.

Rashkind and Miller[14] developed the balloon septostomy for D-transposition of the great vessels in 1966 and in 1971 Portsmann et al[15] reported their success in "plugging" PDAs. With these advances and relative ease of access to the IAS, it was a fait accompli that catheter modalities would evolve to repair defects of the IAS.

King-Mills Cardiac Umbrella— Personal Commentary

I first contemplated device closure of ASD during my cardiology fellowship in the late 1960s. Discussion with colleagues, both cardiologists and heart surgeons, regarding catheter closure of ASDs always led to the same answer, "It's just not feasible."

In 1972, a patient with hydrocephalus and an embolized Pudenz ventriculoperitoneal shunt catheter was transferred for surgical intervention from Wiesbaden, Germany to Wilford Hall Medical Center (Lackland Air Force Base) where I was stationed. The embolized catheter had migrated to the apex of the right ventricle. Upon arrival, the cardiovascular surgeon questioned whether the embolized catheter could be removed during cardiac catheterization since only the distal 1 mm was opaque with the remaining 12 cm floating presumably in the right ventricle (see Fig 4.1). At that time, the four previously reported cases of embolized Pudenz catheter had been surgically removed[16,17]; presumably because the Pudenz catheter is nonopaque, clinicians had not tried catheter removal. Using an 8F catheter and doubled-over guide wire, the Pudenz catheter (see Fig 4.2) was snared and removed without difficulty.[18] This further spurred my interest in interventional procedures because I reasoned, "If septal defects can be created (balloon septostomy) and objects can be retrieved from the heart (snare technique), then why can't we close defects in the atrial septum?"

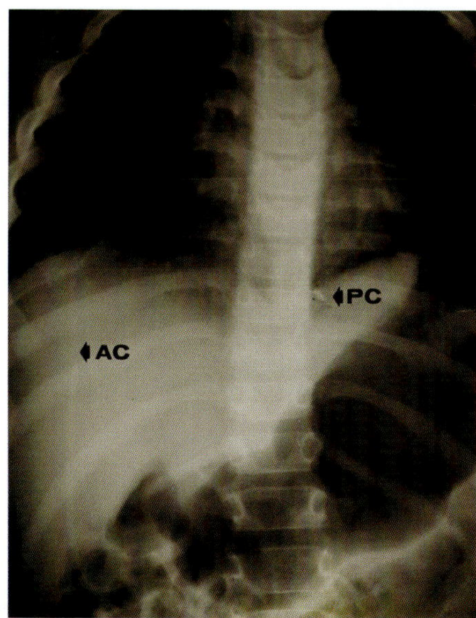

Fig 4.1—Chest x-ray showing opaque tip (P.C.) of Pudenz catheter in the right ventricle. A.C. is the Ames peritoneal catheter. (Courtesy of Dr. Terry Dean King.)

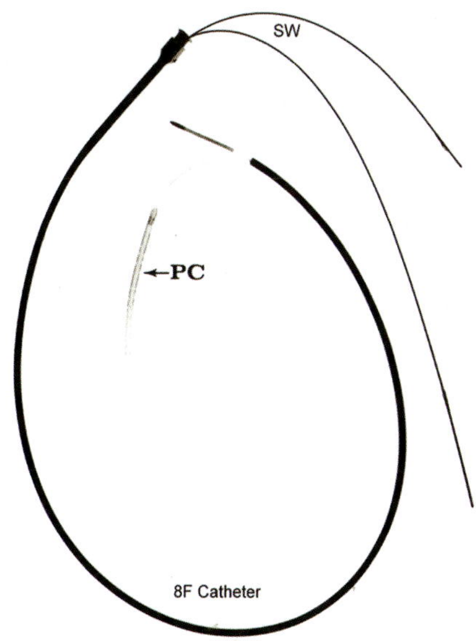

Fig 4.2—8F catheter with snared Pudenz catheter (P.C.) with distal ends of snare wire (SW) visualized at catheter hub. (Courtesy of Dr. Terry Dean King.)

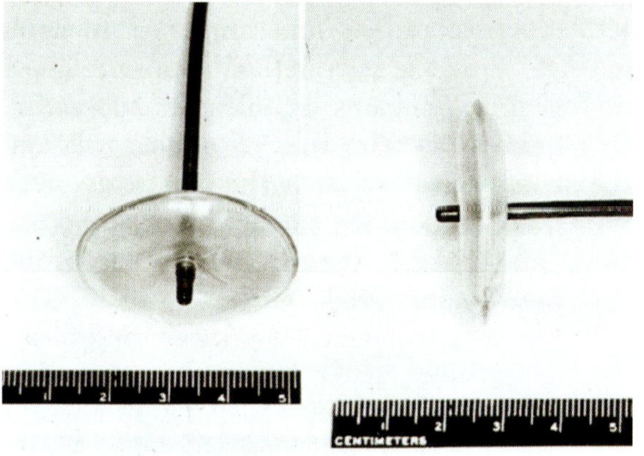

Fig 4.3—Disc-shaped balloon on double lumen cardiac catheter used for closure of VSD. (Reprinted with permission from Mills et al.[19])

Later that same year, during my interview process at the Ochsner Clinic, I met Dr. Noel Mills. I queried him about his thoughts regarding catheter closure of ASDs. To my amazement, he had been trying to develop a catheter with a rubber disc at the distal end (see Fig 4.3) to close post infarct ventricular septal defects (VSDs) in adult patients while in training at New York University Medical Center.[19]

Initially I had envisioned a series of hooks to snare the rim of an ASD and somehow pull it closed. Admittedly, keeping the hooks from grabbing the atrial appendage, mitral valve, and so on was problematic. Early one morning I thought, "What is small enough to pass through a catheter and yet large enough—when in position—to cover a hole?" Then it dawned on me. "Umbrellas!"

In September 1972, Noel Mills and I met with the director of research who agreed to support our efforts to develop a device and technique to close ASDs. The funds came from the Louisiana Heart Association ($10,500), Harvey Pettier Foundation ($25,000), and Kokomo Indiana

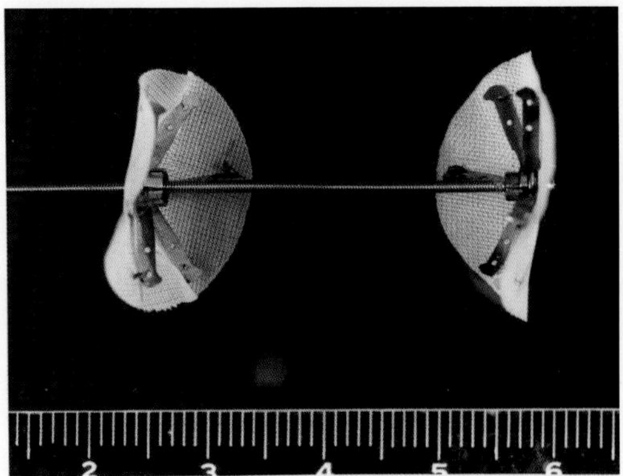

Fig 4.4—Non–self-opening right and left atrial umbrella with six Dacron-covered struts and distal barbs. (Courtesy of Dr. Terry Dean King.)

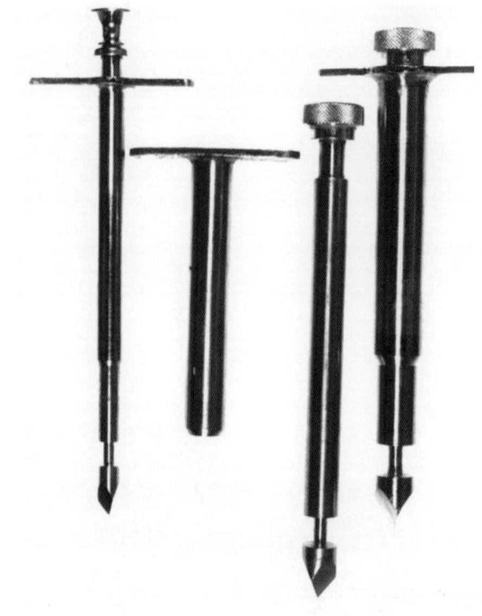

Fig 4.5—Three different size trocars used to create punch ASDs. (Courtesy of Dr. Terry Dean King.)

Fund, but the most cherished funds were given anonymously from hospital employees. The Ochsner Foundation funded the remaining cost.

In early September 1972, I met with a machinist (located by my uncle who was a professor at LSU) in the LSU student union center and drew a crude double umbrella on a napkin. He agreed to assist Noel and me in building the device. Every Friday afternoon the machinist worked with us in the basement of one of the engineering buildings. Finally, a crude device was milled with six stainless steel struts covered with Dacron with distal barbs and a snap lock mechanism as shown in Fig 4.4.

While the device was being developed, several other aspects of our research were pursued. Under the directions of Noel Mills, trocars (see Fig 4.5) were used to create ASDs in mongrel dogs, and with the assistance of a Tulane medical student, hundreds of Fogarty balloon diameters were measured in hopes of being able to size ASDs.[20,21] In that era, because echocardiography was not readily available or of great quality, most patients underwent cardiac catheterization prior to surgery. Between 1973 and 1975 we compared ASDs measured during the patient's catheterization and during the subsequent surgery. We found a very good correlation.[21,22]

We encountered some challenges in our research including scheduling conflicts, heartworms in the animals, and catheter difficulties. We had to use the catheterization laboratory late at night for the experimental animal studies. Early on, we encountered heartworms in the experimental animals that were removed with a snare catheter. This problem was ultimately solved by using Greyhound dogs that were heartworm free and have very large hearts, allowing for easier creation of the punch ASDs. Occasionally, the punch ASD would undergo spontaneous closure. In an attempt to lessen this problem, all research animals were placed on aspirin post-ASD creation. The initial catheters were large and cumbersome. Holding the device in place was difficult and device embolization was an issue.

Despite these challenges, the first cardiac umbrella was successfully implanted in an experimental animal on December 16, 1972 (see Fig 4.6). Ultimately, the experimental closures[23] lead to an interest by Edwards Laboratory in Santa Anna, California. The resulting experimental investigation culminated in receiving the Young Investigator's Award in 1975 at the American Academy of Pediatrics meeting in San Francisco, California. The device developed with Edwards Laboratory was a double umbrella with Dacron-covered struts (see Fig 4.7). This device was used in six patients.

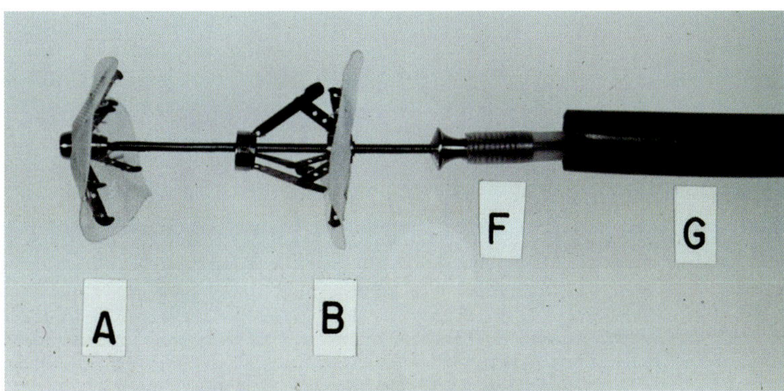

Fig 4.6—Cardiac umbrella used for the first experimental ASD closure. (A) left atrial umbrella, (B) right atrial umbrella, (F) locking catheter and cone, and (G) an outer catheter. (Courtesy of Dr. Terry Dean King.)

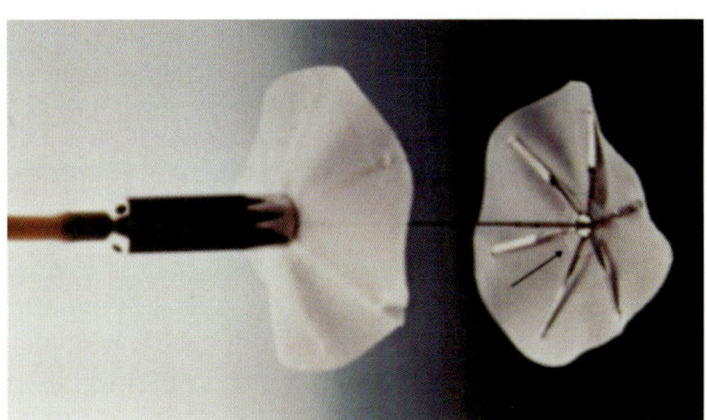

Fig 4.7—Edward's modification of the King-Mills Umbrella, showing left atrial umbrella, right atrial umbrella, obturator wire, and distal capsule. Both umbrellas had silicone rings (arrow) to allow self-opening. (Courtesy of Dr. Terry Dean King.)

Patient selection

The experimental trials led to an Institutional Review Board (IRB) approval to go forward with a clinical trial. Nineteen patients with a clinical diagnosis of secundum ASD were considered as possible candidates for umbrella closure.[24] They ranged in age from 4 years to 76 years. There were five males and fourteen females. Further screening was based on psychiatric aversion to heart surgery, postcerebrovascular accident, poor pulmonary or renal functions, adult ASD with evidence of pulmonary hypertension, and closure of an ASD in association with other nonbypass procedures (eg, PDA). Ten patients were ultimately considered for nonoperative closure and three of this group had associated anomalies that necessitated surgical closure. In the remaining seven patients, the first five underwent successful closure from April 1975 to October 1975. In the last two patients, the device would not seat properly and surgical closure yielded excellent results.

Initial patient

In early 1975, a 17-year-old female was referred for evaluation and possible device closure of an ASD. The patient had refused surgical repair because of scarring issues. On April 8, 1975, after informed consent, the catheterization laboratory was transformed into a hybrid catheterization and operating room suite.

The study revealed a centrally located ASD measured by balloon occlusion at 2.53 cm maximum diameter and a 2:1 shunt. Transcatheter closure was completed using a right femoral vein cut down and a 35-mm double umbrella under fluoroscopy (see Fig 4.8). The Dacron covering on the right atrial umbrella was reduced by about 50% in the first patient only. Total catheterization time was 90 minutes with actual ASD closure time of 7 minutes.[22] Her postoperative course was uneventful. The first patient in the world to undergo nonsurgical closure of an ASD is shown with Dr. King, Dr. Mills, and Sandy Thompson, RN (see Fig 4.9). Within 2 weeks post-closure, she conceived and 9 months later delivered a healthy baby girl.

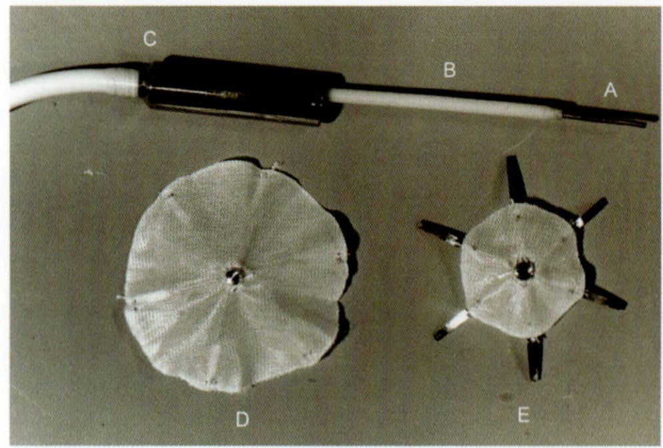

Fig 4.8—King-Mills Umbrella, the device used in closure of ASD in the first patient, 1975: (A) obturator wire, (B) right atrial umbrella catheter, (C) distal capsule and outer catheter, (D) left atrial umbrella, and (E) right atrial umbrella. (Courtesy of Dr. Terry Dean King.)

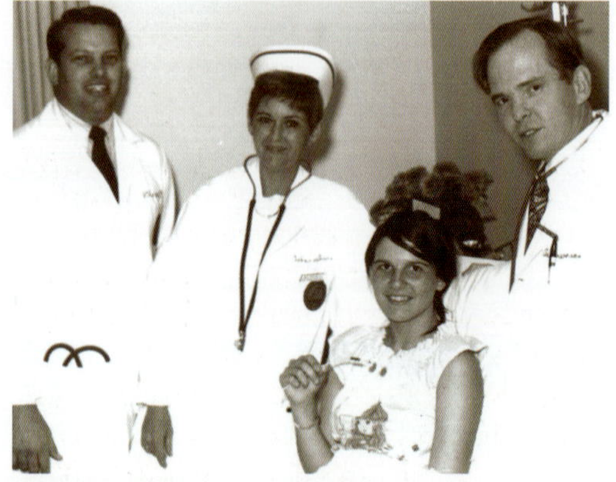

Fig 4.9—Pictured (left to right): Terry Dean King, Sandy Thompson, RN, Suzette (first patient) with ASD device in hand, and Noel L. Mills in April 1975. (Courtesy of Dr. Terry Dean King.)

Subsequently, a 17-year-old male, a 44-year-old male, a 24-year-old female, and a 75-year-old male underwent uneventful transvenous closure of their secundum ASDs. Their clinical courses have been well chronicled in a 27-year follow-up article[25] and a 30-year follow-up was presented at the Pediatric Interventional Cardiology Symposium (PICS) in Buenos Aires in 2005.[26]

Thirty-four-year follow-up

As of December 2009, Patient 1 is 52 years old and is post–left-sided cryptogenic stroke (2006) with full recovery. Echocardiogram at the time of the stroke did not reveal a thrombus site or a shunt. She is on clopidogrel and ezetimibe/simvastatin; she remains in normal sinus rhythm and has never experienced any dysrhythmias. She is the mother of four children and has no exercise limitations (personal communication, December 13, 2009).

Patient 2 is now 52 years old and in perfect health. He is on no medication and races dirt bikes. He has experienced migraines in the past but these were alleviated with caffeine omission and he has never experienced any dysrhythmias (personal communication, December 13, 2009).

Patient 3 turned 79 years old on January 3, 2010. He has experienced atrial fibrillation since 1987 with an unsuccessful ablation in 2005. Due to poor atrial fibrillation control, he underwent AV node ablation and pacemaker implantation in 2007. The AV node ablation procedure was complicated by a low IAS tear which was later closed with a 20-mm AMPLATZER device by Dr. Ziyad M. Hijazi during a live case at the PICS conference in 2008. He is now on aspirin 81 mg, warfarin, amlodipine besylate, and atorvastatin. He has never had a stroke and a recent echocardiogram does not reveal any residual shunt. His energy level is mildly reduced but he walks 1.5 to 2 miles twice per week and rides a stationary bike twice per week for 10 to 15 minutes (personal communication, December 13, 2009).

Patient 4 is now 59 years old and in February 2002 experienced uncontrolled atrial fibrillation and was in early congestive heart failure. Medical treatment with furosemide, diltiazem, and metoprolol relieved her heart failure, and she was discharged on the previously mentioned medications plus simvastatin, potassium, and warfarin. In May 2007, she again experienced atrial fibrillation and underwent successful cardioversion. A transesophageal echocardiogram at the time did not reveal a thrombus. An echocardiogram in December 2008 revealed normal left ventricle measurements, ejection fraction of 60%, and dilated right atrium with peak tricuspid regurgitation of 3.2 m/s, with an estimated pulmonary systolic pressure of 50 mm Hg. No interatrial septal defect was noted and the estimated pulmonary pressure was unchanged from a prior study. There was mild left ventricular hypertrophy and no mention of right ventricular dilatation (personal communication, December 22, 2009). At her last checkup in May 2009, she was in sinus rhythm and her hypertension and hypothyroidism were well controlled. Her current medications are furosemide, potassium, warfarin, and metoprolol. She has never taken digitalis. Her current energy level is excellent and she has remained in normal sinus rhythm since being cardioverted (personal communication, December 13, 2009).

Patient 5 originally presented at 75 years of age in atrial flutter with mild cardiomegaly and increased pulmonary flow. Cardiac catheterization by the adult service revealed a 25-mm ASD. This was closed several days later with 35-mm umbrella device without difficulty. He later developed Hodgkin's disease and expired at age 84 secondary to a cerebral vascular accident. Autopsy confirmed the device-closed ASD and an open inferior 5-mm ASD.

Futher considerations

As one would surmise, this novel approach of transvenous ASD closure produced considerable discussions in the cardiological and surgical arenas. There was some criticism from colleagues, more surgical than cardiological, for attempting an "untried" procedure compared to the well-established "gold standard" of open-heart surgery.

However, the major impediment to further development was the lack of a centering mechanism and not the "barbs," or a "difficult to use" device, or its "sizes" as some have alluded. The need for a centering mechanism was made clear by patients 6 and 7.

Other considerations that lead to our cessation of this endeavor were that one of us (TDK) became interested in politics. However, after a brief stint in Louisiana politics, an offer to develop a much-needed pediatric program in northeast Louisiana was accepted. Therefore, a combination of events and facts resulted in cessation of our research efforts and no further clinical attempts in late 1975. A vignette of his-

torical interest is that Dr. Andreas Gruentzig, an interventional pioneer, obtained several ASD catheters from Noel Mills for experimental use, but were lost with his unfortunate death in a plane crash in October 1985.

Subsequent Devices and Pioneers

Work on interventional closure of ASD essentially lay fallow for a number of years. Rashkind's initial attempts were carried out with a single foam-covered six-ribbed device with hooks at the ends of three ribs. In 1983, eight years after our initial series, Rashkind reported a series of 28 patients in which adequate closure was achieved in 13 patients and inadequate closure in 6 patients. Four patients in the latter group underwent surgical repair with several requiring emergency surgery. Eight patients were not attempted because the defect was deemed too small or too large. One remaining patient could not be accounted for in this article.[27]

Rashkind's attention then shifted to the development of a PDA device. Dr. Chuck Mullins and Dr. Rashkind continued to refine and simplify the PDA device (USCI, Glens Falls, New York). A multicenter clinical trial with the Mullins transseptal sheath and the improved PDA occluder, began in the early 1980s and ultimately received Food and Drug Administration (FDA) panel approval. It was never marketed in the United States.[1]

The Rashkind ASD device underwent modifications in 1985 with the assistance of Drs. James Lock, William Hellenbrand, Larry Latson, and Lee Benson (see Fig 4.10). It was implanted in animal ASD trials using a 16F transseptal sheath. The initial clinical trial under an investigational device exemption was a pilot study at Yale University in early 1987 using the single-sided umbrella device. The procedure was successfully performed by Dr. Hellenbrand and was followed by six more closures either at Yale or Omaha's Children's Hospital.[1]

In 1989, Hellenbrand and Mullins[28] reported single umbrella ASD closure using the

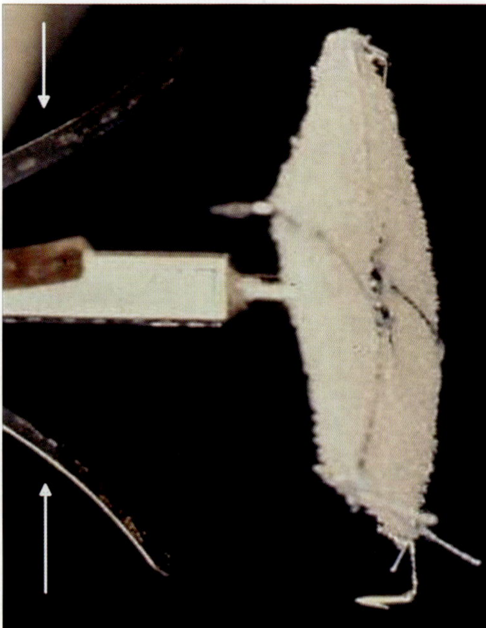

Fig 4.10—Rashkind single disc device with six ribs and alternating hooks (3). Note centering mechanism (arrows) to the left of the disc device. (Courtesy of Dr. Chuck Mullins.)

improved Rashkind ASD device, which had a set of steel guides to help "center" it as the device was withdrawn toward the atrial septum. Three patients were discussed and two of the three had good results; however, the third patient was left with a significantly large shunt that required open-heart surgery. At surgery, the device was attached to the posterior wall of the left atrium.

Their conclusion was that the device had two major problems. First, when opened it could not be removed because of the hooks and would require surgery to remove the device (as in case 3). Secondly, exact positioning of the ASD was a must and therefore would limit the number of patients for this approach. They recommended clinical trials with a double-disc device similar to the ductal occluder device.[28] The Rashkind device and technique were eventually discontinued because of four cases of embolization to the left atrium requiring emergency surgery.[29]

Returning to the Double Umbrella Approach

Clamshell

Rashkind,[27] in his 1983 paper, alluded to a double-disc device which was implanted in a cow septum with complete occlusion and endothelialization at 2 months. As previously mentioned, Hellenbrand and Mullins recommended a double-disc approach.[28] Lock's[30] observations and experiences with the Rashkind ASD "hook" device were not encouraging. This led to a conceptual variation of the Rashkind spring-loaded PDA device. Further work culminated in the development of a double-hinged paired umbrella with four arms that could be folded back on themselves, thus the name Lock Clamshell (USCI Angiographics, Tewksbury, Massachusetts) (see Fig 4.11).

Anecdotally, during a visit to Jim Lock's laboratory, he related that he had thought of the device during a Boston Red Sox baseball game. The arms of the clamshell used spring tension in the mid-arm region, which created a "cone" shape on deployment thus aiding in centering the device. The device had a square-shaped configuration and was covered with Dacron and when implanted needed to be 1.5× to 2× the balloon-sized ASD. This design led to the use of smaller 11F sheaths. Experimental trials in sheep were successful and led to a clinical trial using the new clamshell as reported by Rome et al.[31] The trial included 40 patients who were catheterized with the intent to close their defect. Patient weight was required to be > 8 kg due to the 11F sheath and a device that had to be at least 1.6× the balloon-sized ASD. Attempted closure occurred in 34 patients with defects from 3 to 22 mm and device size 17 to 33 mm. In two cases, early device embolization occurred and one elderly patient expired 1 week postprocedure. Because only the Mullins sheath had crossed the defect when the patient became obtunded, it was presumed to be a non–device-related cerebral embolus. Thirty-one patients were discharged from the hospital

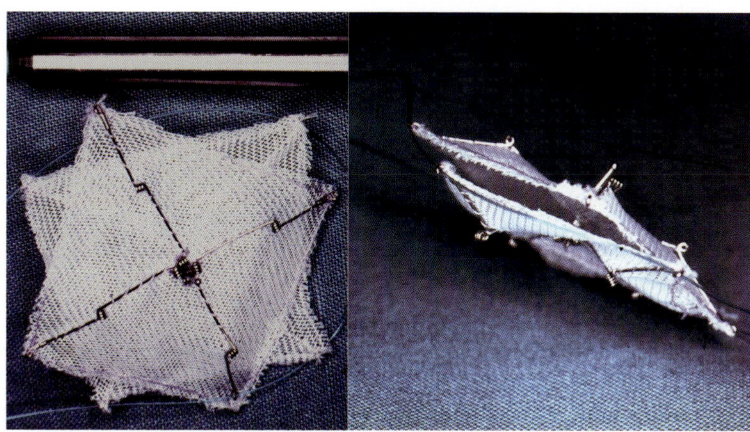

Fig 4.11—Front and side view of Lock's Clamshell device. (Courtesy of Dr. C. Mullins and Dr. J. Lock.)

with implanted clamshells. Despite promising results, the study pointed out a number of limitations including the need for a complete ASD rim and the need for high echocardiographic resolution of the IAS anatomy. Defects > 20 mm or multiple defects were contraindications for device closure. Patient size was a limitation that needed to be addressed with smaller devices and postclosure residual shunts occurred in 10% of patients. Boutin et al[32] reported immediate residual shunts as high as 91% but decreasing to 53% at a mean follow-up of 10 months. Thus, actuarial analysis suggested a gradual closure of residual clamshell shunts over time.

As clinical trials progressed, device arm fractures were being detected. The initial alert came from Japan, followed within a few days by Jim Lock and his group (personal communication, December 21, 2009). In 1992 Bridges et al[33] reported a 30% device arm fracture incidence in one or more arms of the Clamshell device in 36 patients (35 with a PFO and one with an ASD) having Clamshell closure from February 1989 to June 1991. Additionally, Justo et al[34] reported single arm fracture in 56% and multiple fractures in 44%; and Koike et al[35] in 1994 reported a fracture incidence of 82% (9/11) in patients undergoing ASD closure using Clamshell prototypes with arm fracture occurring between 1 week and 12 months after implantation.

By the early 1990s, the Clamshell device had been used in approximately 900 patients.[1] However, the significant number of arm frac-

tures occurring in a high percentage of patients within 1 to 6 months of implantation led to the elective withdrawal of the Clamshell device by the company in 1991.[36] Despite the high percentage of fractures, we are unaware of any known clinical sequelae of the fractures. Ultimately, the device was redesigned using new manufacturing techniques and metal alloy (MP35N) resulting in what is now the CardioSEAL device (Nitinol Medical Technologies, Inc., Boston, Massachusetts). It will be discussed later in this chapter, along with the STARFlex device, as well as Chapter 30.

The "Buttoned" Double-Disk Device and the Center-on-Demand Device

In 1990, Sideris et al[37] first reported their use of the buttoned disk device to close experimental ASDs in piglets. This was followed by a number of modifications to improve its usability, which primarily centered on better visualization and fixation of the buttoning mechanism.[38]

The first four generations had an initial configuration of a single left-sided disc and a "counter occluder" device. The left atrial occluder had a square shape plus the button (actually a string loop knot). The right atrial counter occluder had a rhomboid shape with the buttonhole. The occluder had X-shaped Teflon-coated stainless

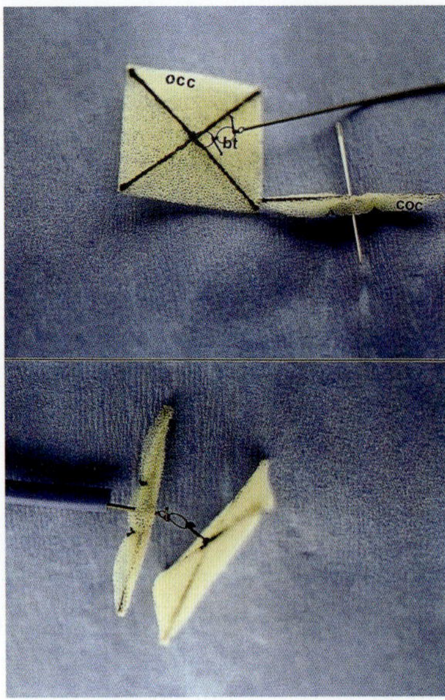

Fig 4.12—Two views of the Sideris button, revealing the occluder button (OCC), counter occluder (COC), and the button connected to the buttoning tie (BT). (Courtesy of Dr. Chuck Mullins.)

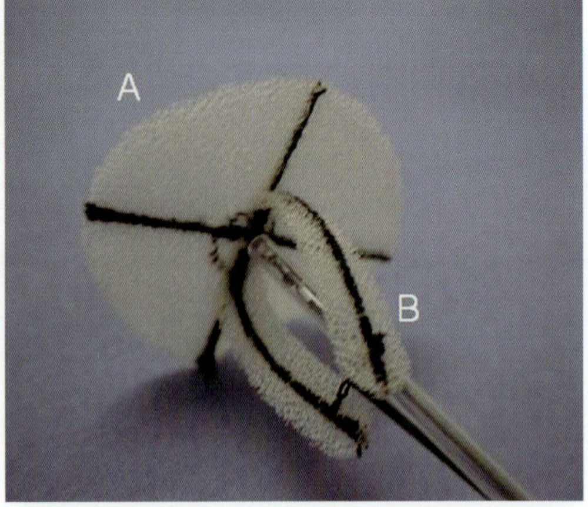

Fig 4.13—Sideris ButtonSeal COD device showing the occluder disc (A) and the centering ring (B). Not shown is the counter-occluder. (Courtesy of Dr. E. Sideris.)

steel wire frames with soft distal tips and was covered with a square, thin, polyurethane foam layer. The counter-occluder was composed of a single strand of Teflon-coated stainless wire skeleton, which was also covered with thin, polyurethane foam covering (see Fig 4.12). These components are connected by "buttoning," which is achieved by pulling the opaque left atrial button (knot) through the buttonhole using gentle traction.[37]

Initially Sideris' devices were implanted using an 8F-long sheath and for larger devices a 9F sheath. The devices were custom made. The device-to-defect ratio was 2.3 to 2.5 due to the lack of self-centering, which ultimately led to a modification of the fourth generation device with that capability. This was achieved by using a centering ring that was attached to two arms of the occluder device—so-named the centering-on-demand buttoned device or COD (see Fig 4.13). This eliminated, to some degree, having to use large devices in a small left atrium. If the defect was small and the centering ring was not needed, it would be folded on the left-sided device before implanting and if used it would be folded on the right side of the IAS. The device then subsequently buttoned. In addition, the occluder disc was changed from a square occluder[39] to a circular configuration[40] as shown in Fig 4.13. The device required a 10 to 12F-long sheath and the stretch diameter-to-device ratio was 1.8. In the first 180 cases, spontaneous unbuttoning of the device was encountered in 13 (7.2%) patients. Modifications of the buttoning mechanism in the fourth-generation device saw a decrease in spontaneous unbuttoning 4/423 (0.9%).[40]

In 2001, Rao and Sideris[40] presented a comprehensive comparison and review from international and US trials of the first four button-device generations and the COD. The first three generations' devices were used during a 3.5-year period ending in February 1993 in 180 patients and 16 institutions worldwide.[40] The successful implantation rate was 92% (166/180). Effective closure (92%) was defined as either no shunt or trivial shunts by echocardiography within 24 hours and was achieved in 92 patients and 62 patients, respectively (154 patients). Unbuttoning occurred in 13 patients (7.2%) and of these (5.5%) 10 had surgical retrieval and closure of their ASD. In the 7-year follow-up, residual shunts were closed surgically in 13 and by catheter in 1 patient. In the remaining patients, the shunt either disappeared or decreased.

The fourth-generation device was implanted during a 4-year period ending in September 1997 in 423 patients at 40 institutions worldwide.[40] The most commonly used devices were 35, 40, and 45 mm and the successful implantation rate was 99.8% (422/423). Unbuttoning diminished to 0.9% and device embolization occurred in only one patient. Four patients had device retrieval and subsequent surgical repair and one patient required urgent surgical retrieval and ASD repair. Effective closure, as previously defined, was 90% (377/417).

Follow-up data are available up to a 5-year period in 333 of 417 patients (80%). During this period reintervention occurred in 21 patients (5%) mainly due to residual shunts. This included 11 patients requiring surgical closure and 9 patients receiving a second device. In the remaining patient, there was a gradual reduction in residual shunt.[40]

Rao reported the COD device was implanted in 65 of 68 patients (95.6%) during an 18-month period ending in July 2000. Device sizes increased from 25 to 60 mm in 5-mm increments and were used to close PFOs or ASDs (~5 mm) to larger ASDs via 10 to 12F sheaths. The device-to-defect ratio was 1.8. Patient ages ranged from 1.5 to 70 years with a median of 11 years. Weight ranged between 10.8 and 100 kg with a median of 24 kg. ASDs measured 5 to 18 mm by echocardiogram and by balloon sizing (stretch diameter) 16.8 ± 6 mm with a range of 9 to 30 mm. The most commonly used devices were 30, 35, and 40 mm. The device was unstable in two patients and in one patient the defect was large without sufficient rim. All three of these patients underwent elective successful surgical closure. The effective closure, as previously defined, was 94% (62/65). One pediatric patient had a suspected thrombus on the occluder disc, which was treated with tissue plasminogen activator (tPA). The clot resolved without complications. At the time of the report a short-term follow-up indicated that no further interventions had been required.

Rao[41] later reported a total of 80 patients (including the 65 patients previously discussed in the Rao and Sideris series) being selected for secundum ASD closure using a COD device. Of this group, 76 (95%) underwent device implantation; their ages ranged from 1.5 to 70 years (median of 9 years) and weight between 9.2 and 100 kg (median 28 kg). Effective closure, as previously defined, was accomplished in 71 patients. Two patients had a deficient rim and the device was unstable in two patients, none of which received device closure. These four patients had elective surgical repair of their defects. The remaining patient was not discussed. The previously mentioned thrombus was the only immediate adversity. Follow-up data for 1 to 12 months revealed no reinterventions and no devices unbuttoned.[41]

As of 2003, the COD was only available under FDA-approved trials in the United States; however it was available outside the United States for general clinical use with local IRB approval. The last buttoned-devices were implanted in the United States in the late 1990s. They were premarketed in 1998 but were never marketed and are now abandoned. The main use of the COD device was to treat aneurysmal ASDs, small ASDs, and PFOs. Approximately 3000 COD and buttoned devices have been used worldwide (personal communication, December 22, 2009).

Metals with Memory— A Technological Leap

In 1932, Arne Ölander[42] was credited with the observation of mechanical recoil in a certain gold-cadmium alloy. Similar observations were noted in certain copper-zinc brasses 6 years later. In 1962, a tremendous breakthrough occurred when William Buehler (United States Naval Ordnance Laboratory) found that an alloy composed of equal parts of nickel and titanium exhibited a strange characteristic and named the material "Nitinol" after the "Nickel-

Titanium Naval Ordinance Laboratory."[42] Further research followed and the uses of this newfound material expanded for use in braces[43] and glasses, as well as many other applications.[42] The property of assuming a distorted shape when squeezed into a catheter and regaining its pre-formed original shape when deployed beyond the catheter lends itself readily to applications for device closure of ASDs. Nitinol (55% nickel and 45% titanium) has now allowed catheter devices to take a "big step" forward from the prior stainless steel era. These alloy materials such as Nitinol, MP35N, and Phynox have proven useful in devices with better centering characteristics and have considerably lessened the risk of stress fractures. From our vantage point, this was a technological leap with limitless possibilities.

Atrial Septal Defect Occluder System (ASDOS)

The need for iatrogenic ASD creation in mitral valve stenosis treatment with balloon valvuloplasty[44] and the absence of a commercially available ASD closure device in Europe led Babic et al[41] to develop the atrial septal defect occluder system (ASDOS). The initial device consisted of two self-opening umbrellas made of stainless steel and covered with preserved pericardium. An Ivalon (polyvinyl alcohol) plug was placed between the umbrellas as shown in Fig 4.14 and was used to aid in centering. Implantation required a long venoarterial wire track and the techniques described by Babic et al.[45] This track utilized a 6F catheter from the arterial approach and initially a 14F sheath from the venous approach. Implantation was accomplished with the serial venous insertion of the left atrial umbrella, followed by the Ivalon plug, and finally the right atrial umbrella. A nylon thread attachment to the right-sided umbrella was used to allow for positioning as desired. The 14F Teflon catheter tip was positioned in the left atrium. The left atrial umbrella was then passed over the long wire into the left atrium where it is expanded. Importantly, a metal ball (metal conus) on the guide wire was used to prevent any distal migration of the left atrial umbrella and also was used to pull the umbrella toward the IAS. The centering Ivalon plug (15 mm) was subsequently pushed into the left atrium. Then, with the sheath in the right atrium, the right-sided umbrella was opened. The two umbrellas with the Ivalon plug between them were locked by a screw mechanism. Positioning was guided initially by left atrial angiography.[45] When optimal positioning was achieved, the long guide wire was removed via the femoral artery.[46] In the initial prototype, once the device was locked in place, it required surgical removal for suboptimal positioning.[41]

In 1990, Babic [45] reported the initial closure of an 18-mm ASD in a 58-year-old female using the preceding prototype. The following year, Babic et al[46] reported the use of a refined experimental prototype in 28 adult patients. Initially, the device frame was stainless steel; however, in the latter cases it was covered with Dacron. Transthoracic and transesophageal echocardiography was used to analyze the anatomy and size of the ASD.

Osypka Company GMbH of Germany licensed the ASDOS system in 1994 for further refinements and evaluation. This version had two self-opening umbrellas made of a Nitinol frame covered with a thin polyurethane membrane. The refined umbrella had five arms and was discoid in shape when deployed (see Fig 4.15). This system used an 11F-long sheath for deployment.

The latest prototype was used experimentally in swine models.[47] These results were followed by further clinical trials. Hausdorf et al[48] reported the use of ASDOS device in 10 pediatric patients with secundum ASDs measuring 10 to 20 mm in diameter. The umbrella sizes ranged from 20 to 40 mm in diameter and the procedure was guided by echocardiography. It was successful in 90% (9/10) of the cases and only one patient had transient atrioventricular block. A trivial shunt was present months later in one patient.

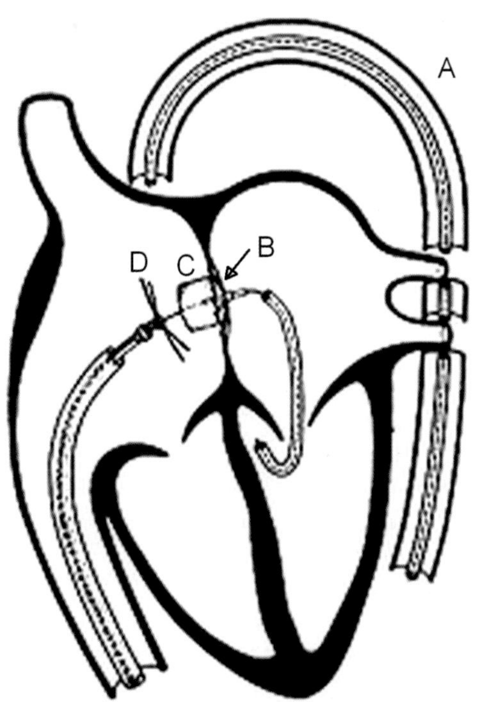

Fig 4.14—ASDOS. Note the venoarterial wire track (A) with left atrial umbrella (B) in place, Ivalon plug (C), and right atrial umbrella (D). (Courtesy of Dr. U. Babic.)

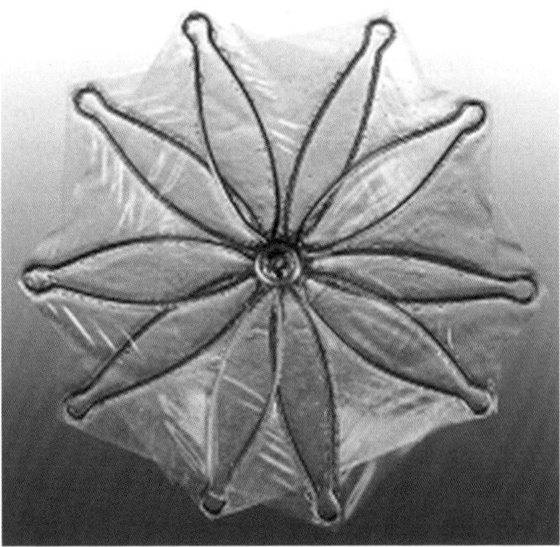

Fig 4.15—En face view of ASDOS device showing the "flower" shape. This new prototype was developed by Osypka Company GMbH in conjunction with Dr. Babic. (Courtesy of Dr. U. Babic.)

In 2000, Babic [49] reviewed the experience with the ASDOS system. Between 1995 and 1998, closure was attempted in 350 patients (ASDOS registry, December 1998) of which 89 had a PFO and 261 had an ASD. The majority of these patients had been in the European multi-institutional study. Three hundred and eighteen patients had successful implants (91%). There were 32 failures (9%), 26 devices retrieved via catheter (7%), 6 devices retrieved by surgery (2%), follow-up surgical extraction in 11 (3%), and 307 implants at the time of reporting. Minor complications were rare with a combined total of 2.8%. Implant-related complications included 3 early embolizations (0.9%), 0 late dislodgments (0%), 3 thromboemboli (0.9%), 6 perforations (1.6%), and 2 suspected infections (0.6%). Embolizations were to the right ventricular outflow tract, the abdominal aorta, and the pulmonary artery.

Immediate postclosure residual shunts (small) remained in 25% to 30% of patients and in a small number of these, the shunt resolved with time. A medium-to-large shunt remained in 8% and were surgically repaired because of no shunt reduction with time. Frame fractures were found in 20% of patients examined by cine-radiography. During the first week postocclusion, a thrombus formation was noted in the majority of patients and in 25% of these patients transesophageal echocardiography revealed a "hamburger-like" thrombus that resolved with time.

Perforation occurred in five patients between 1 day and 8 months postimplant and involved the free atrial wall. Prosthesis endocarditis was assumed in two patients and at surgery the findings were nonconfirmatory for an infection; however, both surgical patients had fatal outcomes.

Babic then asked the question, "What have we learned?" He followed by covering in some detail a number of considerations regarding the anatomy of the IAS and surrounding relationships as well as the texture of the septum. He felt the latter was the most important factor for a successful procedure. In addition, he stressed that occluder diameters must not exceed the short axis of the IAS at end systole. The atrial septal orientation and the ASD location must be fully appreciated because an ASD is a dynamic defect that changes diameter during the cardiac cycles. Individuals with hyper-dynamic defects may not be candidates for catheter closure because the diastolic defect may be larger than the end systolic septal diameter. In addition, he suggested that a vertically aligned IAS with a defect could be difficult to occlude even with a so-called "self-centering" mechanism. Babic understood that modifications to the device might include a Nitinol centering mechanism and making the system more "user friendly." Smaller devices with better centering may lessen the risk of perforation and better locking mechanisms needed to be developed. Providing

a system with a high level of safety is essential to the success of any device.

The ASDOS system obtained European Certification in 1995 and the centralized registry of ASDOS continued until the end of 1999. There were 400 patients registered and since that time another 200 patients have been treated with this device (personal communication, January 2010); however, the certified version has not been used since 2001. An improved investigational prototype has been conceptualized but is not available for clinical use (see Fig 4.16).[41] Babic stated, "Some years ago, it was questionable whether or not an ASD can be closed without surgery. Today, sending a patient with a centrally located ASD to surgery might be regarded as a failure of the current state of the art."[49]

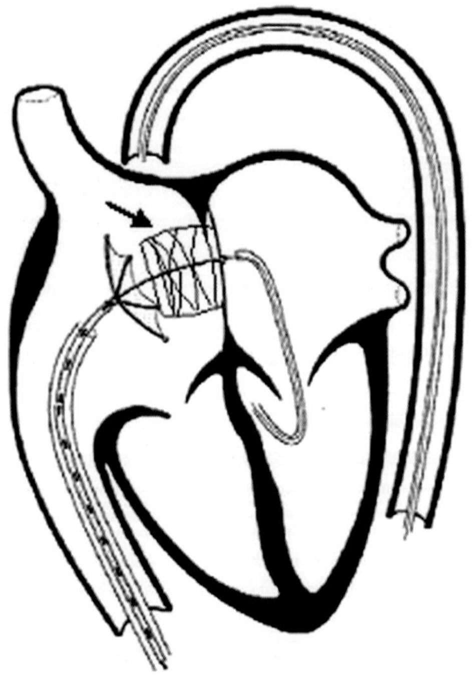

Fig 4.16—ASDOS device as proposed in 2002 with the Nitinol self-centering device (arrow). From Rao and Kern, eds., fig 4.8, p. 42.[41] (Reprinted with permission of Lippincott Williams and Wilkins; and courtesy of Dr. U. Babic.)

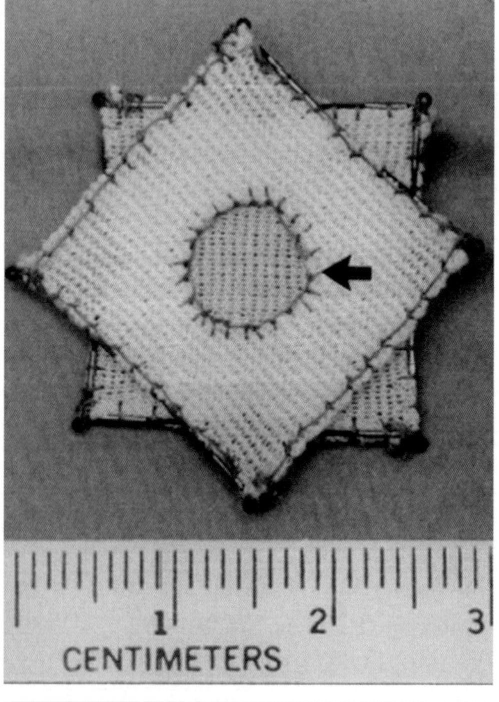

Fig 4.17—En face DAS Angel Wing device. Arrows indicate the left side of the conjoined ring. Not shown is the Guardian Angel. From Das et al with permission.[50]

Angel Wing/
Guardian Angel Device

In 1993, Das et al[50] reported a new ASD device (Angel Wing Das Device, Microvena Corporation, White Bear Lake, Minnesota) that had two Dacron-covered square disks or wings and Nitinol frames with mid-point torsion spring eyelets. A circular hole with a diameter equal to one-half the length of the side of the disc was punched from the right disc with the margins being sewn to the left-sided disc forming a conjoint suture ring, the centering mechanism (see Fig 4.17).

Device sizes ranged from 12 to 40 mm with the most commonly implanted device sizes being 18, 22, 25, and 30 mm squares as determined by the length of each side of the square disk. Delivery catheters were 11F, 12F, or 13F, depending on the device size used. The locking mechanism was formed by a long wire traversing the hollow pusher rod, which was connected to one of the eyelets of the right-sided disk and when deployed, the mechanism was released by the attach-release mechanism in the control handle.[41]

The initial experimental trial using 20 dogs with surgically created ASDs revealed immediate closure in 19 animals, one unsuccessful closure, no shunts in 17 animals, and trivial shunts in 2 animals.[50] No spontaneous embolization occurred and only one strut fracture was noted at 8-months postclosure. Follow-up necropsy studies and tissue studies were performed at 8 weeks in three animals. Those findings revealed endothelial-covered devices enmeshed in mature collagen tissue and only minimal mononuclear cell infiltration. Intentional embolization of four devices occurred in two animals into the right atrium (1) and pulmonary artery (3); all were retrieved with a snare.[50] The investigators felt the animal studies compared favorably with similar studies in the Clamshell[30] and buttoned device[37] and established the feasibility and safety of the device to warrant clinical trials in humans. Dr. Ziyad M. Hijazi implanted the first Angel Wing device on June 7, 1995, in Boston, Massachusetts, in a 16-year-old patient with a cryptogenic stroke (personal communication January 2010).

Rickers et al.[51] reported their experience in 1998 with the Angel Wing. A multicenter study involving eight German institutions enrolled 101 patients with closure attempted in 75 patients. In this study, major adverse events requiring surgical removal occurred in three patients (4%). One patient experienced hemopericardium tamponade 4-months postclosure; one patient experienced a left atrium thrombus 6-months postclosure and the right atrial disc was not fully deployed; and the remaining patient experienced displacement of the left atrial disc with a large residual shunt 9-months postclosure. Based on their experience and follow-up, they felt design modification was mandatory due to the serious complications encountered. In addition, retrieval mechanisms needed to be developed and further randomized clinical trials were pursued to compare device closure with surgical closure, including long-term follow-up data.

In 1999, Banerjee et al[52] reported the results of a US multicenter trial (4) using the Angel Wings ASD closure device in 70 consecutive patients (Phase I clinical trial). Of these, 21 patients had PFOs and 49 patients had a secundum ASD. Deployment was successful in 65 (93%) patients and unsuccessful in 5 who required surgical closure of the defect with device retrieval. Their inclusion criteria included patients with PFO with history of TIA or stroke with no other cause identified and patients with ASDs diameter < 20 mm. The margin of the ASD or PFO must be > 4 mm away from important contiguous structures such as the coronary sinus, the atrioventricular valves, and the pulmonary veins. Device size was based on echocardiographic findings and balloon occlusive diameters. The device-to-balloon occlusive diameter ratio was approximately 1.5 but varied from 2.5 to as small as 1.2. Deployment was guided by transesophageal echocardiography.

At 24-hours postclosure, residual shunt was noted in 11% and only 4% had a large shunt

(> 4 mm color flow width). In a fourth patient, a moderate shunt was noted and resulted from a second ASD in the area of the larger occluded ASD. At 6-month follow-up some degree of residual shunting by TEE was noted in five patients (7.7%).

Attempts at catheter retrieval were deferred due to the relative stiff framework of the Angel Wings device and there were strict policies for surgical retrieval if the device could not easily be retrieved by catheter. Therefore, during clinical trials, device changes were pursued to enhance safety and efficacy.

After the Phase I trial, Phase II was granted by the FDA.[41] Forty-seven patients with secundum ASDs were submitted for closure of their defect. Their defects measured 9.7 ± 4.1 mm by TEE with a median range of 10 mm and 15.9 ± 3.2 mm by balloon occlusion. The device to balloon ratio was 1.59:1. Successful deployment occurred in 44 patients (94% of attempted closures) and there were 3 unsuccessful deployment attempts. Small residual shunts of 1 mm were noted in nine patients and shunts approximately 2 mm were noted in six patients. Paroxysmal atrial fibrillation occurred in two patients, pulmonary embolus occurred in one patient, stroke occurred in one patient, and a small left atrial disc clot was noted in one patient. No deaths occurred in Phase I or Phase II trials.

After initiation of Phase II trials in the United States and the clinical experience in Europe, the decision was made to halt further studies with the intent to reconfigure the device. The new device needed to include round left atrium and right atrium wings, to be retrievable, to be easily repositioned, and to include a self-centering mechanism. The new design was named the Guardian Angel device but since the data presented in 2003 to our knowledge no activity with the proposed new device is available.

Monodisk

The monodisk was described by Pavčnik et al[53] and consisted of a single disk of a stainless steel ring constructed from wire coiled in springlike fashion. This ring was covered with a double layer of nylon mesh and three pieces of braided hollow stainless steel wires were sutured to the back side of the circular device as shown in Fig 4.18. The pusher catheter was connected to the device by three strands of nylon monofilament which were passed through the catheter lumen and looped through the anchoring wires. A 9F sheath was used to compress the device and deliver it to the left atrium.

Once in the left atrium, the self-expanding device, sizes 1.2, 1.6, or 2 cm opened. When the device was positioned against the septum, the nylon monofilament strands were cut allowing the three flexible tubular wires to spring back against the right IAS. The tubular wires also helped center the device. If the device position was not optimal, it would be repositioned prior to cutting the nylon strands. The device was retrievable prior to cutting the strands and the final device position was documented by radiography.

The device was tested on experimentally created ASDs in mongrel dogs. The first dog was the acute model and the remaining four were followed for 6 months. Experiences with handling of the monodisk in the acute animal lead to changing the diameter of the tubular steel from 0.032 to 0.035 inches. Reportedly, all defects were closed and at 6-months postclosure the device was incorporated into the atrial septum by cellular over growth (endothelium). The monodisk was successfully implanted in two patients with secundum ASDs in 1993; however, no clinical trials were planned (personal communication, January 15, 2010).

AMPLATZER Septal Occluder

The AMPLATZER Septal Occluder device is a double disk device (see Fig 4.19) with a self-centering waist and has been used extensively in a wide variety of cardiac defects since the first experimental trial reported by Sharafuddin in1997.[54] The AMPLATZER Septal Occluder

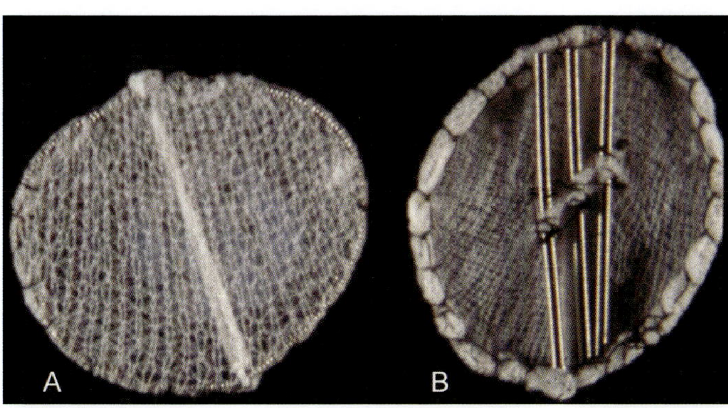

Fig 4.18—Monodisk device showing covered left-sided disc (A) and right side of disc with three braided hollow stainless steel wires (B). (Courtesy of Dr. D. Pavčnik.)

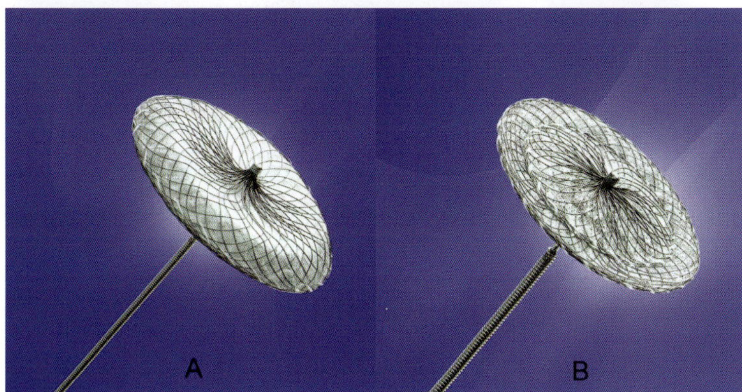

Fig 4.19—AMPLATZER ASO device (A) and PFO occluder device (B). (Courtesy of AGA and Dr. K. Amplatz.)

(AGA Medical Corporation, Plymouth, Minnesota) is made from Nitinol wire mesh that is tightly woven into two disks with a connecting waist between the two disks corresponding to the approximated thickness of the IAS. The device is filled with fluffy Dacron threads (spun bonded polyester), sewn into the prosthesis in a pattern similar to strings of a tennis racquet. The Nitinol device is super elastic with configuration memory that allows placement into a 6 to 8F sheath, pending the device chosen for delivery, and once delivered returns to the preformed configuration. The device size is determined by the waist diameter and ranges from 4 to 40 mm. The disk diameters increase with increasing waist diameters. The device has been used extensively in PFOs, ASDs, and Fontan fenestrations.

The first clinical trial was reported by Masura[55] in 1997 and several have since been documented.[41,56–58] The device was FDA approved in December 2001 and since its inception has been implanted clinically in approximately 13,000 PFOs and 46,000 secundum ASDs. The AMPLATZER Septal Occluder will be discussed in greater detail in Chapter 26.

CardioSEAL/STARFlex

The CardioSEAL occlusion device (Nitinol Medical Technologies, Inc., (NMT, Inc.) Boston, Massachusetts) had its origin in the Rashkind PDA occluder device[27] which led to Lock's[30] Clamshell Septal Occluder (CR Bard Inc., Billerica, Massachusetts) as previously discussed. The manufacturing rights and technology for the Clamshell device was obtained by Nitinol Medical Corporation in 1995.

The CardioSEAL is a self-expanding, double umbrella with arms made from metal alloy (MP35N) and covered with Dacron instead of foam (see Fig 4.20). Four arms in each umbrella radiate out from the disc centers and form a square. There are two hinges or stress coils in

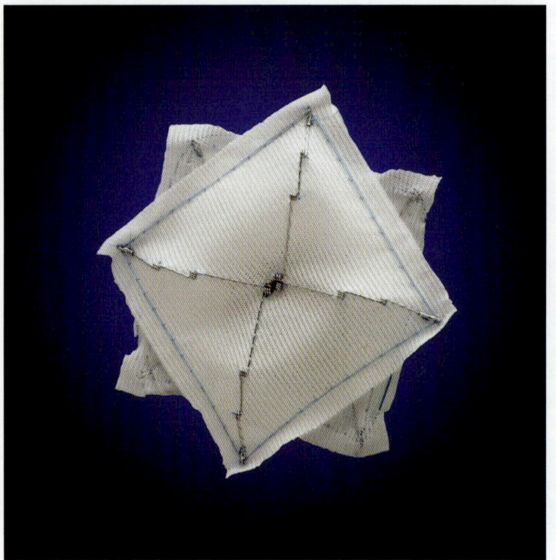

Fig 4.20—CardioSEAL ASD device. Note the two elbows within each supporting arm. (Courtesy of NMT Medical.)

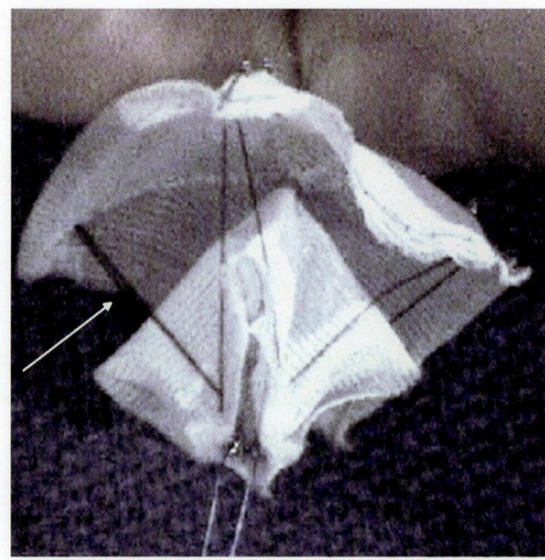

Fig 4.21—STARFlex implant. Note the opened left atrial disc and the microsprings (arrow) that are attached to the umbrella. (Courtesy of NMT Medical.)

each arm to displace stress[36] and overall the device has a "low profile." It is implanted with an 11F sheath and comes in five sizes measured diagonally (17, 23, 28, 33, and 40 mm). Device size should be 1.5× to 2.2× the balloon stretched diameter. It has been tested in experimental clinical trials with initial human implants in late 1996 in the United States, Canada, and in Europe. The device remains under investigation in the United States but was approved for use in the European Common Market and a number of other countries globally in 1997.[36] Since 1988, the CardioSEAL and its predecessor (Clamshell) had been implanted in over 1,000 patients. Residual leaks trended down over time. Arm fractures did occur early but with no adverse clinical consequences.[36]

Further modification of the CardioSEAL led to the STARFlex device in 1998, which utilizes a flexible, auto-adjusting, and self-centering spring mechanism. Microsprings made from Nitinol are attached distally to the struts between the two umbrellas and allow for centering the device. It is available in sizes of 23, 28, 33, and 40 mm (see Fig 4.21). Clinical trials were instituted in North America and European Certification was obtained in 1998. To better occlude larger PFOs and ASDs the STARFlex

was modified further leading to a version with six arms and a device diameter of 38 to 43 mm.[59] These devices are implanted through a 10- to 12F transseptal sheath.

BioSTAR/BioTREK

NMT Medical Inc. further modified and refined these devices which culminated in the BioSTAR Septal Occluder (see Fig 4.22). This device utilizes the STARFlex frame but the Dacron has been replaced with a heparin-coated, acellular, porcine-derived intestinal collagen matrix that allows absorption and replacement of the membrane with human tissue (95%). Total remodeling occurs over approximately 24 months. The metal arms are left behind and are eventually covered with endothelium.[60] The newest device, BioTREK is based on CardioSEAL-BioSTAR technologies but is completely reabsorbable and is currently in preclinical studies. As of January 2010, over 35,000 CardioSEAL, STARFlex, and BioSTAR devices have been implanted (personal communication). Part IV will include further discussion on these devices.

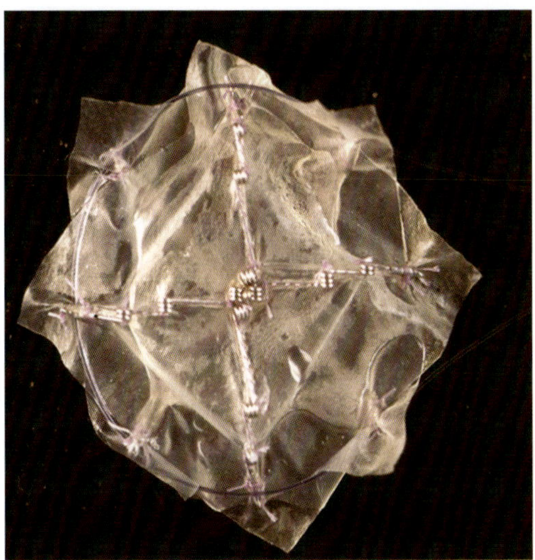

Fig 4.22—BioSTAR. Note the clear bioabsorbable membrane covering the STARFlex frame. (Courtesy of NMT Medical.)

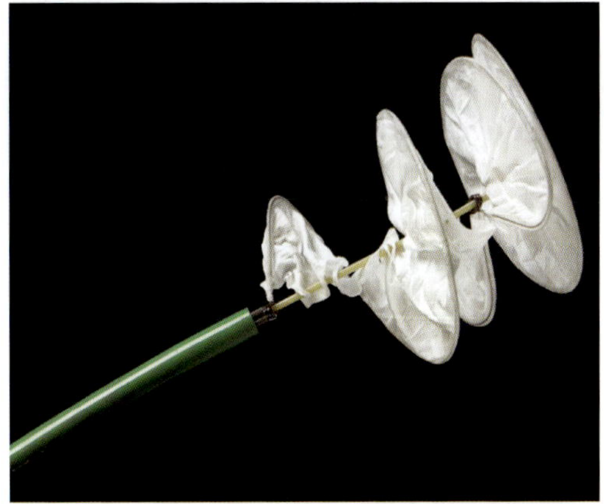

Fig 4.23—HELEX device. (Courtesy of W.L. Gore and Associates.)

HELEX Septal Occluder

The HELEX Septal Occluder (W.L. Gore & Associates, Flagstaff, Arizona) is composed of a single 0.012-inch diameter Nitinol wire covered by an ultrathin membrane of expanded polytetrafluoroethylene (ePTEE). In its occlusive configuration the device forms two round flexible discs that straddle the septum (see Fig 4.23). For delivery, the flexible frame elongates around a central mandrel and is delivered through a 9F catheter. It has a narrow central waist and works well for small defects (eg, PFO), baffle fenestrations, and multiple defects. It is retrievable throughout the procedure even after release from the delivery catheter using the retrieval cord. If fully deployed and/or embolized, it can be retrieved using a snare catheter. In smaller patients, device-to-defect diameter ratio is approximately 1.5 or less and in larger patients who can accommodate large diameter devices, a device-to-defect ratio exceeding 2 can be employed.[41] Both discs are similar in size; therefore, it can be used in patients with right-to-left or left-to-right shunts.

The original animal trial was reported by Zahn et al[61] in 2001, with 100% implanted device success and initial occlusion rate of 88%. At 2-week follow-up, a 100% occlusion rate by transesophageal echocardiography was noted. The first human implantations of the HELEX were performed in Glasgow, Scotland by Dr. Neil Wilson[62] in the summer of 1999 followed shortly by Dr. Horst Sievert[62] in Frankfort, Germany. Since, many studies and trials have been performed with the HELEX device alone or in comparison studies.[63-68] The HELEX Septal Occluder will be discussed in greater depth and detail in Chapter 27.

Detachable Balloon Device

The detachable balloon device (DBD) was reported by Sideris et al in 2000.[69] The balloon device (see Fig 4.24) has the previously described buttoned device locking mechanism but uses a detachable balloon occluder on the left side of the defect. There is a floppy disc on the right side of the defect with the previously described buttoned-type counter-occluder. It also includes a loading wire and needle catheter. The left-sided balloons vary in size and are composed of latex; therefore, latex allergies must be ruled out. The balloons are attached to the needle catheter, which is inserted in a

10-mm-long 5F catheter with several side holes. The needle catheter and the tail of the balloon are tied with a latex tie that will seal the balloon after the needle catheter is removed. The right-sided floppy disc is composed of polyurethane and Nitinol hyperelastic wire and comes in different diameters. The counter-occluder is used to button the device and adds further support.

A long sheath is used to deliver the device to the left atrium and the balloon is inflated with dilute contrast of predetermined volume, which can be varied as desired. The balloon is then withdrawn into the defect and then the sheath is withdrawn into the right atrium exposing the floppy disc. Subsequently, the needle catheter is pulled through the long sheath resulting in detachment of the balloon. A counter-occluder may be passed over the loading wire and buttoned with the balloon occluder. Release of the system is similar to the buttoned device. This device was tested in piglets with promising results; however, human trials were not as favorable.[70] In 2003, Sideris[41] recommended the

current detachable balloon device not be used until better stability was achieved.

Transcatheter Patch

That same year (2000) Sideris et al[71] also reported the use of the transcatheter patch. The transcatheter patch is a variation of this concept with a double balloon support catheter and a double nylon thread. The patch is made from polyurethane foam and constructed to cover the distal balloon of the support catheter (see Fig 4.25). A 2-mm diameter nylon thread loop is attached to the apical internal side of the patch. The nylon loop is attached to the double nylon thread which, if needed, can be used for retraction or retrieval. A radio-opaque thread is sutured to the patch material to provide visualization by fluoroscopy or echocardiography. The balloon/patch diameter is 2 mm larger than the tested occluding diameter of the ASD. The supporting balloons are connected to a triple lumen catheter and each can be independently inflated with dilute contrast material through its own lumen. The central lumen is used for over-the-wire insertion of the device.

After seating of the patch material against the rims of the defect and, if stable, the introducing sheath and balloon catheter along with

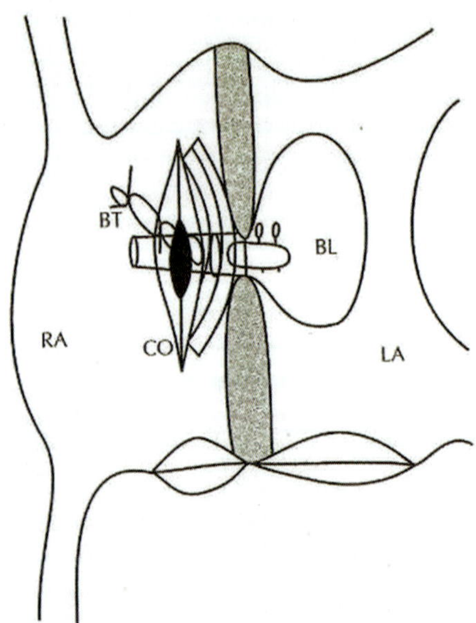

Fig 4.24—Detachable balloon device. A drawing of detachable balloon device correction of atrial septal defect. BL, balloon; BT, button; CO, counter occluder; FD, folding disk; LA, left atrium; RA, right atrium. From Rao & Kern with permission.[41]

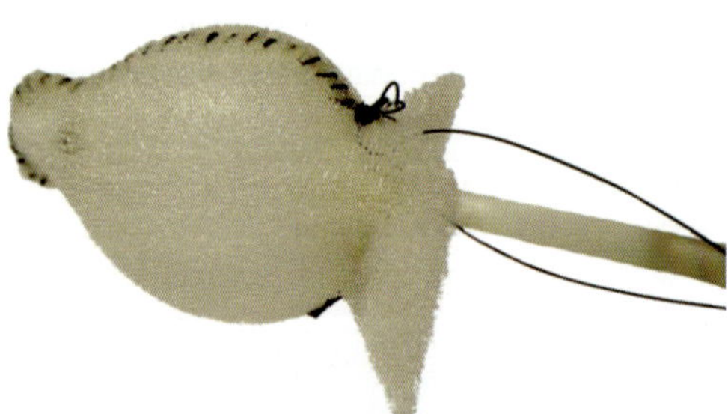

Fig 4.25—Transcatheter patch. It is a frameless, bioabsorbable device. Device apposition is accomplished by balloon inflation. Note the double nylon thread attached to the patch. (Courtesy of Custom Medical Devices.)

the double nylon thread are immobilized by suture and taped to the groin. After 48 hours the patch material is released by first deflating the distal balloon and then the proximal balloon. If the desired results are achieved, the nylon thread is removed in a single strand. Support for this maneuver can be the balloon catheter or the long sheath against the patch as counter tension. The balloon catheter is removed through the sheath and the sheath is extracted.

The transcatheter patch was tested in piglets and then in six humans with promising results. The sleeve patch is primarily for single defects and safer than the single balloon/floppy disk system for larger defects and may have a wider application. A disadvantage of the patch technique is the need for a prolonged hospital stay. The transcatheter patch is approved in the European Union (CE Mark) and has been used in approximately 500 patients (personal communication, December 29, 2009). Chapter 29 includes further information on the wireless devices.

Other Devices

Occlutech Septal Occluder and Occlutech Figulla PFO Flex

In 2003, Occlutech engineers were asked by Professor Hans Figulla (Germany) to develop a new generation of occluders with reduced implanted material. These endeavors lead to the development of the Occlutech Figulla PFO Occluder and the Figulla ASD Occluder (Occlutech GMBH, Jena, Germany) (see Fig 4.26). These devices are double-disc devices composed of self-expanding Nitinol mesh wire. The discs have a low profile and the new Figulla Flex devices have innovative delivery systems. The PFO and ASD Figulla Flex devices received the European CE mark in May 2008. The Figulla ASD and PFO devices have been used in both adult and pediatric patients.[72,73] Please refer to Chapter 28 for further information regarding the Occlutech ASD and PFO devices.

PFO-Star device

Cardia PFO-Star—Cardia's decision to begin PFO closure was personal. A young man well known to the company suffered what was thought to be a PFO-related cryptogenic stoke at the age of 39. This lead to the PFO-star device (STAR) (Cardia, Burnsville, Minnesota), which is a self-opening double umbrella developed for transvenous closure of PFOs. The device is currently in its sixth generation, also known as the ATRIASEPT II and is available in several sizes. The ATRIASEPT II is a self-centering device with Nitinol frames with six arms and Ivalon attached to the outside of the frames (see Fig 4.27).

Several investigators have reported good results using the Cardia devices.[74–80] These devices have been used to close approximately 12,000 PFOs and ASDs (personal communication, January 8, 2010) and will be discussed in greater detail in Chapter 32.

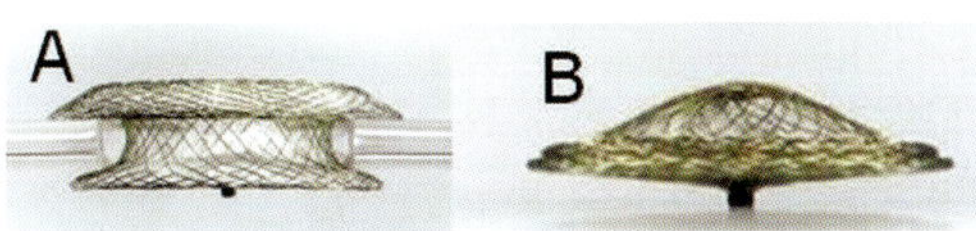

Fig 4.26—Occlutech Figulla ASD Occluder (A) and Occlutech Figulla PFO Occluder (B). (Courtesy of Occlutech International.)

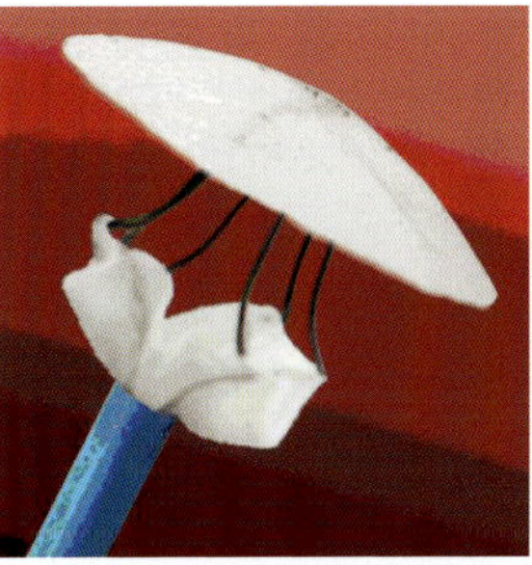

Fig 4.27—ATRIASEPT II with centering mechanism. (Courtesy of Cardia, Inc.)

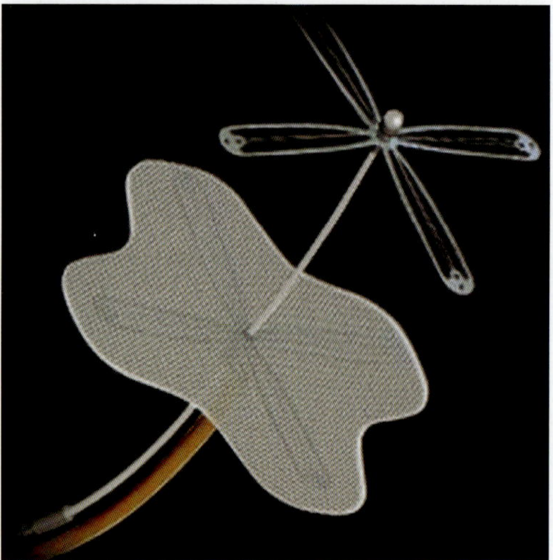

Fig 4.28—Premere device includes flexible, low-profile anchors. Note the adjustable tether connecting the left and right anchors that is intended to adapt to varying septal anatomies. The left atrial side is uncovered to minimize the incidence of thromboembolic complications. (Courtesy of St. Jude Medical, Inc.)

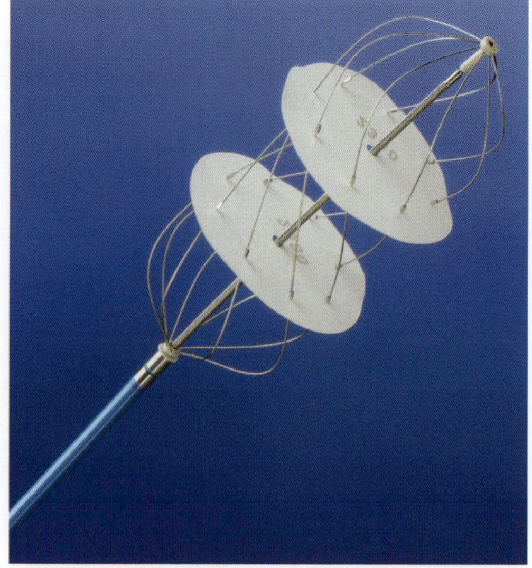

Fig 4.29—Solysafe Septal Occluder consists of a self-centering device with two foldable polyester patches mounted to 8 metal wires of Phynox. (Courtesy of Swissimplant.)

Premere PFO closure system

The Premere occluder (St. Jude Medical, Inc., Minnesota) was designed specifically for PFO occlusion. Clinical trials using the Premere PFO closure system began in 2005.[81] The Premere occluder has two cross-shaped, low-profile Nitinol arms. The left atrial side is uncovered and the right-sided anchor is covered on both sides with a knitted polyester membrane (see Fig 4.28). The Premere Occluder uses a variable length tether that adjusts to the length of the PFO tract.[82] It is not approved for use in the United States at this time, but is available in certain international markets.

Solysafe Septal Occluder

The Solysafe Septal Occluder (Swissimplant AG, Solothum, Switzerland) has been developed by a Swiss-Swedish effort and was first implanted in 2005 in Sweden (see Fig 4.29). The device is a double-patch self-centering occluder with two foldable polyester patches mounted to eight metal wires. Markers are present and due to wire arrangement the device has two stable positions. It can be used for closure of ASDs or PFOs and has been mainly evaluated in adult trials.[83–86] The Solysafe Septal Occluder received the CE Mark in 2007. Further and more complete discussion of the Solysafe Occluder is found in Chapter 33.

Coherex FlatStent EF PFO closure system

The Coherex FlatStent EF PFO Closure System was developed by Coherex Medical Inc., Salt Lake City, Utah (formerly Proximare, Inc.). The device is a laterally ("flat") self-expanding nitinol lattice ("stent") with unique fusion of PFO closure technologies and is the first device developed to treat the PFO tunnel. While not suitable for ASD closure, the development of the FlatStent EF is important historically as it represents the first successful technology to treat PFO that is not, in essence, an ASD device doing double duty. This new direction illustrates the growing clinical importance of

PFO, and the differences between it and ASD, in technology requirements. The FlatStent EF implant leaves a minimal amount of materials exposed in the left atrium therefore reducing, among other known device risks, the risk of thromboembolization.[87] Clinical trials in Europe were in 2007 and the FlatStent EF received the CE Mark in 2009. The Coherex device is not available for investigational use or for commercial distribution in the United States at this time. Chapter 35 discusses the Coherex FlatStent™ EF closure system in more detail.

PFx Closure System

The PFx Closure System (Cierra, California) is a unique nondevice system for closure of a PFO. The PFx-15 closure system is a percutaneous system that employs monopolar radio frequency energy to effect closure of a PFO by welding the tissues of the septum primum and the septum secundum together.[88] The PFx catheter is delivered into the right atrium, the left atrium is not entered, thereby reducing the risk of thromboembolism. Once complete, the catheter-based system is withdrawn, leaving no foreign material behind. Clinical trials began in 2005. However, due to low closure rates, the company discontinued this technology and closed its doors in early 2009.

SeptRx occluder

The SeptRx (Secant Medical, Pennsylvania) was developed to target only the PFO tunnel. It is implanted into the flap of the defect and stretches the defect in anterior-posterior direction leading to an opposition of the septa secundum and primum. The potential advantages are less distortion of the atrial septum and minimization of potential thromboembolic nidus in the left atrium.

HeartStitch

The HeartStitch (Sutura, Inc., Fountain Valley, California) was a transcatheter suture system developed to close septal defects by suturing. The device was delivered into the left atrium and the septum primum and septum secundum were sutured together. Once suturing was complete the device was withdrawn. Although initial experimental results looked promising, this system has been abandoned.

pfm device

The pfm device is currently investigational in South America. Further information regarding the pfm device can be found in Chapter 34.

Summary

The past 40 years has seen tremendous strides in nonsurgical closure of ASDs and PFOs. The technologies and miniaturization capabilities have allowed for improved devices with increasing accuracy, ease of placement, and stability once in place. Beginning with five patients in 1975, thousands upon thousands around the globe have benefitted from the pioneering efforts of physicians, engineers, nurses, and many others who shared in our dream. Those first five patients were pioneers as well and we will be forever grateful for their confidence in our profession. They helped chart a course that is not yet complete.

We have all stood on the shoulders of those before us and thus we need to leave a sound scientific foundation for the pioneers to come. Just because we can do something doesn't mean we should. *Primum non nocere.* Our goal, in these endeavors, has been to alleviate pain, suffering, scars, and as much as possible, anxiety. Device closure must be curative and must not create comorbidities. For us to replace something as outstanding as surgical correction, our results and efforts have to produce results that are superior in every aspect. The wonderment of what the future holds is tantalizing and no longer can we be told, "It's just not feasible," for we know different!

Acknowledgments

Our sincere thanks to my friend Dr. Chuck Mullins for his editorial review of this work. We would also like to express a special thanks to Caroline Carpenter, Jennifer Watson, Brenda Thomason, and Nancy King, for all the time and hard work given in the preparation of this chapter. Their efforts truly made a difference and we are grateful.

References

1. Kapadia S. Patent foramen ovale closure: Historical perspective. *Cardiol Clin.* 2005;23:73–83.

2. Gross R. Surgical management of the patent ductus arteriosus with summary of four surgically treated cases. *Ann Surg.* 1939;110(3):321–356.

3. Gross R, Hufnagel C. Coarctation of the aorta: Experimental studies regarding its surgical correction. *N Engl J Med.* 1945;233:287–293.

4. Crafoord C, Nylin, G. Congenital coarctation of the aorta and its surgical treatment. *J Thorac Surg.* 1945;14:347–361.

5. Cohn R. An experimental method for the closure of interauricular septal defects in dogs. *Am Heart J.* 1947;33:453–457.

6. Murray G. Closure of defects in cardiac septa. *Ann Surg.* 1948;128(4): 843–852.

7. Alexi-Meskishvili V, Konstantinov I. Surgery for atrial septal defect: From the first experiments to clinical practice. *Ann Thorac Surg.* 2003;76:322–327.

8. Dennis C, Spreng D, Nelson G, et al. Development of a pump-oxygenator to replace the heart and lungs: An apparatus applicable to human patients, and application to one case. *Ann Surg.* 1951;134:709–721.

9. Hufnagel C, Gillespie J. Closure of interauricular septal defects. *Bulletin Georgetown University Medical Center.* 1951;4(5):137–139.

10. Lewis F, Taufic M. Closure of atrial septal defects with the aid of hypothermia; Experimental accomplishments and the report of one successful case. *Surgery.* 1953;33(1):52–59.

11. Gross R, Pomeranz A, Watkins E Jr, Goldsmith E. Surgical closure of defects of the interauricular septum by use of an atrial well. *N Engl J Med.* 1952;247:455–460.

12. Gibbon J. Application of a mechanical heart and lung apparatus to cardiac surgery. *Minn Med.* 1954;37(3):171–180.

13. Derra E, Bayer O, Grosse-Brockhoff G. The atrial septal defect and its surgical closure under direct vision during induced hypothermia. *Dutch Medical Worchenschr,* 1955;80(36):1277–1281.

14. Rashkind W, Miller W. Creation of an atrial septal defect without thoracotomy. A palliative approach to complete transposition of the great arteries. *J Am Med Assoc.* 1966;196(11):991–992.

15. Porstmann W, Wierny L, Warnke H, Gertsberger G, Romaniuk P. Catheter closure of patent ductus arteriosus: 62 cases without thoracotomy. *Radiol Clin North Am.* 1971;9(2):203–218.

16. Long D, DeWall R, French L. Unusual complications of ventriculoauriculostomy. Report of two cases. *J Neurosurg.* 1964;21:233–234.

17. Lillehei C, Bonnabeau R Jr, Grossling S. Removal of iatrogenic foreign bodies within cardiac chambers and great vessels. *Circulation.* 1965;32:782–787.

18. King T, Cline R, Wilkinson J, Johnson H, Stanford W. Removal of an embolized Pudenz catheter from the right ventricle using a snare-loop catheter. *South Med J.* 1974;67(6):734–735.

19. Mills N, Vargish T, Kleinman L, Bloomfield D, Reed G. Balloon closure of ventricular septal defect. *Circulation.* 1971;43–44(Suppl. I):111–114.

20. Brodie T, Mills N, Thompson S, King T. Production of experimental atrial septal defects. *Vascular Surg.* 1976;10(5):295–299.

21. King T, Thompson S, Mills N. Measurement of atrial septal defect during cardiac catheterization; Experimental and clinical results. *Am J Cardiol.* 1978;41:537–542.

22. King T, Thompson S, Steiner C, Mills N. Secundum atrial septal defect: Nonoperative closure during cardiac catheterization. *J Am Med Assoc.* 1976;235(23):2506–2509.

23. King T, Mills N. Nonoperative closure of atrial septal defects. *Surgery.* 1974;75(3):383–388.

24. Mason D, ed. *Advances in heart disease.* Vol 2. New York: Grune & Stratton; 1978.

25. Mills N, King T. Late follow-up of nonoperative closure of secundum atrial septal defects using the King-Mills double-umbrella device. *Am J Cardiol.* 2003;92:353–355.

26. King T, Mills N. *Long-term outcome of ASD closure: 30 year follow-up.* Presented at the Pediatric Interventional Cardiac Symposium; Buenos Aries, Argentina; 2005, September.

27. Rashkind W. Transcatheter treatment of congenital heart disease. *Circulation.* 1983;67(4):711–716.

28. Hellenbrand W, Mullins C. Catheter closure of congenital heart defects. *Cardiol Clin.* 1989;7(2):351–368.

29. Rashkind W, Wagner H, Tait M. Historical aspects of interventional cardiology: Past, present, and future. *Texas Heart Inst J.* 1986;13(4): 363–367.

30. Lock J, Rome J, Davis R, et al. Transcatheter closure of atrial septal defects: Experimental studies. *Circulation.* 1989;79(5):1091–1099.

31. Rome J, Keane J, Perry S, Spevak P, Lock J. Double-umbrella closure of atrial defects: Initial clinical applications. *Circulation.* 1990;82 (3): 751–758.

32. Boutin C, Musewe N, Smallhorn J, Dyck J, Kobayashi T, Benson L. Echocardiographic follow-up of atrial septal defect after catheter closure by double-umbrella device. *Circulation.* 1993;88(2):621–627.

33. Bridges N, Hellenbrand W, Latson L, Filiano J, Newburger J, Lock J. Transcatheter closure of patent foramen ovale after presumed paradoxical embolism. *Circulation.* 1992;86(6):1902–1908.

34. Justo R, Nykanen D, Boutin C, McCrindle B, Freedom R, Benson L. Clinical impact of transcatheter closure of secundum atrial septal defects with the double umbrella device. *Am J Cardiol.* 1996;77:889–892.

35. Koike K, Echigo S, Kumate M, et al. Transcatheter closure of atrial septal defect with a prototype clamshell septal umbrella: one year follow-up. *J Cardiol.* 1994;24(1):53–60.

36. Latson L. The CardioSEAL device: History, techniques, results. *J Intervent Cardiol.* 1998;11(5):501–505.

37. Sideris E, Sideris S, Fowlkes J, Ehly R, Smith J, Gulde R. Transvenous atrial septal defect occlusion in piglets with a "buttoned" double-disk device. *Circulation.* 1990;81(1):312–318.

38. Rao P, Berger F, Rey C, et al. Results of transvenous occlusion of secundum atrial septal defects with the fourth generation buttoned device: Comparison with first, second and third generation devices. *J Am Coll Cardiol.* 2000;36(2):583–592.

39. Sideris E, Rao P. Transcatheter closure of atrial septal defects: Role of buttoned devices. *J Invasive Cardiol.* 1996;8(7):289–296.

40. Rao P, Sideris E. Centering-on-demand buttoned device; Its role in transcatheter occlusion of atrial septal defects. *J Intervent Cardiol.* 2001;14(1):81–89.

41. Rao P, Kern M, eds. *Catheter based devices for the treatment of non-coronary cardiovascular disease in adults and children.* Philadelphia: Lippincott; 2003.

42. Ashley S. Metals that remember. *Popular Sci.* 1988;1:78–81, 115.

43. Andreasen G, Wass K, Chan K. A review of superelastic and thermodynamic nitinol wire. *Quintessence Int.* 1985;9:623–626.

44. Babic U, Dorros G, Pejcic P, et al. Percutaneous mitral valvuloplasty: Retrograde, transarterial double-balloon technique utilizing the transseptal approach. *Cathet Cardiovasc Diagn.* 1988;14(4):229–237.

45. Babic U, Grujicic S, Djurisic Z, Vucinic M. Transcatheter closure of atrial septal defects (letter). *Lancet.* 1990;336:566–567.

46. Babic U, Grujicic S, Popovic Z, Djurisic Z, Vucinic M, Pejcic P. Double-umbrella device for transvenous closure of patent ductus arteriosus and atrial septal defect: first experience. *J Intervent Cardiol.* 1991;4(4):283–294.

47. Babic U. The ASDOS device: Technique and Guidelines for use. *J Intervent Cardiol.* 1998;11(5):485–494.

48. Hausdorf G, Schneider M, Franzbach B, Kampmann C, Kargus K, Goeldner B. Transcatheter closure of secundum atrial septal defects with the atrial septal defect occlusion system (ASDOS): Initial experience in children. *Heart.* 1996;75:83–88.

49. Babic U. Experience with ASDOS for transcatheter closure of atrial septal defect and pat-

ent foramen ovale. *Curr Intervent Cardiol Rep.* 2000;2:177–183.

50. Das G, Voss G, Jarvis G, Wyche K, Gunther R, Wilson R. Experimental atrial septal defect closure with a new, transcatheter, self-centering device. *Circulation.* 1993;88(4):1754–1764.

51. Rickers C, Hamm C, Stern H, et al. Percutaneous closure of secundum atrial septal defect with a new self centering device ("angel wings"). *Heart.* 1998;80:517–521.

52. Banerjee A, Bengur R, Li J, et al. Echocardiographic characteristics of successful deployment of the Das Angel Wings atrial septal defect closure device: Initial multicenter experience in the United States. *Am J Cardiol.* 1999;83:1236–1241.

53. Pavčnik D, Wright K, Wallace S. Monodisk: Device for percutaneous transcatheter closure of cardiac septal defects. *Cardiovasc Intervent Radiol.* 1993;16(5):308–312.

54. Sharafuddin M, Gu X, Titus J, Urness M, Cervera-Ceballos J, Amplatz K. Transvenous closure of secundum atrial septal defects: Preliminary results with a new self-expanding nitinol prosthesis in a swine model. *Circulation.* 1997;95:2162–2168.

55. Masura J, Gavora P, Formanek A, Hijazi Z. Transcatheter closure of secundum atrial septal defects using the new self-centering AMPLATZER septal occluder: Initial human experience. *Cathet Cardiovasc Diagn* 1997;42(4): 388–393.

56. Berger F, Ewert P, Björnstad P, et al. Transcatheter closure as standard treatment for most interatrial defects: experience in 200 patients treated with the AMPLATZER Septal Occluder. *Cardiol Young.* 1999;9:468–473.

57. Chan K, Godman M, Walsh K, Wilson N, Redington A, Gibbs J. Transcatheter closure of atrial septal defect and interatrial communications with a new self expanding nitinol double disc device (AMPLATZER septal occluder): multicentre UK experience. *Heart.* 1999;82:300–306.

58. Masura J, Gavora P, Podnar T. Long-term outcome of transcatheter secundum-type atrial septal defect closure using AMPLATZER septal occluders. *J Am Coll Cardiol.* 2005;45(4):505–507.

59. Bayard Y, Ostermayer S, Hein R, et al. Percutaneous devices for stroke prevention. *Cardiovasc Revasc Med.* 2007;8:216–225.

60. Mullen M, Hildick-Smith D, Giovanni J, et al. BioSTAR evaluation study (BEST). A prospective, multicenter, phase I clinical trial to evaluate the feasibility, efficacy, and safety of the BioSTAR bioabsorbable septal repair implant for the closure of atrial-level shunts. *Circulation.* 2006;114:1962–1967.

61. Zahn E, Wilson N, Cutright W, Latson L. Development and testing of the HELEX septal occluder, a new expanded polytetrafluoroethylene atrial septal defect occlusion system. *Circulation.* 2001;104:711–716.

62. Latson L, Zahn E, Wilson N. HELEX septal occluder for closure of atrial septal defects. *Curr Intervent Cardiol Rep.* 2000;2:268–273.

63. Krumsdorf U, Keppler P, Horvath K, Zadan E, Schrader R, Seivert H. Catheter closure of atrial septal defects and patent foramen ovale in patients with an atrial septal aneurysm using different devices. *J Intervent Cardiol.* 2001;14(1):49–55.

64. Sievert H, Horvath K, Zadan E, et al. Patent foramen ovale closure in patients with transient ischemia attack/stroke. *J Intervent Cardiol.* 2001;14(2):261–266.

65. Sievert H. PFO closure in patient with TIA/Stroke. Abstract presented at the 3rd International Workshop on Interventional Pediatric Cardiology; Milan, Italy; 2001, March.

66. Pedra C, Pedra S, Esteves C, et al. Initial experience in Brazil with the HELEX septal occluder for percutaneous occlusion of atrial septal defects. *Arquivos Brasileiros de Cardiologia.* 2003;81(5):435–452.

67. Latson L, Jones T, Jacobson J, Zahn E, Rhodes J. Analysis of factors related to successful transcatheter closure of secundum atrial septal defects using the HELEX septal occluder. *Am Heart J.* 2006;151(5):1129e8–1129e11.

68. Jones T, Latson L, Zahn E, et al. Results of the U.S. multicenter pivotal study of the HELEX septal occluder for percutaneous closure of secundum atrial septal defects. *J Am Coll Cardiol.* 2007;49(22):2215–2221.

69. Sideris E, Kaneva A, Sideris S, Moulopoulos S. Transcatheter atrial septal defect occlusion in piglets by balloon detachable devices. *Cathet Cardiovasc Intervent.* 2000;51(4):529–534.

70. Sideris E, Sideris S, Toumanides S, Moulopoulos S. From disk devices to transcatheter patches: the evolution of wireless heart defect occlusion. *J Intervent Cardiol.* 2001;14(2):211–214.

71. Sideris E, Toumanides S, Alekyan B, Varvarenko V, Stamatelopoulos S, Moulopoulos S. Transcatheter patch correction of atrial septal defects: Experimental validation and early clinical experience. *Circulation.* 2000;102 (Suppl. II):588.

72. Halabi A, Hijazi Z. A new device to close secundum atrial septal defects: First clinical use to close multiple defects in a child. *Cathet Cardiovasc Intervent.* 2008;71:853–856.

73. Krizanic F, Sievert H, Pfeiffer D, Konorza T, Ferrari M, Figulla H. Clinical evaluation of a novel occluder device (Occlutech) for Percutaneous transcatheter closure of patent foramen ovale (PFO). *Clin Res Cardiol.* 2008;97:872–877.

74. Braun MU, Fassbender D, Schoen, S, et al. Transcatheter closure of patent foramen ovale in patients with cerebral ischemia. *J Am Coll Cardiol.* 2002;39(12):2019–2025.

75. Braun M, Gliech V, Boscheri A, et al. Transcatheter closure of patent foramen ovale (PFO) in patients with paradoxical embolism. Periprocedural safety and mid-term follow-up results of three different device occluder systems. *Eur Heart J.* 2004;25:424–430.

76. Schwerzmann M, Windecker S, Wahl A, et al. Percutaneous closure of patent foramen ovale: Impact of device design on safety and efficacy. *Heart.* 2004;90(2):186–190.

77. Meier J, Berger A, Delabays A, et al. Percutaneous closure of patent foramen ovale: Head-to-head comparison of two different devices. *Eurointervention.* 2005;1(1):48–52.

78. Goy J, Stauffer J, Yusoff A, et al. Percutaneous closure of atrial septal defect type ostium secundum using the new INTRASEPT occluder: Initial experience. *Cathet Cardiovasc Intervent.* 2006;67:265–267.

79. Spies C, Strasheim R, Timmermanns I, Schraeder R. Patent foramen ovale closure in patients with cryptogenic thrombo-embolic events using the Cardia PFO occluder. *Eur Heart J.* 2006;27:365–371.

80. Spies C, Reissmann U, Timmermanns I, Schraeder R. Comparison of contemporary devices used for transcatheter patent foramen ovale closure. *J Invasive Cardiol.* 2008;20:442–447.

81. Donti A, Giardini A, Salomone L, Formigari R, Picchio F. Transcatheter patent foramen ovale closure using the Premere PFO occlusion system. *Cathet Cardiovasc Intervent.* 2006;68:736–740.

82. Büscheck F, Sievert H, Kleber F, et al. Patent foramen ovale using the Premere device: The results of the CLOSEUP trial. *J Intervent Cardiol.* 2006;19:328–333.

83. Ewert P, Söderberg B, Dähnert I, et al. ASD and PFO closure with the Solysafe septal occluder—Results of a prospective multicenter pilot study. *Cathet Cardiovasc Intervent.* 2008;71:398–402.

84. Nisli K, Oner N, Aydogan U, Ertugrul T. ASD closure with Solysafe device: First experience in Turkey. *Anatolian J Cardiol.* 2007;7:451–452.

85. Daehnert I, Djukic M, Parezanovic V, et al. Closure of atrial septal defects with the Solysafe occluder. *Cardiol Young.* 2008;18(Supplement 1):13.

86. Kretschmar O, Sglimbea A, Daehnert I, et al. Interventional closure of atrial septal defects with the Solysafe septal occluder—Preliminary results in children [published ahead of print 2009]. *Int J Cardiol.* doi:10.1016/j.ijcard.2009.03.086.

87. Reiffenstein I, Majunke N, Wunderlich N, et al. Percutaneous closure of patent foramen ovale with a novel FlatStent, *Expert Rev Med Devices.* 2008;5(4):419–425.

88. Skowasch M, Leetz M, Buescheck F, et al. The paradigm study: PFO closure without an implant. Abstract presented at the PICS conference; Las Vegas, United States; 2005.

5

PFO Closure for Prevention of Recurrent Stroke and TIA

Ted Feldman

Introduction

The most common indication for patent fore-man ovale (PFO) closure in practice today is for prevention of recurrent stroke or transient ischemic attack (TIA) in patients with a first or second neurologic event, or with brain imaging evidence of embolic events. This practice is built upon a large database demonstrating a strong association between PFO and cryptogenic stroke, especially in patients under the age of 60 years. Numerous indirect pieces of evidence support the association between stroke and TIA and recurrent stroke and TIA outcomes in patients with PFO.

The traditional therapy for this syndrome has been warfarin anticoagulation. There are no data validating improvements in any clinical outcome with warfarin therapy, and more recently aspirin with or without additional antiplatelet therapy has become accepted as first-line therapy for patients with cryptogenic stroke and PFO. Similarly, no evidence exists to support this practice.

Recurrent stroke appears to be diminished by PFO closure in many clinical series, typically using case control or retrospective methods. What are missing from the story are the results of randomized trials of PFO closure for cryptogenic stroke compared to medical therapy. Although these trials are ongoing, it is important to review the database supporting the use of PFO closure devices to treat patients with cryptogenic stroke.

A common misconception in the practice community is that there are "no data to support PFO closure among patients with cryptogenic stroke." This is a striking and disturbing misimpression. There are numerous data, but no randomized trials. In fact, the database to support practice of PFO closure among patients with cerebral embolic events exceeds the evidence base for medical therapy with anticoagulant or antiplatelet drugs for this problem, and may exceed the evidence base used to make strong guideline recommendations for surgical therapy in the valvular heart disease guidelines.[1,2]

PFO and Cryptogenic Stroke

Numerous studies have identified an association with PFO and cryptogenic stroke.[3-12] The prevalence of PFO in the general population ranges between 15% and 25%. Among populations of patients with cryptogenic stroke, studies have shown PFO prevalence between 40% and 60%. Two population-based studies have argued against this association.[13,14] One study in the Mayo Clinic Proceedings published in 2006 examined 1072 residents of Olmstead County and concluded that PFO is not a risk for cryptogenic stroke or TIA in the general population. When one considers that the incidence of cryptogenic stroke in a population of 300,000,000 US citizens is about 50,000 cases per year, the incidence would be 0.1 patient per 1000 population, or 1 patient for every 6000 patients in the United States. Thus, a study of only 1000 patients would have a very small chance of establishing this association even if the frequency of cryptogenic stroke were several fold higher than it actually is. Thus, population studies that do not survey tens of thousands represent the worst kind of beta error, and cannot be used to assert lack of association between PFO and stroke. Further, in this study, the median age of the patients included was over 50 years, as was also the case in a publication by Petty in the *Journal of the American College of Cardiology* in 2006.[14] This study similarly looked at only 585 patients that included only subjects age 45 years or older. Thus, the potential to verify the well-established association between PFO and cryptogenic stroke was not feasible using this methodology, studying much too small a population to make any meaningful association.

PFO and Increased Mortality

Some interesting indirect data points further support the relationship between PFO and adverse outcomes. Konstantinides et al examined the incidence of ischemic stroke, peripheral arterial embolism, and death among patients with pulmonary embolism.[15] Those without a PFO had a low incidence of these major adverse outcomes. Among patients with PFO, the incidence of stroke was sixfold higher, the incidence of peripheral arterial embolism 15-fold higher, and the incidence of death almost twofold higher than among patients without PFO.

Another piece of indirect evidence is the "economy class syndrome." In a 1-year prospective, single center, observational study, 338 patients were surveyed. Patients presenting with a first cerebral ischemic event were studied. Of 338 patients with acute stroke, 42 had a positive travel history (12.4%). These patients were significantly younger than patients with a negative travel history. The frequency of PFO in the positive travel history group (44.8%) was significantly higher than in the non-travel history group (10.8%). Positive travel patients had significantly more cardioembolic and cryptogenic strokes and more often ischemia in the territory of the posterior cerebral artery.[16,17]

A similar observation has been made among patients with pacemaker lead implants.[18] The investigators wondered whether a pacing lead would, as a nidus for thrombus, lead to more systemic embolization among patients with versus without intracardiac shunts. In 202 patients with intracardiac shunts, the relative risk of systemic thromboemboli was 2.6-fold higher than those without a shunt. Aspirin and warfarin were not found protective of embolic events in this study.

Interestingly, the incidence and size of PFO decreases with age. In an autopsy study of 965 normal hearts, Hagan et al found that the overall frequency of PFO was 27.3%.[19] Between ages 1 and 30 years, the incidence was 34%, and then between the ages of 31 and 80 years 25.4%, decreasing to an incidence among patients aged 81 to 99 years of 20%. PFOs do not close spontaneously with age. Thus, the decreasing prevalence with age suggests higher mortality in PFO patients as they age. Another study by Perrenoud et al looked at the prevalence of PFO in an autopsy study of 3430 patients from a geriatric home; the prevalence of PFO was 0.2%.[20] The striking absence of PFO in these older patients would point to the observation that the mechanism of decreased prevalence might be attrition. It suggests a strong association between absence of a PFO and survival to older age. In this older population, the incidence of stroke was twice as high in PFO patients as in non-PFO patients, and the incidence of ischemic brain infarct was similarly almost twice as high (43% versus 25%). Why would complications occur more frequently with age? As hypertension and myocardial ischemia cause changes in intracardiac chamber compliance, and lower extremity venous thrombosis occurs with increasing frequency, the potential for paradoxical embolism increases.

The hospital incidence and case fatality rates of deep vein thrombosis and pulmonary embolism have been studied.[21] The average incidence of deep vein thrombosis alone is about 48 per 100,000, with pulmonary embolism with or without deep venous thrombosis about 23 per 100,000 patients. The incidence rates of deep vein thrombosis and pulmonary embolism increase exponentially with age. The in-hospital case fatality rate of venous thromboembolism is 12%. Among patients discharged from the hospital with these syndromes, the long-term fatality rates are 19%, 25%, and 30% at 1, 2, and 3 years. Extrapolation suggests that there are about 170,000 new cases of clinically recognized venous thromboembolisms in patients treated in short stay hospitals in the United States, and almost 100,000 hospitalizations for recurrent disease.

Thus, the gross number of patients from this group with PFO who would be exposed to risks of thromboembolism represents many tens of thousands of patients annually. This has also been examined in a 20-year cohort study of venous thromboembolism and subsequent hospitalizations due to acute arterial cardiovas-

cular events in a study published in *The Lancet* in 2007.[22] The relative risk of acute myocardial infarction and stroke during follow-up is high. The relative risk of myocardial infarction or stroke is almost 1.5 higher compared to a control population.

Limitations of Medical Therapy

The major therapy for thromboembolic syndromes has been warfarin. The challenges and problems of warfarin therapy are well known.[23–30] Half of patients do not receive or do not take warfarin. Two to three percent (2%–3%) have major and another 18% minor bleeding episodes each year. Major bleeding episodes include a high incidence of intracranial hemorrhage and hospitalizations requiring transfusion. Warfarin-associated intracranial hemorrhage has increased from 5% to 15% of all intracranial hemorrhage over the last 2 decades as utilizing warfarin therapy has become more aggressive. Warfarin has not demonstrated any advantage compared to aspirin in recurrent stroke rate in randomized comparisons. In fact, the very high 8% annual recurrence rate of stroke in both aspirin- and warfarin-treated patients suggests that neither therapy is effective. There have been no trials of warfarin versus placebo in any population of cryptogenic stroke patients.

Real-world use of warfarin in atrial fibrillation patients without contraindications shows that at best about half of patients are treated.[28–30] Numerous reasons including physician hesitancy and patient noncompliance contribute to this problem. Even when warfarin is administered, the adequacy of anticoagulation in atrial fibrillation is poor. Most patients have subtherapeutic INR measurements at some point. In some studies, less than one-quarter of patients are in the therapeutic range at any particular time. This problem is compounded with poor compliance to medical therapy overall. In the CRUSADE Registry, compliance with medical therapy in patients with coronary artery disease suggested that among patients on two medicines such as aspirin and beta blocker, only one-third were compliant after hospital discharge. This is even more difficult in the setting of warfarin therapy where frequent visits to monitor therapeutic effects are needed. Thus, warfarin is often either not prescribed when indicated, often not taken when prescribed, and probably not effective when taken.

Evidence for Reduced Risk of Recurrent Stroke after PFO Closure

The evidence for a decrease in the recurrent stroke and TIA rate among patients with a history of ischemic events who undergo PFO closure comes primarily from a large number of reported nonrandomized, single center experiences.[31–47] The most common methodology in these studies is to compare the event rate in the year prior to closure with the event rate in a year after closure. The event rates prior to closure range between 2% and 26% in the year before closure. Among numerous reports of this type, the range of recurrent event rates in the year after device closure is between 1% and 2.5%. In some individual series, the numbers are quite striking. For example, in the HELEX multicenter registry, the recurrence rate prior to closure was 19%, and in the year afterward 0%.

The strongest evidence to support the concept that closure is effective at reducing recurrent event rates comes from several meta-analyses.[3,48,49] Landzberg reported in 2004 in a summary of 20 studies including 2250 patients the adjusted 1-year stroke and TIA rate prior to closure was 7.07% and after closure 2.71%.[48] Homma reported in a meta-analysis in 2005 of 26 studies including 2534 patients a recurrence rate of 5.55% with surgical closure, 4.86% with medical therapy, and 2.95% after device therapy in terms of events per 100 patient years.[3] Wohrle reported in 2006 on an analysis of 20 studies including 3014 patients.[49] The 1-year recurrence of stroke or TIA rate was 5.2% with medical therapy and 1.3% after device closure.

For the three studies, the proportional decrease in stroke recurrence compared to medical therapy is 62%, 39%, and 75% (Fig 5.1).

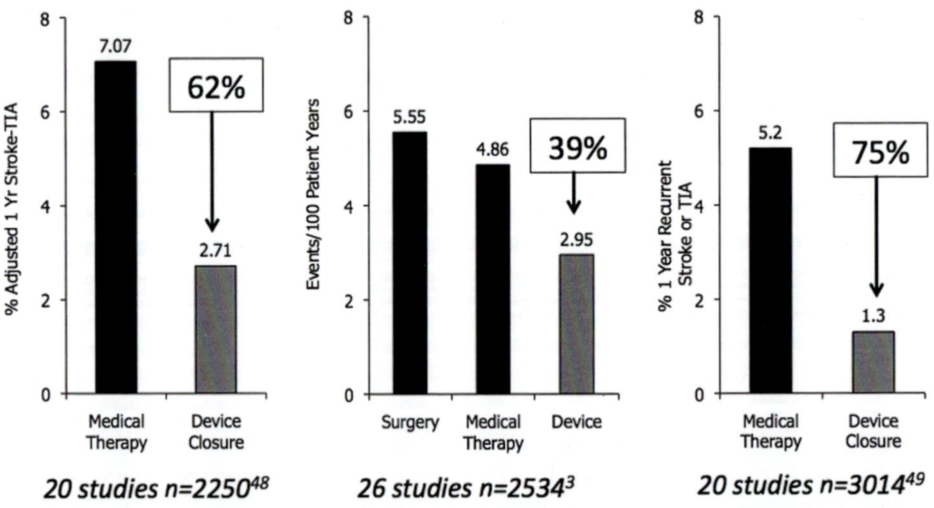

Fig 5.1—Reduced event rate, PFO vs medical therapy. The strongest evidence to support the concept that closure is effective at reducing recurrent event rates comes from several meta-analyses. These date are nonrandomized, but are clearly highly consistent and it is difficult to interpret them as reflecting anything other than a meaningful reduction in recurrent stroke or TIA rates after device closure.

These data are nonrandomized, but are clearly highly consistent and it is difficult to interpret them as reflecting anything other than a meaningful reduction in recurrent stroke or TIA rates after device closure.

These studies are all nonrandomized and important limitations should be considered. TIA is considered a combined end point with stroke. It is entirely possible that many of these TIA events represent migraine headache. Thus, the reduction in stroke rates may be skewed if TIA represents a large part of the population. The studies summarized in these meta-analyses take place over many years, and include many different devices. The rates of shunt closure are not well documented. This particular limitation would bias in favor of masking a treatment effect if it were there, because residual shunts from some of the very early generation devices would not have been effective in reducing stroke rates. Some methodologic issues strengthen the conclusion that the meta-analyses reflect real outcomes.

The methodologies for the individual studies that are lumped together in the meta-analyses vary, and this is another criticism of the validity of these meta-analyses. Nonetheless, in numerous studies with thousands of patients at a wide variety of centers using an array of devices, the results are totally consistent and are highly concordant with the experience we all have in practice, that the utility of device closure for preventing recurrent events appears to be high.

For those who will not accept the nonrandomized evidence as it is, randomized trials are ongoing. We are all hopeful that randomized trials will provide clear answers to any uncertainties that remain regarding the utility of device closure for preventing recurrent events. There are risks in the randomized trials as well, including an important bias to refer the highest risk patients directly for device closure, leaving a lower risk, low event rate, "muddy" population in the randomized trials. This may lead to event rates in the trials that are lower than were utilized to make power calculations for trial sample size, which can result in important errors. That is, there is some potential to overlook a real finding if event rates in the randomized trials turn out to be similar in control and treatment groups due only to lower-than-expected real event rates.

Some ongoing trials will include only patients with positive brain imaging studies, and this methodology has promise to result in a highly relevant and event-rich population, in whom a firm conclusion will be reached.

References

1. Committee on Management of Patients with Valvular Heart Disease. ACC/AHA guidelines for the management of patients with valvular heart disease: a report of the American College of Cardiology/American Heart Association Task Force on Practical Guidelines. *J Am Coll Cardiol.* 1998;32:1486–1588.

2. Bonow RO, Carabello BA, Chaterjee K, et al. ACC/AHA 2006 guidelines for the management of patients with valvular heart disease: a report of the American College of Cardiology/American Heart Association Task Force on Practice Guidelines (Writing Committee to Develop Guidelines for the Management of Patients With Valvular Heart Disease). *J Am Coll Cardiol.* 2006;48:e1–148. *Circulation.* 2005;112 Suppl I:I402–408.

3. Homma S, Sacco RL. Patent foramen ovale and stroke. *Circulation.* 2005;112:1063–1072.

4. Lechat P, Mas JL, Lascault G, et al. Prevalence of patent foramen ovale in patients with stroke. *N Engl J Med.* 1988;318:1148–1152.

5. Webster MW, Chancellor AM, Smith HJ, et al. Patent foramen ovale in young stroke patients. *Lancet.* 1988;2:11–12.

6. Cabanes L, Mas JL, Cohen A, et al. Atrial septal aneurysm and patent foramen ovale as risk factors for cryptogenic stroke in patients less than 55 years of age. A study using transesophageal echocardiography. *Stroke.* 1993;24:1865–1873.

7. De Belder MA, Tourikis L, Leach G, Camm AJ. Risk of patent foramen ovale for thromboembolic events in all age groups. *Am J Cardiol.* 1992;69:1316–1320.

8. Di Tullio M, Sacco RL, Gopal A, Mohr JP,

Homma S. Patent foramen ovale as a risk factor for cryptogenic stroke. *Ann Intern Med.* 1992;117:461–465.

9. Hausmann D, Mügge A, Becht I, Daniel WG. Diagnosis of patent foramen ovale by transesophageal echocardiography and association with cerebral and peripheral embolic events. *Am J Cardiol.* 1992;70:668–672.

10. Hart RG, Miller VT. Cerebral infarctions in young adults: a practical approach. *Stroke.* 1983;14:110–114.

11. Jones EF, Calafiore P, Donnan GA, Tonkin AM. Evidence that patent foramen ovale is not a risk factor for cerebral ischemia in the elderly. *Am J Cardiol.* 1994;74:596–599.

12. Overell JR, Bone I, Lees KR. Interatrial septal abnormalities and stoke: a meta-analysis of case-control studies. *Neurology.* 2000;55:1172–1179.

13. Meissner I, Khandheria BK, Heit JA, et al. Patent foramen ovale: Innocent or guilty? Evidence from a prospective population-based study. *J Am Coll Cardiol.* 2006;47:440–445.

14. Petty GW, Khandheria BK, Meissner I, et al. Population-based study of the relationship between patent foramen ovale and cerebrovascular ischemic events. *Mayo Clin Proc.* 2006 May;81(5):602–608.

15. Konstantinides S, Geibel A, Kasper W, Olschewski M, Blumel L, Just H. Patent foramen ovale is an important predictor of adverse outcome in patients with major pulmonary embolism. *Circulation.* 1998;97:1946–1951.

16. Isayev Y, Chan RK, Pullicino PM. "Economy class" stroke syndrome? *Neurology.* 2002;58:960–961.

17. Heckmann JG, Stadter M, Reulbach U, Duetsch M, Nixdorff U, Ringwald J. Increased frequency of cardioembolism and patent foramen ovale in patients with stroke and a positive travel history suggesting economy class stroke syndrome. *Heart.* 2006;92(9):1265–1268.

18. Khairy P, Landzberg MJ, Gatzoulis MA, et al. Transvenous pacing leads and systemic thromboemboli in patients with intracardiac shunts: a multicenter study. *Circulation.* 2006;113:2391–2397.

19. Hagen PT, Scholz DG, Edwards WD. Incidence and size of patent foramen ovale during the first 10 decades of life: an autopsy study of 965 normal hearts. *Mayo Clin Proc.* 1984;59:17–20.

20. Perrenoud J, Bustos D, Herrmann F, Michel JP. Patent foramen ovale and survival in old age. *Age Ageing.* 2000;29(5):460–461.

21. Anderson FA Jr, Wheeler HB, Goldberg RJ, et al. A population-based perspective of the hospital incidence and case-fatality rates of deep vein thrombosis and pulmonary embolism. The Worcester DVT Study. *Arch Intern Med.* 1991 May;151(5):933–938.

22. Sorensen HT, Horvath-Puho E, Pedersen L, Baron JA, Prandoni P. Venous thromboembolism and subsequent hospitalisation due to acute arterial cardiovascular events: a 20-year cohort study. *Lancet.* 2007;370:1773–1779.

23. Glazer NL, Dublin S, Smith NL, et al. Newly detected atrial fibrillation and compliance with antithrombotic guidelines. *Arch Intern Med.* 2007;167(3):246–252.

24. DiMarco JP, Flaker G, Waldo AL, et al; AFFIRM Investigators. Factors affecting bleeding risk during anticoagulant therapy in patients with atrial fibrillation: observations from the Atrial Fibrillation Follow-up Investigation of Rhythm Management (AFFIRM) study. *Am Heart J.* 2005;149(4):650–656.

25. Flaherty ML, Kissela B, Woo D, et al. The increasing incidence of anticoagulant-associated intracerebral hemorrhage. *Neurology.* 2007;68(2):116–121.

26. Homma S, Sacco RL, Di Tullio MR, Sciacca RR, Mohr JP, and PICSS Investigators. Atrial anatomy in non-cardioembolic stroke patients: Effect of medical therapy. *J Am Coll Cardiol.* 2003;42:1066.

27. Mohr JP, Thompson JL, Lazar RM, et al. A comparison of warfarin and aspirin for the prevention of recurrent ischemic stroke. *N Engl J Med.* 2001;345:1444–1451.

28. Bungard TJ, Ghali WA, McAlister FA, et al. Physicians' perceptions of the benefits and risks of warfarin for patients with nonvalvular atrial fibrillation. *CMAJ.* 2001;165(3):301–302.

29. Bungard TJ, Koshman SL, Tsuyuki RT. Patient preferences for ongoing warfarin management after receiving care by an anticoagulation management service. *Am J Health Syst Pharm.* 2008; 65(16):1498–1500.

30. Bungard TJ, Ackman ML, Ho G, Tsuyuki RT. Adequacy of anticoagulation in patients with atrial fibrillation coming to a hospital. *Pharmacotherapy.* 2000 Sep;20(9):1060–1065.

31. Windecker S, Wahl A, Chatterjee T, et al. Percutaneous closure of patent foramen ovale in patients with paradoxical embolism: long-term risk of recurrent thromboembolic events. *Circulation.* 2000;101:893–898.

32. Mohr JP, Homma S. Patent cardiac foramen ovale: stroke risk and closure. *Ann Intern Med.* 2003;139:787–788.

33. Krumsdorf U, Ostermayer S, Billinger K, et al. Incidence and clinical course of thrombus formation on atrial septal defect and patient foramen ovale closure devices in 1,000 consecutive patients. *J Am Coll Cardiol.* 2004;43: 302–309.

34. Ende DJ, Chopra PS, Rao PS. Transcatheter closure of atrial septal defect or patent foramen ovale with the buttoned device for prevention of recurrence of paradoxic embolism. *Am J Cardiol.* 1996;78:233–236.

35. Hung J, Landzberg MJ, Jenkins KJ, et al. Closure of patent foramen ovale for paradoxical emboli: intermediate-term risk of recurrent neurological events following transcatheter device placement [In Process Citation]. *J Am Coll Cardiol.* 2000;35:1311–1316.

36. Wahl A, Meier B, Haxel B, et al. Prognosis after percutaneous closure of patent foramen ovale for paradoxical embolism. *Neurology.* 2001;57:1330–1332.

37. Beitzke A, Schuchlenz H, Gamillscheg A, Stein JI, Wendelin G. Catheter closure of the persistent foramen ovale: mid-term results in 162 patients. *J Intervent Cardiol.* 2001;14:223–229.

38. Martin F, Sanchez PL, Doherty E, et al. Percutaneous transcatheter closure of patent foramen ovale in patients with paradoxical embolism. *Circulation.* 2002;106:1121–1126.

39. Braun MU, Fassbender D, Schoen SP, et al. Transcatheter closure of patent foramen ovale in patients with cerebral ischemia. *J Am Coll Cardiol.* 2002;39:2019–2025.

40. Bruch L, Parsi A, Grad MO, et al. Transcatheter closure of interatrial communications for secondary prevention of paradoxical embolism: single-center experience. *Circulation.* 2002;105: 2845–2848.

41. Windecker S, Wahl A, Nedeltchev K, et al. Comparison of medical treatment with percutaneous closure of patent foramen ovale in patients with cryptogenic stroke. *J Am Coll Cardiol.* 2004;44:750–758.

42. Schuchlenz HW, Weihs W, Berghold A, Lechner A, Schmidt R. Secondary prevention after cryptogenic cerebrovascular events in patients with patent foramen ovale. *Int J Cardiol.* 2005;101:77–82.

43. Chatterjee T, Petzsch M, Ince H, et al. Interventional closure with AMPLATZER PFO occluder of patent foramen ovale in patients with paradoxical cerebral embolism. *J Intervent Cardiol.* 2005;18:173–179.

44. Fischer D, Fuchs M, Schaefer A, et al. Transcatheter closure of patent foramen ovale in patients with paradoxical embolism. Procedural and follow-up results after implantation of the STARFlex® occluder device with conjunctive intensified anticoagulation regimen. *J Interv Cardiol.* 2008;21:183–189.

45. Wahl A, Tai T, Praz F, et al. Late results after percutaneous closure of patent foramen ovale for secondary prevention of paradoxical embolism using the AMPLATZER PFO Occluder without intra-procedural echocardiography: effect of device size. *JACC Cardiovasc Intervent.* 2009 Feb;2(2):116–123.

46. Wahl A, Krumsdorf U, Meier B, Sievert H, Ostermayer S, Billinger K, Schwerzmann M, Becker U, Seiler C, Arnold M, Mattle HP, Windecker S. Transcatheter treatment of atrial septal aneurysm associated with patent foramen ovale for prevention of recurrent paradoxical embolism in high-risk patients. *J Am Coll Cardiol.* 2005;45:377–380.

47. Windecker S, Meier B. Patent foramen ovale

and cryptogenic stroke: to close or not to close? Closure: what else! *Circulation,* Nov 2008;118:1989–1997.

48. Landzberg MJ, Khairy P. Indications for the closure of patent foramen ovale. *Heart (British Cardiac Society).* 2004;90(2):219–224.

49. Wohrle J. Closure of patent foramen ovale after cryptogenic stroke. *Lancet.* 2006;368:350–352.

6

PFO Closure and Migraines

Jonathan Tobis and Swarnendra Verma

Introduction

The connection between patent foramen ovale (PFO) and migraine headaches is a fascinating and instructive topic. Taken from an historical perspective, it contains lessons about how long-held beliefs within the field of medicine can be overturned in paradigm shifts. The concept of closing a PFO holds out the potential for reducing some of the suffering that patients with migraine headaches endure. This chapter will make the argument of why that may be the case.

The basic hypothesis is that migraine, especially migraine with visual aura or other transient neurologic deficits (TNDs), may be triggered by chemicals that ordinarily are metabolized during passage through the lungs. However, if there is a right-to-left shunt, these chemicals avoid the metabolic alteration that would normally occur in the lungs, and gain access to the arterial circulation in a higher concentration so that when they reach the brain, they stimulate receptors in susceptible individuals which produces the cerebral phenomena experienced as a migraine headache. There is no obvious reason why a right-to-left shunt would be associated with induction of migraine headaches. This hypothesis evolved from observations that closure of a PFO for other reasons, such as decompression illness in divers or to prevent cryptogenic stroke, resulted in relief of migraine headaches.

Generation of the Hypothesis

M. Del Sette and colleagues at the University of Genova, Italy, initially reported in 1998 on the association of strokes, migraine with aura,

Transcatheter Closure of ASDs and PFOs: A Comprehensive Assessment. © 2010 Ziyad M. Hijazi, Ted Feldman, Mustafa H. Abdullah Al-Qbandi, and Horst Sievert, editors. Cardiotext Publishing, ISBN: 978-0-9790164-9-3.

and right-to-left shunting.[1] Right-to-left shunting was diagnosed with transcranial Doppler using an agitated saline solution. The prevalence of right-to-left shunting was 16% in normal controls as compared with 41% in patients who had migraine with aura, p<0.005. This was similar to the incidence of right-to-left shunting in patients with cryptogenic stroke (35%). They suggested that the mechanism of stroke in patients with migraine and aura might be due to the high frequency of right-to-left shunting. Anzola and coworkers in Brescia, Italy, used transcranial Doppler in 113 patients referred for migraine with aura compared with 53 patients referred for migraine without aura and 25 age-matched controls. The prevalence of PFO was 48% in patients who had migraine and aura, 23% in migraine without aura patients, and 20% in control subjects, p=0.002.[2] Peter Wilmshurst described the beneficial effect of PFO closure on migraine headache in professional divers who had decompression illness or

in people with cryptogenic stroke.[3] Of 37 people who had their PFO closed and were available for follow-up, a history of migraine with aura was present in 16 and migraine without aura in 5 (total 21/37 or 57%). In those with migraine with aura, 7/16 claimed to have complete relief of migraine and 8 of the remaining 9 reported an improvement in frequency and severity of migraines. Of those people who had a history of migraine without aura, 3/5 claimed that their migraines were abolished. There was no beneficial effect in frequency of migraine episodes in only a small minority of patients, 3/37 or 8%. These reports stimulated subsequent observations from 9 laboratories around the world that described similar findings, which are summarized in Table 6.1.

Because the migraine headache improves after the passageway is closed, the conclusion is that there must be something that is no longer getting through. The possible causative agents include a variety of chemicals that otherwise

STUDY	Prevalence # Migraine / #Closed / (%)		% Migraine Improved or Cured	Length of Follow-up (months)
Wilmshurst (2000)	21/37	(59%)	86%	30
Morandi (2003)	17/62	(27%)	88%	6
Schwerzmann (2004)	48/215	(22%)	81%	12
Post (2004)	26/66	(39%)	65% (cured)	6
Reisman (2005)	57/162	(35%)	70%	12
Azarbal, Tobis (2005)	37/89	(42%)	76%	18
Giardini (2005)*	35/131	(27%)	91%	20
Kimmelstiel (2007)	24/41	(59%)	83%	3
Papa (2009)	28/76	(37%)	82%	12
TOTAL	293/879	(31%)	80%	13

Table 6.1—Observational Studies of the Prevalence of Migraine in Patients Referred for PFO Closure and the Effect of the Procedure on Migraine *This study focused explicitly on migraine headache with aura.

would be metabolized in passage through the lungs; alternatively, particles such as platelet plugs could enter the cerebral circulation or perhaps the induction of migraine is caused by the sudden change in oxygen saturation due to venous blood entering the left atrium through the PFO. There are many proponents of the particulate embolic hypothesis for the induction of migraine. Particles could cause stroke or TIA in specific areas of the brain, but why should embolic material, which would be distributed randomly, stimulate repetitive phenomenon such as a migraine headache? It appears more reasonable to suspect that some chemical enters the brain and then triggers a neural receptor to produce the phenomenon of migraine headache. This concept is more consistent with the observation that there are certain foods such as nuts, chocolate, alcohol, or red wine that can trigger a migraine in susceptible individuals.[4–8]

In epidemiological studies of migraine, the prevalence in the general population is reported as 12% with a 3:1 predominance of migraine in women versus men; that is, approximately 18% of women have migraine and 6% of men have migraine.[9] In observational studies of people with PFO, the prevalence of migraine is reported to be considerably higher at 30% to 50%.[1,10,11] When the PFO is closed either by surgery or percutaneously, many patients report a profound effect on their frequency of migraine. Of those who had migraine with aura, approximately 60% report complete abolition of their headaches and the TNDs that constituted their aura. An additional 15% state that although they still develop migraine, the frequency is reduced by 50% as measured by the number of headache days per month. A value of 50% reduction in headache days is frequently used to justify the clinical effectiveness of a new anti-migraine medication. Therefore the total frequency of significant benefit is reported as approximately 75% of people who have migraine and aura. In people who have migraine without aura the response is less predictable, but 30% of our patients without aura still claimed that their headaches were completely alleviated following PFO closure.[12]

The individual histories are extremely dramatic and are one of the more impressive phenomena that we have observed in over 30 years of clinical medicine. People with frequent severe migraine or even chronic daily headache, associated with confusion, partial blindness, and inability to function at work or socially, claim that the migraine headache and neurologic symptoms are completely gone within a few days of PFO closure. The neurologic community however remains very skeptical of these anecdotal descriptions as none of these claims have been confirmed by a randomized clinical trial.

In addition to the usual concerns about the validity of observational studies, the difficulty with these reports on the reduction of migraine following closure of a PFO is that migraine is a very subjective experience that is impossible to measure objectively. Moreover, there is a significant psychological component to migraine sufferers that is typical of anyone who has chronic pain. These people frequently take multiple medications and tend to overuse pain medications due to the intensity and frequency of their discomfort. It is therefore recognized that the only way to prove a connection between PFO and migraine would be to perform a randomized clinical trial where the patient and the neurologist, who would document the effects, are blinded to whether the patient received PFO closure or a sham procedure.

The MIST Trial

The hypothesis that PFO is causally related to migraine headache was tested in a randomized blinded controlled study in England using the STARFlex device (NMT, Inc. Boston, Massachusetts).[13] To identify patients who would be enrolled in the study, 432 people with migraine and aura were screened for a right-to-left shunt by using an intravenous injection of agitated saline during transthoracic echocardiographic imaging. An important observation from this screening procedure was that the majority

(60%) of these people with migraine and aura had evidence of a right-to-left shunt. Most of these shunts were due to PFO, but pulmonary shunts or atrial septal defects (ASDs) were also observed. Because the frequency of PFO in the general population is reported as 20%, this threefold higher incidence of right-to-left shunt in people who have migraine with aura is certainly suggestive that the two conditions may be related. The MIST trial (Migraine Intervention with STARFlex Technology) ultimately randomized 163 people who complained of migraine with aura. Of these, 73 were assigned to medical therapy and 74 were designated to have PFO closure using the STARFlex device. In contradistinction to all of the previous observational reports, the final conclusion of the MIST trial was that there was no significant beneficial effect of PFO closure on the frequency of migraine compared with placebo.[13]

Unfortunately, the MIST trial is mired in controversy.[14] Peter Wilmshurst, one of the original principal investigators of this trial, claims that up to 35% of the people assigned to receive the STARFlex device had large residual shunts by transthoracic echocardiography.[14,15] This assertion has been refuted by the sponsor of the trial, NMT Inc., but they have not published the results of a review of the echocardiograms by a core laboratory. In addition, they could restudy the patients assigned to the device arm with a transthoracic echocardiogram or transcranial Doppler with an echo contrast study to assess the frequency of persistent shunts. The obvious concern is that if there is a large percentage of patients who had persistent shunts, this could explain some of the lack of effect on the frequency of migraine headaches observed in this trial. It would also suggest that this particular device is not very effective in completely closing the right-to-left shunt.

Current Clinical Trials

In the United States, there have been three attempts to perform a randomized clinical trial to test the hypothesis that PFO closure will reduce the frequency and severity of migraine headaches. The MIST II trial was similar to the clinical trial performed in England, sponsored by NMT Inc. Given the negative results of their English trial, the company decided to discontinue this randomized trial in the United States. A second clinical trial, called The Effect of Septal Closure of Atrial PFO on Events of Migraine with Premere (ESCAPE) was sponsored by St. Jude Medical, Inc. to test their Premere device for PFO closure. After enrolling 56 subjects (out of a planned 492 patients), this study was closed due to difficulty in enrolling patients and perhaps due to concerns about the device itself.[16,17]

The PREMIUM trial, sponsored by AGA Medical Inc., is currently the only randomized clinical trial evaluating PFO closure in patients with migraine headache (Gov. Trials #NCT00355056). This study assesses the AMPLATZER PFO occluder device in patients who have migraine with or without visual aura. Similar to the MIST trial, it is a randomized controlled study where the patient and the neurologist are blinded. All of the patients are brought to the catheterization laboratory and receive an intracardiac echo instead of a transesophageal study, which is more uncomfortable for the patient. The atrial septum is probed with a guide wire prior to randomization to prove that a PFO is present and that it can be crossed without the need to perform a transseptal puncture, which would increase the risk of complications due to the procedure. A higher-than-expected complication rate was another criticism leveled at the MIST trial. The patients are then randomized to either have their PFO closed with the AMPLATZER device or to a sham procedure. All of the patients remain on their baseline medical therapy of prophylactic drugs that are not changed throughout the 1-year period of analysis. Acute rescue medications and medications to relieve pain are permitted. Several methods are used to ensure that the patients and the neurological evaluation team are blinded to treatment assignment.

Similar to the MIST and ESCAPE trials, the PREMIUM trial also has had significant difficulty enrolling patients. This is partly due to the constraints placed upon the trial by the FDA, which allows only the most severe patients to be treated. Although this limitation is reasonable to justify the inherent risk of implanting a permanent cardiac device in an otherwise healthy young individual, it has been difficult to identify patients who meet all of the strict inclusion criteria. In addition, the PFO clinical trials, whether for migraine or to prevent cryptogenic stroke, are hampered by the fact that other devices that are approved for ASD or VSD closure can be used by physicians via an off-label route to close a PFO. This results in patients "shopping around" for a physician who is willing to close their PFO rather than undergoing the uncertainty of randomization. The recent decision of the FDA to permit patients who are assigned to the control group to receive the AMPLATZER PFO occluder at the end of the 1-year observation period may significantly aid in encouraging patients to enroll in the PREMIUM trial.

What Is a Migraine?

The change in the concept of the etiology of migraine headache constitutes an example of a paradigm shift in our understanding of medical physiology. Until the 1990s, the training in medical schools was that migraine was a "vascular headache." The concept was that the headache was induced by intense cerebral arterial spasm. This produced relative ischemia in the brain that accounted for the visual aura or other TNDs. The vasospasm was then followed by vasodilation of the cerebral vessels. It was reasoned that the throbbing component to migraine headaches was due to the blood pulsating through the dilated arteries. The only problem with this conceptualization was that there was no data in animals or humans to prove that this was correct.

When newer methodologies were developed which could image brain perfusion and metabolism in humans, the understanding of migraine changed dramatically.[18] More recent studies with positron emission tomography (PET) and functional magnetic resonance (MR) imaging demonstrate the opposite of the original concept of migraine.[19-24] Initially there is vasodilation of the cerebral vessels, then constriction. This is associated with a wave of neuronal depression, which spreads over the cerebral cortex and corresponds to the transient deficit of neurologic function associated with the aura of migraine. This wave of cortical depolarization begins in the optical cortex and proceeds at approximately 3 to 5 mm per minute up to the motor and sensory cortices. This new concept of migraine has been confirmed in elegant experiments using a mouse transgenic model of migraine.[25,26]

One subset of migraine is a genetic variant called familial migraine with hemiplegia. People in these families develop severe migraine headache associated with transient hemiplegia. There is no permanent deficit and no evidence of stroke on MRI. The gene for this familial condition has been cloned and inserted into a transgenic mouse. Phenotypically, these mice develop transient hemiplegia, and imaging of the mouse brain reveals the spreading wave of cortical depression. Therefore migraine is now conceptualized as an interaction between the cerebral vasculature and neurogenic centers in the brain that are stimulated to induce the physiology of a migraine headache. The potential role a PFO could play in this physiology is that it acts as the passageway for potential chemical triggers to get to the appropriate neural receptors in the brain. The neurologic depression that spreads over the cerebral cortex produces the TNDs that the patient experiences as aura. This is usually visual dysfunction with zigzag white lines, star bursts of light, or scintillating scotoma, but can also manifest as a variety of neurologic symptoms such as paresthesias, motor weakness, diminished thought processing, or global amnesia.

The presence of these TNDs makes it difficult to distinguish between a migraine with aura and a transient ischemic attack (TIA). Both migraine and TIA can present with a transient neurologic deficit without leaving any trace in the brain as assessed by the most sensitive current methods of imaging with MRI. In addition, the TNDs due to migraine can occur without any cephalalgia, which makes it more difficult to ascribe this to a migraine. This has important implications for clinical trials of cryptogenic stroke if TIA is used as an end point and it is assumed that all TNDs are due to embolic phenomena. In the observational studies of migraineurs, it has been reported that PFO closure not only reduces migraine headache but also the associated TNDs.[12] In the clinical trials for stroke, if PFO closure is effective for preventing migraine, the group with device closure would theoretically have fewer events than the group on medical therapy, which could still be having migraine with TNDs. That is, it would appear as if PFO closure is preventing TIAs when in fact it is preventing TNDs due to migraine. Of course, from the patient's point of view, they would be pleased as long as the symptoms are diminished, but from a mechanistic perspective, it would be helpful to be able to distinguish between an embolic TIA due to a small thrombus versus a chemically induced migraine with TND.

Association of PFO, Migraine, and Cryptogenic Stroke

A more complete discussion of PFO and cryptogenic stroke is presented in another chapter of this book. However, cryptogenic stroke occurs with increased frequency in migraineurs and therefore needs to be discussed here as well. Cryptogenic stroke is defined as stroke of unknown etiology after an extensive workup for standard causes of stroke has been performed. Typically this definition is reserved for people < 60 years of age, above which it is assumed that atherosclerosis is present and is the most likely etiology of the stroke. As the origin of the clot is usually not found unless a deep vein thrombosis is present, it is hypothesized that one etiology of cryptogenic stroke is a venous thrombus (per-

haps from peripheral or pelvic varicose veins) that bypasses the lungs via a PFO and enters the arterial circulation. Occasionally, it can be documented by echocardiography that a large thrombus is trapped in a PFO, so clearly this mechanism of paradoxical embolism from the venous to the arterial circulation can occur. The venous clots that produce cryptogenic stroke are usually < 3 mm in diameter (based on the size of the cerebral vessels that they occlude). The problem is that once the clot passes to the brain, it is not possible to prove how it got there. Although this mechanism is now more generally accepted based on all of the observational studies with cryptogenic stroke and PFO closure, it is still necessary to obtain the results of current randomized clinical trials to prove this connection. If it can be demonstrated that by closing the PFO, compared with medical therapy, the recurrence rate of cryptogenic stroke decreases, then we will have more certainty in this proposed mechanism as well as data to support the benefit of percutaneous closure of PFO.[27–29]

The relevant issue to this discussion of migraine and PFO is the increased risk of cryptogenic stroke in people with migraine headache, especially migraineurs with aura. Based on a meta-analysis of 6 case-control studies, the relative risk of ischemic stroke for migraine without aura is 1.8 (range 1.06–3.15), whereas migraineurs with aura have a 2.3 greater risk.[30–44] In addition, the risk for ischemic stroke in women with migraine using oral contraceptives is increased 8.7 (range 5.05–15.05). Based on these epidemiologic studies, it is recommended that women with migraine should not take oral contraceptives. The dose of estrogen in transdermal patches may be associated with a lower incidence of ischemic stroke, but this has not been fully evaluated. In the Women's Health Study, there were 3577 women with migraine at baseline, and of these, 40% had migraine with aura. The greatest association between ischemic stroke and migraine was observed in younger women, < 50 years old, HR = 6.2 (95%CI 2.3–16.2).[32] In addition, these findings were independent of the usual risk factors for atherosclerosis: women with the lowest Framingham risk score had a greater risk of ischemic stroke (age-adjusted HR 3.9, 95%CI 1.9–8.1).

A population-based study in The Netherlands used MRI to assess 134 people with migraine without aura and 161 people who had migraine with aura compared with 140 matched controls.[45] Although the total percentage of patients with an ischemic infarct was not increased in migraine patients versus controls (5% versus 8.1%), when the data were analyzed by vascular supply, there was an increased incidence of posterior circulation infarcts in migraineurs with aura (8.1% versus 0.7% in controls). The absolute number of strokes was small, but the relative risk of posterior circulation strokes was significant (13 versus 1).

The longest prospective study occurred in Iceland with the Age Gene/Environment Susceptibility (AGES)-Reykjavík study in which 4689 people (57% women, mean age 51 years) were followed an average of 25 years, and then received a brain MRI. A total of 12.2% of the participants had migraine and 63% of them were identified as having migraine with aura. Those people who had migraine with aura had an increased risk of subsequent infarct lesions on MRI (OR 1.4; 95% CI 1.1–1.8). These results were predominantly due to an association of migraine with aura and cerebellar lesions among women (OR 1.9; 95% CI 1.4–2.6).[46] Unfortunately, this large epidemiologic study did not assess the presence of right-to-left shunting in these people, so we do not know the relative frequency of PFO in those migraineurs who developed stroke versus the migraineurs who did not develop a stroke or were not found to have a PFO, in the control population.

In the past, it was assumed that aura associated with migraine was due to the intense arterial constriction that produced ischemia and was thought to be the cause of the TND. The assumption was that if the arterial constriction was severe enough and long enough, it would account for the cerebral infarcts observed in migraineurs. Now that our understanding of the etiology of TNDs and the time course of vasoconstriction in migraine has completely changed, the etiology of stroke in migraine is also subject to a new analysis. As it appears that

the majority of people with migraine and aura have a right-to-left shunt, our hypothesis is that the cause of stroke in migraineurs is predominantly due to a paradoxical embolism through a PFO. This is consistent with the high frequency of migraine in those people who present with cryptogenic stroke and are found to have a PFO. In people who present with cryptogenic stroke, the frequency of migraine headache is approximately 30% to 50%.[47] Future epidemiologic studies of migraine and stroke need to include a sensitive screening method for determining whether a right-to-left shunt is present in those migraineurs who develop stroke. The question is, in a population of migraineurs who develop stroke, what is the frequency of transient right-to-left shunting across the circulation?

This hypothesis is also consistent with the increased risk of stroke in migraineurs who take birth control pills or hormone replacement therapy. Estrogen increases the risk of venous thrombosis. The presence of migraine, especially with visual aura, suggests that a PFO may be present. This combination of increased risk for venous thrombosis and a pathway through the PFO may permit a paradoxical embolism to occur and produce the cryptogenic strokes seen in migraineurs. If this hypothesis is corroborated by data on the incidence of PFO in migraineurs with stroke, then it will not only affect our understanding of the mechanism of stroke in migraineurs, but will also suggest that prophylactic closure of PFO should be evaluated in a randomized trial to test whether it is an effective method of treatment for prevention of stroke in migraineurs. The difficulty of this type of study is that the absolute risk of stroke in migraineurs is small. Therefore, a large number of people would need to be treated with PFO closure and followed over many years to show an effect.

Migraine and Cerebral White Matter Lesions

In addition to MRI lesions consistent with ischemic stroke, migraineurs have a higher incidence of nonspecific lesions that involve myelinated white matter neurons. These abnormalities are usually 2 to 5 mm in diameter and are described as white matter lesions (WML). They can be seen anywhere along the white matter tracts of the cerebrum, cerebellum, or even the brain stem, especially the pons.[48] They correspond to myelin degradation which is replaced by water and therefore show up as white spots or hyperintensities on FLAIR or T2 sequences on MRI studies. The differential diagnosis of these lesions is disconcerting and includes multiple sclerosis, vasculitis, and lacunar strokes.

In the 3-City Study from France, 1643 people older than 65 years had WML on MRI and were followed for 5 years.[49] The risk of subsequent stroke was associated with the volume of the WML and was 5× higher for the highest quartile of WML volume. Of note, WML were not predictive of other cardiovascular events, suggesting that the etiology of WML may be different from atherosclerosis.

It is not known what causes WML in migraineurs or what their significance is. It is not known whether the lesions are due to some metabolic disturbance associated with the physiology of migraine or whether they represent an insult due to embolic material. These lesions have also been seen in patients with PFO who do not have a history of migraine headache. This suggests that these lesions may be caused by chemicals or particulate matter such as platelet plugs that bypass the lungs and enter the brain circulation via a right-to-left shunt.

In opposition to this theory that WML are due to paradoxical embolism of chemicals or particulate material, is the observation that migraineurs without PFO also have WML on MRI. Blasco and co-authors from Spain looked at brain MRIs in 44 migraine patients with (12) and without aura (32). Of the 44 patients, 29 (66%) had WML, but only 7 (24%) of the people with WML had a right-to-left shunt. The frequency of right-to-left shunting by TCD was not statistically different among those migraineurs with WML versus those without WML (both groups 50%).[50] This study was underpowered

and thus unable to provide conclusive answers, but it suggests that either right-to-left shunting is unrelated to WML, or there may be multiple causes for WML in migraine.

Another study with twice the number of patients arrived at the same conclusion. Del Sette and co-workers at the University of Genova, Italy studied 80 patients who had migraine with aura. MRI images were obtained in all patients and right-to-left shunting was determined by transcranial Doppler.[51] The mean age of the patients was 37 ± 11 years with a mean duration of migraine of 16 ± 12 years; the mean number of migraine attacks without aura was 43 ± 70 per year, and the mean number of migraine attacks with aura was 28 ± 55 per year. The frequency of WML was high at 61%, but the presence of WML did not correlate with any clinical migraine characteristic. The number and volume of WML increased with age (r=0.25, p<0.05). Of relevance to the present discussion, there was no difference in the total volume or number of WML between patients with or without right-to-left shunting. They conclude that WML in migraineurs may only be an expression of age-related gliosis or scar formation, and that the presence of WML should not be used as a criterion for closing a PFO in patients with migraine.

The results of the Genova group were extended to 185 patients (77% women) in the ongoing Shunt Associated Migraine (SAM) study, which included five other neurology groups in Italy and Belgium.[52] The incidence of periventricular WML was similar in patients with and without right-to-left shunts, and the incidence of deep WML was actually less in patients with a right-to-left shunt (p=0.045).

We also do not understand the natural history of WML in people with or without migraine headache. The Italian group headed by Carlo Vigna reported an interesting study in these patients.[53] This was not a randomized trial but an observational study of 82 people with severe migraine and PFO. All of these people had WML on MRI. The patients were offered PFO closure. In the 53 people who elected to have their PFO closed, the frequency of migraine headaches was significantly reduced from 32 ± 9 in the 6 months before closure to 7 ± 7 in the 6 months following closure (p<0.001). This was compared to the 29 people who elected not to have their PFO closed in whom there was no significant reduction in migraine headaches from 36 ± 13 to 30 ± 21. We anticipate that there will be follow-up MRI studies in these patients, which may elucidate the long-term effect of PFO closure on migraineurs with WML. This study also raises the issue whether there is a subpopulation of migraineurs who are more likely to respond to PFO closure. Certainly in this study, migraineurs with WML had a high response rate to PFO closure. Whether this is because the PFO is causally related to the migraine headache, or whether the WML are an indication of greater responsiveness to PFO closure, is still not known.

Another concern related to the presence of WML in migraine is whether there is any long-term cognitive dysfunction in these people. Although a variety of studies have produced conflicting results,[54–69] two large and well-controlled studies did not find any evidence for cognitive impairment in migraineurs. The first study came from the Danish twin registry[70] and the second was part of the prospective Baltimore Epidemiologic Catchment Area Study[71] which compared 204 migraine patients with 1244 nonmigraineurs. In this study, it is reassuring to note that migraineurs, including those with aura, had less decline in cognitive function tests compared with nonmigraineurs.

Is It the PFO or Will Any Right-to-Left Shunt Suffice?

Is there something unique about a pathway through the atrial septum with the presence of a PFO, or are migraines associated with any mixture of venous blood directly with the arterial circulation? The best natural experiment to test this hypothesis would be in adults with congenital heart disease. These people have a variety of abnormal connections in the circulation but can be generally categorized as having a right-to-left shunt, a left-to-right shunt, or no shunt. To test this hypothesis, adults were chosen because they would have lived long enough to have the possibility of experiencing migraine headache, which usually begins in the teenage years or early 20s. UCLA has a specialized Adults with Congenital Heart Disease Clinic that has followed over 2000 patients. Of these, 800 people were available and contacted by phone. A history of migraine headaches was obtained with the MIDAS questionnaire.[72] The frequency of migraine in this population was compared with a control population that was matched by gender. In the control population, the frequency of migraine was 11%, which is consistent with previously published epidemiologic studies.[9] However, in people with a diagnosis of right-to-left shunt (such as Tetralogy of Fallot, pulmonary or tricuspid atresia, etc.) the prevalence of migraine headache was 52% (p<0.001). In those people with a primary diagnosis of left-to-right shunt (such as ASD, VSD, or PDA), the prevalence of migraine headache was 44% (p< 0.001).

Unexpectedly, in people with a congenital heart lesion that does not normally have a shunt (such as bicuspid aortic valve, Marfan's syndrome, aortic dilatation, etc.), the prevalence of migraine headaches was also elevated at 38% (p<0.001). The next study will assess whether the congenital heart disease patients without an obvious shunt by standard echo/Doppler (which does not include an echo contrast/bubble study) actually have a higher incidence of PFO to explain the high frequency of migraine headache. In addition, people who had a history of migraines and had surgical correction of their congenital heart disease as an adult, reported a dramatic reduction in the frequency of their migraine headaches as documented by the MIDAS questionnaire. This frequency of reduction in migraine after closure of the shunt was similar to that observed in migraineurs with cryptogenic stroke who have their PFO closed percutaneously.[73]

There are also rare examples (1% of our cases) of pulmonary arteriovenous malformation (AVM) in patients who do not have a PFO, who may present with cryptogenic stroke and migraine headache. The migraine may also be reduced or eliminated when the arterial AVM is closed. Thus it appears that it is the presence of persistent right-to-left shunting or intermittent right-to-left shunting (in the case of predominant left-to-right shunts such as ASDs) that is associated with migraine headaches as distinguished from something unique about a PFO.

Exacerbation of Migraine Headache Following PFO or ASD Closure

Another interesting phenomenon that may be relevant to our eventual understanding of migraine triggers is the observation that some people develop migraine headache for the first time, or have exacerbation of pre-existing migraine with aura, after an atrial connection is closed. This apparently paradoxical phenomenon has been observed with either PFO or ASD closure with certain devices, but has not been described following surgical closure. This implies that it is something particular to the devices and not closure of the shunt that is culpable. We reported on 7 patients who complained of new onset or exacerbation of migraine with aura associated with closure of PFO (2 cases) or ASDs (5 cases, 2 with a large device [38 mm]).[74] All of these patients received AMPLATZER devices, which are made of Nitinol, an alloy of nickel (55%) and titanium (45%). Nickel allergy was assessed by using the TRUE skin patch test.[74] The 2 patients who had a PFO closure device were allergic to nickel, as were 3 of the 5 ASD patients. The 2 patients with the large 38-mm AMPLATZER devices did not demonstrate nickel allergy on skin patch testing.

The migraine episodes in these patients were notable for the prominent component of visual aura. The other fascinating observation was the remarkable sensitivity of the headache and visual aura to treatment with clopidogrel. Although aspirin was often also used, it did

not appear to have the same beneficial effect as clopidogrel. The typical scenario was that aspirin and clopidogrel were used as standard treatment immediately following AMPLATZER device insertion. The clopidogrel was stopped 1 to 3 months following the procedure. Within a few days, the patients complained of migraine with aura. Restarting the clopidogrel alleviated the symptoms within hours and stopping the clopidogrel for a few days would reinitiate the complaints of migraine headache. After 4 to 12 months, these symptoms dissipated even when the clopidogrel was stopped.

Our hypothesis to explain these observations is that allergy to nickel in susceptible individuals or excessive inflammation on the larger AMPLATZER devices induces platelet aggregation and activation with release of serotonin on the left atrial side of the device. Serotonin or perhaps other chemicals or mediators of inflammation such as chemokines then travel to the brain without being metabolized through the pulmonary circulation, and trigger migraine in susceptible individuals. The clopidogrel may be inhibiting platelet activation on the left atrial side of the device or perhaps is acting directly on nociceptive ADP receptors in the brain. Eventually the device gets covered with fibrous scar tissue and the inflammatory stimulus is no longer exposed to blood. It is interesting to note that we have not observed any postclosure migraines in 60 patients who received a HELEX device (W.L. Gore, Inc., Flagstaff, Arizona). The HELEX device is made of Teflon (tetrafluoroethylene), which also covers the rim of Nitinol wire so less nickel is exposed to the bloodstream.[75]

Sensitivity of Testing for Patent Foramen Ovale

Epidemiologic studies of cryptogenic stroke or migraine describe the frequency of right-to-left shunting and draw conclusions based on the relative prevalence. The literature on this subject is confusing because of the wide discrepancy of results concerning the association of a PFO and these disease states.[76] It is reminiscent of the proverb of the blind men describing an elephant based on a small sampling area. The results vary widely depending on whether they are touching the trunk, belly, hair, or the tail. We suspect the same is true of epidemiologic studies and PFO; there is a wide variation in description due to sampling errors based on the group being studied. In addition, the sensitivity of techniques for determining the presence of a PFO varies widely.

A common method for detecting PFO is to perform transthoracic echo imaging using an agitated saline bubble injection from a brachial vein as the contrast medium. This is easy to perform and uses standard echocardiography equipment. However the sensitivity of this technique is less than that reported with transesophageal echo because some people do not have a good thoracic echo window.[77] Transesophageal echo is more invasive and uncomfortable for many patients, but is more specific for making the diagnosis of a PFO.[78] However, a transesophageal echo may miss the diagnosis of PFO in about 10% of patients because they cannot cooperate and perform an adequate Valsalva maneuver either because they are sedated or because it is difficult to perform with a tube passing through the oropharynx into the esophagus. There are several reports of increased sensitivity for detecting right-to-left shunts using transcranial Doppler.[78–80] This equipment is less readily available but is not expensive and the technique can be learned quickly. We suggest that transcranial Doppler should be the preferred screening method for large populations to identify right-to-left shunting in epidemiologic studies of migraine or stroke. If the specific question is whether a PFO is present, then a subsequent transesophageal echo could be obtained.

There are also subtle issues with the technique of performing transcranial Doppler or any screening test for right-to-left shunt. The sensitivity of the agitated saline bubble study is improved if 1 cc of blood is withdrawn and added to the mixture. The serum protein makes an emulsion of fine bubbles that do not dissipate as quickly as when saline alone is used. In addition, it is necessary for the right atrium to be filled with the echocontrast bubble solution so that the area adjacent to the septum is opacified. Blood flows from the superior vena cava away from the septum. Blood from the inferior vena cava follows the fetal circulation and is directed toward the fossa ovalis by the residual eustachian valve. It has been demonstrated that TCD studies performed in the cath lab with injections from the femoral vein are more sensitive than TCD performed with injections through veins located in the arm.[81] Because the PFO is oriented in an inferior-superior direction, to ensure complete filling of the right atrium, some authors also recommend performing the TCD in a sitting position to optimize sensitivity.[82]

The Genetics of Migraine and PFO

Are migraine and PFO related only by a mechanical passageway and the metabolic influence of some chemical trigger, or is there some genetic predisposition for both conditions? Peter Wilmshurst was the first to document an association of migraine headaches and septal defects, in families who had either an ASD or a PFO.[83] His group used contrast echocardiography to detect right-to-left shunts in 71 relatives of 20 probands who had either a large PFO or an ASD. The occurrence of atrial shunts was consistent with an autosomal dominant inheritance. When the proband had migraine with aura and an atrial shunt, 15 of the 21 (71%) first-degree relatives with a right-to-left shunt also had migraine with aura, compared with 3 of 14 (21%) without a significant shunt (p<0.02).

Perhaps the atrial defect is an independent bystander that permits some chemical to pass through and triggers the migraine in these susceptible families. But the demonstration of both migraines and atrial defects persisting in several generations implies that there is a genetic component to both the susceptibility of migraine headaches as well as the development of cardiac septal defects. It is possible that the same gene could be active in both the heart and brain or that separate genes are closely related on a section of a chromosome. It is anticipated that future research may identify the gene or genes, which could have a significant impact on the treatment of both migraines and PFO.

An intriguing study that demonstrates the potential connection between genetic determinants of cardiac structure and predisposition to migraine was provided by Zicari and co-workers from the University of Siena, Italy.[84] They studied 21 patients with the syndrome of CADASIL (cerebral autosomal dominant arteriopathy with subcortical infarcts and leukoencephalopathy). This familial disease manifests with recurrent strokes, dementia, and migraine with aura. Transcranial Doppler studies demonstrated the presence of right-to-left shunting in 15 of the 21 patients (71%), although there was no correlation between the clinical presentation or the amount of MRI changes and the presence of right-to-left shunting. CADASIL is due to a mutation in the Notch3 gene that regulates cell differentiation in vascular smooth muscles in the brain, as well as during the development of the cardiovascular system.[85] Lacunar strokes and subsequent leukoencephalopathy are produced by degeneration of the vascular smooth muscles, leading to arterial wall thickening and luminal narrowing in the small penetrating arteries of the brain. Notch3 is also expressed in cardiac tissue during embryogenesis and regulates the morphogenesis of cardiac valves and septa. Although CADASIL is an unusual genetic disorder, it demonstrates how the predisposition to migraine and cardiac morphogenesis producing a PFO could be related genetically.

The Influence of Estrogen on Migraine Headaches

The lifetime risk of having migraine is 40% for women and 20% for men. Thus women are twice as likely to develop migraine headaches at some time in their lives compared with men. Approximately 50% of women state that migraines are more frequent or are typically induced in the perimenstrual time frame. Several studies have demonstrated that the onset of migraine is associated with the decrease in estrogen blood level that occurs during the luteal phase.[86–88] In addition, the administration of 1.5-mg estradiol gel can postpone the development of migraine in these susceptible women. There was no absolute level of estrogen that was associated with the induction of migraine, suggesting that it is the withdrawal of estrogen rather than a specific blood level that is the trigger.[89] However, there are other reports that estrogen can induce migraine in susceptible women.[90] It is not known whether it is the fall in estrogen alone that induces migraine, or whether other chemicals such as prostaglandins, which also fluctuate throughout the menstrual cycle, also play a role in triggering the migraine.

Migraine without aura commonly improves or is eliminated after menopause whereas migraine with aura is not reduced by menopause.[91,92] Surgical oophorectomy also improves or eliminates migraine.[93] However, in one study, 9% of women reported worsening of migraine following menopause.[94] The potential origin of the responsible chemicals is also intriguing. In a survey of 986 hysterectomized women with one or both ovaries present compared with 5636 women with both ovaries and uterus intact, the prevalence of moderate to severe migraine was higher in hysterectomized women with both ovaries, than in women with ovaries and uterus intact (15% vs. 9%, p<0.001).[95] A somewhat contradictory observation reported that the prevalence of migraine is lowest in women who have had a hysterectomy with bilateral oophorectomy at 16%, compared with hysterectomy alone 29%, and hysterectomy with unilateral oophorectomy at 36% (but this did not reach statistical significance, p=0.3).[93]

The effect on migraine of estrogen replacement during menopause is also an important clinical question. In the Women's Health Study, there were 21,788 postmenopausal women, of whom 30% had never used hormone replacement therapy (HRT), and 48% were current users.[96] Of these women, 8% complained of migraine within the preceding year. By multivariate analysis, the use of HRT was associated with a 42% increased risk of having migraine. However this was not a trial of HRT randomized for the presence of migraine, and it is possible that many of these postmenopausal women were given HRT as a treatment for their headaches.[97]

PFO, Migraine, and Arterial Spasm

It has been postulated that there may be a connection between migraine and coronary arterial spasm. This concept was initially described in the 1960s due to an apparent higher incidence of migraine headache in patients who manifested Prinzmetal's angina.[98] Although this concept initially received some support, it lost favor due to the concern that the angina was secondary to medical treatment of the migraine headache with ergotamine, which subsequently produced coronary arterial spasm. With the new observations about PFO, we believe that there is reason to resurrect this hypothesis that there could be a connection between migraine headache and coronary artery spasm. The unifying hypothesis would be that there is some chemical that normally gets metabolized in the lungs that can pass through the PFO and induce coronary artery spasm, whereas other chemicals, if they bypass the lungs through the PFO, could induce migraine. For example, acetylcholine has been shown to induce paradoxical coronary artery spasm in susceptible individuals who may have underlying endothelial dysfunction.[99]

In the vast majority of people with PFO who present with paradoxical embolism, a cerebral event is the presenting symptom. Systemic, noncerebral, paradoxical embolism occurs with far less frequency, accounting for 5% to 10% of all paradoxical embolisms.[100] Although uncommon, these events have been described as a cause of acute myocardial infarction (MI), renal infarction, and limb ischemia. It is not known

why the overwhelming majority of paradoxical embolism associated with PFO present as strokes. Blood flow to the cerebral vessels only accounts for 15% of the cardiac output[101] yet of the patients we have seen who had presumed paradoxical embolism, 95% (219/231) had cerebral emboli. Presumably there are other emboli to different parts of the body that may be asymptomatic, such as to the kidneys or spleen.

There were 12 patients who presented with embolic events other than stroke, which presumably were the result of embolization of thrombus from right-to-left shunting through a PFO.[102] Patients in our series who presented with acute MI were found to have regionally depressed wall motion on echocardiography or left ventriculogram, yet no evidence of obstructive epicardial coronary disease was found on angiography. In many of these cases, evidence of the thrombus was documented by angiography. However, this is not always the case, which raises the possibility of another cause for the infarction. The following is an instructive case history of a person who had a PFO and long-standing migraine headaches who presented with a life-threatening MI.

An Unusual Case of PFO, Migraine, and Myocardial Infarction

A 49-year-old woman with a 30-year history of migraine headache presented to an outside hospital with progressive chest pain. The initial ECG was normal without ST elevation or depression. While being evaluated in the emergency department, she suffered a cardiac arrest and required cardiopulmonary resuscitation and defibrillation. She was rushed to cardiac catheterization, which showed no evidence of occlusive thrombus in the coronary arteries. The angiograms were interpreted later as demonstrating coronary artery spasm (Fig 6.1A), although such a diagnosis could not be proven definitely because intracoronary vasodilators were not used and intravascular ultrasound (IVUS) imaging was not obtained at the time to rule out other entities such as dissection. Eventually an automatic implantable cardioverter-defibrillator (AICD) was implanted, and she was referred to our institution for evaluation of her unusual coronary presentation. Because of the history of migraine, a TEE was performed which demonstrated a PFO. Her symptoms improved with treatment with nitrates and cyproheptadine, a serotonin antagonist. Six months after the cardiac arrest, successful closure of her PFO was performed. Coronary angiography obtained during the closure procedure demonstrated no evidence of atherosclerotic disease (Fig 6.1B). Intravascular ultrasound revealed no dissection or atherosclerotic plaque (Fig 6.1C).

As distinguished from the mechanism of thrombotic embolism to the coronary arteries as a cause of MI in the presence of a PFO, the patient presented here is particularly unusual. Because there was no evidence of obstruction or thromboembolism to the coronary arteries at the time of the patient's MI, we suspect that the event was the result of intense coronary spasm and not a paradoxical embolus. We hypothesize that a vasospastic substance, such as serotonin or acetylcholine, can bypass degradation in the lungs and enter the arterial system through a

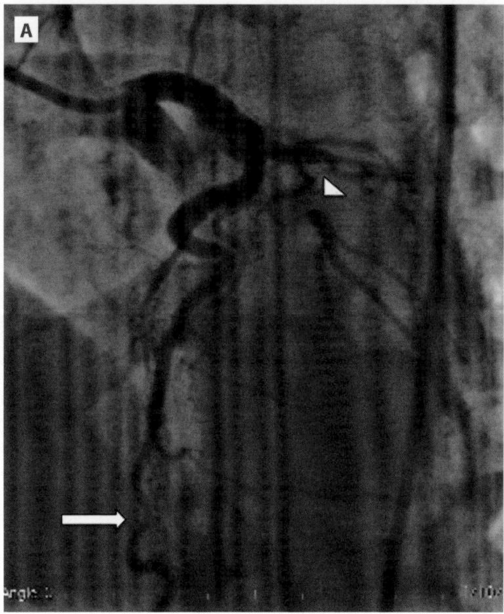

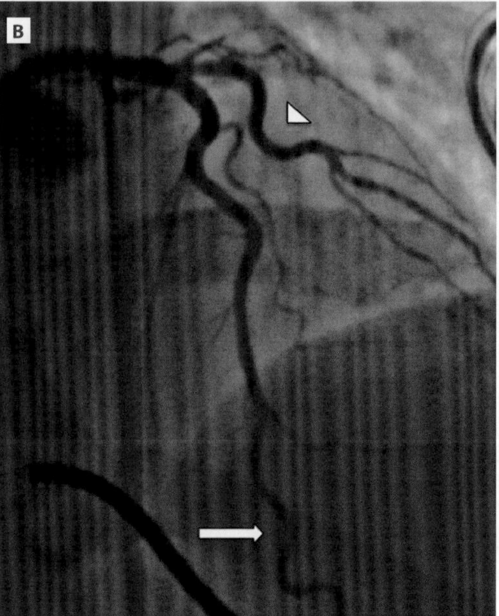

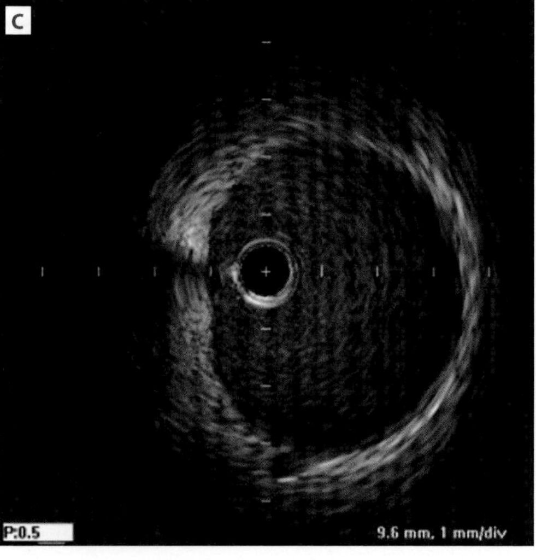

Fig 6.1—A: Left coronary angiography reveals a long segment of diffuse narrowing in the diagonal branch of the left anterior descending artery (LAD) (arrowhead), as well as a shorter segment in the distal LAD (arrow). The other coronary arteries have no evidence of atherosclerotic disease. The diagonal artery was treated with balloon dilatation only. B: Angiography repeated 6 months later demonstrates no evidence of coronary disease or spasm in the previously stenosed vessels. The patient received an AICD for her episode of cardiac arrest (dark electrode at base of picture). C: Intravascular ultrasound in the LAD reveals no evidence of atherosclerotic disease or arterial dissection.

PFO in a higher concentration than would occur in the absence of a PFO. The substance could then trigger intense arterial spasm in a coronary vessel producing an infarction, Prinzmetal's angina, or ischemia with ventricular arrhythmia.

There are isolated reports of patients who have single or recurrent MIs due to coronary spasm, but we do not know the frequency of right-to-left shunting in these patients. There is not a large series of patients who present with coronary artery spasm. Perhaps with increased awareness, physicians can combine patient observations to help elucidate whether coronary spasm is associated with the intermittent right-to-left shunt of a PFO.

Migraine and Increased Cardiovascular Mortality

There are several large epidemiologic studies that describe an increased incidence of cardiovascular events in men and women who have migraine (Table 6.2). The Physicians Health Study followed 20,084 male physicians to assess the risk of developing disease and correlated that with baseline clinical characteristics.[103] Of these men, 7.2% had a history of migraine headache. The mean age of these physicians was 56 years and they were followed for a mean of 15.7 years. In these men with migraine, there was a 24% increased risk for cardiovascular disease events. This included a 42% increase in MI, a 12% increase in ischemic stroke, and a 7% increase in cardiovascular death compared with men who did not have migraine at baseline. These increased risks were independent of the standard Framingham risks for developing cardiovascular disease, which suggests that migraine is not associated with an increase in the usual risk factors for atherosclerosis.

The Women's Health Study followed 27,840 women to evaluate the association between lifestyle, risk factors, and subsequent clinical outcomes. A history of migraine headaches was reported in 5125 of these individuals (18.4%). These women were all age 45 and older, and were followed for a mean of 10 years. In the women

	Physicians' Health Study (2007)	Women's Health Study (2006)	Women's Health Study (2009)*
Total # of Participants	20,084	27,840	27,840
Gender	Male	Female	Female
% with Migraine	7.2%	18.4%	5.2%
Age	56 (mean)	45 & older	45 & older
Follow-up	15.7 years	10 years	11.9 years
↑ risk of CVD	24%	42%	115%
↑ risk of MI	42%	41%	108%
↑ risk of ischemic stroke	12%	22%	91%
↑ risk of CV death	7%	63%	133%

Table 6.2—Increased Risk of Stroke or Myocardial Infarction in Men and Women with Migraine Headache. Increased risks are relative to individuals without any history of migraine headache. * Refers to women with Active Migraine Headaches with Aura (MHA). Abbreviations: CVD, cardiovascular disease; CV, cardiovascular; MI, myocardial infarction.

with migraine, there was a 42% increased risk for cardiovascular disease events. This included a 41% increase in MI, a 22% increase in ischemic stroke, and a 63% increase in cardiovascular death compared with women who did not have migraine at baseline.[32]

The migraine patients were analyzed separately, according to the presence or absence of aura. Women who had migraine with aura had an even greater increase in the risk for cardiovascular events. In women with migraine and aura, there was a 115% increased risk for cardiovascular disease events. This included a 108% increase in MI, a 91% increase in ischemic stroke, and a 133% increase in cardiovascular death compared with women who did not have any type of migraine at baseline.[104]

Although it is unknown why these men and women with migraine have an increased risk for stroke, MI, and death, it is intriguing to hypothesize that a large number of these people, especially those with migraine and aura, may have an associated PFO. This would provide a pathway for cryptogenic stroke, paradoxical embolism to the coronaries for MI, or a conduit for chemical substances that might induce coronary spasm with ischemia-induced arrhythmias or MI.

Is There a Specific PFO-Associated Type of Migraine Headache?

Until a randomized controlled trial demonstrates a significant benefit of PFO closure to reduce migraine headaches, this field will remain clouded in controversy. One main area of focus for the neurologists and cardiologists interested in this issue is the question of whether there is a subset of patients with migraine that might be more responsive to PFO closure. Although the observational studies have reported dramatic reduction in the frequency of migraine in a large portion of the patients, there are still 25% of patients who do not respond to PFO closure. Similarly, although

the majority of patients with migraine and aura appear to have evidence for a right-to-left shunt, not all patients with migraine and aura have a PFO. Because we are implanting a permanent cardiac device in relatively young individuals, it would be preferable if we could identify those patients with migraine who are more likely to respond positively to PFO closure.

Peter Goadsby, Mark Reisman, Brian Whisenant, and others have attempted to define a patient population of migraineurs that have responded to PFO closure with a dramatic reduction in the frequency of migraine headaches. They hypothesize that a common feature is patients who have migraine with aura that can be manifested with either visual field defects, or other TNDs, which may occur intermittently with or without headache. They will test this hypothesis in a randomized clinical trial using the Coherex FlatStent (Salt Lake City, Utah) device to percutaneously close PFO. As distinct from prior migraine trials, the patients will need to have at least 5 migraine days per month, but there will be no upper limit of migraine frequency. It had previously been thought that patients who have chronic daily headache would not respond to PFO closure, but observational reports suggest that some patients with daily headache may respond as well as those migraineurs who have episodic headache. Another potential target population that may respond favorably to PFO closure is migraineurs with WML as described previously in the study by Vigna et al.[105]

The Controversy Continues

As this book was being prepared for publication, two articles appeared in *Circulation Cardiovascular Interventions* under the heading of "Controversies in Interventional Cardiology: Is Patent Foramen Ovale Closure Indicated For Migraine?".[106] Many of the observations described in this chapter are reviewed in these point-counterpoint articles. The authors recognize that certain patients have a dramatic response to PFO closure with either reduction or complete elimination of migraine headache, but without a positive result from a randomized prospective trial, this area is still encumbered by hypothesis without confirmation. It is everyone's fervent hope that future research and the results of randomized clinical trials will help elucidate the subset of patients for which PFO closure can be helpful in reducing the significant suffering associated with migraine headaches. This field is progressing rapidly. Hopefully in the near future we will have many more answers to the questions raised in this chapter concerning the relationship of migraine headaches and PFO.

References

1. Del Sette M, Angeli S, Leandri M, et al. Migraine with aura and right-to-left shunt on transcranial Doppler: A case-control study. *Cerebrovasc Dis.* 1998;8(6):327–330.

2. Anzola GP MM, Guindani M, Rozzini L, Dalla VG. Potential source of cerebral embolism in migraine with aura: a transcranial Doppler study. *Neurology.* May 12 1999;52(8):1622–1625.

3. Wilmshurst PT, Nightingale S, Walsh KP, Morrison WL. Effect on migraine of closure of cardiac right-to-left shunts to prevent recurrence of decompression illness or stroke or for haemodynamic reasons. *Lancet.* 2000;356(9242):1648–1651.

4. Lassen LH TL, Olesen J. Histamine induces migraine via the H1-receptor. Support for the NO hypothesis of migraine. *Neuroreport.* 1995; 15:1475–1479.

5. Olesen J IH, Thomsen LL. Nitric oxide supersensitivity: a possible molecular mechanism of migraine pain. *Neuroreport.* Aug 1993;4(8): 1027–1030.

6. Olesen J TL, Iversen H. Nitric oxide is a key molecule in migraine and other vascular headaches. *Trends Pharmacol Sci.* May 1994;15(5): 149–153.

7. Lassen L, Haderslev P, Jacobsen V, Iversen H, Sperling B, Olesen J. CGRP may play a causative role in migraine. *Cephalalgia.* 2002;22(1):54–61.

8. Schytz HW BS, Wienecke T, Kruuse C, Olesen J, Ashina M. PACAP38 induces migraine-like attacks in patients with migraine without aura. *Brain.* 2009;132(1):16–25.

9. Diamond S, Bigal ME, Silberstein S, Loder E, Reed M, Lipton RB. Patterns of diagnosis and acute and preventive treatment for migraine in the United States: Results from the American Migraine Prevalence and Prevention Study. *Headache J Head Face Pain.* 2007;47(3):355–363.

10. Sztajzel R, Genoud D, Roth S, Mermillod B, Le Floch-Rohr J. Patent foramen ovale, a possible cause of symptomatic migraine: A study of 74 patients with acute ischemic stroke. *Cerebrovasc Dis.* 2002;13(2):102–106.

11. Schwedt T, Demaerschalk B, Dodick D. Patent foramen ovale and migraine: a quantitative systematic review. *Cephalalgia.* 2008;28(5):531–540.

12. Azarbal B, Tobis J, Suh W, Chan V, Dao C, Gaster R. Association of interatrial shunts and migraine headaches: Impact of transcatheter closure. *J Am Coll Cardiol.* 2005;45(4):489–492.

13. Dowson A, Mullen MJ, Peatfield R, et al. Migraine Intervention With STARFlex Technology (MIST) Trial: A prospective, multicenter, double-blind, sham-controlled trial to evaluate the effectiveness of patent foramen ovale closure with STARFlex septal repair implant to resolve refractory migraine headache. *Circulation.* 2008;117(11):1397–1404.

14. Tobis J. Management of patients with refractory migraine and PFO: Is MIST I relevant? *Cathet Cardiovasc Intervent.* 2008;72(1):60–64.

15. Wood S. Disputed echo results from MIST I require regulatory attention, article states *theheart.org [Internet].* 2008. http://www.theheart.org/article/864751.do Accessed Dec 15, 2009.

16. Carroll JD, Carroll EP. Is patent foramen ovale closure indicated for migraine?: PFO closure is not indicated for migraine: "Don't Shoot First, Ask Questions Later." *Circ Cardiovasc Interv.* October 1, 2009;2(5):475–481.

17. Wood S. NOMAS: Just a 2% overlap for PFO and migraine; St Jude shuts down ESCAPE trial. *theheart.org [Internet].* 2008. http://www.theheart.org/article/910063.do. Accessed Dec 4, 2009.

18. Tfelt-Hansen PC. History of migraine with aura and cortical spreading depression from 1941

and onwards. *Cephalalgia.* 2009; Sep 9 [Epub ahead of print].

19. Cutrer FM ODA, Sanchez del Rio M. Functional neuroimaging: enhanced understanding of migraine pathophysiology. *Neurology.* 2000;55(9):S36–45.

20. Charles A, Brennan K. Cortical spreading depression & new insights and persistent questions. *Cephalalgia.* 2009;29(10):1115–1124.

21. Schwedt TJ, Dodick DW. Advanced neuroimaging of migraine. *Lancet Neurol.* 2009;8(6):560–568.

22. Afridi SK, Giffin NJ, Kaube H, et al. A positron emission tomographic study in spontaneous migraine. *Arch Neurol.* August 1, 2005;62(8):1270–1275.

23. Matharu MS, Bartsch T, Ward N, Frackowiak RSJ, Weiner R, Goadsby PJ. Central neuromodulation in chronic migraine patients with suboccipital stimulators: a PET study. *Brain.* January 1, 2004;127(1):220–230.

24. Cao Y AS, Nagesh V, Patel SC, Welch KM. Functional MRI-BOLD of brainstem structures during visually triggered migraine. *Neurology.* Jul 9 2002;59(1):72–78.

25. Brennan KC, Beltran-Parrazal L, Lopez-Valdes HE, Theriot J, Toga AW, Charles AC. Distinct vascular conduction with cortical spreading depression. *J Neurophysiol.* June 1, 2007;97(6): 4143–4151.

26. Brennan KC, Romero-Reyes M, Valdés HEL, Arnold AP, Charles AC. Reduced threshold for cortical spreading depression in female mice. *Ann Neurol.* 2007;61(6):603–606.

27. Closure I Website. [Internet Website]. http://www.closurei.com/. Accessed Dec 30, 2009.

28. RESPECT PFO Clinical Trial Website. [Internet Website]. http://amplatzer.com/us/Respect/index.html. Accessed Dec 30, 2009.

29. Stroke Trials Registry. [Internet Website]. http://www.strokecenter.org/trials/TrialDetail.aspx/?tid=946. Accessed Dec 30, 2009.

30. Stang PE, Carson AP, Rose KM, et al. Headache, cerebrovascular symptoms, and stroke: The Atherosclerosis Risk in Communities Study. *Neurology.* May 10, 2005;64(9):1573–1577.

31. Becker C, Brobert GP, Almqvist PM, Johansson S, Jick SS, Meier CR. Migraine and the risk of stroke, TIA, or death in the UK (CME). *Headache J Head Face Pain.* 2007;47(10):1374–1384.

32. Kurth T, Gaziano JM, Cook NR, Logroscino G, Diener H-C, Buring JE. Migraine and risk of cardiovascular disease in women. *JAMA.* July 19, 2006;296(3):283–291.

33. Paemeleire K. Brain lesions and cerebral functional impairment in migraine patients. *J Neurol Sci.* 2009;283(1–2):134–136.

34. MacClellan LR, Giles W, Cole J, et al. Probable migraine with visual aura and risk of ischemic stroke: The stroke prevention in young women study. *Stroke.* September 1, 2007;38(9):2438–2445.

35. Kurth T, Schurks M, Logroscino G, Gaziano JM, Buring JE. Migraine, vascular risk, and cardiovascular events in women: prospective cohort study. *BMJ.* August 7, 2008;337(aug07_1): a636.

36. Henrich JB, Horwitz RI. A controlled study of ischemic stroke risk in migraine patients. *J Clin Epidemiol.* 1989;42(8):773–780.

37. Tzourio C IS, Hubert JB, et al. Migraine and risk of ischaemic stroke: a case-control study. *BMJ.* Jul 31 1993;307(6899):289–292.

38. Tzourio C, Tehindrazanarivelo A, Iglesias S, et al. Case-control study of migraine and risk of ischaemic stroke in young women. *BMJ.* April 1, 1995;310(6983):830–833.

39. Carolei A MC, De Matteis G. History of migraine and risk of cerebral ischaemia in young adults. The Italian National Research Council Study Group on Stroke in the Young. *Lancet.* Jun 1 1996;347(9014):1503–1506.

40. Chang CL, Donaghy M, Poulter N. Migraine and stroke in young women: case-control study. *BMJ.* January 2, 1999 1999;318(7175):13–18.

41. Nightingale AL, Farmer RDT. Ischemic stroke in young women: A nested case-control study using the UK General Practice Research Database. *Stroke.* July 1, 2004;35(7):1574–1578.

42. Kurth T, Slomke MA, Kase CS, et al. Migraine, headache, and the risk of stroke in women: A prospective study. *Neurology.* March 22, 2005;64(6):1020–1026.

43. Scher AI, Terwindt GM, Picavet HSJ, Verschuren WMM, Ferrari MD, Launer LJ. Cardiovascular risk factors and migraine: The GEM

population-based study. *Neurology.* February 22, 2005;64(4):614–620.

44. Etminan M, Takkouche B, Isorna FC, Samii A. Risk of ischaemic stroke in people with migraine: systematic review and meta-analysis of observational studies. *BMJ.* January 8, 2005;330(7482):63.

45. Kruit MC, van Buchem MA, Hofman PA, et al. Migraine as a risk factor for subclinical brain lesions. *JAMA.* Jan 28 2004;291(4):427–434.

46. Scher AI, Gudmundsson LS, Sigurdsson S, et al. Migraine headache in middle age and late-life brain infarcts. *JAMA.* June 24, 2009;301(24):2563–2570.

47. Rundek T, Elkind MSV, Di Tullio MR, et al. Patent foramen ovale and migraine: A cross-sectional study from the Northern Manhattan Study (NOMAS). *Circulation.* September 30, 2008;118(14):1419–1424.

48. Kruit M, Buchem MV, Launer L, Terwindt G, Ferrari M. Migraine is associated with an increased risk of deep white matter lesions, subclinical posterior circulation infarcts and brain iron accumulation: the population-based MRI CAMERA study. *Cephalalgia.* 2010;30(2):129–136.

49. Buyck JF, Dufouil C, Mazoyer B, et al. Cerebral white matter lesions are associated with the risk of stroke but not with other vascular events: The 3-City Dijon Study. *Stroke.* July 1, 2009;40(7):2327–2331.

50. Bosca M TJ, Bosca I, Lago A. Study of the relationship between white matter lesions in the magnetic resonance imaging and patent foramen ovale. *Neurologia.* Oct 23 2008;23(8):499–502.

51. Sette MD, Dinia L, Bonzano L, et al. White matter lesions in migraine and right-to-left shunt: a conventional and diffusion MRI study. *Cephalalgia.* 2008;28(4):376–382.

52. Adami A, Rossato G, Cerini R, et al. Right-to-left shunt does not increase white matter lesion load in migraine with aura patients. *Neurology.* July 8, 2008;71(2):101–107.

53. Vigna C, Marchese N, Inchingolo V, et al. Improvement of migraine after patent foramen ovale percutaneous closure in patients with subclinical brain lesions: A case-control study. *JACC.* 2009;2(2):107–113.

54. Zeitlin C, Oddy M. Cognitive impairment in patients with severe migraine. *Br J Clin Psychol.* 1984 Feb 1984;23(1):27–35.

55. Le Pira F LF, Zappalà G, Morana R, Panetta MR, Reggio E, Reggio A. Relationship between clinical variables and cognitive performances in migraineurs with and without aura. *Funct Neurol.* Apr–Jun 2004;19(2):101–105.

56. Hooker W, Raskin N. Neuropsychologic alterations in classic and common migraine. *Arch Neurol.* 1986;43(7):709–712.

57. Mulder E, Linssen W, Passchier J, Orlebeke J, Geus E. Interictal and postictal cognitive changes in migraine. *Cephalalgia.* 1999;19(6):557–565.

58. Calandre E, Bembibre J, Arnedo M, Becerra D. Cognitive disturbances and regional cerebral blood flow abnormalities in migraine patients: their relationship with the clinical manifestations of the illness. *Cephalalgia.* 2002;22(4):291–302.

59. Waldie KE, Hausmann M, Milne BJ, Poulton R. Migraine and cognitive function: A life-course study. *Neurology.* September 24, 2002;59(6):904–908.

60. Riva D, Aggio F, Vago C, et al. Cognitive and behavioural effects of migraine in childhood and adolescence. *Cephalalgia.* 2006;26(5):596–603.

61. Pira FL, Zappalà G, Giuffrida S, et al. Memory disturbances in migraine with and without aura: a strategy problem? *Cephalalgia.* 2000;20(5):475–478.

62. Scherer P BH, Baum K. Alternate finger tapping test in patients with migraine. *Acta Neurol Scand.* Dec 1997;96(6):392–396.

63. Sinforiani E FS, Mancuso A, Manzoni GC, Bono G, Mazzucchi A. Analysis of higher nervous functions in migraine and cluster headache. *Funct Neurol.* Jan–Mar 1987;2(1):69–77.

64. Pearson A, Chronicle E, Maylor E, Bruce L. Cognitive function is not impaired in people with a long history of migraine: a blinded study. *Cephalalgia.* 2006;26(1):74–80.

65. Leijdekkers ML PJ, Goudswaard P, Menges LJ, Orlebeke JF. Migraine patients cognitively impaired? *Headache.* May 1990;30(6):352–358.

66. Jelicic M, Boxtel MPJv, Houx PJ, Jolles J. Does migraine headache affect cognitive function in the elderly? Report from the Maastricht Aging

Study (MAAS). *Headache J Head Face Pain.* 2000;40(9):715–719.

67. Haverkamp F, Hönscheid A, Müller-Sinik K. Cognitive development in children with migraine and their healthy unaffected siblings. *Headache J Head Face Pain.* 2002;42(8):776–779.

68. Bell BD, Primeau M, Sweet JJ, Lofland KR. Neuropsychological functioning in migraine headache, nonheadache chronic pain, and mild traumatic brain injury patients. *Arch Clin Neuropsych.* 1999;14(4):389–399.

69. Palmer J, Chronicle E. Cognitive processing in migraine: a failure to find facilitation in patients with aura. *Cephalalgia.* 1998;18(3):125–132.

70. Gaist D PL, Madsen C, Tsiropoulos I, et al. Long-term effects of migraine on cognitive function: a population-based study of Danish twins. *Neurology.* Feb 22 2005;64(4):590–591.

71. Kalaydjian A ZP, Swartz KL, Eaton WW, Lyketsos C. How migraines impact cognitive function: findings from the Baltimore ECA. *Neurology.* Apr 24, 2007;68(17):1417–1424.

72. Truong T, Slavin L, Kashani R, et al. Prevalence of migraine headaches in patients with congenital heart disease. *Am J Cardiol.* 2008;101(3):396–400.

73. Papa M, Gaspardone A, Fracasso G, et al. Usefulness of transcatheter patent foramen ovale closure in migraineurs with moderate to large right-to-left shunt and instrumental evidence of cerebrovascular damage. *Am J Cardiol.* 2009;104(3):434–439.

74. Wertman B, Azarbal B, Riedl M, Tobis J. Adverse events associated with nickel allergy in patients undergoing percutaneous atrial septal defect or patent foramen ovale closure. *J Am Coll Cardiol.* 2006;47(6):1226–1227.

75. Reddy BT, Patel JB, Powell DL, Michaels AD. Interatrial shunt closure devices in patients with nickel allergy. *Cathet Cardiovasc Intervent.* 2009;74(4):647–651.

76. Tobis J, Azarbal B. Does patent foramen ovale promote cryptogenic stroke and migraine headache? *Tex Heart Inst J.* 2005;32(3):362–365.

77. Blum A RS, Farbstein Y. Transesophageal echocardiography vs. transthoracic echocardiography in assessing cardio-vascular sources of emboli in patients with acute ischemic stroke. *Med Sci Monit.* September 2004;10(9):521–523.

78. Zito C, Dattilo G, Oreto G, et al. Patent foramen ovale: Comparison among diagnostic strategies in cryptogenic stroke and migraine. *Echocardiography.* 2009;26(5):495–503.

79. Sastry S, MacNab A, Daly K, Ray S, McCollum C. Transcranial Doppler detection of venous-to-arterial circulation shunts: Criteria for patent foramen ovale. *J Clin Ultrasound.* 2009;37(5):276–280.

80. Mangiafico SAC, Davide B, Tamburino CB. Transcranial color Doppler is essential to quantify right-to-left shunt severity. *J Cardiovasc Med (Hagerstown).* Dec 2009;10(12):890.

81. Hamann GF S-KD, Fröhlig G, Strittmatter M, et al. Femoral injection of echo contrast medium may increase the sensitivity of testing for a patent foramen ovale. *Neurology.* 1998;50(5):1423–1428.

82. Lao AY, Sharma VK, Tsivgoulis G, Malkoff MD, Alexandrov AV, Frey JL. Effect of body positioning during transcranial Doppler detection of right-to-left shunts. *Eur J Neurol.* 2007;14(9):1035–1039.

83. Wilmshurst PT, Pearson MJ, Nightingale S, Walsh KP, Morrison WL. Inheritance of persistent foramen ovale and atrial septal defects and the relation to familial migraine with aura. *Heart.* November 1, 2004;90(11):1315–1320.

85. Niessen K, Karsan A. Notch signaling in the developing cardiovascular system. *Am J Physiol Cell Physiol.* July 1, 2007;293(1):C1–11.

86. Zacur H. Hormonal changes throughout life in women. *Headache.* Oct 2006;46(2):49–54.

87. Lay CL, Broner SW. Migraine in women. *Neurol Clin.* 2009;27(2):503–511.

88. Martin VT LR. Epidemiology and biology of menstrual migraine. *Headache.* Nov–Dec 2008;48(3):124–130.

89. MacGregor EA, Frith A, Ellis J, Aspinall L, Hackshaw A. Incidence of migraine relative to menstrual cycle phases of rising and falling estrogen. *Neurology.* 2006;67(12):2154–2158.

90. Martin V, Wernke S, Mandell K, et al. Medical oophorectomy with and without estrogen add-back therapy in the prevention of

migraine headache. *Headache J Head Face Pain.* 2003;43(4):309–321.

91. Freeman EW SM, Lin H, Gracia CR, Kapoor S. Symptoms in the menopausal transition: hormone and behavioral correlates. *Obstet Gynecol.* Jan 2008;111(1):127–136.

92. Mattsson P. Hormonal factors in migraine: A population-based study of women aged 40 to 74 years. *Headache J Head Face Pain.* 2003;43(1):27–35.

93. Wang S-J, Fuh J-L, Lu S-R, Juang K-D, Wang P-H. Migraine prevalence during menopausal transition. *Headache J Head Face Pain.* 2003;43(5):470–478.

94. Neri I GF, Nappi R, Manzoni GC, Facchinetti F, Genazzani AR. Characteristics of headache at menopause: a clinico-epidemiologic study. *Maturitas.* Jul 1993;17(1):31–37.

95. Oldenhave A JL, Everaerd WT, Haspels AA. Hysterectomized women with ovarian conservation report more severe climacteric complaints than do normal climacteric women of similar age. *Am J Obstet Gynecol.* Mar 1993;168(3):765–771.

96. Misakian AL, Langer RD, Bensenor IM, et al. Postmenopausal Hormone Therapy and Migraine Headache. *Journal of Women's Health.* 2003;12(10):1027–1036.

97. MacGregor EA. Estrogen replacement and migraine. *Maturitas.* 2009;63(1):51–55.

98. Prinzmetal M KR, Merliss R, Wada T, Bor N. Angina pectoris. I. A variant form of angina pectoris; preliminary report. *Am J Med Sci.* Sep 1959;27:375–388.

99. Ludmer PL SA, Shook TL, Wayne RR, Mudge GH, Alexander RW, Ganz P. Paradoxical vasoconstriction induced by acetylcholine in atherosclerotic coronary arteries. *N Engl J Med.* Oct 1986;315(17):1046–1051.

100. Crump R, Shandling AH, Van Natta B, Ellestad M. Prevalence of patent foramen ovale in patients with acute myocardial infarction and angiographically normal coronary arteries. *Am J Cardiol.* 2000;85(11):1368–1370.

101. Kirsch TD, Lipinski CA. Head injury. In: Tintinalli JE, Kelen GD, Stapczynski JS, Ma OJ, Cline DM, eds. *Tintinalli's Emergency Medicine: A Comprehensive Study Guide.* New York: McGraw-Hill, 2002, 25:6e.

102. Dao CN, Gevorgyan R, Cua B, Perlowski A, Tobis JM. PFO and paradoxical embolism producing events other than stroke: Department of Medicine (Cardiology Division), David Geffen School of Medicine at UCLA; 2009.

103. Kurth T, Gaziano JM, Cook NR, et al. Migraine and risk of cardiovascular disease in men. *Arch Intern Med.* April 23, 2007;167(8):795–801.

104. Kurth T, Schurks M, Logroscino G, Buring JE. Migraine frequency and risk of cardiovascular disease in women. *Neurology.* August 25, 2009;73(8):581–588.

106. Reisman M, Fuller CJ. Is patent foramen ovale closure indicated for migraine?: Patent foramen ovale closure for migraine. *Circ Cardiovasc Interv.* October 1, 2009;2(5):468–474.

PART II

Imaging and Assessment

7

Imaging to Guide ASD and PFO Closure: TTE and TEE

Sinai C. Zyblewski and Girish S. Shirali

Introduction

Transcatheter closure of an atrial septal defect (ASD) or patent foramen ovale (PFO) requires precise delineation of the defect size, location, morphology, and the surrounding atrial septal tissue. Echocardiography remains the diagnostic gold standard for interatrial communications and plays an important role in the planning, guidance, and follow-up of a successful transcatheter device closure. With advances in echocardiography technology, the imaging options extend beyond the traditional two-dimensional transthoracic echocardiograms (2D TTE) and two-dimensional transesophageal echocardiograms (2D TEE). More recent technologies include three-dimensional transthoracic (3D TTE), three-dimensional transesophageal (3D TEE), and intracardiac echocardiography (ICE). Each modality contributes uniquely to the preparation and guidance of transcatheter closure of ASDs and PFOs.

The Precatheterization Assessment

A detailed transthoracic or transesophageal echocardiogram prior to the catheterization is a crucial initial step in planning the transcatheter closure of an ASD or PFO. In children and adults with a favorable body habitus, a TTE can be easily performed. In adults with poor acoustic windows, a TEE may be the preferred modality. The goals of this precatheterization echocardiogram include determining whether the defect is amenable to transcatheter closure, identifying the number of defects, confirming

Transcatheter Closure of ASDs and PFOs: A Comprehensive Assessment. © 2010 Ziyad M. Hijazi, Ted Feldman, Mustafa H. Abdullah Al-Qbandi, and Horst Sievert, editors. Cardiotext Publishing, ISBN: 978-0-9790164-9-3.

the absence of other structural heart disease, and obtaining a baseline assessment of cardiac structures that may be affected by the transcatheter procedure.

Identification of the ASD amenable to transcatheter device closure

ASDs are classified according to their location relative to the fossa ovalis and their embryonic origins. Interatrial communications amenable to transcatheter device closure are restricted to secundum ASDs and PFOs. In children and infants, the subcostal view is the most effective for diagnosis and classification of interatrial communications because it places the ultrasound beam perpendicular to the plane of the atrial septum. However, adults often have inadequate acoustic windows for this view so TEE has become the more accepted diagnostic examination in this age group. In patients who require a TEE, the diagnostic findings are optimally seen at the 0°, 30°, and 90° views.

The foramen ovale represents a normal interatrial communication that is present throughout fetal life. Functional closure of the foramen ovale occurs postnatally when left atrial pressure exceeds right atrial pressure; however, in 25% to 30% of people, anatomic closure does not occur. This results in a potential interatrial channel for air or blood to shunt through when right atrial pressure exceeds left atrial pressure.[1] By TTE, the PFO is characterized by a flap and color Doppler confirms the presence of shunting across the communication (Fig 7.1). Peripheral contrast-enhanced echocardiography may aid in the diagnosis with the visualization of shunting of agitated saline bubbles across the atrial septum.

A secundum ASD is the result of the deficiency of the septum primum and is characterized by dropout of the mid-atrial septum on echocardiography (Figs 7.2 and 7.3). Left-to-right shunting at the atrial level is confirmed by pulsed wave Doppler. The pulsed wave Doppler profile has a characteristic pattern. Blood shunting from left-to-right usually begins in mid-systole and the velocity progressively decreases until early diastole. When atrial contraction occurs, the left-to-right velocity increases again. There may be a brief right-to-left shunt in early ventricular systole.

Interatrial communications not suitable for transcatheter device closure include primum defects, sinus venosus defects, and defects involving the coronary sinus. The primum defect is located anterior to the fossa ovalis and is characterized by a deficiency in the lower septum that is just cephalad to the atrioventricular valves (Fig 7.4). The sinus venosus defect is located posterior and superior to the fossa ovalis and usually occurs in conjunction with anomalous connection of the right pulmonary veins (Fig 7.5). The interatrial communication

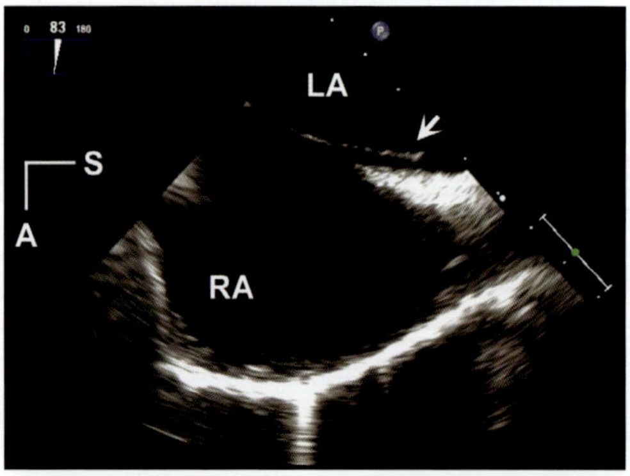

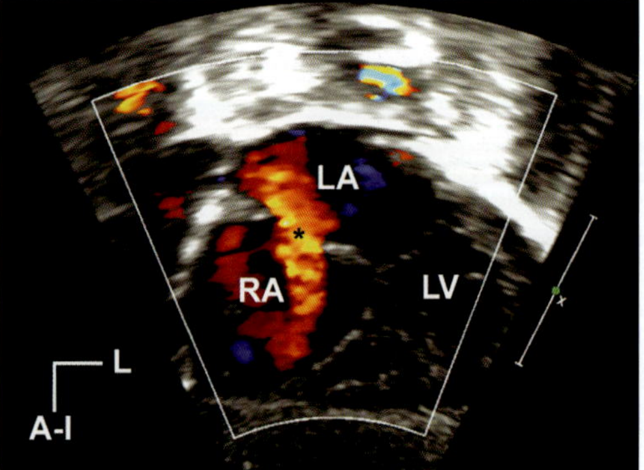

Fig 7.1—Two-dimensional transesophageal bicaval view. It demonstrates a flap of tissue with a patent foramen ovale (arrow). As in this instance, such defects are frequently tunnel-like and tortuous. Abbreviations: LA, left atrium; RA, right atrium; S, superior; A, anterior.

Fig 7.2—Two-dimensional transthoracic subxiphoid long-axis view at the base of the heart. It demonstrates a moderate-sized central secundum atrial septal defect (asterisk) with left-to-right flow. Abbreviations: LA, left atrium; RA, right atrium; LV, left ventricle; A-I, antero-inferior; L, left.

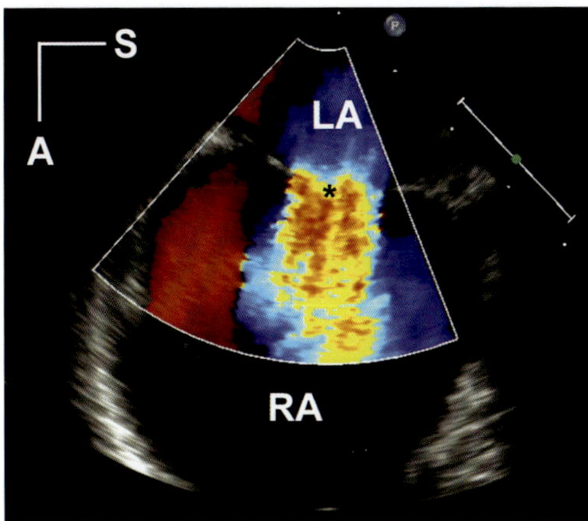
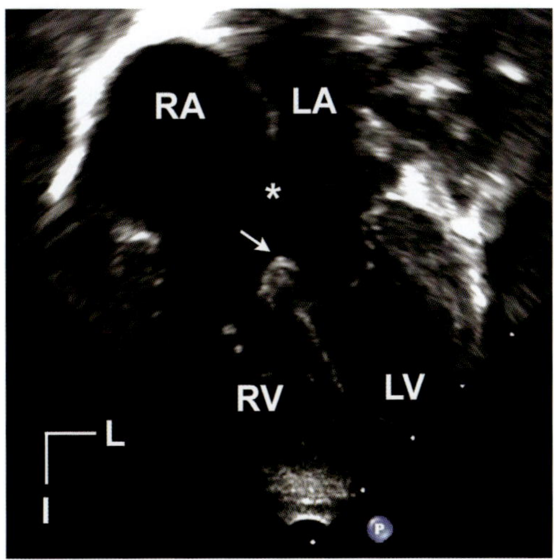

Fig 7.3—Two-dimensional transesophageal bicaval view, rotated rightwards to evaluate the atrial septum in a plane perpendicular to the ultrasound beam. It demonstrates a central secundum atrial septal defect (asterisk) with left-to-right flow. Abbreviations: LA, left atrium; RA, right atrium; A, anterior; S, superior.

Fig 7.4—This two-dimensional transthoracic apical four-chamber view demonstrates a large primum atrial septal defect (asterisk). The lower rim of the defect consists of the atrioventricular valves. Normal offset of the atrioventricular valves is lost, with both the right and left atrioventricular valves sharing a common hinge (arrow). Abbreviations: LA, left atrium; LV, left ventricle; RA, right atrium; RV, right ventricle; I, inferior; L, left.

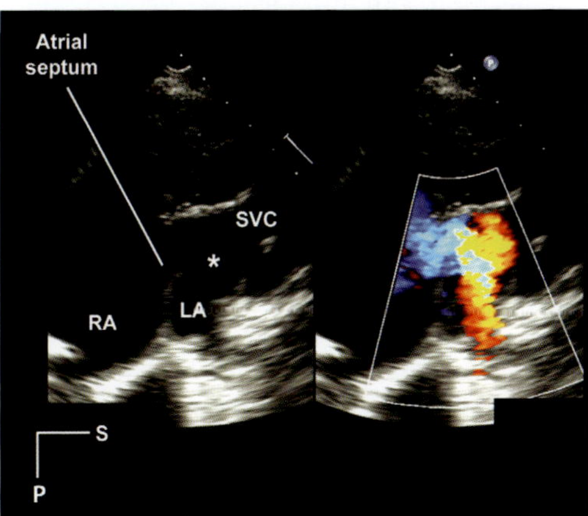
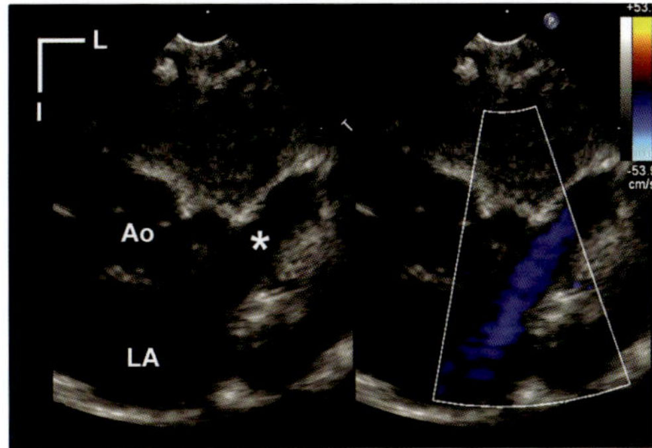

Fig 7.5—This two-dimensional transthoracic high right parasternal view demonstrates a sinus venosus defect. The superior vena cava (SVC) overrides the atrial septum. This type of defect is almost always associated with anomalous drainage of one or more of the right pulmonary veins into the superior vena cava or the adjacent superior aspect of the right atrium (RA). Such defects are not candidates for device closure. Abbreviations: P, posterior; S, superior.

Fig 7.6—Two-dimensional transthoracic high parasternal short-axis view. The transducer has been rotated slightly clockwise and tilted inferiorly. It demonstrates a left-sided superior vena cava (asterisk) that drains directly into the left atrium (LA). In this defect, the orifice of the coronary sinus itself provides for communication between the two atria. Abbreviations: I, inferior; L, left.

occurs just below the junction of the superior vena cava (SVC) and right atrium, and on echocardiography, the SVC appears to override the atrial septum. The sinus venosus defect is best visualized from the transthoracic subcostal and high right parasternal views or from the 0° and 90° transesophageal views. Defects involving the coronary sinus are characterized by a communication at the level of the orifice of the coronary sinus and are often associated with an unroofed coronary sinus and connection of a persistent left SVC to the left atrium (Fig 7.6).

Identification of other important structures

In addition to evaluating the interatrial communication, the precatheterization echocardiogram should be used to comprehensively assess other cardiac structures. In settings of a moderate- or large-sized ASD, right-sided chamber dilation is expected. However, if the right-sided enlargement seems disproportionate to the size of the interatrial communication, a thorough evaluation for additional pretricuspid left-to-right shunts should be pursued (ie, additional atrial communications, pulmonary vein anomalies). The discovery of other defects such as anomalous pulmonary veins, cleft mitral valve, or ventricular septal defect may require surgical intervention and preclude transcatheter device closure of an ASD.

The heart catheterization and transcatheter device closure may potentially distort or disrupt specific cardiac structures so it is important to establish a good baseline examination. Specifically, atrial inflows and outflows should be fully evaluated including the systemic venous return, pulmonary venous return, and coronary sinus drainage (Fig 7.7). The tricuspid and mitral valves should be interrogated for regurgitation or abnormal valve leaflet motion. The aortic valve should also be assessed for baseline function, especially if the aortic rim is small and there is potential for the device to splay on the aortic root.

Transcatheter Device Closure with Two-Dimensional TEE Guidance

The availability of echocardiographic imaging in the catheterization laboratory is an essential component of an ASD/PFO closure program. Transesophageal or intracardiac echocardiography provides images that are unique and complementary to fluoroscopy. While transthoracic echocardiographic guidance has been described for transcatheter ASD closure, TEE and ICE are the preferred modalities in the catheterization suite due to better acoustic windows and easier accessibility in light of sterile drapes and rotating gantrys.[2-7]

Measurement of the rims

The relation and distance of the secundum ASD/PFO to adjacent cardiac structures is particularly important for planning device implantation. At our institution, the measurement of rims for device size selection is performed in the catheterization lab by TEE. In a large multicenter trial of 442 patients who underwent transcatheter closure of an ASD, the most common reasons for technical failure of device placement were insufficient atrial rims or a defect that was too large for the available device.[8] In a review of a registry of complications for the AMPLATZER Septal Occluder, 28 cases of hemodynamic compromise were reported between 1998 and 2004. Twenty-five out of the

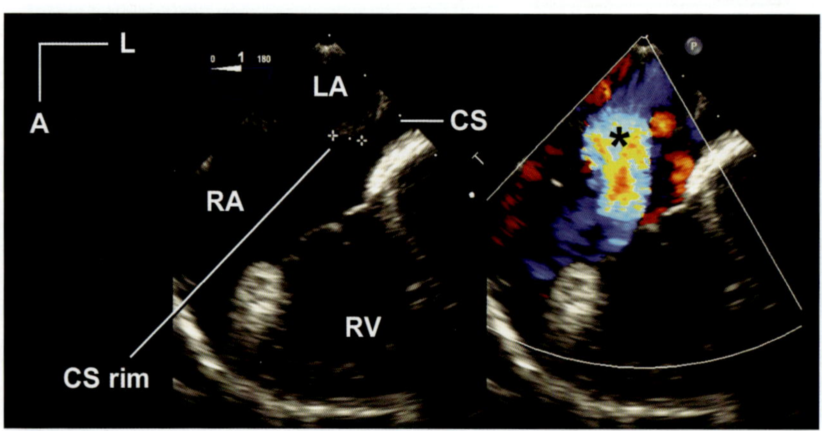

Fig 7.7—This two-dimensional transesophageal four-chamber view demonstrates a low secundum atrial septal defect (right panel, asterisk) with left-to-right flow. Cursors mark the coronary sinus (CS) rim. Abbreviations: A, anterior; L, left.

28 (89%) patients had a deficient aortic and/or superior rim.[9] For the purposes of clarity, nomenclature of the rims is designated according to the structure to which they relate.[10,11] Rims should be measured from the closest edge of the defect to the designated rim structure. The superior rim abuts the superior wall of the right atrium. The superior cavoatrial junction (SVC) rim is located posterior-superiorly and is bordered by the superior vena cava near the right upper pulmonary vein. The inferior cavoatrial junction (IVC) rim is located posterior-inferiorly, adjacent to the inferior vena cava (Figs 7.8–7.10). The mitral and tricuspid valvar (MV and TV) rims are positioned inferiorly and bordered by the septal hinge points of the atrioventricular valves (Fig 7.11). The aortic rim is related to the aorta and abuts the anterior-superior septum (Fig 7.12). If more than one defect is present, the rim between the defects should be evaluated to determine sufficiency for separate device closure.[12]

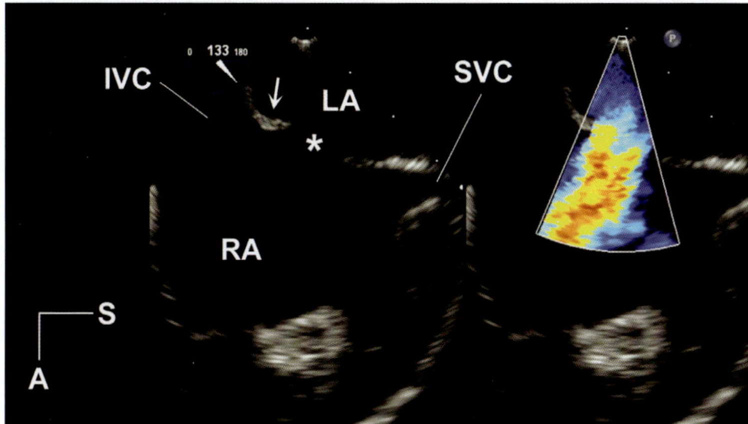

Fig 7.8—This two-dimensional transesophageal bicaval view is obtained between 90° and 130°. It demonstrates a secundum atrial septal defect (asterisk). Both the superior (SVC) and inferior vena cava (IVC) are clearly demonstrated. The inferior aspect of the defect is clearly seen (arrow). Abbreviations: LA, left atrium; RA, right atrium; A, anterior; S, superior.

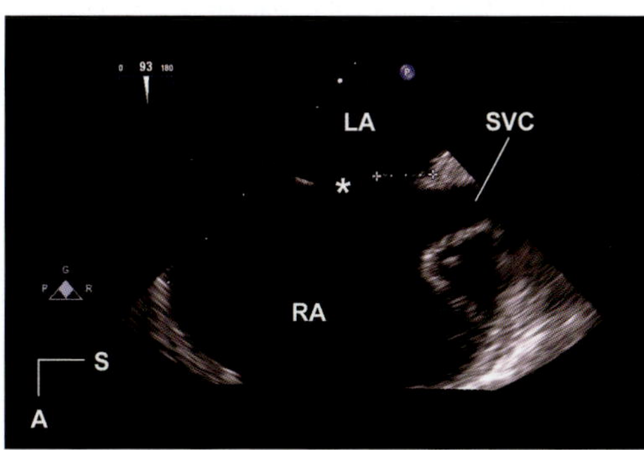

Fig 7.9—Two-dimensional transesophageal bicaval view. The probe has been withdrawn to examine the junction of the superior vena cava (SVC) and the right atrium (RA). The atrial septal defect is marked by an asterisk. The length of the SVC rim of the defect has been measured between the superior rim of the defect and the SVC-RA junction. Abbreviations: A, anterior; S, superior.

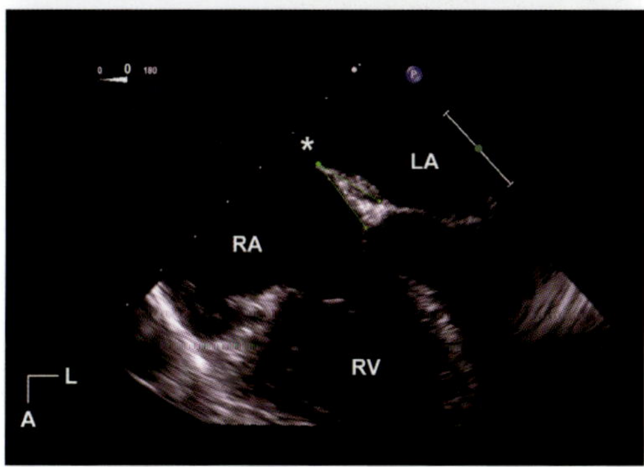

Fig 7.10—This two-dimensional transesophageal four-chamber view demonstrates a secundum atrial septal defect (asterisk). Measurements of the rims to the mitral and tricuspid valve septal hinges are shown. Abbreviations: LA, left atrium; RA, right atrium; RV, right ventricle; A, anterior; L, left.

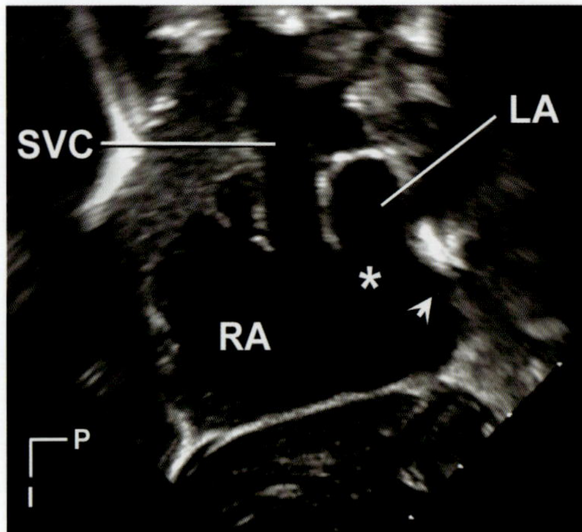

Fig 7.11—Two-dimensional transthoracic subxiphoid short-axis view at the base of the heart. It demonstrates a large secundum atrial septal defect (asterisk), with no posteroinferior rim (arrowhead). Abbreviations: LA, left atrium; RA, right atrium; SVC, superior vena cava; I, inferior; P, posterior.

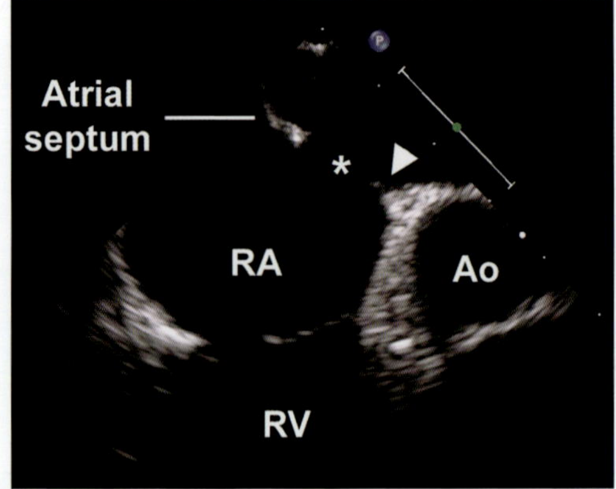

Fig 7.12—This two-dimensional transesophageal view at 30° demonstrates a secundum atrial septal defect (asterisk). The arrowhead points to the aortic rim. Abbreviations: Ao, aorta; RA, right atrium; RV, right ventricle.

The SVC and IVC rims are best visualized in the biatrial long-axis view at approximately 90° to 100° with some clockwise rotation and color flow mapping. The mid-esophageal four-chamber view at 0° to 20° is generally used for evaluating the MV and TV rims. The distances from the defect to both the mitral and tricuspid valves should be measured. The aortic rim is typically best seen at the short-axis view at 30° to 40°. The right upper pulmonary vein drainage can be interrogated from either the mid-esophageal four-chamber view at 0° to 20° with clockwise rotation and also from the biatrial long-axis view at approximately 90° to 100°. To view the coronary sinus, a low esophageal position at 0° is most effective.

Sizing the defect

Views for defect sizing can range from between 0° to 120° but typically are optimal between 20° and 70°[5] (Fig 7.13). A complete search for the plane with the maximal diameter should be performed. In addition to measuring the size of the actual defect, the entire atrial septal length should be measured in multiple planes. Historically, sizing of the defect was performed using a balloon stretched diameter.[5,6,13] More recently,

a modified balloon sizing technique has been described that avoids overstretching the defect and oversizing the device.[14] The modified balloon sizing technique employs the inflation of a sizing balloon just until there is color Doppler TEE confirmation that the balloon successfully occludes the defect without residual shunts. This modified technique does not inflate the balloon to the point of creating a waist in the balloon. The diameter of the inflated balloon across the defect is then measured by echo-

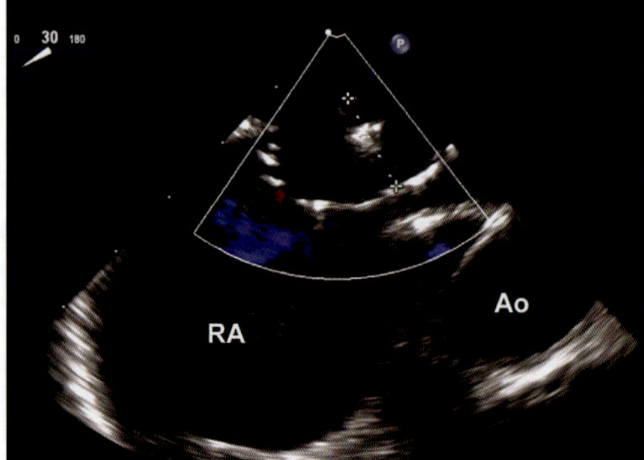

Fig 7.13—This two-dimensional transesophageal view at 30° can be used to visualize and guide balloon sizing of the atrial septal defect. The image demonstrates the sizing balloon that has been inflated just until it has completely occluded the defect with no residual shunt. Cursors mark the measurement of the balloon diameter. Abbreviations: Ao, aorta; RA, right atrium.

cardiography using the caliper. Both 2D and 3D TEE measurements of the ASD correlate well with the balloon occlusive diameter technique measurements.[15] Balloon sizing remains popular but does not necessarily have to be performed, especially with the advent of real-time 3D TEE.[16]

ASD/PFO sizing by 2D TEE has its limitations. As now demonstrated by 3D echocardiography, the defects are often nonuniform in diameter and have dynamic changes in shape.[17–19] In addition, as the right atrial size increases secondary to the interatrial shunt, the plane of the atrial septum can become distorted and difficult to accurately image by 2D TEE.[13]

Device deployment

A major advantage of TEE is that it provides continuous monitoring of device position during deployment. As the delivery catheter is passed over the guide wire into the left atrium, it is important to visualize the catheter crossing through the defect of interest and to ensure that it is in the main body of the left atrium. The catheter has the potential to become entangled in the left atrial appendage, mitral valve, or the Chiari network.[13]

Dislodgment of the device most commonly occurs during withdrawal of the left atrial disc against the septum just prior to deployment of the right atrial disc.[7] If the left atrial disc is positioned properly, it should assume a flat, streamlined appearance against the septum prior to the release of the right atrial disc. If the left atrial disc is pulled prematurely against the septum before the waist is expanded, the disc edge may prolapse into the right atrium (Fig 7.14). If the left atrial disc is not pulled sufficiently against the septum, the right atrial disc may be inadvertently deployed into the left atrium.

After both the left and right atrial discs have been deployed, TEE confirms the presence of atrial septal tissue between both discs (Fig 7.15). Until the device is released, the right atrial disc may not completely flatten. Minimizing the tension on the cable attached to the right atrial disc will allow the disc to flatten enough

to perform an assessment for residual shunts and disturbance of surrounding structures (Fig 7.16). Device assessment from multiple views should be performed to ensure that the device is not interfering with atrial inflows (ie, SVC, IVC, right upper pulmonary vein, coronary sinus) and outflows (ie, mitral and tricuspid valves) (Fig 7.17). Device stability can be confirmed by

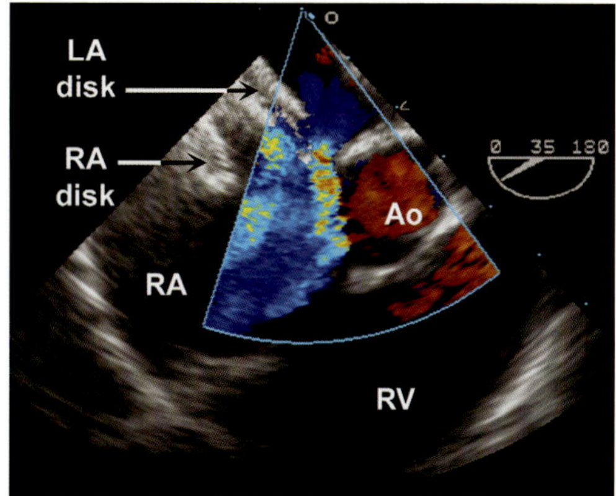

Fig 7.14—This two-dimensional transesophageal view at 35° during device deployment demonstrates that the left atrial disc has slipped into the right atrium through the anterior portion of the defect. The aliased blue color flow immediately behind the aorta represents the resulting atrial level communication. If the device were to be released in this position, the result would be suboptimal, with a residual shunt and an inadequately anchored device. Abbreviations: Ao, aorta; RA, right atrium; RV, right ventricle.

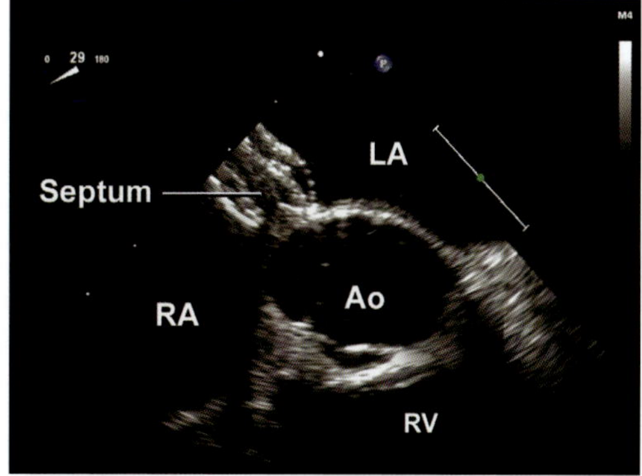

Fig 7.15—This two-dimensional transesophageal view at 30° was obtained after both discs have been expanded, before releasing the device. The atrial septum is clearly seen between the right and left atrial discs of the device. Abbreviations: Ao, aorta; LA, left atrium; RA, right atrium; RV, right ventricle.

performance of the "Minnesota wiggle" which entails gently pushing and pulling on the delivery catheter while it is still attached to the right atrial disc.

It is not unusual to visualize a trivial shunt (< 1 mm) on color flow mapping while the delivery catheter is attached to the right atrial disc.

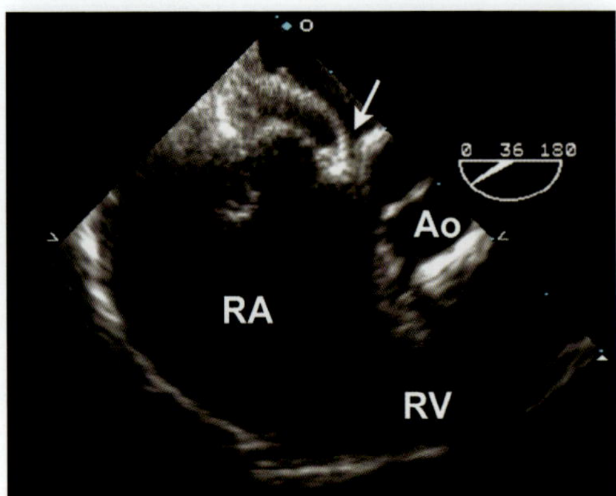

Fig 7.16—This two-dimensional transesophageal view between 30° and 40° is used to test the stability of the device using the "Minnesota wiggle," wherein the device assembly is alternately pushed in and pulled out. In this image, the assembly is being pulled. The anterior inferior portion of the left atrial disc of the device appears to slip past the plane of the atrial septum into the right atrium. This is an indication that the device probably needs to be upsized. Abbreviations: Ao, aorta; RA, right atrium; RV, right ventricle.

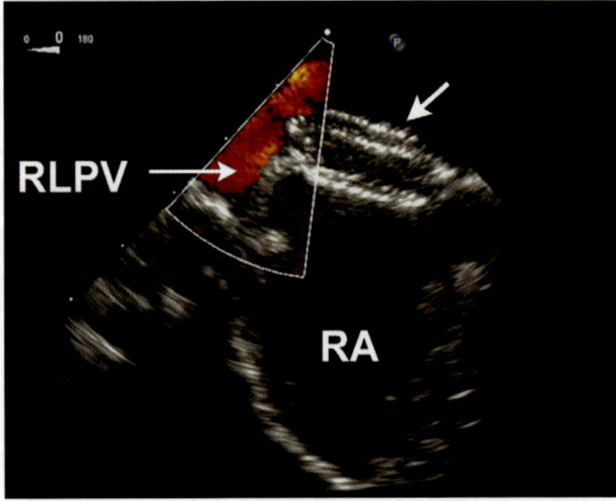

Fig 7.17—In this two-dimensional transesophageal four-chamber view, the probe has been rotated rightwards to evaluate whether the left atrial disc of the device (arrow) is impinging on the right lower pulmonary vein (RLPV). In this patient, there is no such impingement. The vein is widely patent and flow in it is laminar.

These trivial shunts typically disappear once the device is fully released and the right atrial disc completely flattens against the septum. However, 2% to 14% of patients who undergo ASD or PFO closure with an AMPLATZER device are found to have a residual shunt at their 6-month follow-up visit.[5,6,11,20] In a large multicenter trial where 442 patients underwent transcatheter closure of a secundum ASD, 1.5% had a residual shunt (> 1 mm) at their 12-month follow-up visit.[8]

Transcatheter Closure with Three-Dimensional Echocardiography Guidance

The advent of real-time three-dimensional (3D) echocardiography has provided superior and unique views of the atrial septum. Specifically, it is especially useful in delineating the static and dynamic shape of septal defects, the spatial relationship of the septal defect to other cardiac structures, and the distance between multiple defects. Previously, the clinical utility of 3D echocardiography was limited by lengthy acquisition and processing time, motion artifacts, facility resources, and specialized operator skills.[21] More recently, improvements in transducer technology have allowed the acquisition of high-quality real-time 3D echocardiography. The capability of acquiring real-time images without offline reconstruction has facilitated wider acceptance of this modality in the catheterization lab.

Three-dimensional transesophageal echocardiography

A miniaturized, fully sampled matrix array probe has been coupled with a transesophageal probe, which allows the acquisition of high-quality real-time 3D transesophageal images. The fully sampled matrix array transducer is capable of three types of data acquisition: (1) narrow-angled acquisition (live 3D);

(2) 3D zoom; and (3) wide-angled full-volume acquisition.[22]

Narrow-angled acquisitions allow real-time 3D imaging without the need for ECG gating. This mode displays a pyramidal volume of approximately 30° × 60° and the image can be rotated to visualize the structure from multiple angles. This mode is most ideal for imaging structures that are in the far zone of the ultrasound beam. Narrow-angled acquisitions do not permit color Doppler imaging.

The 3D zoom mode displays a smaller, magnified pyramidal volume that can be manually adjusted to focus on the region of interest. This mode also allows image rotation so it can be visualized from multiple angles. The 3D zoom mode is preferable for structures in the near zone of the ultrasound beam. Because structures can be imaged at a near-perpendicular angle to the ultrasound beam, this mode is ideal for evaluating the interatrial septum. The 3D zoom mode does not allow color Doppler imaging.

The third mode, wide-angled full-volume acquisition, requires ECG gating and results in a large pyramidal volume. This mode is appropriate for structures that are in either the far or near zone of the ultrasound beam and also allows color Doppler imaging. The wide-angled full-volume mode provides important information during the precatheterization assessment but is less practical for the dynamic environment of the catheterization lab for several reasons. This mode requires that data acquisition be performed over 4 to 7 cardiac cycles. And although the full-volume data sets allow the simultaneous visualization of multiple structures, this often requires further processing (online or offline), which may be too time consuming during an intervention.

The contributions of real-time 3D transesophageal echocardiography (RT3D-TEE) in the catheterization lab are valuable and its utilization is becoming more widespread and popular.[12,16,18,19,23,24] At our institution, we found the most effective strategy to be the concomitant use of RT3D-TEE and simultaneous biplane imaging (X plane).[19] For real-time demonstra-

tion of cardiac structures and catheters, the narrow-angled acquisition and 3D zoom modes are most commonly used.[18] We also find that having two operators helps facilitate the speed of the study; one operator manipulates the transesophageal probe while the other operates the machine and focuses on maximizing image quality.

RT3D-TEE provides excellent anatomic details of the atrial septum. Specifically, the 3D zoom mode allows an en face view of the atrial septum, which is unavailable with 2D TEE (Fig 7.18). This unique perspective provides excellent details of the morphology and size of the septal defect. The specific details include noting the ellipsoidal shape, the dynamic changes in the defect shape, the specific location in the septum, the relationship to other cardiac structures, and the evaluation of multiple defects (Fig 7.19).

RT3D-TEE provides intraprocedural information clearly and quickly. During defect closure, RT3D-TEE is especially useful for confirming the passage of the delivery sheath

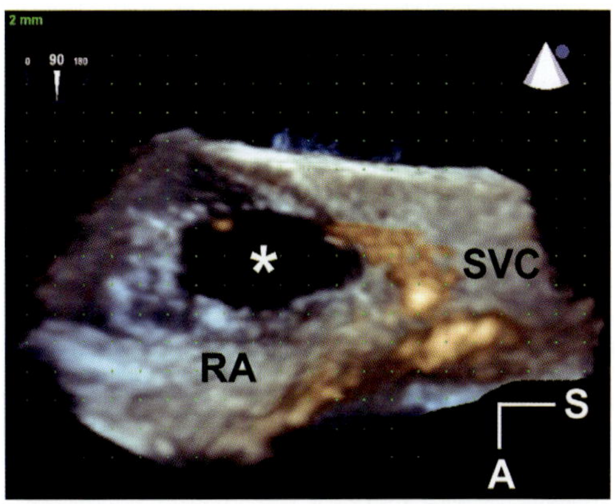

Fig 7.18—Three-dimensional transesophageal acquisition from the bicaval (90°) view. The free walls of the atria have been cropped. The viewing perspective is from the right atrium, looking leftwards. A moderate-sized central defect is seen (asterisk). A measurement grid (green dots) has been superimposed on the display. Any two adjacent horizontally or vertically oriented points on this display are 2 mm apart. This provides a means to make real-time judgments of distance during device deployment. Abbreviations: RA, right atrium; SVC, superior vena cava; A, anterior; S, superior.

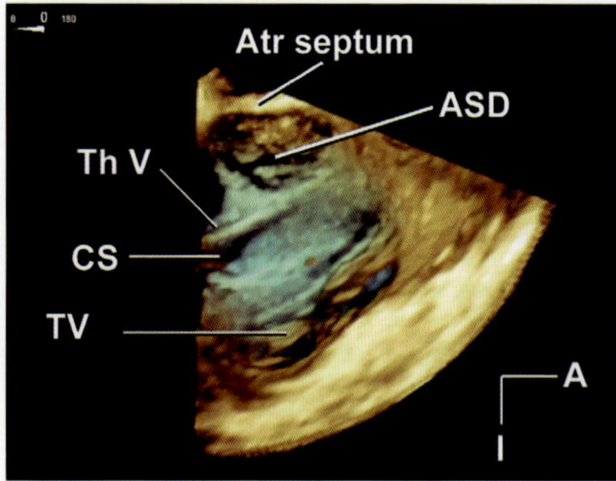

Fig 7.19—Three-dimensional transesophageal acquisition from the four-chamber view. The free walls of the right atrium and the right atrial appendage have been cropped. The viewer's perspective is from the front of the heart, looking back. Note the irregularly T-shaped atrial septal defect (ASD). The proximity of the posterior-inferior portion of the defect to the coronary sinus (CS) is evident. The Thebesian valve (Th V) is clearly seen. The tricuspid valve (TV) is closed in this systolic frame. Abbreviations: A, anterior; I, inferior.

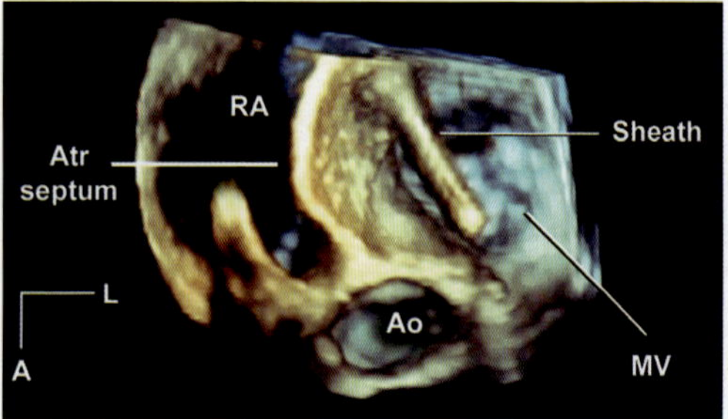

Fig 7.20—Three-dimensional transesophageal acquisition from the four-chamber view. The superior walls of both atria have been cropped, and the image has been tilted so that the viewing perspective is from above downwards. In this holographic image, structures in the far field appear blue, and those in the near field appear sepia-toned. A sheath is seen coursing from the right atrium (RA) into the left atrium across the atrial septum (Atr septum) through a patent foramen ovale. This image was acquired during ventricular systole; hence, the mitral valve, which is colored blue, is closed. The sheath points anteriorly and leftwards toward the left atrial appendage. This image demonstrates the potential role of three-dimensional transesophageal imaging in guiding interventions. Abbreviations: A, anterior; L, left.

across the septum (Fig 7.20). RT3D-TEE is especially advantageous when there are multiple defects.[16,18,19,23,25] The spatial relationship between multiple defects can be delineated with superb clarity and precision (Fig 7.21). RT3D-TEE also provides a better image of the catheters so it minimizes the risk of passing two separate catheters through the same defect. Live 3D imaging allows the continuous visualization of the left atrial disc and its relation to the left atrial wall and appendage. After the device has been deployed, the left atrial en face septal view provides a nice perspective to evaluate the appropriate entrapment of septal rim around the device (Fig 7.22).

Three-dimensional transthoracic echocardiography

In those patients who have a contraindication to TEE or who are at high risk for general anesthesia, transcatheter device closure with real-time 3D transthoracic echocardiography (RT3D-TTE) remains an alternative option.[26–28] Chen et al described the use of RT3D-TTE guidance

in 29 patients who underwent transcatheter AMPLATZER Septal Occluder device closure of a secundum ASD. All 29 patients received only local anesthesia. All defect closures were uneventful and the imaging was adequate enough to monitor the various stages of deployment and result in 100% successful device deployment.[26] The parasternal and subcostal approaches provide appropriate images to visualize the atrial septum, measure the defect, guide the catheter for device deployment, and assess device position.[26–28]

Limitations to three-dimensional echocardiography

There are limitations to real-time 3D echocardiography. Additional training is required to master the optimization of the image quality. There is occasional tissue dropout secondary to low gain settings that can mimic a true anatomic defect. In 3D zoom mode, the frame rate

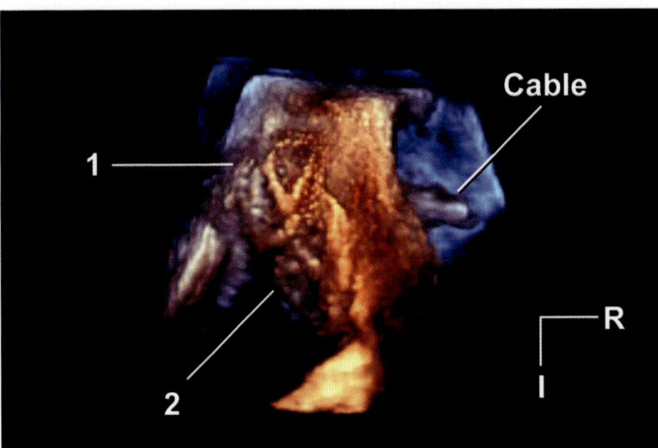

Fig 7.21—This three-dimensional transesophageal acquisition is oriented so that the viewer's perspective is above and behind the heart, looking down and forwards. The anterior, posterior, and superior walls of the atria have been cropped. This patient had multiple atrial septal defects. The left atrial discs of two devices are seen. Device 1 is still attached to the delivery cable, while device 2 has already been released. Note the overlapping portions of the two devices. Abbreviations: I, inferior; R, right.

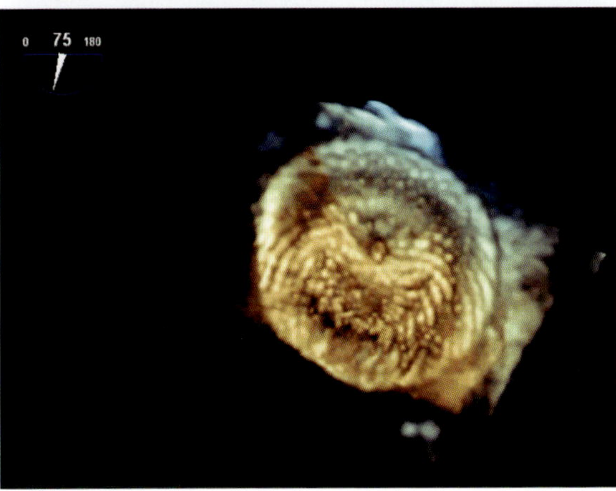

Fig 7.22—Three-dimensional transesophageal acquisition from the four-chamber view. The free walls of the left atrium have been cropped to help visualize all the margins of the AMPLATZER atrial septal defect occluder. Parts of the circumference of the right atrial disc are seen in the background.

can drop low enough to make the moving image appear less smooth. In large near-field defects, it can be difficult to consistently visualize the entire device in live 3D mode. In these cases, lateral electronic steering of the image allows rapid evaluation of the entire defect without actual manual manipulation of the probe. There are also limitations related to patient size and body habitus. Currently, a pediatric-sized 3DTEE probe is not commercially available so its use is limited to patients > 15 kg. For 3D transthoracic imaging, the acoustic window can greatly affect the quality of the image acquisitions.

Despite these limitations, RT3D echocardiography provides useful and additive information. The image quality is superior to 2D echocardiography and it offers a more thorough assessment of the cardiac anatomy and pathology. In summary, RT3D echocardiography is extremely valuable in guiding transcatheter device closures of atrial septal defects and may become the imaging modality of choice.

References

1. Hagen PT, Scholz DG, Edwards WD. Incidence and size of patent foramen ovale during the first 10 decades of life: an autopsy study of 965 normal hearts. *Mayo Clin Proc.* 1984;59(1):17–20.

2. Kardon RE, Sokoloski MC, Levi DS, et al. Transthoracic echocardiographic guidance of transcatheter atrial septal defect closure. *Am J Cardiol.* 2004;94(2):256–260.

3. Kleinman CS. Echocardiographic guidance of catheter-based treatments of atrial septal defect: transesophageal echocardiography remains the gold standard. *Pediatr Cardiol.* 2005;26(2):128–134.

4. Koenig P, Cao Q-L. Echocardiographic guidance of transcatheter closure of atrial septal defects: is intracardiac echocardiography better than transesophageal echocardiography? *Pediatr Cardiol.* 2005;26(2):135–139.

5. Figueroa MI, Balaguru D, McClure C, Kline CH, Radtke WA, Shirali GS. Experience with use of multiplane transesophageal echocardiography to guide closure of atrial septal defects using the AMPLATZER device. *Pediatr Cardiol.* 2002;23(4):430–436.

6. Mazic U, Gavora P, Masura J. The role of transesophageal echocardiography in transcatheter closure of secundum atrial septal defects by the AMPLATZER septal occluder. *Am Heart J.* 2001;142(3):482–488.

7. van der Velde ME, Perry SB, Sanders SP. Transesophageal echocardiography with color Doppler during interventional catheterization. *Echocardiography.* 1991;8(6):721–730.

8. Du ZD, Hijazi ZM, Kleinman CS, Silverman NH, Larntz K. Comparison between transcatheter and surgical closure of secundum atrial septal defect in children and adults: results of a multicenter nonrandomized trial. *J Am Coll Cardiol.* 2002;39(11):1836–1844.

9. Amin Z, Hijazi ZM, Bass JL, Cheatham JP, Hellenbrand WE, Kleinman CS. Erosion of AMPLATZER septal occluder device after closure of secundum atrial septal defects: review of registry of complications and recommendations to minimize future risk. *Cathet Cardiovasc Intervent.* 2004;63(4):496–502.

10. Shrivastava S, Radhakrishnan S. Echocardiographic anatomy of atrial septal defect: "nomenclature of the rims." *Indian Heart J.* 2003;55(1):88–89.

11. Balaguru D, Anderson RH, Rosenthal GL, Cook AC, Radtke WA, Shirali GS. Predictors of residual defects following closure of defects in the oval fossa using the AMPLATZER device: echocardiography recapitulates morphometry. *Cardiol Young.* 2003;13(4):352–360.

12. Cao Q-L, Radtke W, Berger F, Zhu W, Hijazi ZM. Transcatheter closure of multiple atrial septal defects. Initial results and value of two- and three-dimensional transoesophageal echocardiography. *Eur Heart J.* 2000;21(11):941–947.

13. Cooke JC, Gelman JS, Harper RW. Echocardiologists' role in the deployment of the AMPLATZER atrial septal occluder device in adults. *J Am Soc Echocardiogr.* 2001;14(6):588–594.

14. Carlson KM, Justino H, O'Brien RE, et al. Transcatheter atrial septal defect closure: modified balloon sizing technique to avoid overstretching the defect and oversizing the AMPLATZER septal occluder. *Catheter Cardiovasc Intervent.* 2005;66(3):390–396.

15. Zhu W, Cao Q-L, Rhodes J, Hijazi ZM. Measurement of atrial septal defect size: a comparative study between three-dimensional transesophageal echocardiography and the standard balloon sizing methods. *Pediatr Cardiol.* 2000;21(5):465–469.

16. Taniguchi M, Akagi T, Watanabe N, et al. Application of real-time three-dimensional transesophageal echocardiography using a matrix array probe for transcatheter closure of atrial septal defect. *J Am Soc Echocardiogr.* 2009;22(10):1114–1120.

17. Pepi M, Tamborini G, Bartorelli AL, et al. Usefulness of three-dimensional echocardiographic reconstruction of the AMPLATZER septal occluder in patients undergoing atrial septal closure. *Am J Cardiol.* 2004;94(10):1343–1347.

18. Perk G, Lang RM, Garcia-Fernandez MA, et al. Use of real time three-dimensional transesophageal echocardiography in intracardiac catheter based interventions. *J Am Soc Echocardiogr.* 2009;22(8):865–882.

19. Baker GH, Shirali G, Ringewald JM, Hsia TY, Bandisode V. Usefulness of live three-dimensional transesophageal echocardiography in a congenital heart disease center. *Am J Cardiol.* 2009;103(7):1025–1028.

20. Hijazi ZM, Cao Q-L, Patel HT, Rhodes J, Hanlon KM. Transesophageal echocardiographic results of catheter closure of atrial septal defect in children and adults using the AMPLATZER device. *Am J Cardiol.* 2000;85(11):1387–1390.

21. Marx GR, Fulton DR, Pandian NG, et al. Delineation of site, relative size and dynamic geometry of atrial septal defects by real-time three-dimensional echocardiography. *J Am Coll Cardiol.* 1995;25(2):482–490.

22. Sugeng L, Shernan SK, Salgo IS, et al. Live

3-dimensional transesophageal echocardiography initial experience using the fully-sampled matrix array probe. *J Am Coll Cardiol.* 2008;52(6):446–449.

23. Arcidiacono C, Gaio G, Butera G, Carminati M. Percutaneous closure of multiple secundum atrial septal defects using 3 AMPLATZER atrial septal occluder devices: evaluation by live transthoracic 3-dimensional echocardiography. *Circ Cardiovasc Imaging.* 2008;1(2):e15–e16.

24. Lodato JA, Cao Q-L, Weinert L, et al. Feasibility of real-time three-dimensional transoesophageal echocardiography for guidance of percutaneous atrial septal defect closure. *Eur J Echocardiogr.* 2009;10(4):543–548.

25. Lopez L, Ventura R, Welch EM, Nykanen DG, Zahn EM. Echocardiographic considerations during deployment of the HELEX Septal Occluder for closure of atrial septal defects. *Cardiol Young.* 2003;13(3):290–298.

26. Chen FL, Hsiung MC, Hsieh KS, Li YC, Chou MC. Real time three-dimensional transthoracic echocardiography for guiding AMPLATZER septal occluder device deployment in patients with atrial septal defect. *Echocardiography.* 2006;23(9):763–770.

27. Mehmood F, Vengala S, Nanda NC, et al. Usefulness of live three-dimensional transthoracic echocardiography in the characterization of atrial septal defects in adults. *Echocardiography.* 2004;21(8):707–713.

28. Roman KS, Nii M, Golding F, Benson LN, Smallhorn JF. Images in cardiovascular medicine. Real-time subcostal 3-dimensional echocardiography for guided percutaneous atrial septal defect closure. *Circulation.* 2004;109(24):e320–e321.

8

Imaging to Guide ASD and PFO Closure: Intracardiac Echocardiography

Mustafa H. Abdullah Al-Qbandi, Qi-Ling Cao, and Ziyad M. Hijazi

Introduction

Intracardiac echocardiography (ICE) is increasingly being used to guide percutaneous interventional procedures, principally the closure of interatrial septal defects.[1-3] Since its introduction to guide device closure of atrial septal defect (ASD) and patent foramen ovale (PFO) in the early 2000s,[4] its use in congenital heart disease has become well established. The main advantages of ICE over transesophageal echocardiography (TEE) during closure of ASD and PFO include no need for general anesthesia, better views of the left atrium, better views of the posteroinferior part of the septum, shorter procedure times, and the ability of the interventional cardiologist to perform the interventional procedure as well as the imaging part of the procedure without needing an expert echocardiographer for transesophageal echocardiography.

The principal disadvantage is the additional cost of the imaging catheter, although this can be offset by improved turnaround times in a busy catheterization laboratory and reduced personnel costs (anesthesia and echocardiography).[5-7] Table 8.1 lists the important advantages/disadvantages of each imaging modality.

ICE systems currently commercially available include the AcuNav catheter manufactured by Siemens Medical Systems and distributed by Biosense Webster, California; the ViewFlex catheter (St. Jude Medical, Minnesota) and the Ultra ICE catheter (Boston Scientific, Boston, Massachusetts). Most operators currently use the AcuNav ICE catheter. It is available as an 8 or 10F catheter, multifrequency (5–10 MHz), 64-elements, linear phased array, ultrasound catheter that can perform pulsed and color Doppler imaging. The control handle has three knobs: a posterior/anterior knob, a right/left

TEE (Transesophageal echocardiography)	ICE (Intracardiac echocardiography)
Requires general anesthesia	Sedation only
Fluoroscopic time may be prolonged	Fluoroscopic time may be shortened
Not patient friendly! More stress to patient	Less stress to patient
Requires a separate operator	One operator can do both intervention and imaging
Difficulty in visualization of posteroinferior rim	Excellent for visualization of the posteroinferior rim
Only one femoral venous access	Need a second femoral venous puncture
Less cost	Higher cost?
Multiple use of the probe	Limited use of catheter
Temperature sensing	No temperature sensing. Cooling effect of blood on the catheter
TEE probe sometimes interferes with balloon sizing during fluoroscopy	Probe is in right atrium and is small with no interference during fluoroscopy
Esophageal injury	Vascular injury

Table 8.1—Advantages/Disadvantages of TEE and ICE

knob, and a locking knob (Fig 8.1 demonstrates the AcuNav catheter with its control handle and the tip). It is capable of tissue penetration of up to 14 cm, thereby allowing imaging of the left atrial structures from a position in the right atrium.

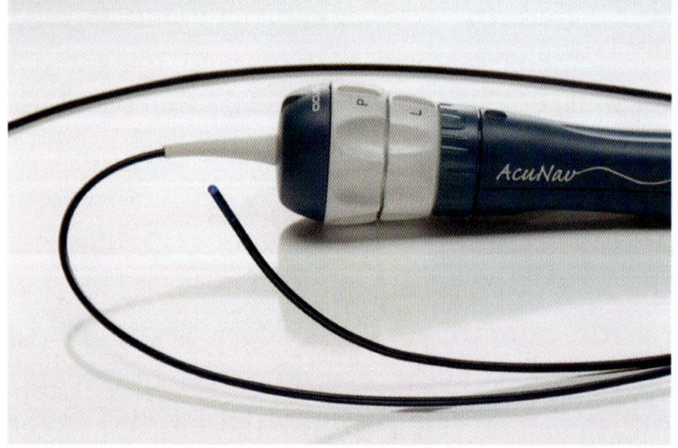

Fig 8.1—The AcuNav Intracardiac Echocardiographic (ICE) Catheter. Note, the control handle with the three knobs.

Imaging Protocol for ASD/PFO Device Closure

We reported the protocol of image guidance during ASD/PFO closure (4) and it is summarized here.

Under local anesthesia, venous access is usually obtained via the same femoral vein (if the patient's weight is > 35 kg) and from the contralateral vein (if the weight is < 35 kg) and, while under continuous fluoroscopic guidance, the catheter is gently advanced to the mid-right atrium.

Most patients undergoing device closure of their defect (ASD/PFO) have already undergone complete transthoracic echocardiographic and/or TEE evaluation of their defect and associated structures. Nonetheless, we believe that ICE also can be used to fully evaluate the defect and surrounding structures. For patients with an ASD, the size of the defect via two-dimensional (2D) imaging as well as the measurement of surrounding rims is obtained. Transcranial Doppler (TCD) can be performed with ICE after injecting agitated saline microbubbles for patients with a PFO in order to confirm the presence of a right-to-left shunt.

The first view to obtain is what is called "neutral" or "home" view. In the proper alignment in this view, the ICE catheter is parallel to the spine with the transducer portion facing the tricuspid valve (see Fig 8.2). The corresponding schematic sketch of the area visualized, the fluoroscopic (AP view), and echocardiographic images obtained with the ICE catheter in this position are shown in Figure 8.2 (left, middle, and right). In this position the tricuspid valve, right ventricular inflow and outflow, and the long axis of the pulmonary valve are well seen. The aortic valve may also be seen (short axis) in this view. The septum is not well seen in this view. However, on occasions the anterior portion of the septum can be seen and if color Doppler is turned on, one may see the shunt (Fig 8.2 right top/bottom). This view is important to assess the tricuspid valve function.

While the catheter is in the neutral position, rotating the posterior-anterior knob slightly posterior and the right-left knob slightly rightward, the transducer will face the interatrial septum (Fig 8.3 left, middle, and right). This view is called the septal view. In this position, the resulting fluoroscopic image showing the position of the ICE catheter appears in Fig 8.3 (middle). The schematic sketch and echocardiographic images via ICE are shown in Fig 8.3 (left, right top/bottom). In this view, the entire length of the atrial septum and the defect, the coronary sinus, and the pulmonary veins are well seen. The latter can be seen in more or less detail depending on the exact location of the transducer.

After advancing the ICE catheter into a more cephalad location toward the superior vena cava (SVC), a view can be obtained which can be referred to as the SVC or "long-axis view" (Fig 8.4 left, middle, and right). The resulting schematic sketch, fluoroscopic images showing the position of the catheter as well as corresponding echocardiographic images, are shown in Fig 8.4. In this plane, the transducer faces the interatrial septum and the SVC can be seen as it relates to the right atrium. The interatrial septum is shown in a superior/inferior plane and

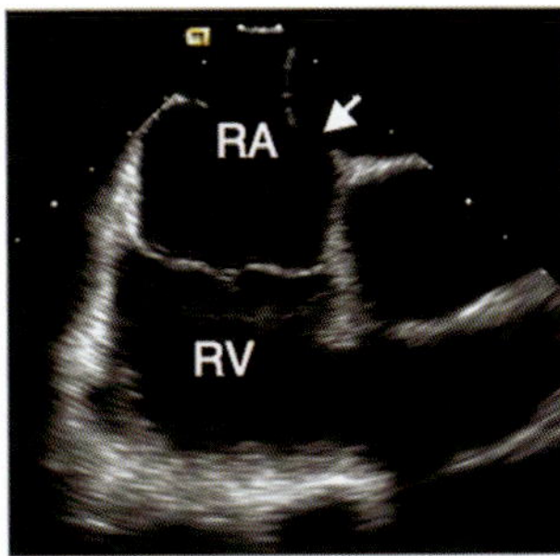

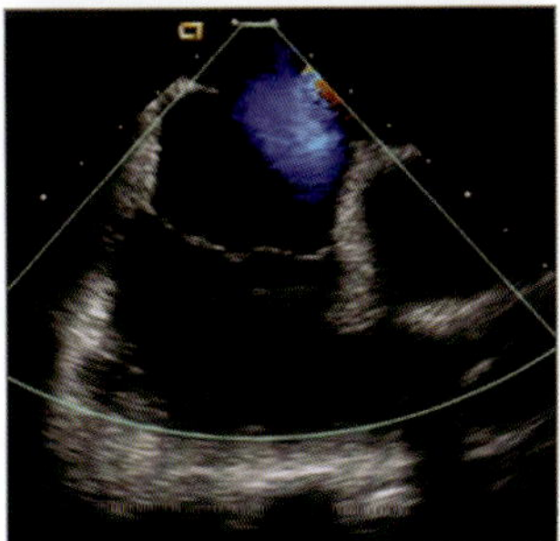

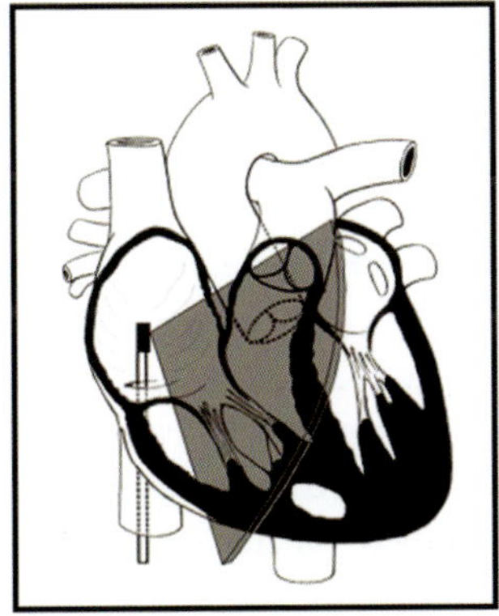

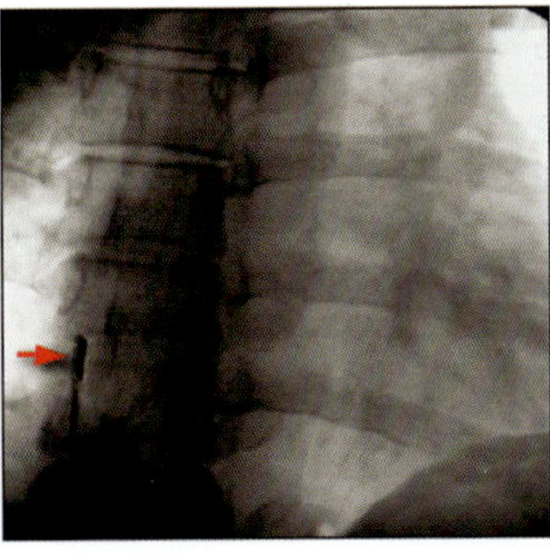

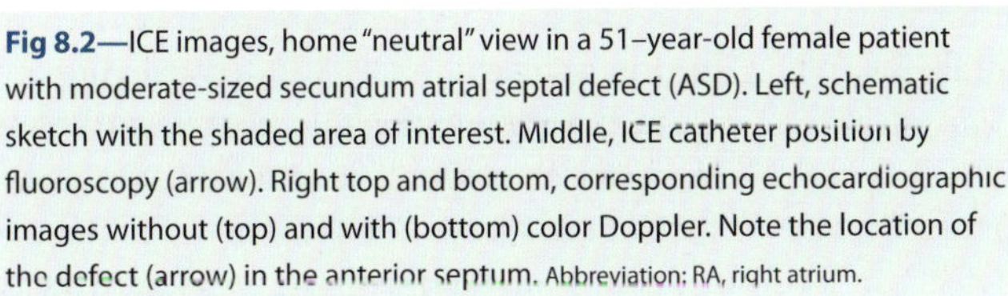

Fig 8.2—ICE images, home "neutral" view in a 51–year-old female patient with moderate-sized secundum atrial septal defect (ASD). Left, schematic sketch with the shaded area of interest. Middle, ICE catheter position by fluoroscopy (arrow). Right top and bottom, corresponding echocardiographic images without (top) and with (bottom) color Doppler. Note the location of the defect (arrow) in the anterior septum. Abbreviation: RA, right atrium.

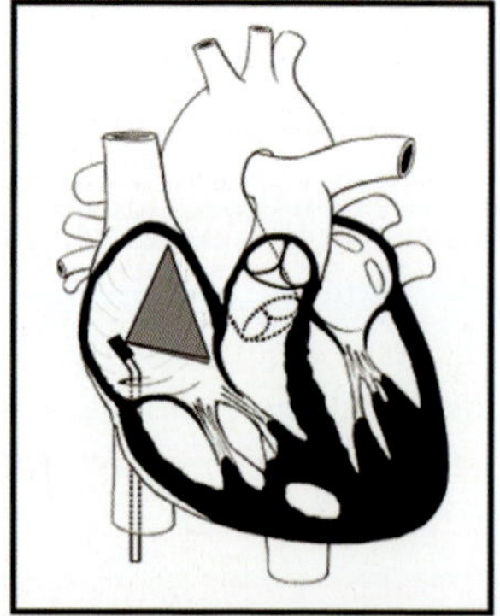 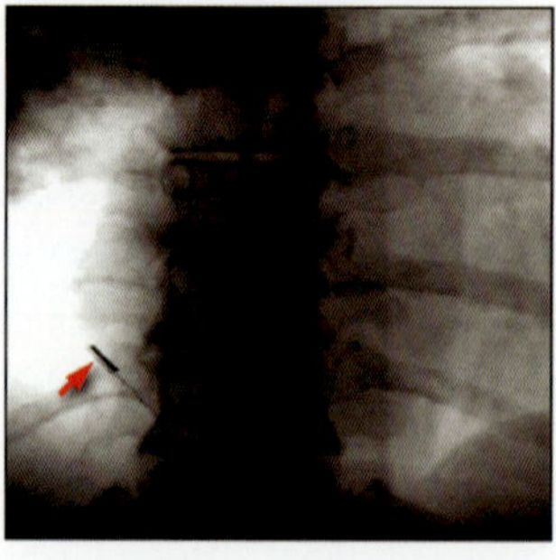 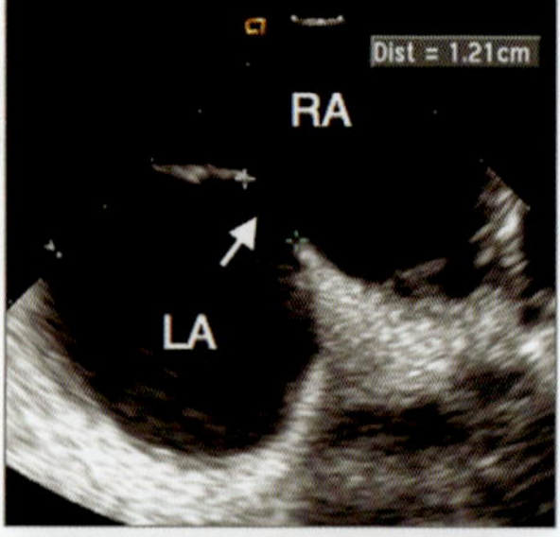

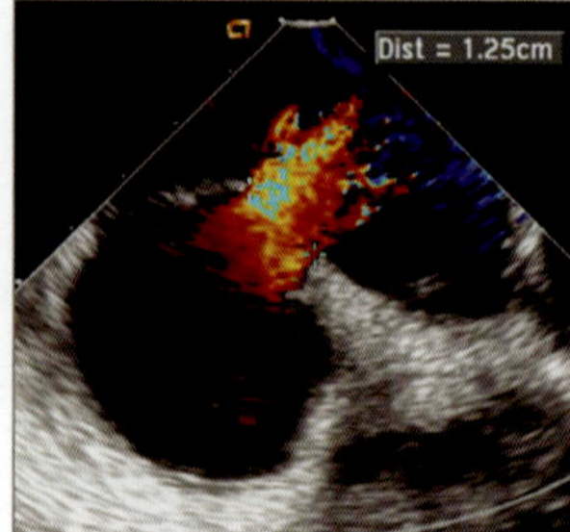

Fig 8.3—ICE images, septal view. Left, sketch of the area of interest. Middle, fluoroscopic image of ICE catheter and right corresponding echocardiographic images showing the defect (arrow). RA: right atrium; LA: left atrium.

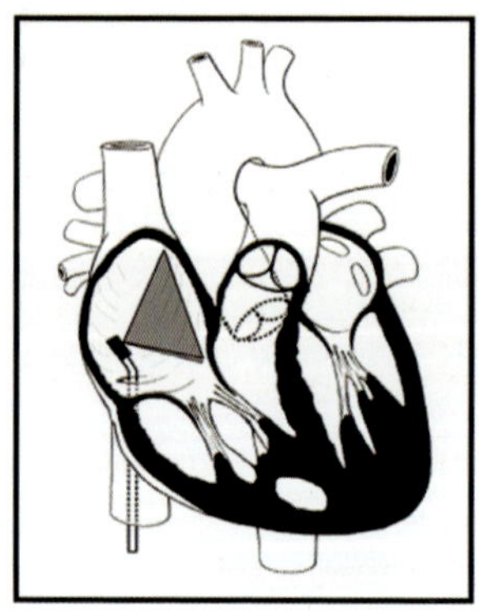 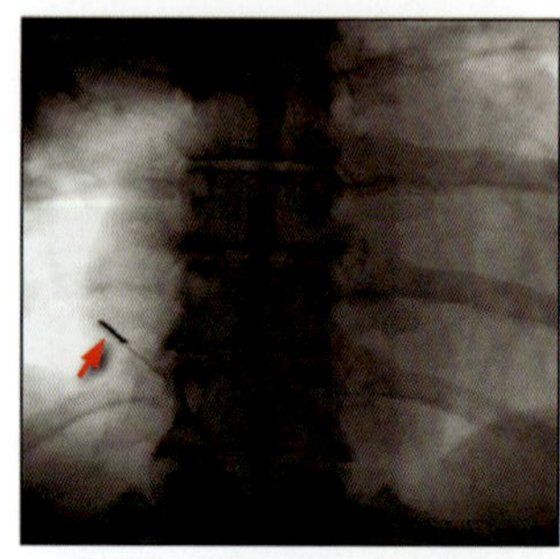

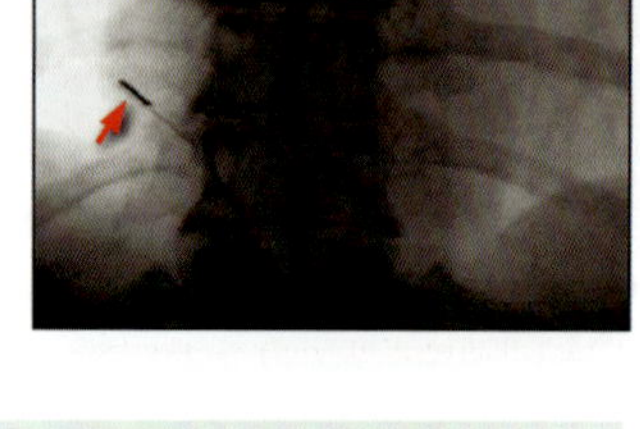

Fig 8.4—ICE images, bicaval "long axis/SVC" view. Left, sketch of the area of interest. Middle, fluoroscopic image of ICE catheter (arrow). Right, corresponding echocardiographic images showing the defect (arrow).

corresponds to the TEE long-axis view. Greater portions of the SVC can be seen as the ICE catheter is further advanced in this flexed position toward the SVC with slightly more rightward flexion. Greater portions of the inferior septum can similarly be imaged by withdrawing the ICE catheter toward the inferior vena cava. A defect in the interatrial septum (ASD/PFO) can be well profiled, and the superior and inferior rims as well as the diameter of the defect can be measured. In this view, both the right and left pulmonary veins may also be imaged, depending on the exact angle of the imaging plane. The imaging angle can be manipulated with clockwise and counterclockwise rotation as well as flexion/anteflexion to achieve these views.

After placing the ICE catheter into a locked position, the entire handle with the catheter shaft at the sheath hub is rotated clockwise until it sits in a position with the transducer near the

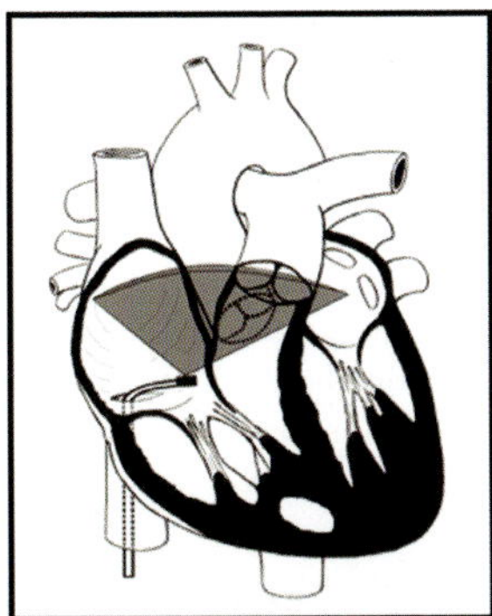
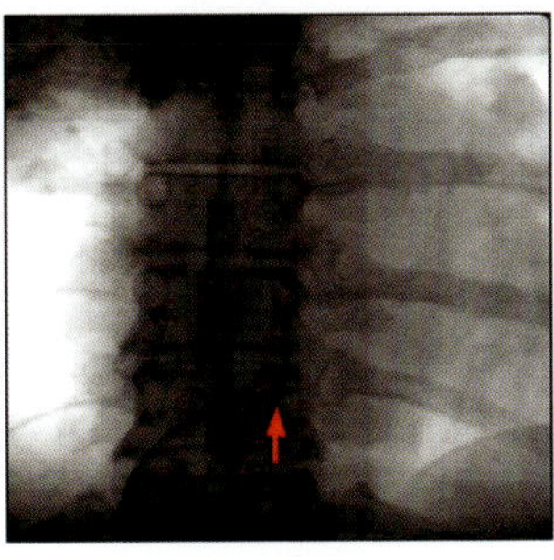
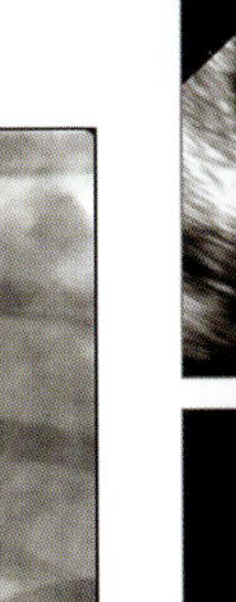
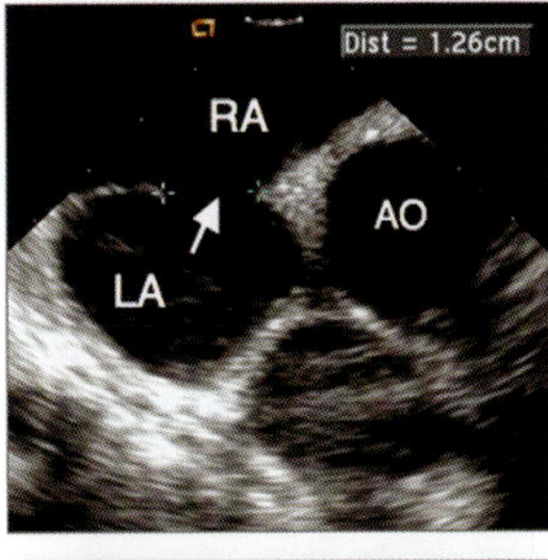

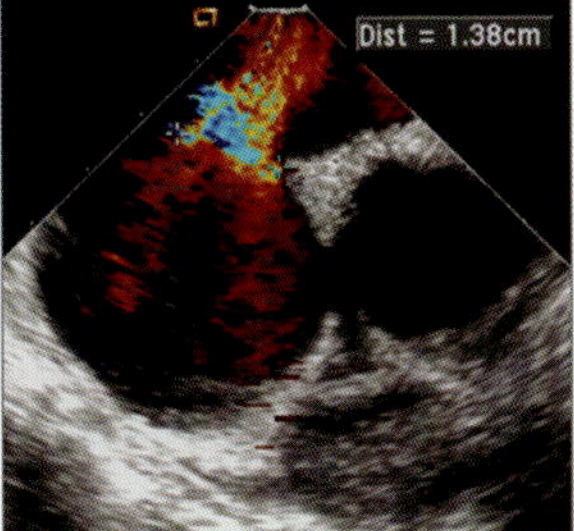

Fig 8. 5—ICE images, short-axis view. Left, sketch of the area of interest. Middle, fluoroscopic image of ICE catheter (arrow) and right corresponding echocardiographic images showing the defect (arrow). Abbreviations: RA, right atrium; LA, left atrium.

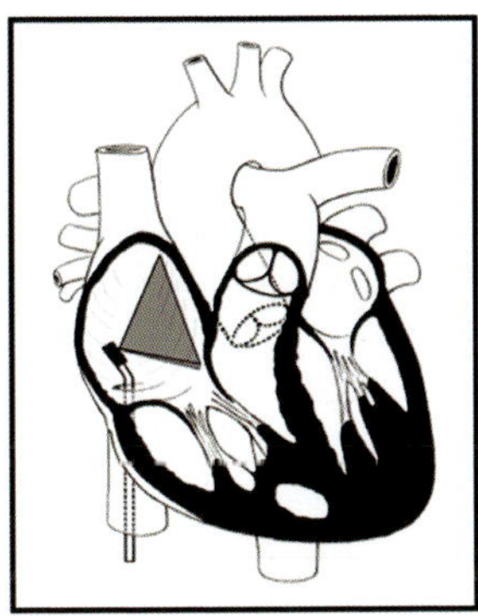
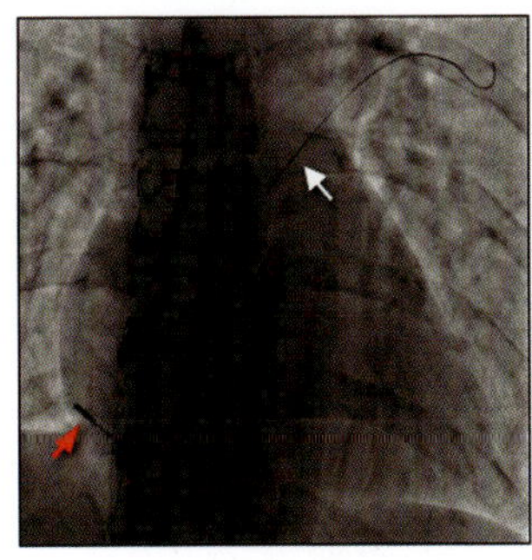
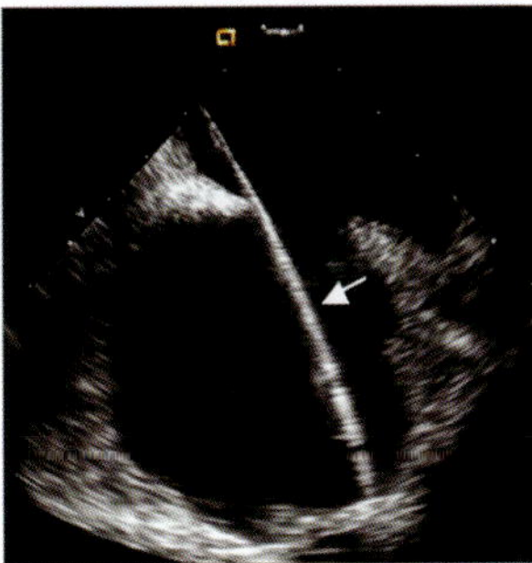

Fig 8. 6—ICE images, long-axis view during passage of the guide wire through the ASD. Left, sketch of the area of interest. Middle, fluoroscopic image of ICE catheter position (red arrow) and the guide wire in the left upper pulmonary vein (white arrow). Right, corresponding echocardiographic image showing the guide wire in left atrium (arrow).

tricuspid valve annulus, and inferior to the aorta (Fig 8.5 left, middle, and right). Minor adjustments of the posterior/anterior knob with less posterior flexion and more leftward rotation in the right-left knob can demonstrate the short-axis view. A schematic sketch, fluoroscopic image showing the catheter position, and corresponding echocardiographic images are shown in Fig 8.5. In this view, visible anatomic structures include the aortic valve in short axis and the interatrial septum. This view is very similar to the basal short-axis view obtained by TEE and is known as the "short-axis view." However, the right atrium is shown in the near-field and the left atrium is in the far-field, which is opposite of what is seen with TEE.

After imaging the intracardiac anatomy and assessing the defect(s) and the rims as previously described, ICE imaging can be used to visualize the guide wire crossing the defect (Fig 8.6 left, middle, and right), then measure the "stop-flow" diameter of the defect using the sizing balloon (Fig 8.7 left, middle, and right). The balloon can be viewed in either short- or long-axis view (Fig 8.7 right). After the defect was balloon sized, the appropriate device was

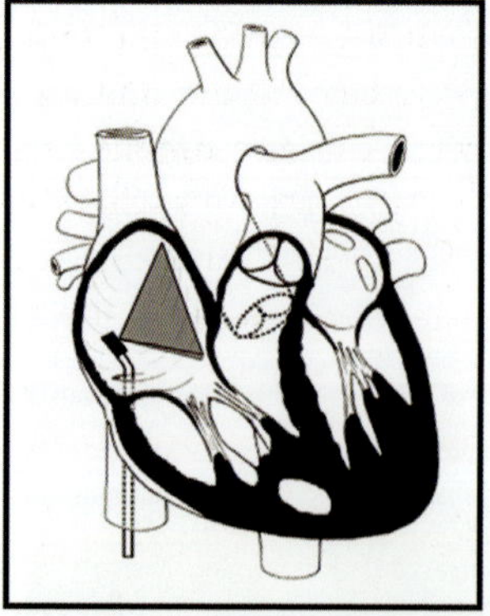 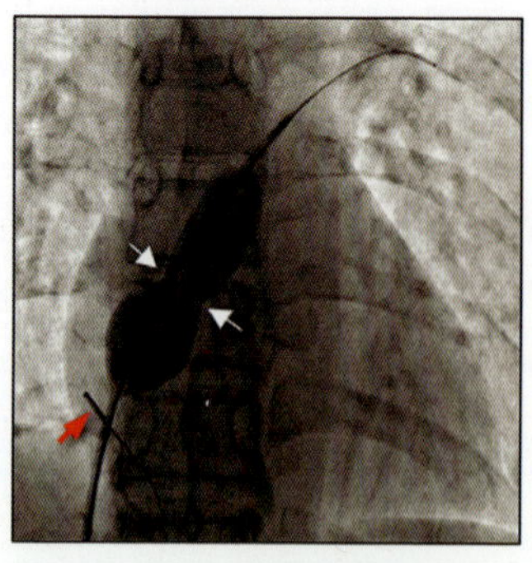 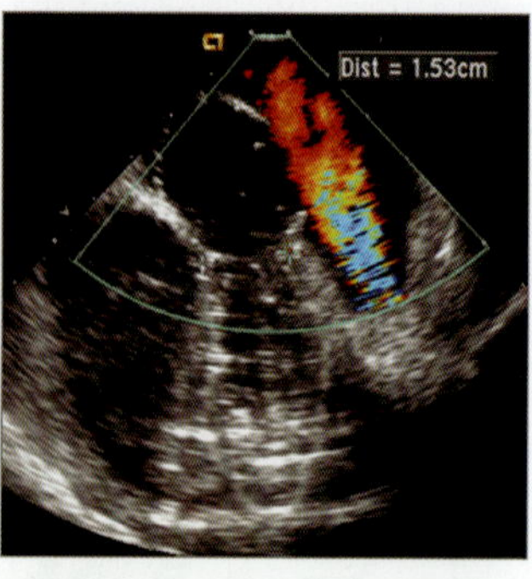

Fig 8.7—ICE images during balloon sizing. Left, sketch of the area of interest. Middle, fluoroscopic image of ICE catheter position (red arrow) showing the balloon sizing (arrows). Right, corresponding echocardiographic image during stop-flow measurement by a balloon.

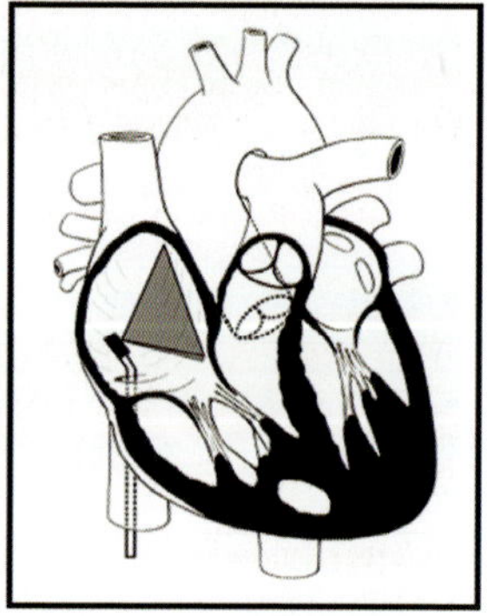

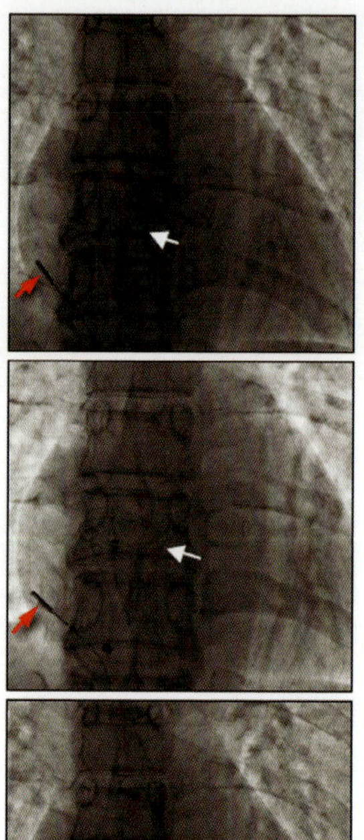 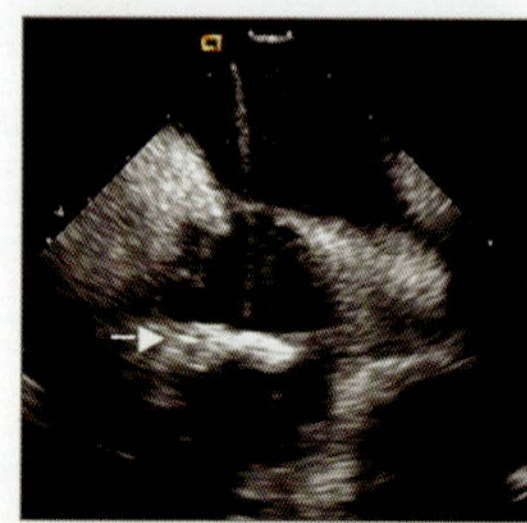

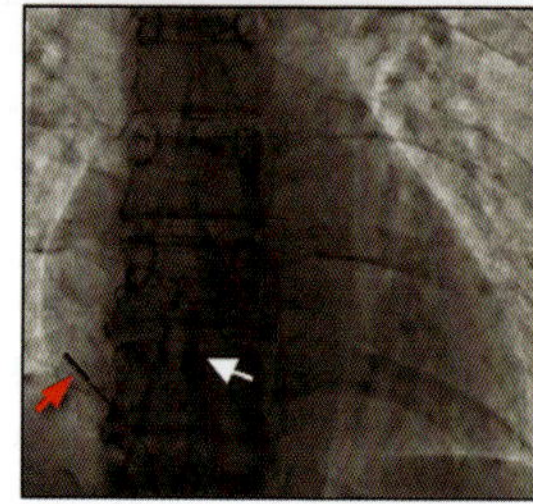 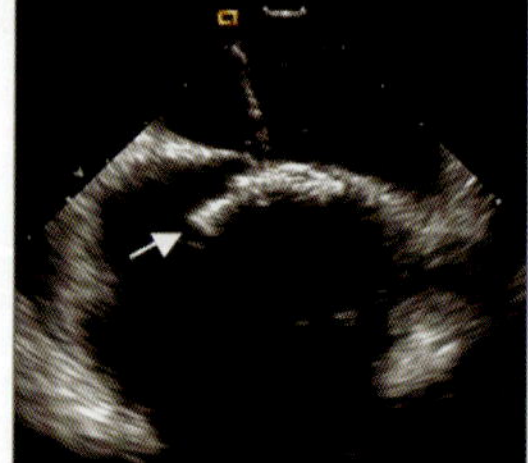

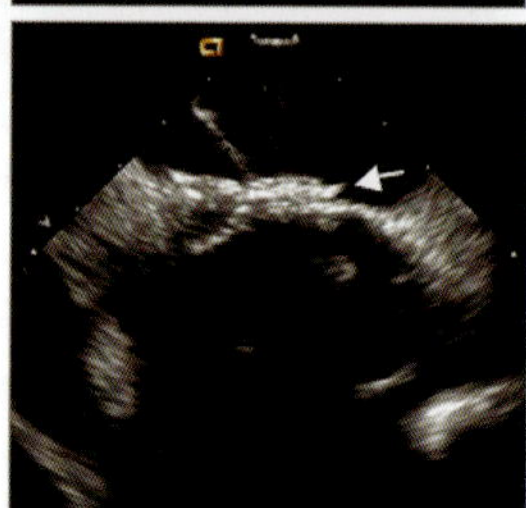

Fig 8.8—ICE images during various stages of deployment of the HELEX device. Red arrows denote position of the ICE catheter. White arrows denote the HELEX device. The fluoroscopic images' quality for the HELEX device is not as good.

loaded into the delivery sheath. Figure 8.8 demonstrates various steps for the implantation of the HELEX device. After the device has been deployed, ICE can assess the position and whether there is residual shunt/defect (Fig 8.9).

For PFO, evaluation of the defect, presence of right-to-left shunt, and closure steps can be monitored with ICE in a similar fashion to ASD closure.

ICE catheter can be positioned in the home view that evaluates the tricuspid valve function. Figure 8.10 (left, middle, and right) shows the schematic sketch as well as fluoroscopic position of the ICE catheter, and the corresponding echocardiographic images. Then the ICE catheter is flexed posteriorly with slight rightward rotation of the right/left knob to obtain the septal view. Figure 8.11 (left, middle, and right) demonstrate the schematic sketch, fluoroscopic image of the ICE catheter position, and corresponding echocardiographic images in a patient with PFO. Notice the length of PFO tunnel can be measured nicely in this view (Fig 8.11 right top). In this position, further advancement of the ICE catheter cephalad will get the bicaval or SVC view (Fig 8.12 left, middle, and right). Again, in this view one can measure the length of the tunnel (Fig 8.12 right top). Clockwise rotation of the entire control handle until the transducer tip is over the tricuspid valve and

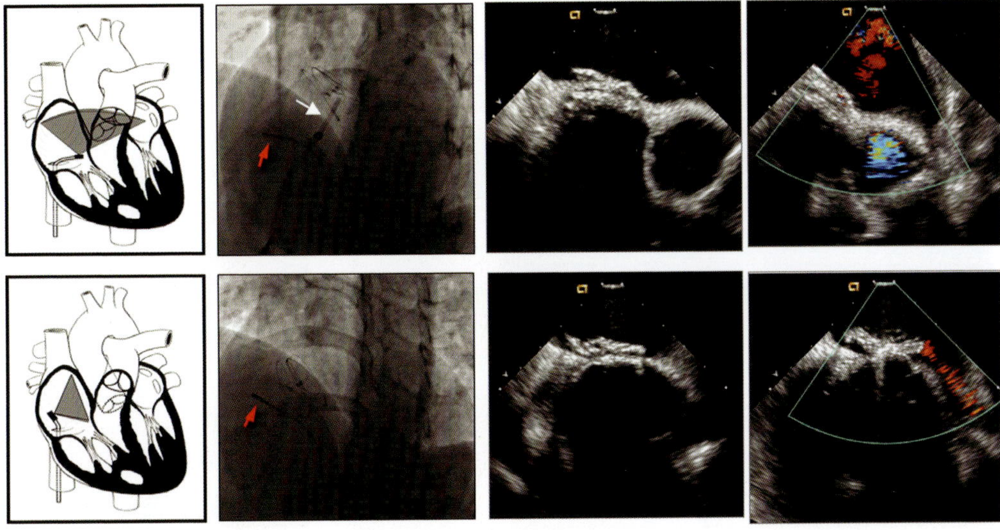

Fig 8.9—ICE images after the device has been released demonstrating good device position and no residual shunt.

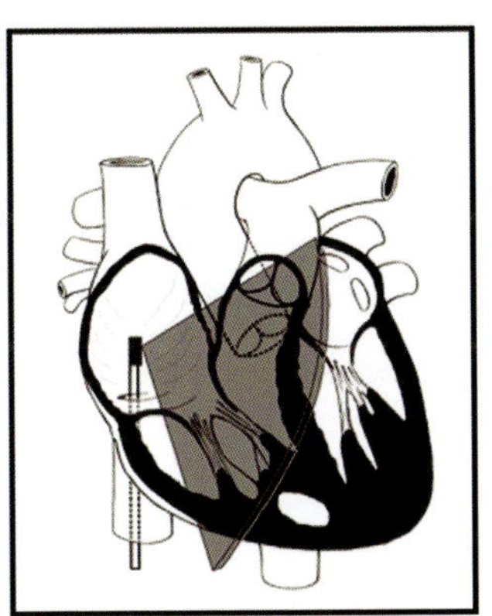

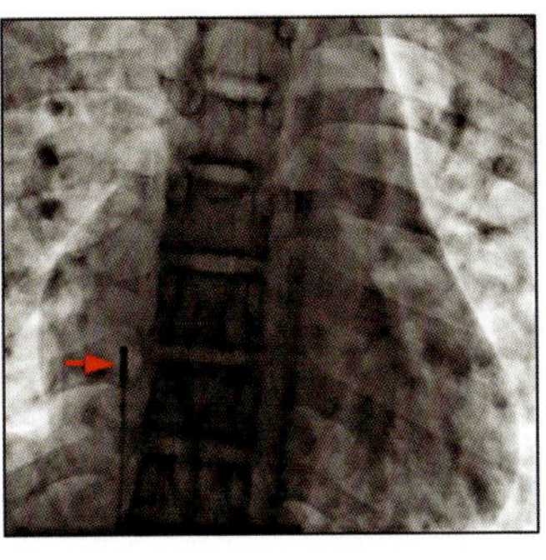

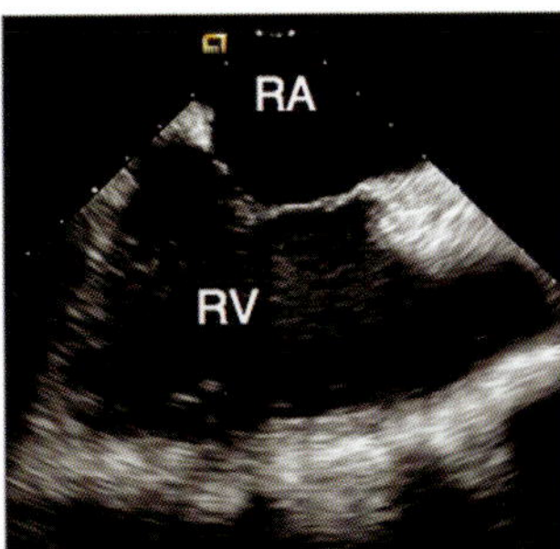

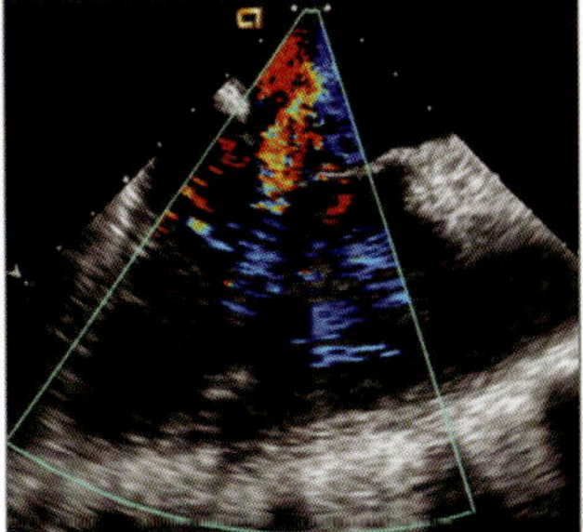

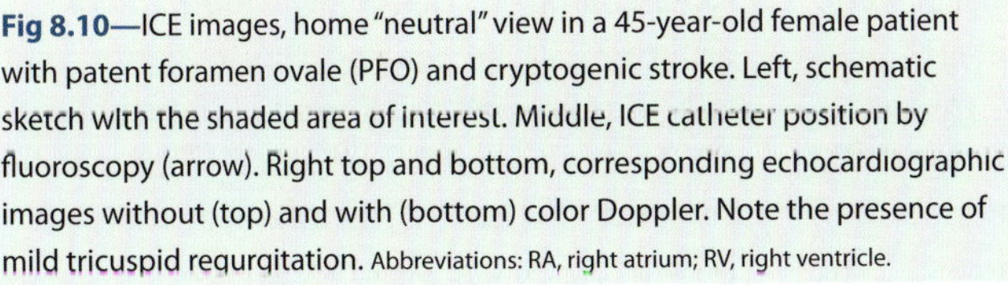

Fig 8.10—ICE images, home "neutral" view in a 45-year-old female patient with patent foramen ovale (PFO) and cryptogenic stroke. Left, schematic sketch with the shaded area of interest. Middle, ICE catheter position by fluoroscopy (arrow). Right top and bottom, corresponding echocardiographic images without (top) and with (bottom) color Doppler. Note the presence of mild tricuspid regurgitation. Abbreviations: RA, right atrium; RV, right ventricle.

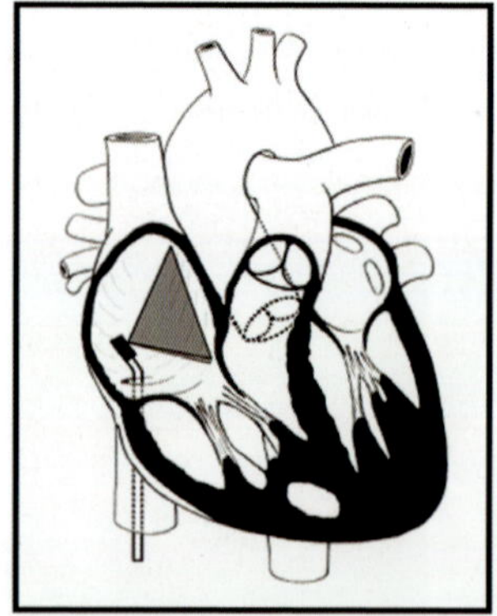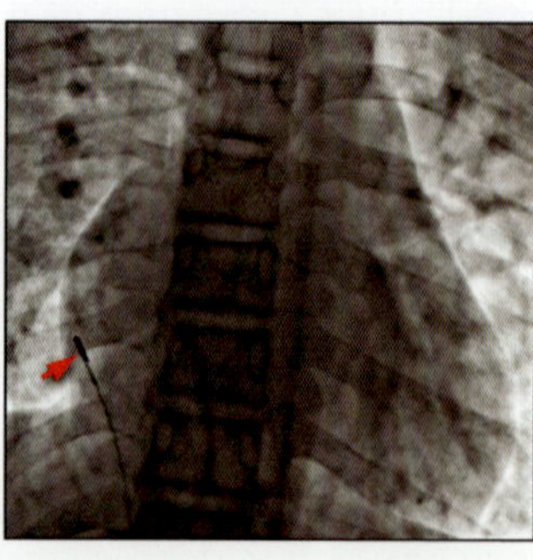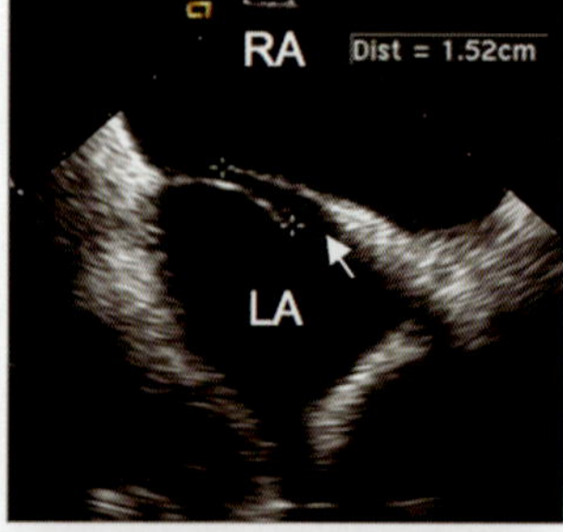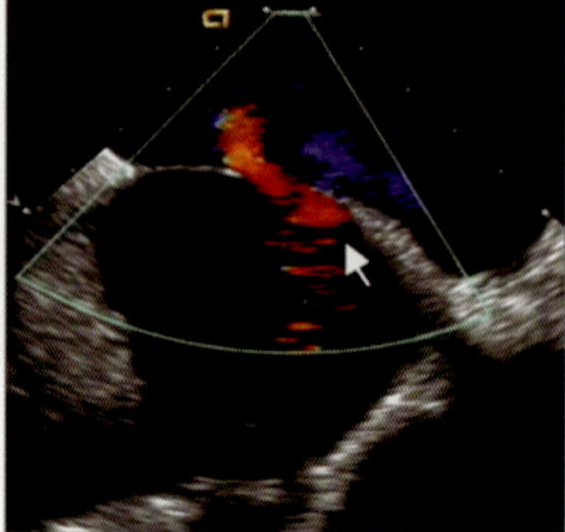

Fig 8.11—ICE images, septal view. Left, sketch of the area of interest. Middle, fluoroscopic image of ICE catheter. Right, corresponding echocardiographic images showing the defect (arrow) and the tunnel (asterisk). Abbreviations: RA, right atrium; LA, left atrium.

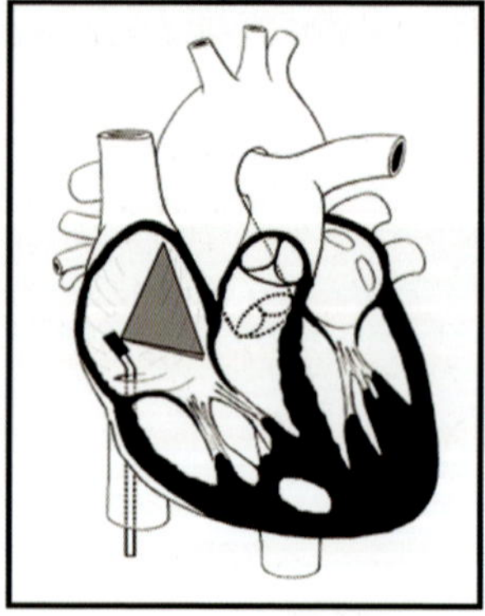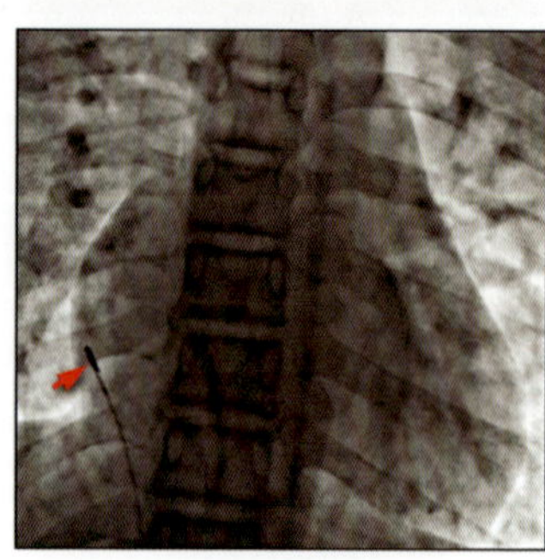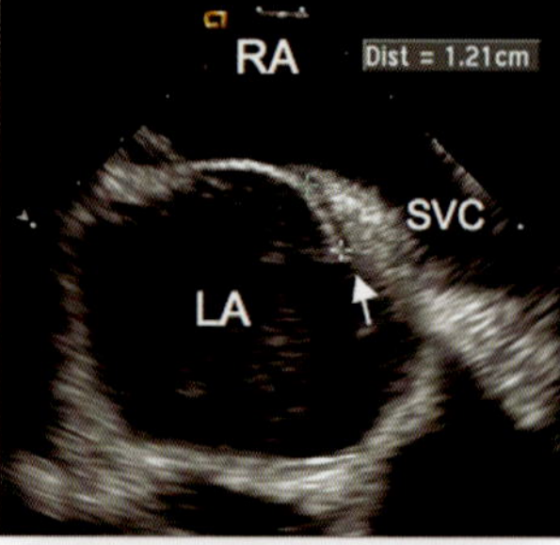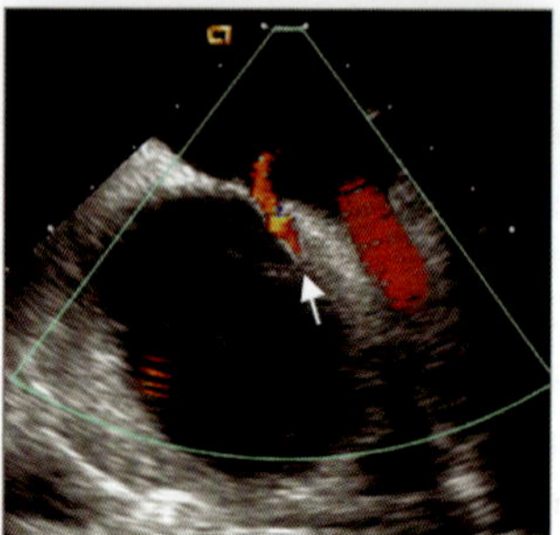

Fig 8.12—ICE images, bicaval "long-axis/SVC" view. Left, sketch of the area of interest. Middle, fluoroscopic image of ICE catheter (arrow). Right, corresponding echocardiographic images showing the defect (arrow). Abbreviations: RA, right atrium; LA, left atrium; SVC, superior vena cava.

beneath the aortic valve with less rightward rotation (more leftward) of the right/left knob will obtain the short-axis view. Figure 8.13 (left, middle, and right) represents the short-axis view in schematic sketch (left), the fluoroscopic image of the ICE catheter position (middle), and the corresponding echocardiographic images without and with color Doppler (right top and bottom). This view is similar to what we get with TEE in the short-axis view, except by ICE the near-field chamber is the right atrium in contrast to the left atrium by TEE. Once the anatomy of the PFO is assessed, the next step is to perform the contrast bubble study and as

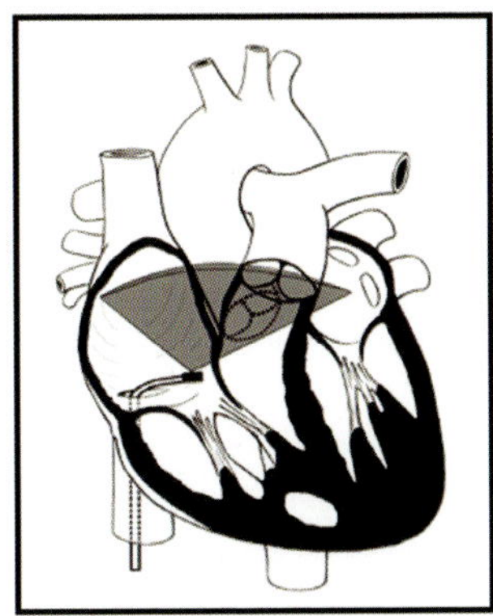
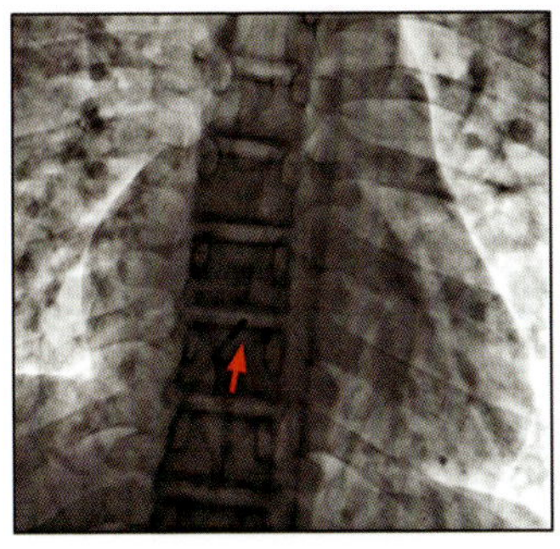
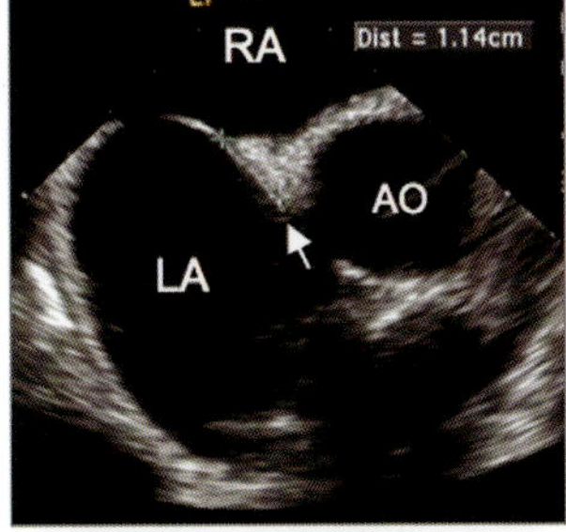
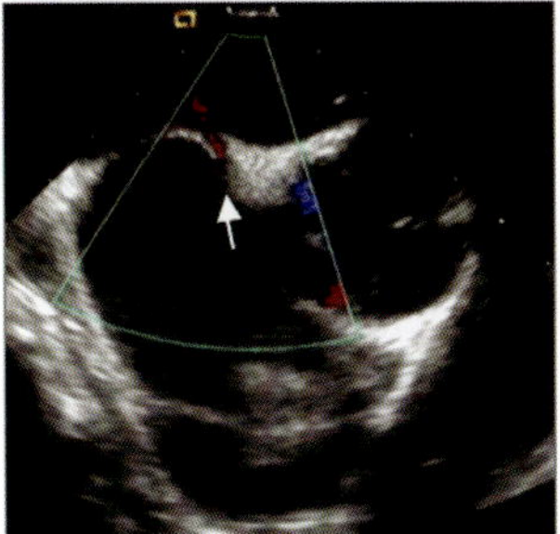

Fig 8.13—ICE images, short-axis view. Left, sketch of the area of interest. Middle, fluoroscopic image of ICE catheter (arrow). Right, corresponding echocardiographic images showing the defect (arrow), asterisk denote the tunnel. Abbreviations: RA, right atrium; LA, left atrium.

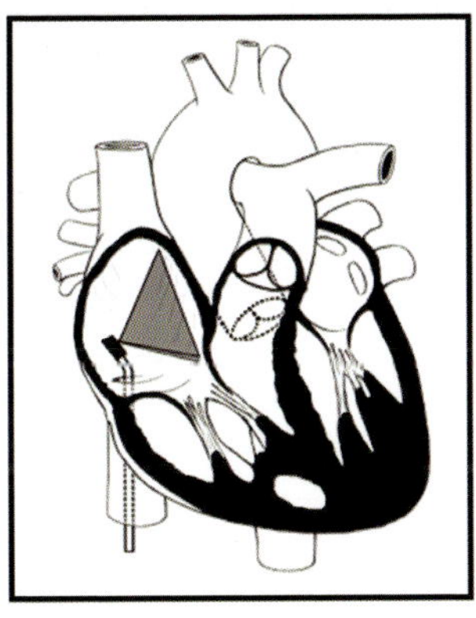
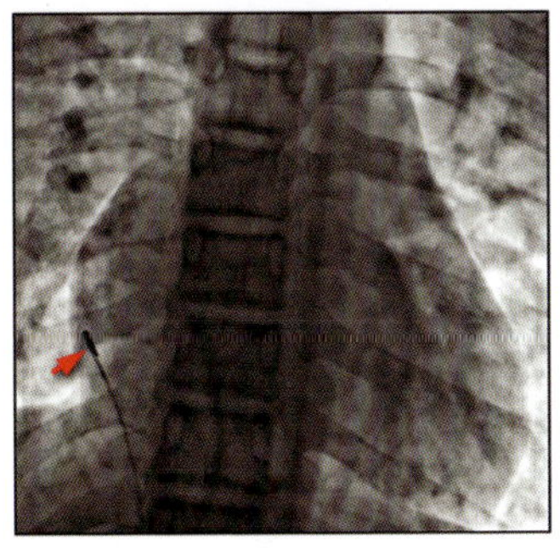
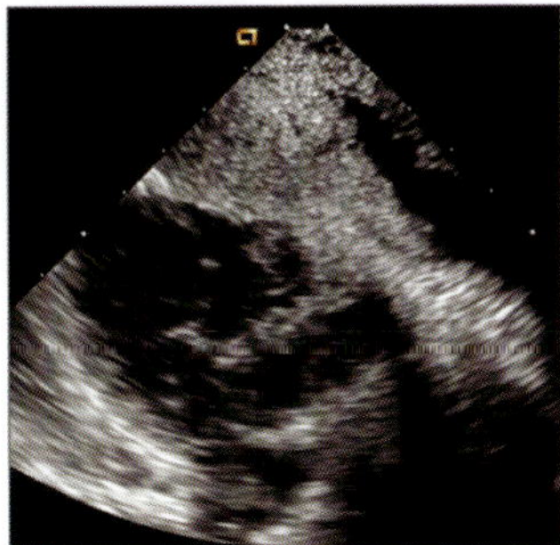

Fig 8.14—ICE images during contrast bubble injection. Left, sketch of area of interest in long-axis view. Middle, ICE catheter position (red arrow). Right, corresponding echocardiographic image showing right-to-left shunt.

mentioned previously, combine this with TCD (it has superior sensitivity). Figure 8.14 (left, middle, and right) demonstrates the schematic sketch, the fluoroscopic image of the ICE catheter position, and the echocardiographic image in the long-axis view demonstrating the right-to-left shunt.

Once the anatomic assessment is over, the PFO is crossed using a multipurpose catheter and a guide wire is positioned in the left upper pulmonary vein. This can be monitored via ICE (Fig 8.15 left, middle, and right). Some opera-

tors perform balloon sizing of the PFO. Using the HELEX device, balloon sizing is essential and this can be monitored using ICE (Fig 8.16 left, middle, and right). The appropriate device size is chosen and steps of deployment are somewhat similar to those of ASD device closure. Figures 8.17 and 8.18 demonstrate steps for implantation of the HELEX device. Once the device has been released, repeat ICE assessment in short- and long-axis views is done (Fig 8.19) and repeat contrast bubble study is performed to assess for residual shunt (Fig 8.20).

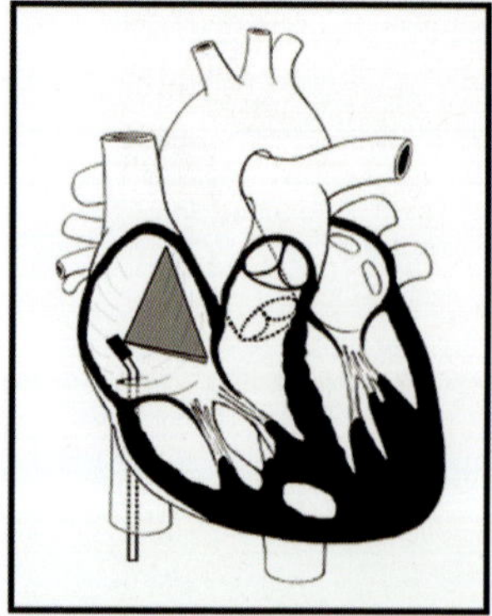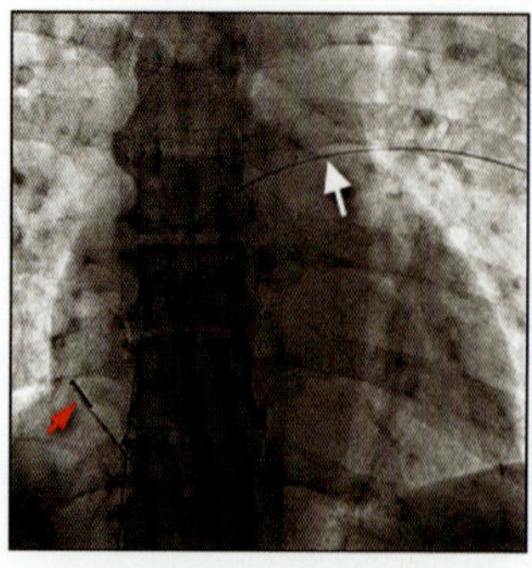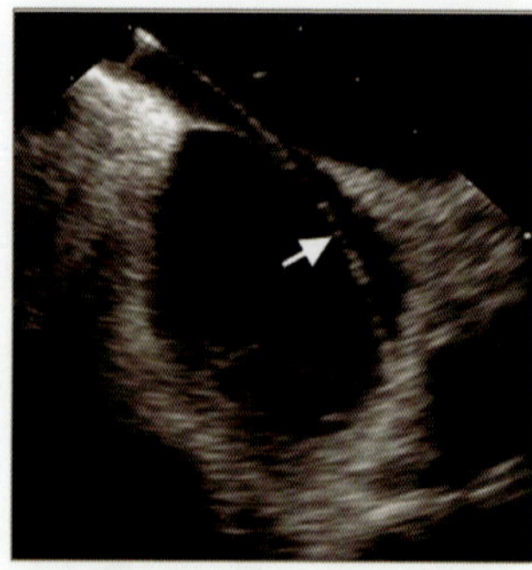

Fig 8.15—ICE images, long-axis view during passage of the guide wire through the PFO. Left, sketch of the area of interest. Middle, fluoroscopic image of ICE catheter position (red arrow) and the guide wire in the left upper pulmonary vein (white arrow). Right, corresponding echocardiographic image showing the guide wire in left atrium (arrow).

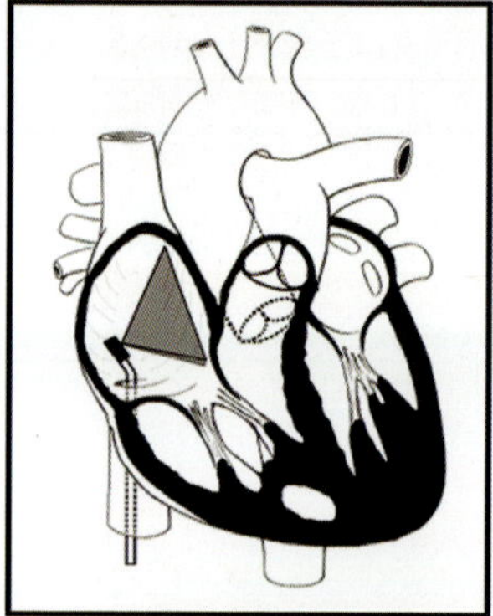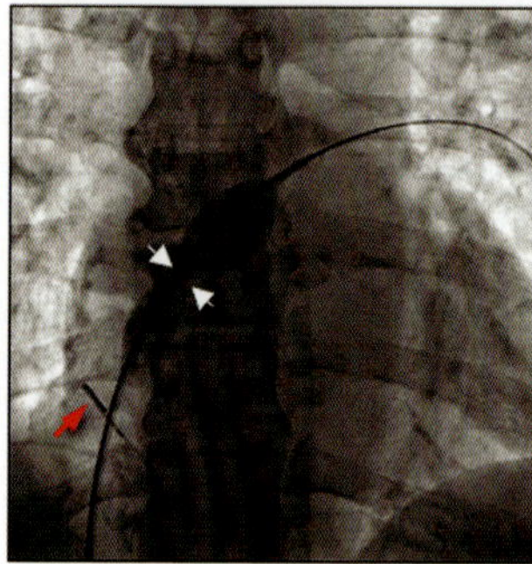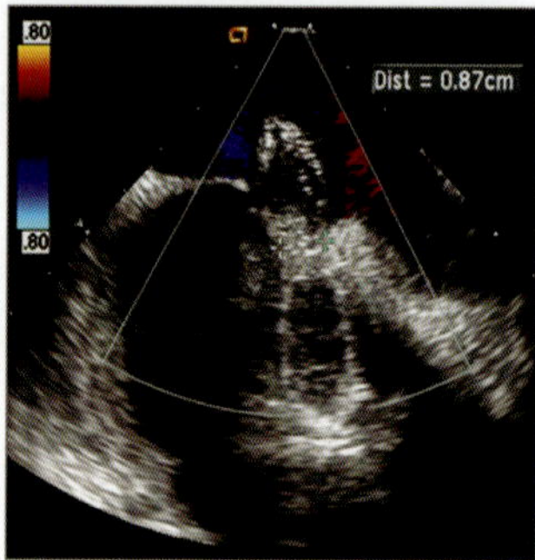

Fig 8.16—ICE images during balloon sizing. Left, sketch of the area of interest. Middle, fluoroscopic image of ICE catheter position (red arrow) showing the balloon sizing (arrows). Right, corresponding echocardiographic image during stop-flow measurement by a balloon (asterisk).

Although ICE can be performed safely with careful manipulation, the reported procedural adverse events rate is 1% to 3%.[5,8,9] Adverse events include arrhythmias, allergic reactions from latex exposure to the sterile sleeve used to cover the handle and connecting cable, groin hematoma, and pericardial effusion. In addition, there are reports of retroperitoneal bleeding and venous perforation. Therefore, safety may be improved by advancing the probe under fluoroscopic guidance or using a long sheath positioned in the high inferior vena cava. Despite these potential adverse events, the important advantages include the probe's proximity to intracardiac structures (especially the inferior atrial septum), the absence of any air or tissue interference with the catheter in the right atrium, and its maneuverability to achieve almost any orthogonal view. These strengths make it an ideal adjunct imaging tool for the invasive cardiologist in the congenital catheterization laboratory because it permits more accurate assessment of the atrial septal defect and real-time guidance of intervention in combination with fluoroscopy. Limitations remain, however, including the absence of multiplane views when compared to TEE, the current probe cost, and the probe size limiting manipulation as well as resulting in the need of an additional 8 to 11F sheath. Despite these limitations, it is generally agreed that ICE is on the cutting edge of an evolving paradigm in which multiple imaging tools can improve the safety and overall outcome of ASD/PFO device closure[10–12]

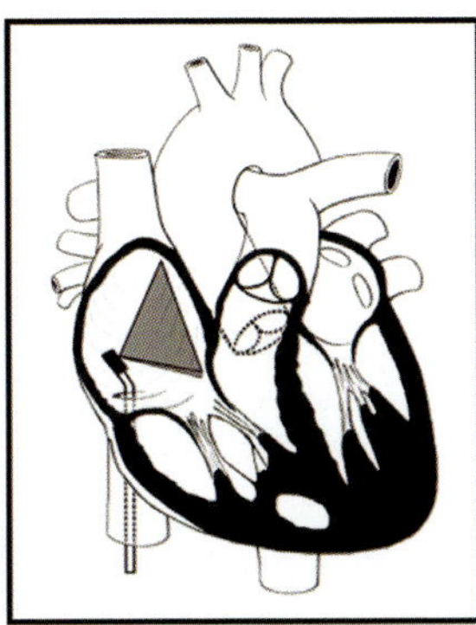

Fig 8.17—ICE images during various stages of deployment of the HELEX device. Red arrows denote position of the ICE catheter. White arrows denote the HELEX device. The fluoroscopic images' quality for the HELEX device is not as good.

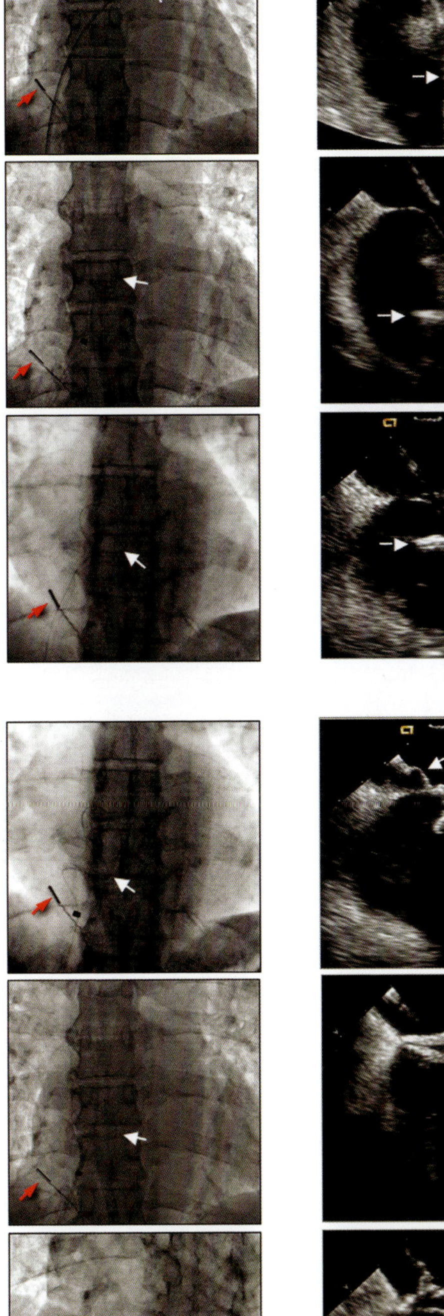

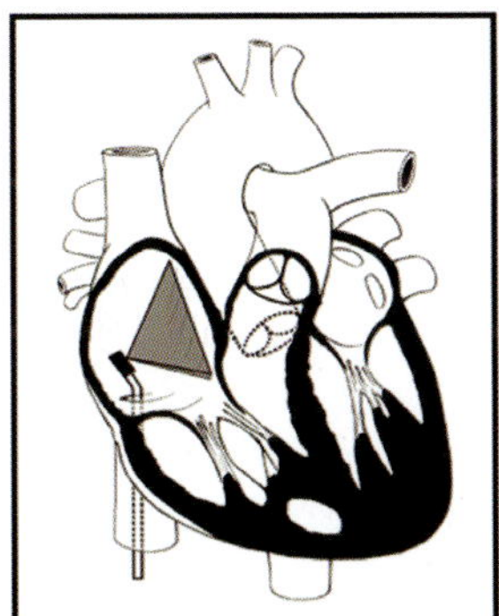

Fig 8.18—ICE images during final stages of device deployment demonstrating good device position.

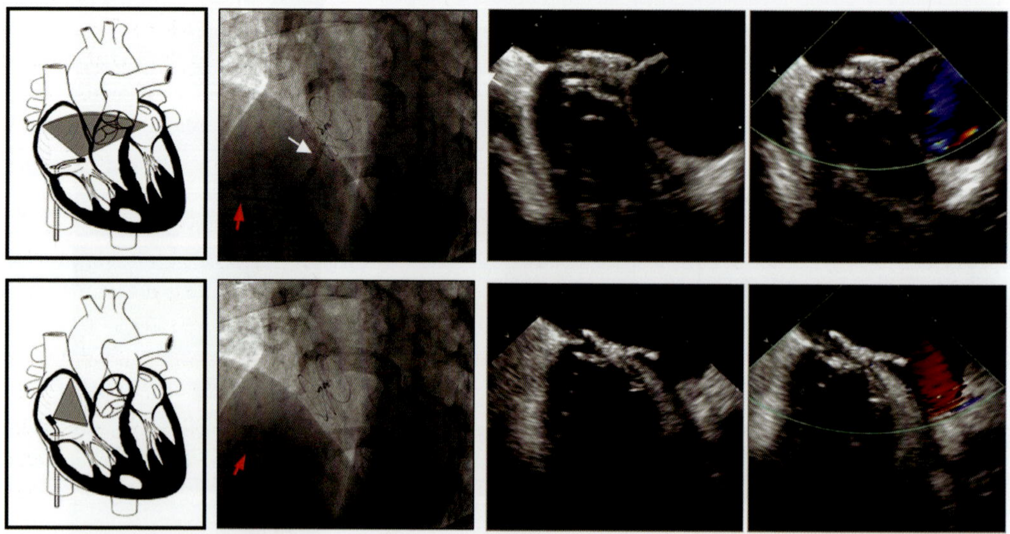

Fig 8.19—ICE images after the device has been released, demonstrating good device position and by color no shunt.

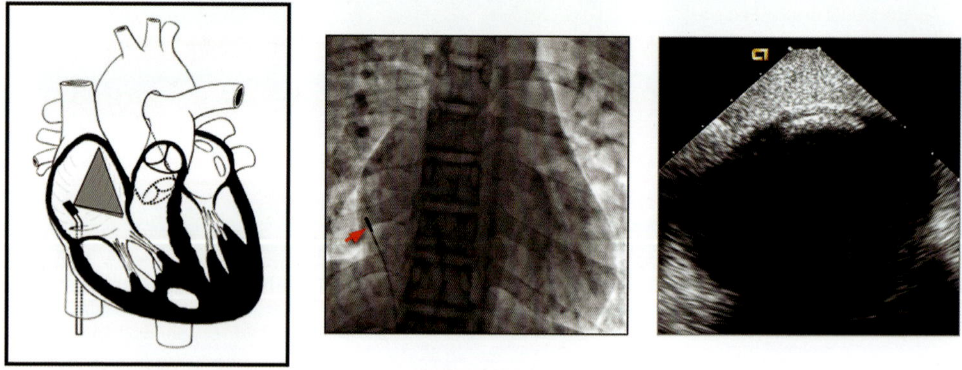

Fig 8.20—ICE images after device has been released with contrast bubble study, showing no right-to-left shunt.

References

1. Fu M, Hung JS, Lo PH, Wu CJ, Chang KC, Lau KW. Intracardiac echocardiography via the transvenous approach with use of 8F 10-MHz ultrasound catheters. *Mayo Clin Proc.* 1999;74:775–783.

2. Mullen MJ, Dias BF, Walker F, Siu SC, Benson LN, McLaughlin PR. Intracardiac echocardiography guided device closure of atrial septal defects. *J Am Coll Cardiol.* 2003;41:285–292.

3. Patel A, Cao Q-L, Koenig PR, Hijazi ZM. Intracardiac echocardiography to guide closure of atrial septal defects in children less than 15 kilograms. *Cathet Cardiovasc Interv.* 2006;68:287–291.

4. Barker PCA. Intracardiac echocardiography in congenital heart disease. *J Cardiovasc Trans Res.* 2009;2:19–23.

5. Hijazi Z, Wang Z, Cao Q-L, Koenig P, Waight D, Lang R. Transcatheter closure of atrial septal defects and patent foramen ovale under intracardiac echocardiographic guidance: feasibility and comparison with transesophageal echocardiography. *Cathet Cardiovasc Interv.* 2001;52:194–199.

6. Awad SM, Cao Q-L, Hijazi ZM. Intracardiac echocardiography for the guidance of percutaneous procedures. *Curr Cardiol Rep.* 2009;11:210–215.

7. Hijazi ZM, Shivkumar K, Sahn DJ. Intracardiac echocardiography during interventional and electrophysiological cardiac catheterization. *Circulation.* 2009;119:587–596.

8. Hijazi Z, Wang Z, Cao Q-L, Koenig P, Waight D, Lang R. Transcatheter closure of atrial septal defects and patent foramen ovale under intracardiac echocardiographic guidance: feasibility and comparison with transesophageal echocardiography. *Cathet Cardiovasc Intervent.* 2001;52:194–199.

9. Koenig PR, Abdulla RI, Cao Q-L, Hijazi ZM. Use of intracardiac echocardiography to guide catheter closure of atrial communications. *Echocardiography.* 2003;20:781–787.

10. Bartel T, Konorza T, Arjumand J, et al. Intracardiac echocardiography is superior to conventional monitoring for guiding device closure of interatrial communications. *Circulation.* 2003;107:795–797.

11. Bartel T, Konorza T, Neudorf U, et al. Intracardiac echocardiography: an ideal guiding tool for device closure of interatrial communications. *Eur J Echocardiogr.* 2005;6:92–96.

12. Bartel T, Konorza T, Barbieri V, Erbel R, Pachinger O, Muller S. Single-plane balloon sizing of atrial septal defects with intracardiac echocardiography: an advantageous alternative to fluoroscopy. *J Am Soc Echocardiogr.* 2008;21:737–740.

9

CT Evaluation
of the Interatrial Septum in ASDs

Robert A. Quaife and John D. Carroll

Introduction

Over the past two decades, cardiac imaging has benefited from advances in multidetector computed tomography (MDCT) technology allowing improved spatial and temporal resolution. This technology has developed into an important method to assess patients with congenital heart disease. Initial detection, follow-up, and treatment of ASDs remain largely performed by transthoracic echocardiography or transesophageal echocardiography (TTE and TEE).[1] Limitations with regard to spatial resolution and lack of a full field of view to evaluate associated anomalies renders echocardiography less comprehensive than one might expect.[1–9]

The advent of closure devices has resulted in the majority of ASDs now being closed percutaneously. Successful percutaneous closure of ASDs depends heavily on defect anatomy,[10] including the definition of specific rims (infero-

posterior, near the inferior vena cava and antero-superior, around the aorta) both providing the tissue on which the closure device is secured. Inadequate rim tissue by echocardiography has been defined as a predictor of poor procedural success.[10,11] In large ASDs, a position adjacent to structures such as the pulmonary veins or coronary sinus may significantly limit placement of occluder devices due to potential vascular obstruction or occlusion[7,12,13] and recognition is very important. Thus, full characterization of the defect anatomy and surrounding architecture is highly desirable for optimal patient triage and subsequent successful device deployment in those triaged to percutaneous therapy. CT angiography (CTA) is a high-resolution and wide-field view technique that allows detailed resolution, assessment, and spatial orientation of ASDs and their adjacent anatomic structures.[6–14]

Transcatheter Closure of ASDs and PFOs: A Comprehensive Assessment. © 2010 Ziyad M. Hijazi, Ted Feldman, Mustafa H. Abdullah Al-Qbandi, and Horst Sievert, editors. Cardiotext Publishing, ISBN: 978-0-9790164-9-3.

125

Atrial Embryology and Anatomy by Cardiac CT

ASDs result from the variable growth and arrest of septum primum and septum secundum during embryological development.[1] Therefore, a review of normal atrial anatomy by cardiac CT is essential to understanding the aberrant formation of ostium secundum and primum in ASDs. Partition of the developing atrial chamber begins with caudal growth of a thin, curtainlike crescentic membranous rim of tissue from the roof of the atrium called septum primum (Fig 9.1, primum). The free wall of this septum extends caudally toward the fusing dorsal and ventral endocardial cushions. The gap or hole formed between the advancing free edge of septum primum and the endocardial cushions is called ostium primum. Thereafter, small perforations develop in septum primum that will eventually coalesce to form a second hole or interatrial communication called ostium secundum. Further extension of septum primum and fusion of the free edge of septum primum with the endocardial cushion occur and the ostium primum becomes obliterated. However lack of fusion of the septum primum with the endocardial cushion results in primum ASD.

A thick muscular rim of tissue called septum secundum develops adjacent to the septum primum in the roof of the right atrium (Fig 9.1, secundum). This thick rim of tissue extends caudally toward the endocardial cushions, similar to septum primum, ultimately covering ostium secundum like a curtain. Failure of the secundum tissue to migrate to the endocardial cushions results in the various positions of secundum ASDs. Occasionally the dissolution of the septum primum is more aggressive resulting in a fenestrated ASD (Fig 9.1, fenestration). Normal developmental arrest of septum secundum results in a small hole called foramen ovale. While septum secundum develops, there is degeneration and regression of the septum primum, resulting in a small ovoid flap of tissue that becomes the one-way valve of the foramen ovale (allowing right-to-left flow; Fig 9.1, PFO). Figure 9.1 shows examples of the different septal components and accompanying defects identified by cardiac CT.[1]

Cardiac CT Methodology

Initial application of CT technology applied to ASDs was demonstrated using Ultrafast CT to detect interatrial shunt.[3–5] This methodology had temporal resolution of approximately 50 ms per frame, thereby stopping cardiac motion. Progressive development of CT imaging systems resulted in multidetector equipment with faster gantry rotation speed (necessary to stop cardiac motion), increased numbers of detectors, and dual source CT scanners all allowing improved temporal and spatial resolution in cardiac CT. Imaging of ASDs requires a minimum of 40- to 64-row detector system with new 256- or 320-row CT able to acquire all information in 1 to 4 heart beats.

The advent of high flow rate and multiphase contrast injectors has allowed minimization of contrast artifacts and differential chamber [4–8] concentrations that occur with cardiac CT. Delivery of an adequately dense contrast bolus to opacify the cardiac chambers while at the same time reducing beam hardening artifact emanating from the superior vena cava requires fast power injection of the contrast bolus with washout by saline chaser injection. Importantly, reducing the concentration or creating a gradient of the contrast level compared to other structures or chambers is important for the accurate evaluation of ASD. To achieve the desired opacification of chambers, the rate of injection and percentage of contrast needs to be varied. It is possible to change the concentration by either diluting the contrast or reducing the rate of injection. The development of high-concentration contrast agents (350–370 mg/mL) has also dramatically improved the image quality. These agents combined with differential chamber contrast concentration provide iden-

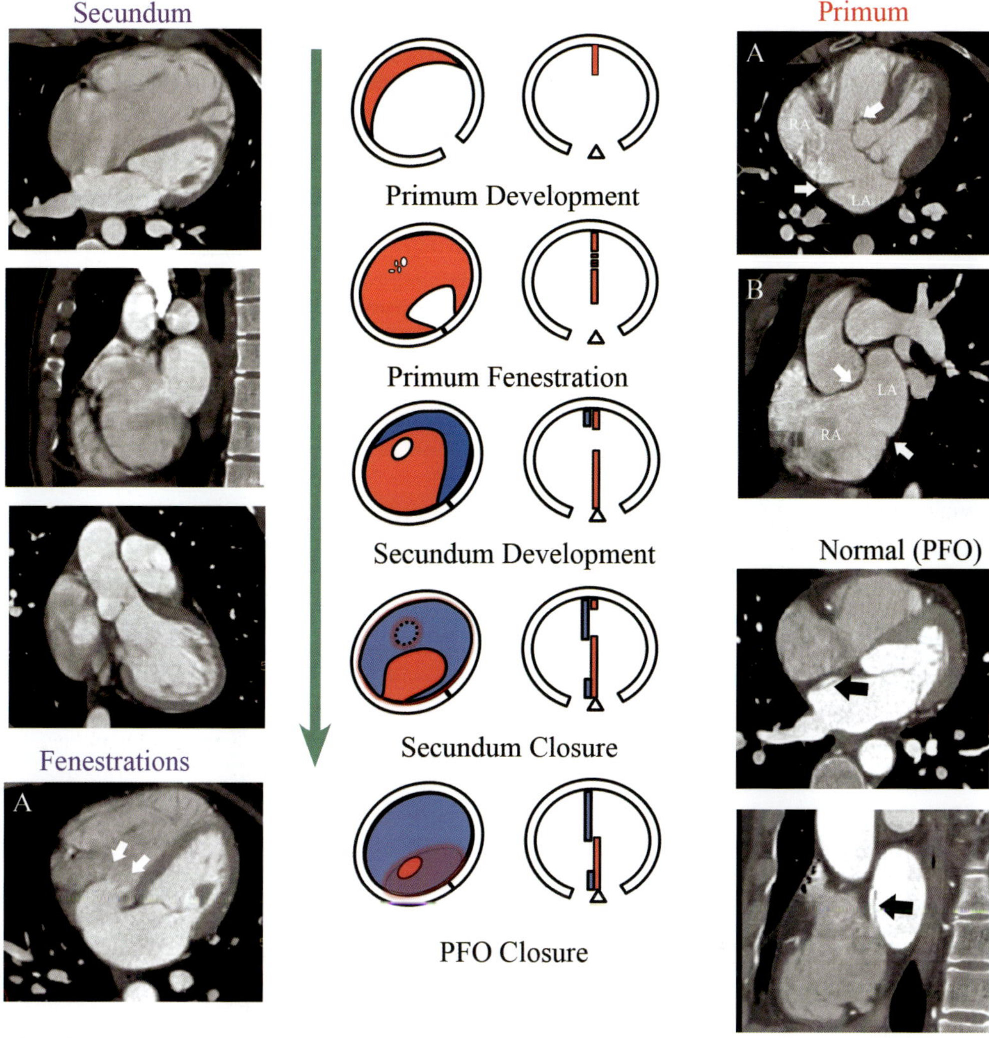

Fig 9.1—The spectrum of atrial septal abnormalities as illustrated by CTA imaging. Development of the primum and secundum septae are shown with associated ASD defects.

tification of the shunts and delineation of fine structures such as the septum primum.

Optimal acquisition protocols require 64 row or greater CT scanner with a gantry rotation time of 420 ms or faster, tube voltages of 80-100-120 kVp, and tube current of upwards of 800 mAs. Most current systems have radiation dose reduction methods that should be applied whenever possible. These include ECG phase dose modulation or "Step and Shoot" sequential axial imaging technologies. The dynamic nature of ASD size may need to be assessed throughout the cardiac cycle. Consideration of patient size is required to properly tailor tube current and voltage to deliver the minimum radiation dose to the patient necessary to answer the clinical question. This is especially important in young individuals who, because of their disease, have often been subjected to multiple procedures using ionizing radiation.

Elimination of motion artifacts is of the utmost importance in obtaining high-quality cardiac images. Cardiac motion is least significant during end systole and mid to late diastole making electrocardiographic gating a requirement of any cardiac CT exam. The use of oral or intravenous beta blockers to slow heart rate also helps to limit cardiac motion and improve image acquisition. However, care must be used in patients with pulmonary hypertension or reduced ventricular function, or cardiac conduction abnormalities (ie, heart block with VSD or TOF).

In a typical cardiac exam using a 64-slice scanner, approximately 75 mL of iodinated contrast (Iopamidol—Isovue; 370 mg/mL) is injected in the right antecubital vein at 5 mL/s followed by a 30- to 50-mL saline chaser also delivered at 3 to 4 mL/s. However, the site of injection such as right or left antecubital veins or possibly the leg may be important for the identification of different intracardiac shunts.[3-7]

Information regarding the potential right-to-left direction of ASD shunting can be determined by performing a dynamic contrast-enhanced cardiac exam. Funabashi et al were able to demonstrate shunt directionality in VSD, ASD, and PDA by comparing the density of right and left chamber at 5 and 30 seconds postcontrast injection.[6] Similarly, Gade et al showed shunt directionality utilizing a triple phase contrast protocol using 60 cc of iodixanol followed by 40 cc of dilute iodixanol (50:50 with saline), then followed by a 50 cc saline flush.[7] Furthermore, the orientation of a contrast jet on dynamic contrasted cardiac CT can be helpful in the differentiation of secundum ASD from patent foramen[8] and other complex congenital heart disease.

Postprocessing of the CT data set is important in order to select those images that will yield the least cardiac motion. Typically, axial data sets are reconstructed retrospectively from 0% to 90% of the R-R interval at between 0.8- to 1.0-mm slice thickness with 50% slice overlap (0.8/0.4 or 1/0.5 mm). Data may then be evaluated in multiplanar reformat images (MPR) or maximum intensity projections (MIP) image sets in orthogonal views which provide the basis for assessment of CHD (Fig 9.2).

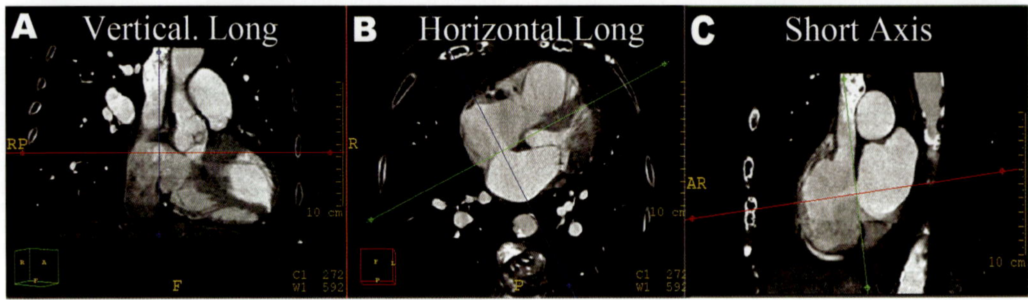

Fig 9.2—Three standard CTA orthogonal planes for assessing the interatrial septum, which are key to accurate sizing.

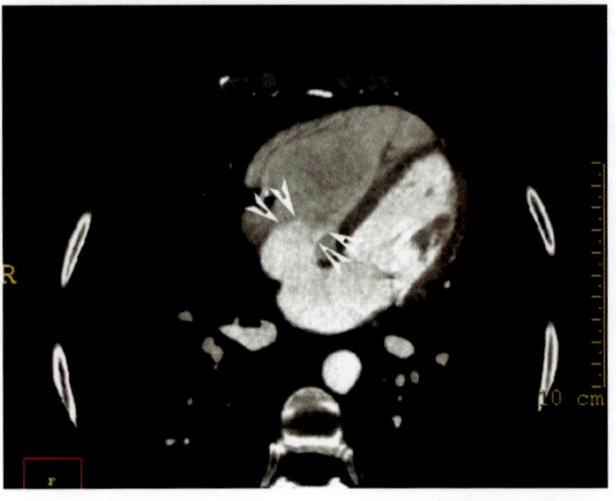

Fig 9.3—Fenestrated septum. CTA of a fenestrated ASD with the arrows pointing to discrete contrast jets. Note the left atrial aneurysm bulging into the right atrial.

Analysis of CT Images

CT images possess significantly greater information than just the two-dimensional data shown in axial image sets. Reorientation into orthogonal, modified axial (panel B), sagittal (panel A), and coronal or short-axis images (panel C) ASD planes (Fig 9.2) are critically important. MPR images of the ASD are used to obtain the orientation, location, and maximum diameter for ASD. MPR images are used to characterize the type of ASD, any fenestrations (Fig 9.3), and location in relationship to other structures. It is important to assess these structures throughout the cardiac cycle in the short-axis or sagittal oblique images planes (Fig 9.4) because the relative stretch of the defect is related to differential flow between the atria during diastole and systole. Measurement of the maximum diameter (axial and sagittal) and total area can be performed at maximal size throughout the cardiac cycle using CT analysis software. Characterization of the edges of the interatrial septal defect or rims such as the antero-superior and infero-posterior rims (Fig 9.5) is important to determine the feasibility of percutaneous defect closure. The orientation and relationship of the IVC to both the right and left atrium should also be determined by orienting the MPR image sets to obtain the best interatrial septal projection (Fig 9.6).

One of the major advantages of CTA is its ability to provide high-resolution images of

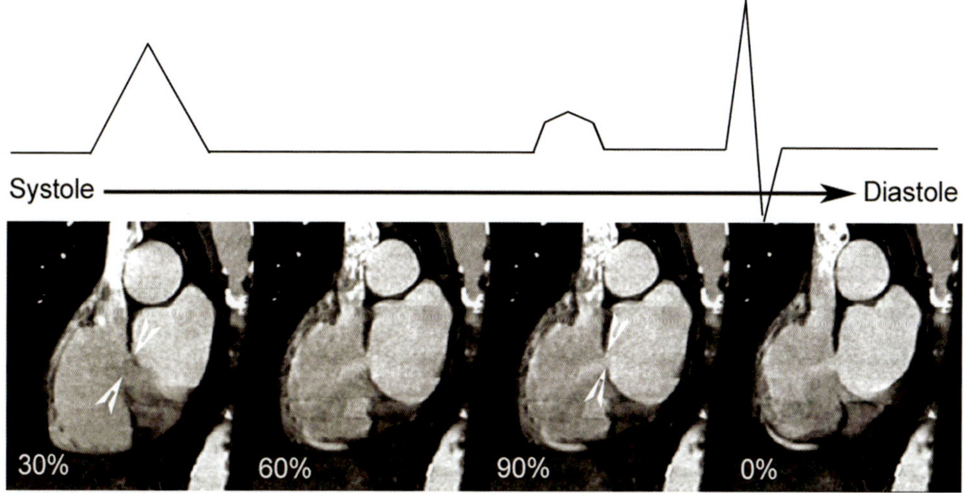

Fig 9.4—Variable shunting during the cardiac cycle through a secundum ASD.

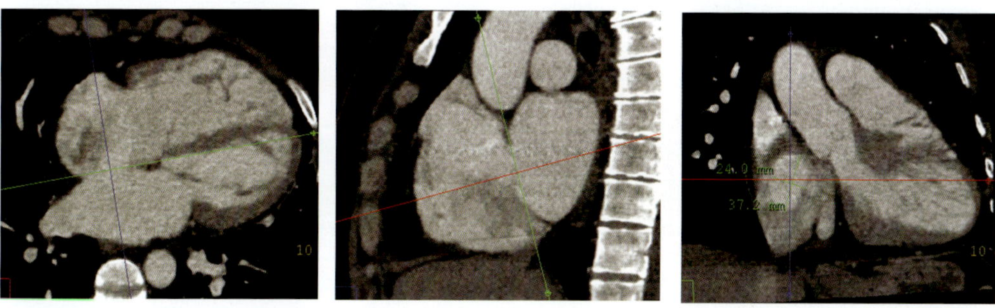

Fig 9.5—Characterization of the edges of the interatrial septal defect or rims by CTA. Note the central ASD, with clear rim tissue. Lines represent orthogonal views from the esophagus.

the pulmonary veins, coronary sinus, and specific ASD morphologic characteristics (eg, rim dimensions and tissue quality). This information is invaluable in clarifying the feasibility of percutaneous defect closure with occluder devices.[9] Patients who may be clearly identified by CTA include those with anomalies of the pulmonary veins, defects close to the coronary sinus, and defects with deficiencies of the inferior rim that may be poorly visualized by TEE.

Single-plane imaging modalities such as TEE are limited in their capacity to thoroughly evaluate ASDs with deficient inferior rims.[10-13] The angulation of TEE planes, despite multiplane technology, is still limited by the esophageal location (Fig 9.5). Furthermore oblong defects may be cut tangentially resulting in misinterpretation of size of the defect and/or the presence or absence of rims are a key factor for procedural success. Shown in Figure 9.6 is an example of the distortion of the defect size by orientation related to the standard bicaval imaging plane. Importantly, CTA views the adjacent structure such as the coronary sinus [14,15] with a full field of view and may better define percutaneous versus surgical candidates when compared to TEE.

We have shown that CTA in a spectrum of ASD size is an accurate method of determining defect size, which is critical in preprocedural planning.[9] Measurements obtained by CTA in either the axial or sagittal projections appeared to correlate with the maximum diameter determined by invasive balloon sizing by

ICE.[16,17] Although comparable to balloon sizing in evaluating ASD size, CTA offers the added advantage of providing operators an insight into procedural success. This is especially true where TEE appears to miss the atrial inferior rim; CTA appears in this small study to clearly define this architectural characteristic (see Fig 9.6). The use of CTA in selected cases, such as in large (15 mm) or inferiorly positioned ASDs, potentially would reduce attempts at percutaneous closure with a low chance of success and triage them to surgical closure.

CTA also affords the ability to understand the dynamic nature of the interatrial septum. Clearly, the accuracy of defect measurement as determined by 2D modalities such as echocardiography is subject to this limitation. This has prompted operators to use balloon sizing as the definitive modality in the defect dimension assessment. Our study confirms that gated CTA provides both the ability to assess the dynamic characteristics of the atrial septum as well as visualize the associated changes of the defect orifice throughout the cardiac cycle (Fig 9.4). These dynamic changes likely explain the enhanced correlation of defect size and area measurement when the nonuniform shape (Fig 9.6) of the particular defects is considered.[9] Additionally, secondary to the enhanced spatial and temporal resolution, CTA permits the identification and 3D characterization of fenestrated ASDs (Fig 9.3), and absent posterior inferior rims (Fig 9.5 vs. Fig 9.6) which can be challenging to close percutaneously.

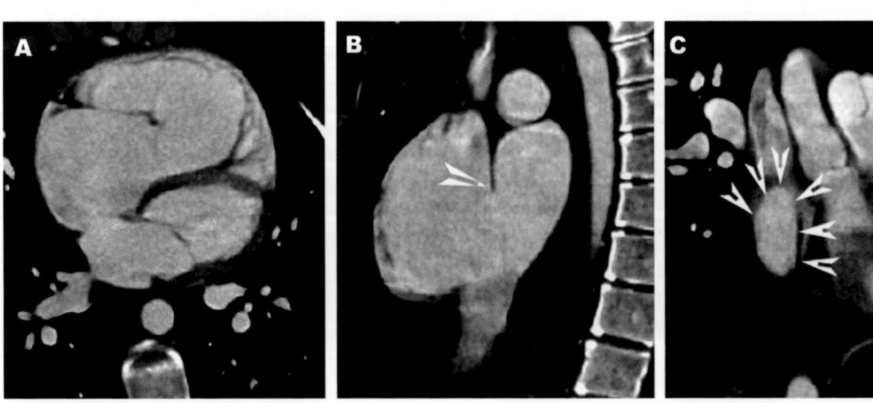

Fig 9.6—Absent posterior rim. CTA visualization of a secundum ASD with an absent posterior rim.

CTA has some similarities and differences to cardiac magnetic resonance imaging (CMRI) that should be understood in assessing patients with defects of the interatrial septum. Previous studies using CMRI have demonstrated a reasonable correlation (Pearson's r=0.69) between CMRI-derived ASD sizing and location with those derived from balloon sizing and fluoroscopy respectively.[18-20] The utility of CMRI however is limited by significant data scatter rather than a close correlation. An explanation for this disparity is nonisotropic voxel resolution present with CMRI which restrict the modality's ability to adequately image thin interatrial septal walls. CTA, on the other hand, has isotropic voxels of approximately 0.4 mm (absolute) and 0.6 mm functional size thereby possessing higher spatial resolution and an enhanced ability to resolve thin structures.[7] Although CMRI has enhanced temporal resolution, when coupled with ECG-gated multisegment/multiphase acquisition, CTA appears to yield equivalent results to CMRI. For these reasons, CTA is becoming an important diagnostic modality for structural heart disease imaging in adults.[6,7,9]

CTA to Plan Catheter-Based Defect Closure

Assessment of size, shape, and location are key to proper patient selection and allow a preprocedure assessment of likely device size but also has potential value in other technical issues. For example, CTA determination of the actual 3D orientation of interatrial defect may allow selection of the delivery catheter shape that is important in the alignment of the left atrial disc to the plane of the defect. We routinely assess the RAO and caudal coordinates of the x-ray system to visualize en face closure devices immediately postinsertion. This assessment of the defect plane has shown an excellent correlation to the interatrial septum orientation predicted by CTA with the positions obtained by fluoroscopy (Fig 9.7).[9] Knowledge of the plane of the interatrial septum is critical to an efficient percutaneous ASD closure as specific delivery catheter shapes are needed to provide the correct left atrial disc alignment during deploy-

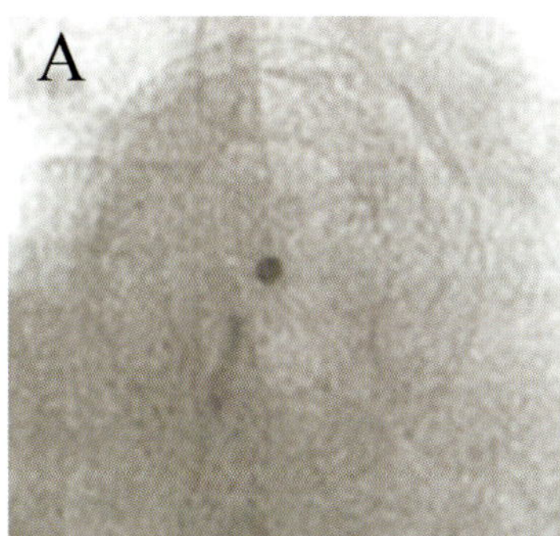

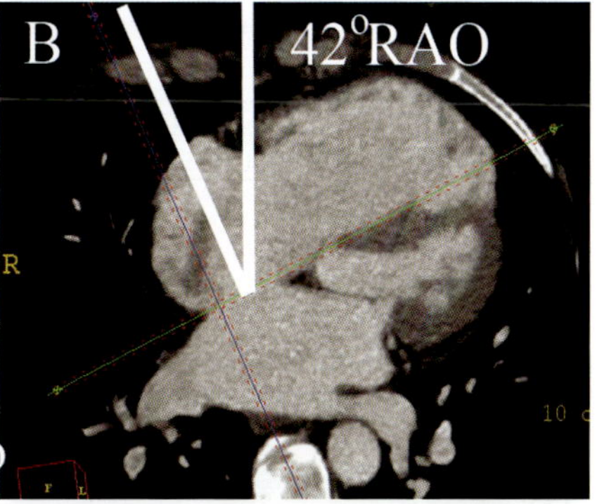

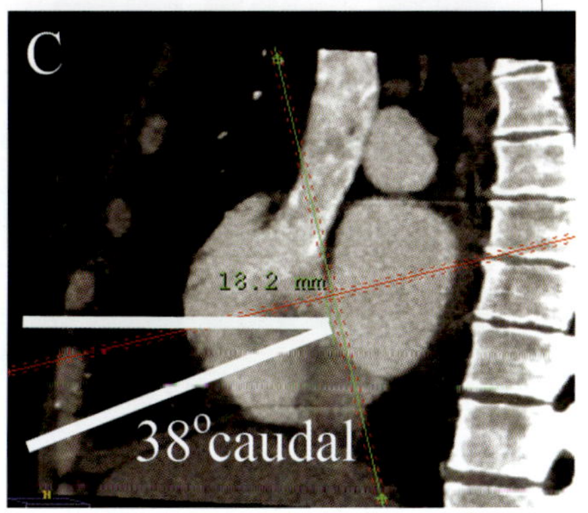

Fig 9.7—Determination of the plane of the septum. A: En face AMPLATZER device. Postclosure the markers on the device are aligned in an RAO-Caudal gantry position. B (CTA image [axial]) and C (Saggital) CTA images are analyzed to extract the plane of the defect; axial image for RAO and sagittal image for caudal tilt.

ment.[21] Indeed, special catheter shapes such as the Hausdorf-Lock sheath (Cook Incorporated, Bloomington, Indiana) are often required to overcome the poor device alignment and CTA theoretically can provide the ability to select the correct catheter shape preprocedurally, replacing the current trial-and-error method used intraoperatively (Fig 9.8). Further studies are needed to see whether these patient-specific 3D anatomical features, which are easily determined by CTA, can be used to improve device closure procedures and avoid device-anatomy size mismatch or misalignment that lead to complications such as device embolization and erosion.[22,23]

Use of CTA to Assess Device-Related Issues Postimplantation

Multiple clinical issues may arise in the postprocedure period that require imaging to clarify or exclude causes. Patients with chest pain, pericardial effusion, residual leaks, device erosion, and arrhythmias are encountered in clinical practice and both echocardiography and CTA are assessment tools. CTA visualization of devices and their orientation within the complex 3D interface of the interatrial septum and surrounding structures is superb and useful for troubleshooting.[24,25]

Use of CTA During Procedures: Coregistration with Fluoroscopy

Most commonly fluoroscopy is used with various forms of echocardiography to guide the closure of interatrial defects. An alternative imaging strategy is to use the preprocedural CTA along with fluoroscopy. The CTA image is first segmented to show the relevant structures and then imported into an imaging workstation that is part of many advanced cardiac catheterization systems. At the beginning of the procedure the CTA and fluoroscopy are coregistered such that they precisely overlay each other and are identically scaled. Subsequent deployment of the device using live fluoroscopy with the CTA overlay allows approximate knowledge of the plane of the defect and the rim tissue. This technology continues to improve with

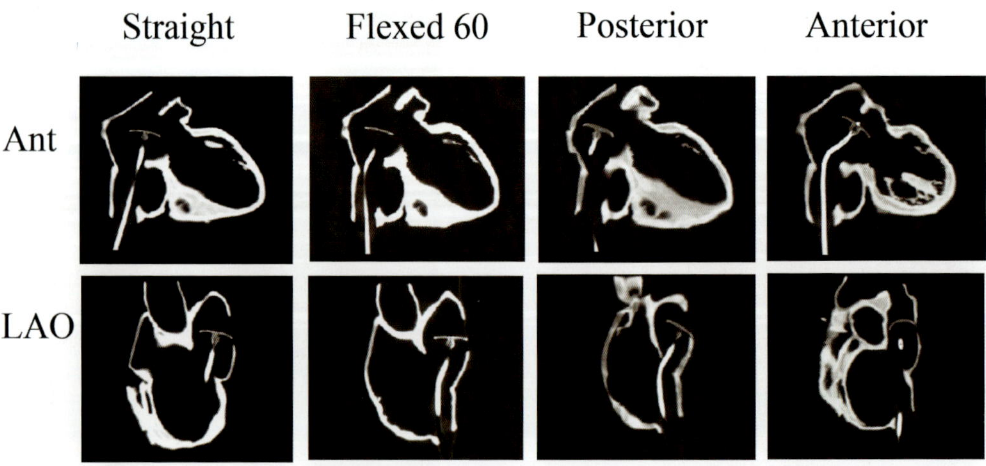

Fig 9.8—CTA-derived model used to assess modifiable delivery system shape relative to plane of defect. Catheter position is simulated in panel for the anterior (Ant) and left anterior oblique (LAO) image planes.

enhancements in the registration process, importation of dynamic images from CTA, and improvements in image display (Fig 9.9). While this approach is often used in the electrophysiology lab, its use in the structural heart disease interventional lab remains for the most part investigative.[26]

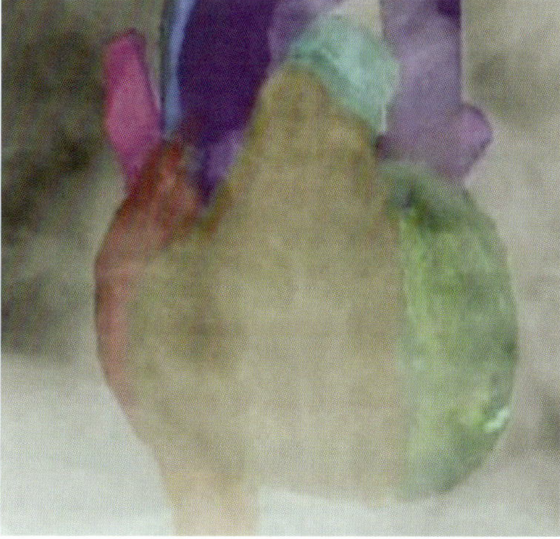

Fig 9.9—CTA and fluoroscopy coregistration. A fluoroscopic image is shown with an overlay of a segmented CTA image that was acquired preprocedure. The colors allow clearer chamber identification.

Advanced Image Processing of CTA Images and Presentation as Physical Models

Appreciation of the size and shape of interatrial abnormalities as well as the relationship to surrounding structures is not intuitive especially to adult cardiologists learning device closure. On the other hand an accurate physical model of a patient's heart enables an efficient and intuitive approach to not only understanding the patient-specific anatomy but also to plan and simulate an interventional procedure.

Starting in 2007 the 3D Lab in the Interventional Cardiology section at the University of Colorado, in collaboration with Dr. Robert Quaife, head of the Advanced Cardiac Imaging service at the University of Colorado Hospital have taken routine CTA studies and transformed them into the rapid prototyping data form of an STL file. The STL file can subsequently be used by a variety of commercially available 3D printing technologies to create a physical model. The initial methodology and clinical applications have been fully described in several publications.[27–29]

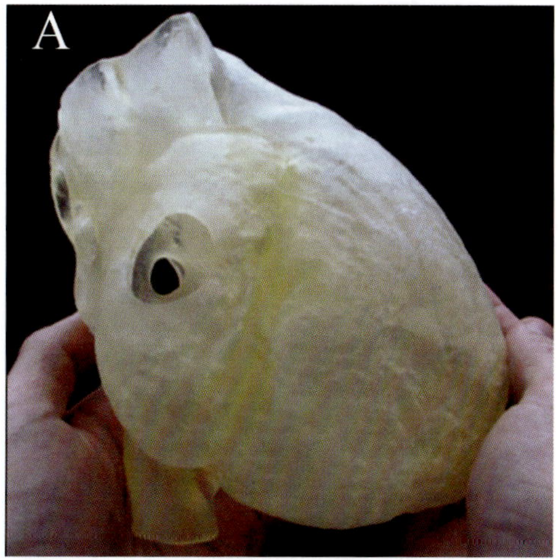

Right atrial view (anterior)

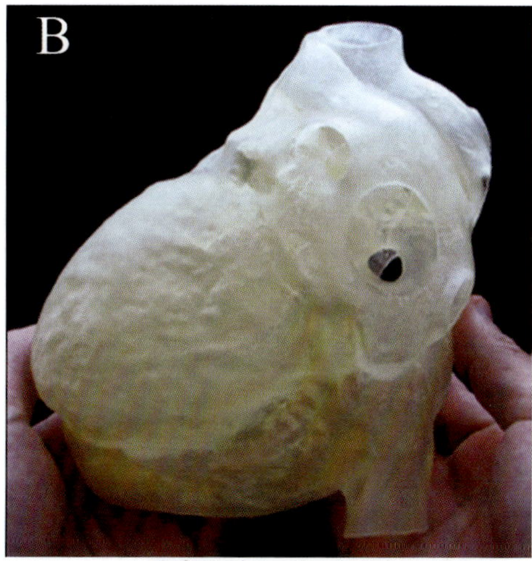

Left atrial view (posterior)

Fig 9.10—Physical model of small secundum ASD. A, View of defect through window in anterior right atrial wall. B, View of defect through window in posterior left atrial wall

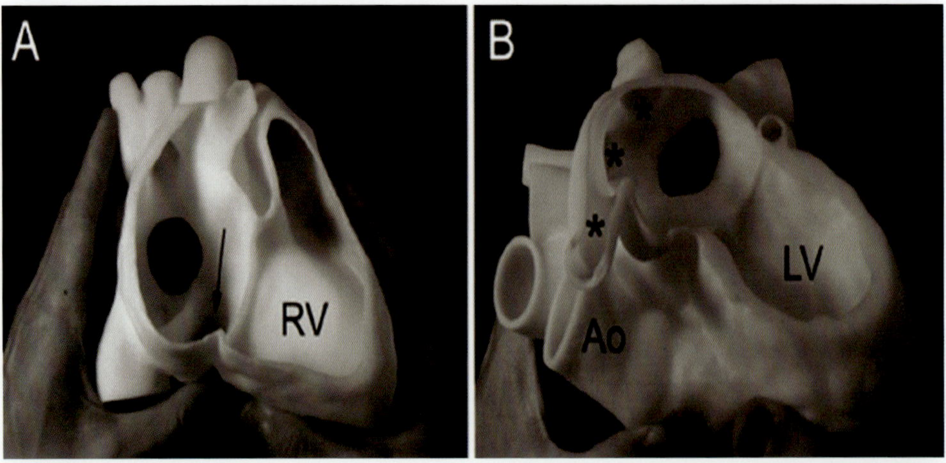

Fig 9.11—CT planning for device deployment. Physical model of ASD to clarify 3D relationships. Panel A demonstrates location of the ASD relative to the coronary sinus ostium (arrow). Panel B demonstrates the location of the ASD relative to the pulmonary veins (asterisks).

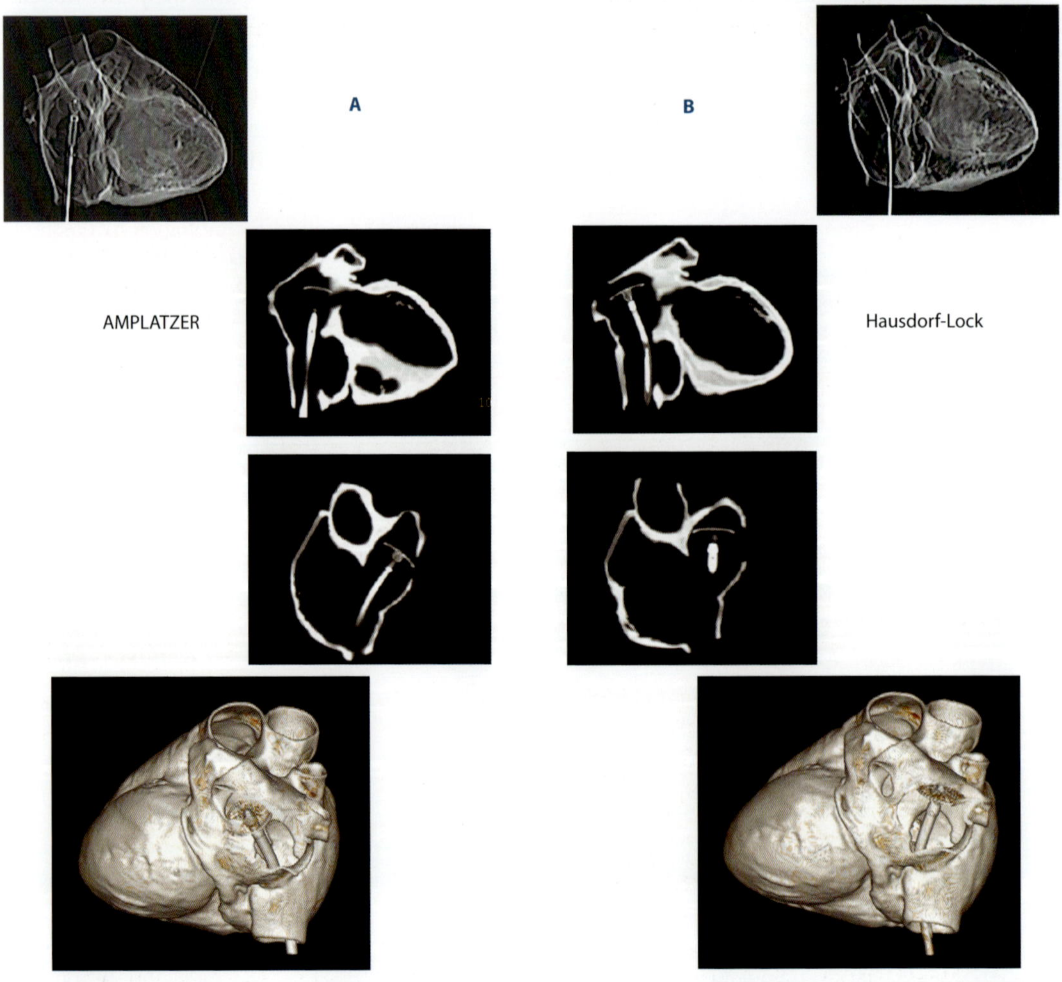

Fig 9.12—CTA-derived model used to assess delivery system shape relative to plane of defect. Two delivery systems were used; the AGA delivery catheter and the Hausdorf-Lock shape.

The first step of identifying all surfaces of the heart is changing but CT yields data which can be graphically displayed that clearly visualize the interatrial defect and surrounding structures (Fig 9.10). Subsequently a physical model is created. Figure 9.11 shows a model created with viewing windows in the walls of the right and left atria to observe the atrial septal defect.

Models can more clearly help physicians understand the 3D relationships of structures contiguous to the interatrial septum. Figure 9.11 shows a model that clarifies the defect's relationship to the coronary sinus, Eustachian ridge, and pulmonary veins.

The models can also be used to show how different delivery catheter shapes are appropriate or inappropriate to the different ASD sizes, shapes, and spatial orientation of the plane of the defect. In Figs 9.12 and 9.13, examples are shown of different delivery systems placed in models that then undergo imaging by an ex vivo CTA.

Finally models are useful for simulation of device placement. In Fig 9.14 it becomes apparent that a large residual shunt would result of placement of a septal occluder in this large oval-shaped defect.

Conclusions

CTA is an important imaging modality to understand and use in the course of both routine patient care but also in research and training for transcatheter closure of interatrial septal defects. Whereas echocardiography may be the workhorse of simple ASD imaging and guid-

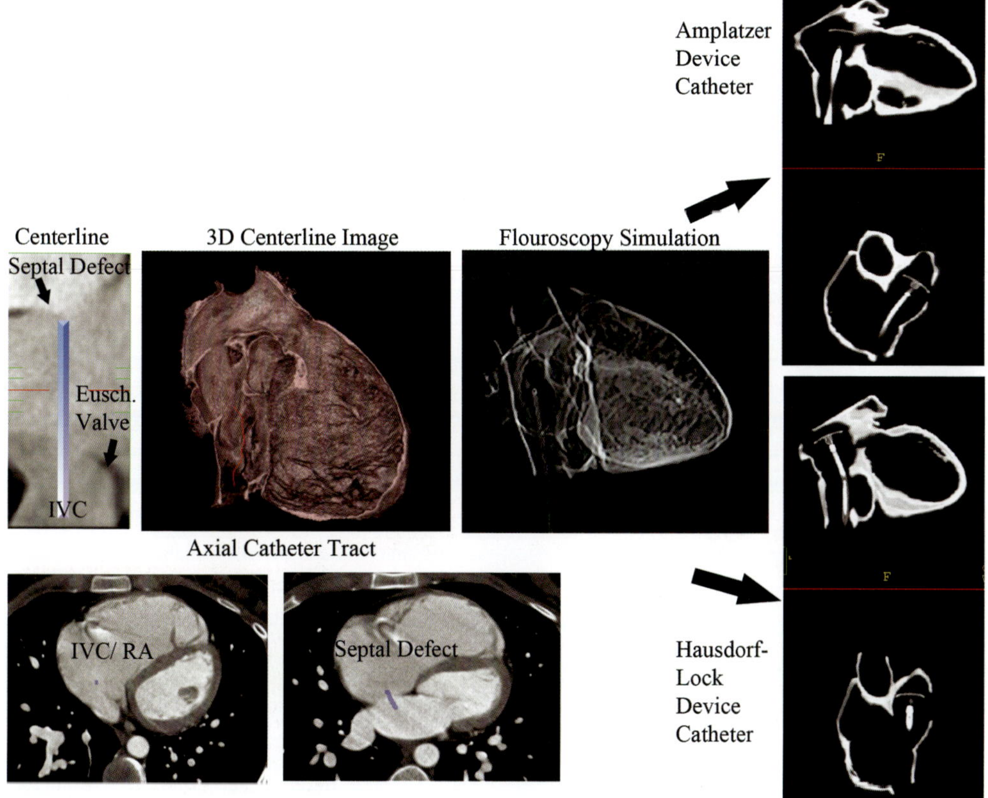

Fig 9.13—CTA planning for device deployment. Shown on the left is a centerline, catheter simulation (blue) of the inferior vena cava (IVC) to the defect. Two axial images are shown with the corresponding 3D volumetric CT images. Then using a model, fluoroscopic and catheter position/projections with the left atrial disk deployed are simulated for this patient and this specific ASD.

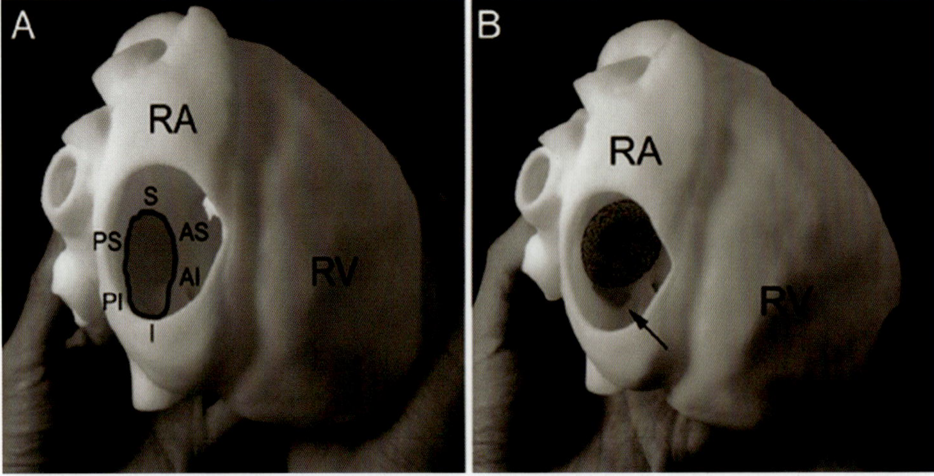

Fig 9.14—Physical model to assess device-defect mismatch. Panel A demonstrates a large, oval-shaped ASD with labeled rims (S, superior; AS, anterior septal; AI, antero-inferior; I, inferior; PI, postero-inferior; PS, postero-superior). Panel B demonstrates placement of a large AMPLATZER ASO with inability to appose the inferior rim (arrow).

ance for closure, CTA is essential in more complex anatomy, when echocardiography fails, and in advanced imaging applications such as image coregistration, rapid prototyping, and whole heart modeling.

Acknowledgments

Michael Kim, MD, James Chen, PhD, and Adam Hansgen have been partners in the development of the rapid prototyping approach to understanding interatrial defects.

References

1. Brickner ME, Hillis LD, Lange RA. Congenital heart disease in adults. First of two parts. *N Engl J Med.* 2000;342(4):256–263.

2. Steiner RM, Reddy GP, Flicker S. Congenital cardiovascular disease in the adult patient: imaging update. *J Thorac Imaging.* 2002 17(1):1–17.

3. AboulHosn J, French WJ, Buljubasic N, Matthews RV, Budoff MJ, Shavelle DM. Electron beam angiography for the evaluation of percutaneous atrial septal defect closure. *Catheter Cardiovasc Interv.* 2005;65(4):565–568.

4. Lipton, MJ, Higgins CB, Farmer D, Boyd DP. Cardiac imaging with a high-speed Cine-CT Scanner: preliminary results. *Radiology.* 1984;152(3):579–582.

5. Skotnicki R, MacMillan RM, Rees MR, et al. Detection of atrial septal defect by contrast-enhanced ultrafast computed tomography. *Cathet Cardiovasc Diagn.* 1986;12(2):103–106.

6. Funabashi N, Asano M, Sekine T, Nakayama T, Komuro I. Direction, location, and size of shunt flow in congenital heart disease evaluated by ECG-gated multislice computed tomography. *Int J Cardiol.* 2006;112(3):399–404.

7. Gade CL, Bergman G, Naidu S, Weinsaft JW, Callister TQ, Min JK. Comprehensive evaluation of atrial septal defects in individuals undergoing percutaneous repair by 64-detector row computed tomography. *Int J Cardiovasc Imaging.* 2007;23(3):397–404.

8. Kim YJ, Hur J, Choe KO, et al. Interatrial shunt detected in coronary computed tomography angiography: differential features of a patent foramen ovale and an atrial septal defect. *J Comput Assist Tomogr.* 2008;32(5):663–667.

9. Chen MY, Quaife RA, Groves BM, Carroll JD. Cardiac computed tomographic angiography pre-procedural planning for percutaneous atrial septal defect closure. Presented at the 2006 AHA Scientific Sessions. 2006.

10. Berger F, Ewert P, Abdul-Khaliq H, Nurnberg JH, Lange PE. Percutaneous closure of large atrial septal defects with the AMPLATZER Septal Occluder: technical overkill or recommendable alternative treatment? *J Interv Cardiol.* 2001;14(1):63–67.

11. Knirsch W, Dodge-Khatami A, Valsangiacomo-Buechel E, Weiss M, Berger F. Challenges encountered during closure of atrial septal defects. *Pediatr Cardiol.* 2005;26(2):147–153.

12. Hijazi ZM, Cao Q-L, Patel HT, Rhodes J, Hanlon KM. Transesophageal echocardiographic results of catheter closure of atrial septal defect in children and adults using the AMPLATZER device. *Am J Cardiol.* 2000;85(11):1387–1390.

13. Schwinger ME, Gindea AJ, Freedberg RS, Kronzon I. The anatomy of the interatrial septum: a transesophageal echocardiographic study. *Am Heart J.* 1990;119(6):1401–1405.

14. Harper RW, Mottram PM, McGaw DJ. Closure of secundum atrial septal defects with the AMPLATZER septal occluder device: techniques and problems. *Cathet Cardiovasc Intervent.* 2002;57(4):508–524.

15. Hein R, Buscheck F, Fischer E, et al. Atrial and ventricular septal defects can safely be closed by percutaneous intervention. *J Interv Cardiol.* 2005;18(6):515–522.

16. Bartel T, Konorza T, Neudorf U, et al. Intracardiac echocardiography: an ideal guiding tool for device closure of interatrial communications. *Eur J Echocardiogr.* 2005;6(2):92–96.

17. Hijazi ZM. Catheter closure of atrial septal and ventricular septal defects using the AMPLATZER devices. *Heart Lung Circ.* 2003;12 (suppl 2):S63–S72.

18. Piaw CS, Kiam OT, Rapaee A, et al. Use of non-invasive phase contrast magnetic resonance imaging for estimation of atrial septal defect size and morphology: a comparison with trans-esophageal echo. *Cardiovasc Intervent Radiol.* 2006;29(2):230–234.

19. Berbarie RF, Anwar A, Dockery WD, Grayburn PA, Vallabhan RC, Schussler JM. Dramatic RV volume reduction following atrial septal defect closure demonstrated by multi-slice CT volume rendering. *Clin Cardiol.* 2006;29(8):372.

20. Durongpisitkul K, Tang NL, Soongswang J, Laohaprasitiporn D, Nanal A. Predictors of successful transcatheter closure of atrial septal defect by cardiac magnetic resonance imaging. *Pediatr Cardiol.* 2004;25(2):124–130.

21. Gupta A, Kapoor G, Dalvi B. Transcatheter closure of atrial septal defects. *Expert Rev Cardiovasc Ther.* 2004;2(5):713–719.

22. Webb GD, Smallhorn JF, Therrien J, Redington AN. Left to right shunts. In: Libby P, Bonow RO, Mann DL, Zipes DP, eds. *Braunwald's Heart Disease: A Textbook of Cardiovascular Medicine.* 8th ed. St. Louis: WB Saunders;2007:1577.

23. Webb G, Gatzoulis MA. Atrial septal defects in the adult: recent progress and overview. *Circulation.* 2006;114(15):1645–1653.

24. Zaidi AN, Cheatham JP, Raman SV, Cook SC. Multislice computed tomographic findings in symptomatic patients after septal occluder device implantation. *J Intervent Cardiol.* 2009;22:92–96.

25. Carroll JD. Device Erosion. *CCI.* 2009;73:931–932.

26. Garcia J, Eng MH, Chen SY, Carroll JD. Image guidance of percutaneous coronary and structural heart disease interventions using a computed tomography and fluoroscopic integration vascular disease management. 2007;4(3):89–87.

27. Kim M, Hansgen AR, Wink O, Quaife RA, Carroll JD. Rapid prototyping—A new tool in understanding and treating structural heart disease. *Circulation.* 2008;117:2388–2394.

28. Carroll JD. The Future of image guidance of cardiac interventions. *Cathet Cardiovasc Intervent.* 2007;70:783.

29. Kim MS, Hansgen AR, Carroll JD. Use of rapid prototyping in the care of patients with structural heart disease. *Trends Cardiovasc Med.* 2008;18(6):210–216.

10

Cardiac Magnetic Resonance Assessment of ASDs and PFOs: Relation to Device Closure, Pre and Post

Mark A. Fogel

Introduction

The use of cardiac magnetic resonance (CMR) in the evaluation of congenital heart disease has played an increasingly important role in modern medicine. Although the patient who comes for evaluation of the atrial septum generally has undergone echocardiography already, CMR can offer a number of unique contributions as well as overlapping capabilities to this assessment. This chapter will focus on these contributions as they apply to the atrial septum and congenital heart disease.

Advantages/Disadvantages of CMR as It Relates to the Atrial Septum

CMR is a broad-based noninvasive tool to assess the cardiovascular system including the atrial septum and does not expose the patient to ionizing radiation (which places the patient at risk for future neoplastic disease[1,2]). Because of its tomographic nature, there are no overlapping structures to obscure regions of interest as may occur in angiography and it is not limited to acoustic windows as in echocardiography. Patient size is nearly never a problem for imaging. There are no artifacts from calcifications, patches, or prosthetic valves as in echocardiography and three-dimensional (3D) reconstruction of images are routine. No contrast agents are needed to visualize luminae, cavities, and valves as is the case, again, in angiography.

Anatomically, the thin, detailed nature of the components of the atria and atrial septum require special techniques and experience to image by CMR but the effort is certainly worthwhile for the additional information that can be obtained. The atrial chambers and venous connections are identified effortlessly by CMR; however, the smaller structures of the septum

Transcatheter Closure of ASDs and PFOs: A Comprehensive Assessment. © 2010 Ziyad M. Hijazi, Ted Feldman, Mustafa H. Abdullah Al-Qbandi, and Horst Sievert, editors. Cardiotext Publishing, ISBN: 978-0-9790164-9-3.

and walls such as the pectinate muscles and crista terminalis cannot always be identified (although most of the times, this is not necessary). Accurate assessment of these thin structures requires creative use of many different forms of CMR techniques. Although anatomic evaluation with static dark or bright blood imaging can visualize the atrial septum or lack thereof, these techniques cannot be used alone. The full battery of technology necessary to make an accurate diagnosis regarding the atria and atrial septum may include bright blood cine imaging, the use of presaturation bands with cine imaging, phase contrast velocity encoded imaging for anatomy and flow assessment, and imaging in numerous appropriate prescribed planes.

In evaluating anatomy, one of the powers of CMR is its wide field of view, allowing for associated lesions of the atrial septum to be assessed. For example, the anatomy of valves can be easily evaluated using either steady-state free precession (SSFP) or spoiled gradient echo techniques both en face or in long-axis views as in the case of an endocardial cushion defect associated with an ostium primum atrial septal defect (ASD). In addition, valve function can be assessed utilizing cine CMR[3] and phase encoded velocity mapping[3,4] which is more robust and gives more useful and quantitative information than the information obtained using echocardiography or cardiac catheterization (see following). Sequences utilizing gadolinium as a magnetic contrast agent can create a 3D image of the associated findings with atrial septal pathology[5] such as partial anomalous pulmonary venous connections as in the case of sinus venosus ASDs. Postoperatively, increased fibrous scar tissue on a patch associated with an ASD closure may easily be visualized utilizing delayed enhancement.[6]

As it relates to the atrial septum and ASDs, a distinct advantage of CMR is the capability of assessing ventricular volumes and mass independent of geometric assumptions because of its tomographic nature.[7] This is accomplished utilizing cine CMR with contiguous short-axis images from base to apex. Multiple publications used to validate echocardiographic techniques use CMR as the gold standard,[8,9] and it is generally accepted that CMR is the method of choice for this evaluation. This is extremely useful in assessing the volume overload physiology of interatrial communications and its associated anomalies (eg, partial anomalous pulmonary venous connections). Phase encoded velocity mapping is a CMR technique that can measure flow across the cross-sectional area of a blood vessel ("through plane") or image velocity in the plane of the image ("in-plane" velocity mapping) similar to Doppler echocardiography. Though plane imaging is useful in evaluation of the pulmonary to systemic flow ratio (Qp/Qs),[10] cardiac index or atrioventricular valve insufficiency, and in-plane imaging is useful in identifying ASDs.

A unique capability of functional evaluation using CMR is that in nearly all imaging strategies, the image is an average of many heartbeats (unlike echocardiography and angiography) and therefore, may better reflect the long-term functioning of the cardiovascular system.[11] The image itself is actually an average, embedding the function of the ventricle or the flow in the main pulmonary artery over the course of 15 seconds to 2 minutes. The healthcare provider does not have to view many heartbeats and do this averaging "in his/her head" as in echocardiography and angiography. In addition, quantitative data from CMR usually have internal checks; for example, Qp/Qs using cine CMR (in the absence of valve regurgitation) should be the same as with velocity mapping or flows in the branch pulmonary arteries should equal flow in the main pulmonary artery. This common practice of internal checks makes CMR a highly accurate quantitative tool to assess physiology and function.

CMR has a few limitations. Patients with coils, pacemakers, or pacemaker wires cannot be imaged because of the effects from and on the magnetic field. Devices such as those used for ASD closure yield a localized artifact so the details of the device itself cannot be imaged. Sternal wires may give some artifacts near the region of interest. Patients need to remain motionless in the scanner so infants, small children, and uncooperative subjects need to be sedated. For those who aren't sedated, claustrophobia may be an issue although this is rare. With new imaging sequences, arrhythmias generally are not a problem anymore but occasionally may preclude successful imaging.

Protocol and Techniques Utilized to Evaluate the Atrial Septum, ASDs, and Associated Anomalies

A generalized protocol must be employed to effectively assess the atrial septum, ASD, and associated anomalies although each exam must be tailored to the individual. This generalized approach to CMR assessment is not the only one but the author feels it is one that can be useful in most instances and is most efficient at being comprehensive and diagnostic in the least amount of time.

After localizing the heart in the chest, the first procedure performed is acquiring anatomic data, which gives a basic survey of the cardiovascular system; acts as localizers themselves for future anatomic, physiologic, and functional imaging; and ensures that there are no artifacts to contend with near the regions of interest. A full, volumetric, contiguous axial data set from the diaphragm to the thoracic inlet is obtained generally using "static" SSFP (eg, true-FISP) which is a "bright blood technique"—the blood vessels and cavities of the heart are bright and the myocardium and other tissues are gray. This type of imaging is acquired in diastole so the diastolic dimensions of the right atrium (RA), right ventricle (RV), and pulmonary arteries can be evaluated. These axial images form the basis of examining the anatomy and identifying the spectrum of diseases associated with atrial septal pathology such as partial or total anomalous pulmonary venous connection or endocardial cushion defects. Evaluation of postoperative ASDs such as in hypoplastic left

heart syndrome can also be performed. A final reason why this is performed first is that if the patient becomes unstable or if there are technical difficulties with the scanner or computers, a full volumetric, anatomic data set has already been obtained.

The axial images are stacked one atop the other by specialized software called multiplanar reconstruction, which allows any plane of interest to be reconstructed. Exact slice orientations and positions can be obtained for future imaging during the scan. This procedure also allows for inspection of the anatomy from multiple views from just the set of axial images. So, the atrial septum and ASD can be sliced in multiple views to visualize the salient points of the anatomy.

Dark blood imaging is another imaging technique performed for anatomy (Fig 10.1); this form of static imaging is used sparingly because it is time consuming. One or two images can be obtained in a breathhold. As the name suggests, blood from cavity and vessels are black while soft tissue is signal intense. It can be performed in a number of different ways with T1 weighting, T2 weighting, using spin echo, turbo spin echo, double or triple inversion recovery, etc. This can be used to visualize ASDs or associated pathology.

Cine CMR is generally the next technique applied (Figs 10.2 and 10.3) and is tailored to the lesion under study. It is one of the "workhorses" of CMR, used to visualize cardiac motion, turbulent blood flow (a signal void or blackness in the image is created) and assess ventricular volumes. In general, when examining the atrial septum and ASDs, the structures and lesions are visualized in two orthogonal planes (eg, a four-chamber view and a sagittal view) with contiguous cine slices covering the entire septum. Turbulence (or lack thereof) can be noted crossing the atrial septum as "black" on the image. This is more noticeable on the gradient echo type of cine CMR than the SSFP type and if an interatrial communication is suspected but not visualized on SSFP cine, the gradient echo type with longer echo times (TE 7–10 ms) should be done. In addition, the technique of

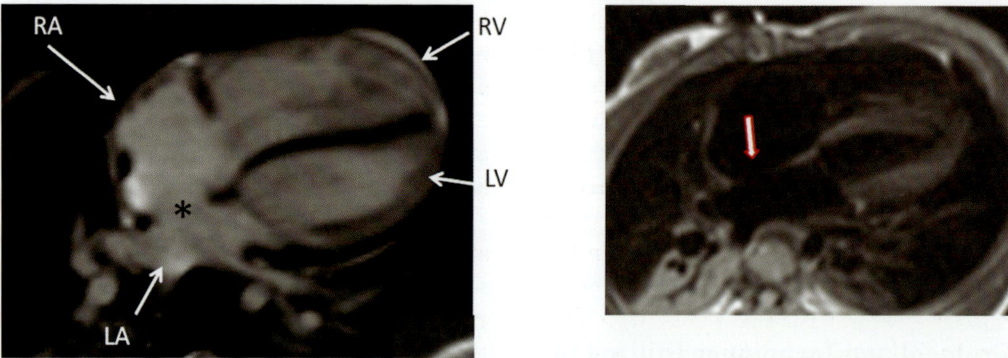

Fig 10.1—Secundum atrial septal defect. The left and right panels are steady-state free precession and double inversion dark blood imaging respectively of a secundum atrial septal defect (star in upper left and arrow in lower right) in a 16-month-old child. Both images are of the four-chamber view. Noted the mild right ventricular (RV) dilatation. Abbreviations: LA, left atrium; LV, left ventricle; RA, right atrium.

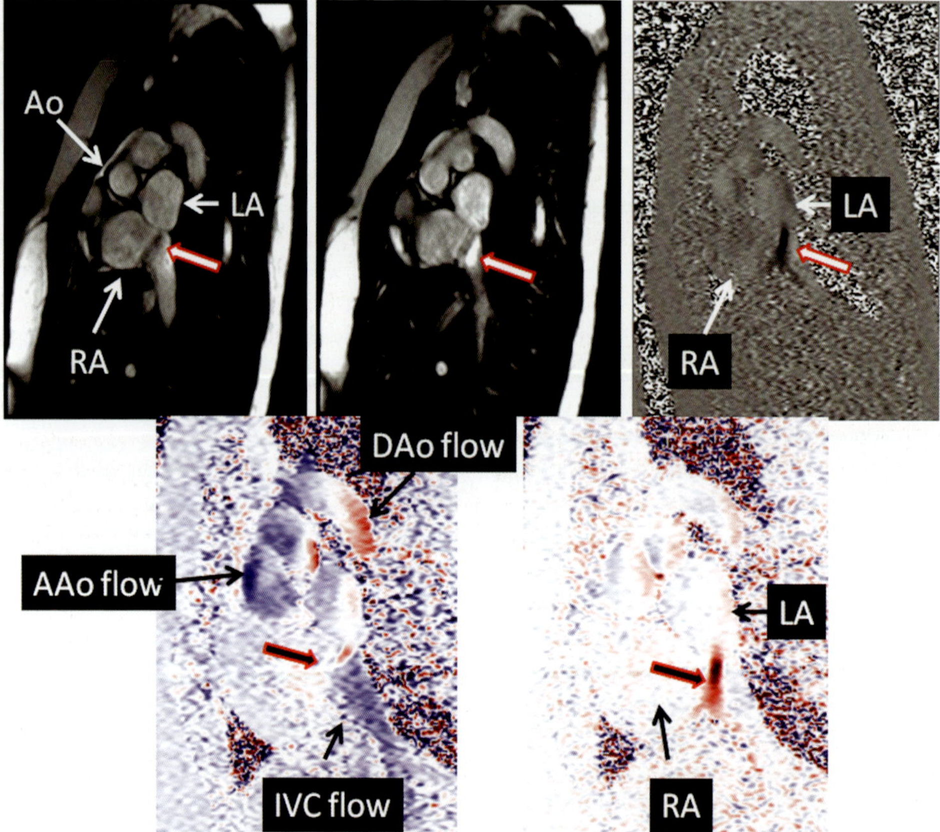

Fig 10.2—Cine and in-plane phase encoded velocity mapping of a small secundum atrial septal defect (ASD). Even small ASDs can be visualized by CMR. The upper left and middle panels are off-axis sagittal cine images of a small secundum ASD from a 3-year-old; note the turbulence on cine (arrows). The upper panel is an in-plane phase encoded velocity map in the same orientation as the upper left and middle panels where flow inferiorly is labeled "dark" and flow superiorly is labeled "white." Arrow denotes flow from the left atrium (LA) to the right atrium (RA). Just as in color flow echocardiography, cardiac magnetic resonance can color code flow; the lower right and left panels are color-coded in-plane velocity maps in the same orientation as the upper panels. Flow toward inferiorly is red and superiorly is blue; note the left-to-right flow (arrow) designated as red while flow in the inferior vena cava (IVC) and ascending aorta (AAo) is blue (opposite flow from the ASD flow). Flow in the descending aorta (DAo), as expected, is red and is directed inferiorly.

presaturation blood tagging (in which the spins of the protons in a region where a tag is laid down are destroyed and hence, the blood from this area is "black"), dark regions of flow across an ASD can been visualized in the bright areas of the atrial cavity if flow is from the dark region to the bright region (eg, left-to-right flow where the presaturation tag is on the left atrium). If flow is from the bright to dark regions, bright blood flow will be visualized across the ASD to enter the dark areas (eg, right-to-left flow where the presaturation tag is on the left atrium). See Fig 10.10 for primum ASD in the following text

as an example of presaturation tagging. Utilization of in-plane velocity mapping to visualize flow across the ASD will be discussed later.

ASDs and atrial pathology can be associated with a number of atrioventricular valve lesions. To visualize these, an RV long-axis view and four-chamber view through the valve are obtained. From these cines, evaluation of tricuspid valve regurgitation or stenosis can be assessed. Cine CMR is the technique used to visualize leaflets and their attachments, which is especially important in cases of endocardial cushion defects or Ebstein's anomaly. An en

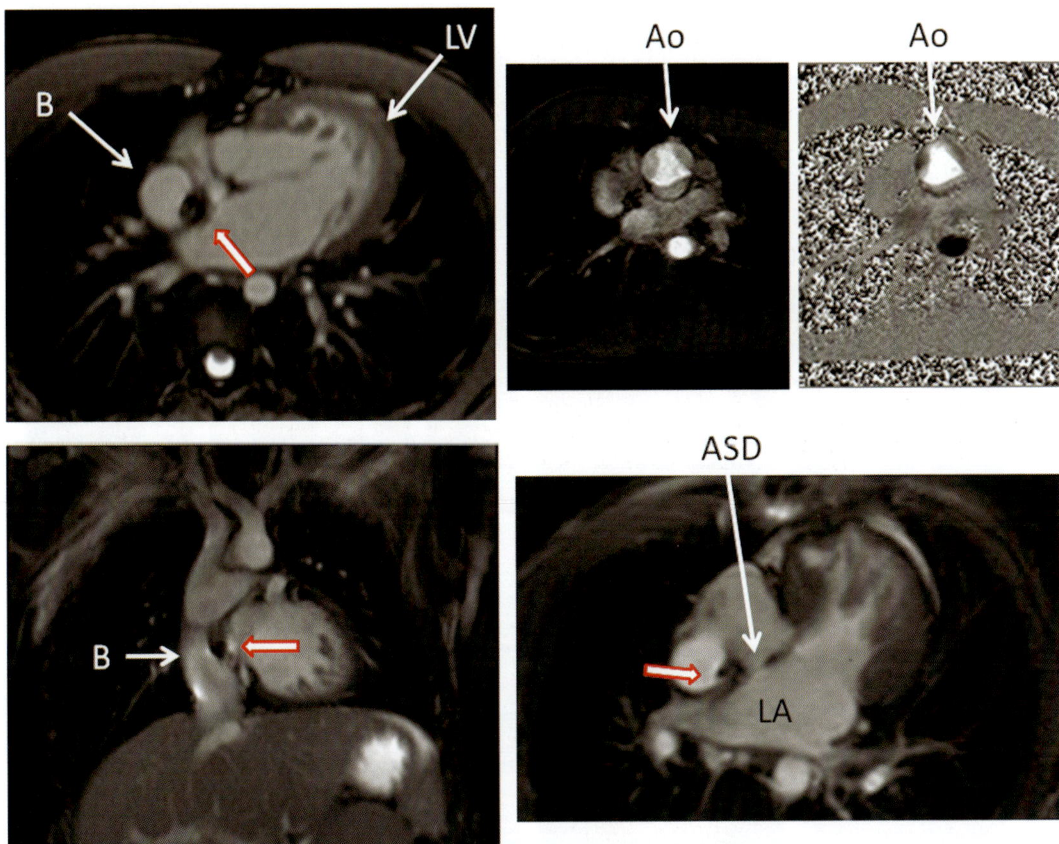

Fig 10.3—Tricuspid atresia with atrial septal defect (ASD) after Fontan and closure of fenestration with a CardioSEAL device. This is an 18-year-old, single ventricle patient with a lateral wall tunnel Fontan baffle with a fenestration (communication between the systemic and pulmonary venous pathways), which was closed by a CardioSEAL device. The right images are steady-state free precession images in the axial (top) and coronal (bottom) planes demonstrating the Fontan baffle (B) in cross-section (top) and in long axis (bottom). The CardioSEAL device artifact is show by the arrow. Note the absence of a right ventricle. The lower right panel is also a steady-state free precession image in systole in the "three-chamber" view demonstrating the ASD and the CardioSEAL device artifact (arrow). The upper middle and right panels are anatomic (middle) and phase (right) images of the aortic (Ao) valve; the phase encoded velocity mapping technique allows for measurement of cardiac index and pulmonary to systemic flow ratios (Qp/Qs). Abbreviation: LV, left ventricle.

face view of the valve is used to obtain morphologic information of leaflet size and coaptation; although SSFP imaging can be utilized for this purpose, the author prefers gradient echo images with a high flip angle that increases the signal of inflowing blood and highlight the leaflet edges.

Cine CMR is also utilized to evaluate ventricular volumes, mass, ejection fraction, and cardiac index[3,12–14] which are significant parameters in the setting of ASDs and their associated lesions. After obtaining four-chamber and long-axis views of the ventricles, a set of contiguous cine CMR slices are performed in short axis from base to apex (usually 8 to 12 slices, thickness depending upon the length of the ventricles) at a temporal resolution of ~25 to 50 ms, depending upon the heart rate. The endocardial borders of each slice are contoured at end-diastole and end-systole and measuring the areas,

end-diastolic and end-systolic ventricular volumes can be obtained (the product of the areas and slice thickness, summed across all slice levels). Stroke volume, cardiac output, and ejection fraction are calculated in the usual fashion. The difference in left ventricular (LV) and RV stroke volumes, in the absence of valve regurgitation will yield the Qp/Qs. By contouring the epicardial borders of the ventricles at end diastole and subtracting end-diastolic volume, ventricular mass can be obtained. Myocardial tagging can be used if regional wall motion is an issue; this technique will not be discussed in this chapter.

Gadolinium is a magnetic contrast agent and although it is not used directly in routine practice to image the atrial septum, it is used to create 3D models of the associated abnormalities with atrial septal pathology such as the partial anomalous pulmonary venous connections (Fig 10.4). This type of imaging is next

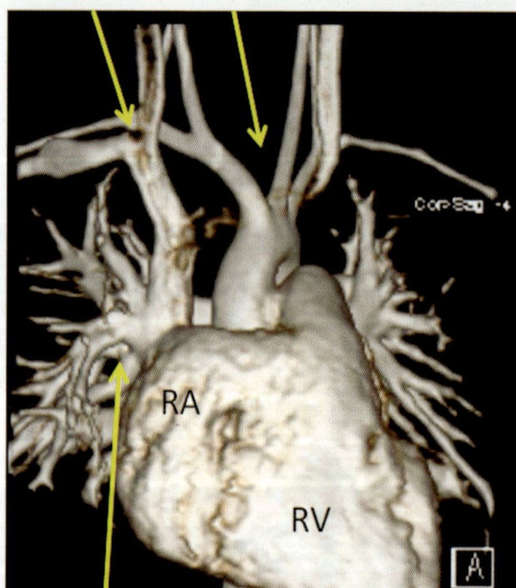
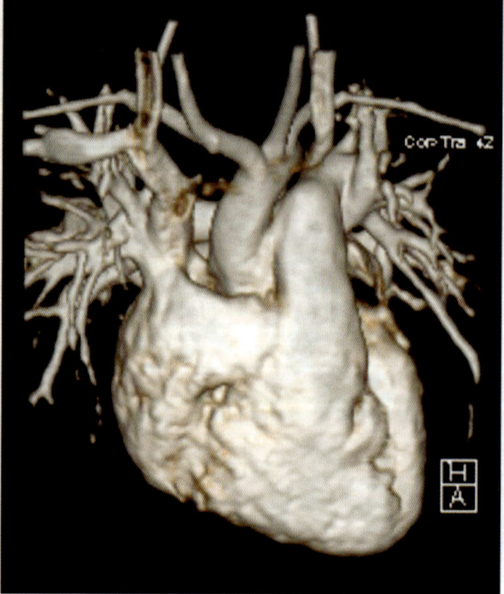

Fig 10.4—Three-dimension reconstruction of partial anomalous pulmonary venous connection of the right upper (RUPV) and right middle pulmonary veins (RMPV) associated with sinus venosus ASD of the superior vena cava type (SVC). The left panel is an anterior view and the right panel is the same view tipped toward the transverse view. Note the connection of the RUPV and RMPV to the SVC just above the SVC-right atrial (RA) junction. Abbreviations: Ao, aorta; RV, right ventricle.

performed after cines. Gadolinium accumulates in scar tissue and using a technique called delayed enhancement or viability imaging, this scar tissue can be visualized as a signal intense region on the image (Fig 10.5).[15] Viability imaging is usually done 10 minutes after gadolinium administration and while that time passes, velocity mapping is typically performed (see following). A recent study[6] has demonstrated that delayed enhancement "lights up" surgical patches as well and although there is some speculation about the mechanism, it is unknown why this is the case (see Fig 10.5). This may also be used to evaluate for scar tissue in the myocardium postoperatively.[15] Specialized gadolinium techniques can also evaluate myocardial

perfusion,[16] which may be important in lesions associated with ASDs and PFOs such as tricuspid atresia.

Velocity mapping (Figs 10.2, 10.3, and 10.6–10.8) is a CMR technique that uses the phase information in the image to measure velocity and flow.[17-19] In the through-plane version (Fig 10.3), velocity is measured perpendicular to the imaging plane and flow can be calculated; the in-plane version (Figs 10.2, 10.7, and 10.8) measures velocity in the plane of the image similar to echocardiography. On the image, directionality is encoded as either white or black and the amount of "whiteness" or "blackness" represents the degree of velocity and flow although it could be color coded similar to echocardiog-

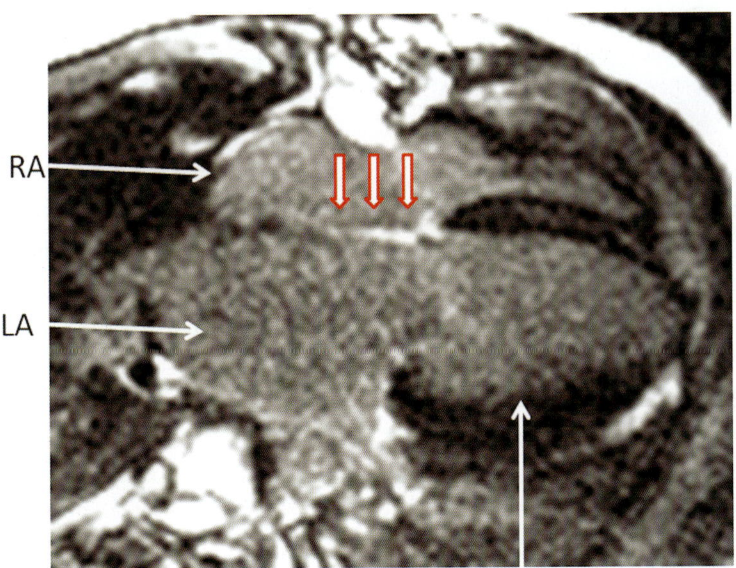

Fig 10.5—Delayed enhancement (viability imaging) and patch material. This is a four-chamber view delayed enhancement image from a 3-year-old with a complete common atrioventricular canal after repair. The atrial and ventricular septal defects were closed with a patch. It is presumed that fibrous tissue is formed over the patch, which accumulated gadolinium approximately 10 minutes after injection and shows up as "white" on the image. This can be used to positively identify the patch area where an atrial septal defect was closed.[6]

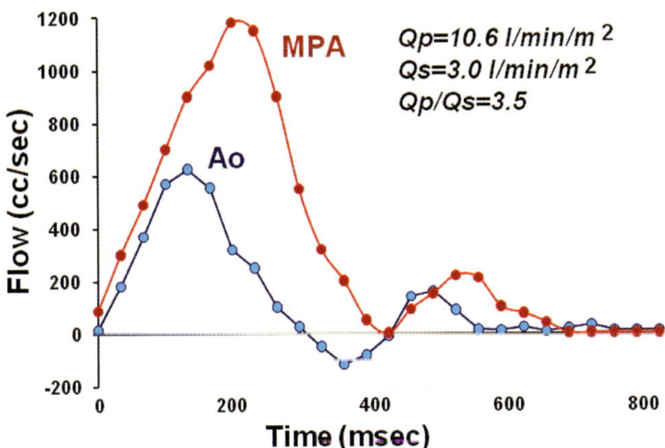

Fig 10.6—Flow-time curves. This graph plots the flow-time curves across the aortic valve (Ao) and main pulmonary artery (MPA) in a patient with a large secundum type atrial septal defect. The pulmonary flow (Qp) to systemic flow (Qs) ratio is elevated to 3.5. Abbreviations: cc, cubic centimeters; l/min/m², liters/minute/meter squared; msec, milliseconds; sec, seconds.

raphy (Fig 10.2). In the context of atrial septal pathology, velocity mapping is mostly used to (1) measure Qp/Qs[29] (Fig 10.6) and (2) visualize ASD flow including the anatomic delineation of the lesion (Fig 10.2). In a study of 44 patients, an en face view of the ASD using velocity mapping correlated well with final device size for closure and importantly, added additional information which changed management in 20% when compared with echocardiography alone.[20] It can also be utilized to obtain RV pressure estimates with a tricuspid regurgitation jet similar to Doppler echocardiography as well as measuring tricuspid regurgitant fractions in combination with ventricular volumes via cine CMR. Velocity

mapping is a very powerful tool, not only to measure flows, but also as an internal check to validate the CMR measures of physiology (see previous).

CMR of Specific Atrial Septal Defects

Secundum ASD (Figs 10.1, 10.2)

Defects in the atrial septum can be detected by CMR from early infancy through adulthood and the most common type of ASD is the secundum form, which is the result of a deficiency in

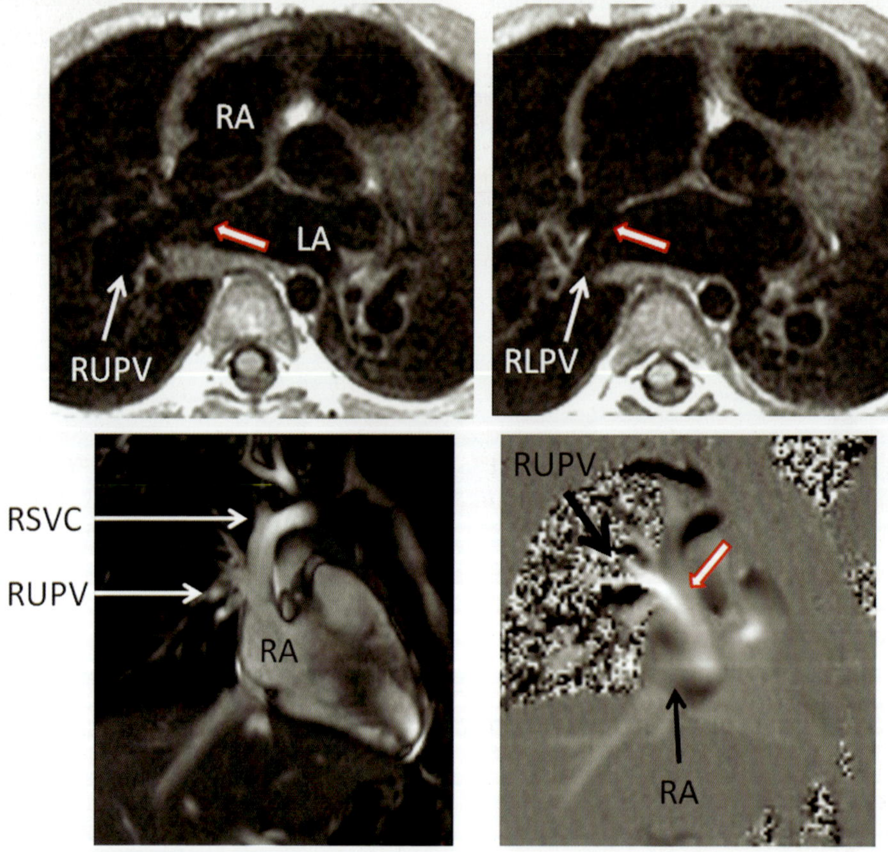

Fig 10.7—Sinus venosus atrial septal defect (ASD). Upper panels are two axial dark blood images of a sinus venosus ASD of the superior vena cava type (arrows) in a 5-year-old. The right upper pulmonary vein (RUPV) can be easily seen to straddle the atrial septum and be directed to the right atrium (RA). The right lower pulmonary vein (RLPV) is seen to connect normally to the left atrium (LA). The left lower panel is a cine image in an off-axis coronal view demonstrating the RUPV inserting at the right superior vena cava (RSVC)–RA junction. The right lower panel is an in-plane phase encoded velocity map in the same orientation as the left lower panel where flow is encoded "white" going right to left and "black" going the opposite way; note the RUPV flow directed toward the RA.

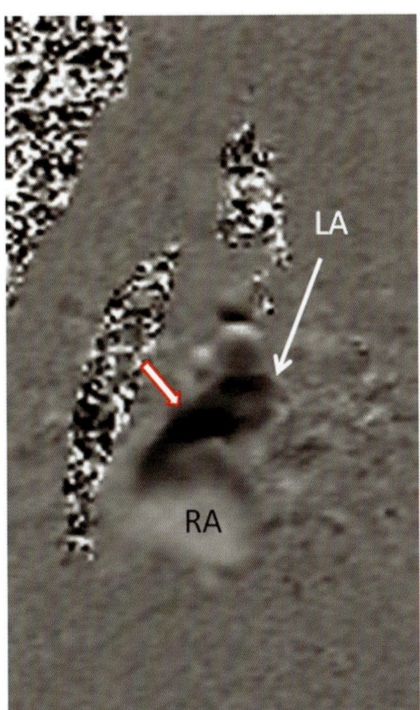

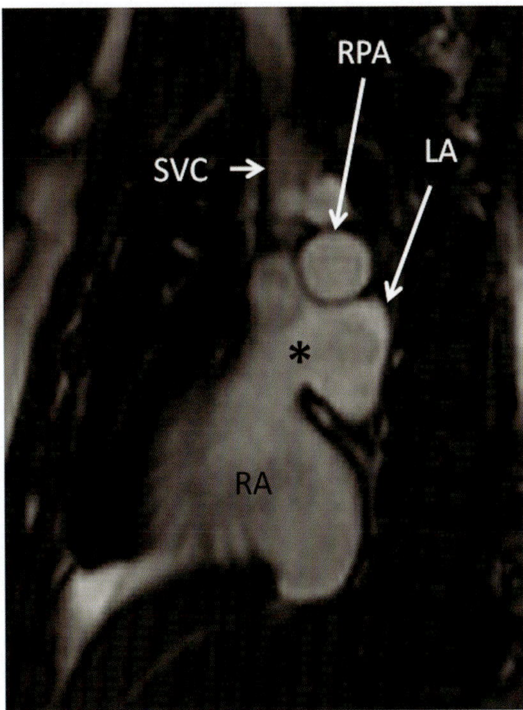

Fig 10.8—Sinus venosus atrial septal defect (ASD) of the superior vena cava (SVC) type. The right panel is an off-axis sagittal cine of a large sinus venosus ASD of the SVC type (star). The left panel is an in-plane phase encoded velocity map in the same orientation as the right panel where flow is encoded "white" going posteriorly (ie, toward the left atrium [LA]) and "black" going the opposite way (ie, toward the right atrium [RA]); note the left-to-right flow. Abbreviation: RPA, right pulmonary artery.

septum primum. CMR is used to determine the presence, dimensions, and margins of the defect along with the degree of shunting and effects on ventricular volume and cardiac function. CMR also allows for the evaluation of associated lesions, such as anomalous pulmonary veins or other simple or more complex congenital heart defects.

Using either static SSFP or dark blood techniques (Figs 10.1 and 10.2) to obtain a full axial volume data set covering the entire heart and great vessels, the atrial septum is initially localized. Axial images usually identify obvious defects. Combining multiple imaging methods, ASD size and margins can be measured accurately. In this plane, the atrial septum is easily localized and most significant secundum defects can be seen. There can, however, be normal thinning of the septum in the region of the fossa ovalis and with low signal intensity in

some techniques, there may be signal dropout, even when no ASD is present resulting in a false positive diagnosis if this was used alone. Caution should be used initially and further imaging is always mandatory to confirm the presence of the secundum ASD.

In the standard four-chamber or axial views, multiple contiguous slices with bright blood cine SSFP or gradient echo cine images can reveal the location of the ASD with the largest dimensions generally in the four-chamber view. Maximal flow across an ASD occurs in late systole or in early diastole during the rapid-filling period. As secundum ASDs are not perfectly round, the maximal diameter may occur in planes other than the four-chamber or axial ones. Orthogonal views are mandatory; however, bright blood cine and phase contrast in-plane imaging in multiple views with contiguous slices are utilized to determine the shape and maximal diameter. As noted earlier, the jet across the septum creates a signal void on cine, defining the width of the defect. When the shunt flow or signal void is difficult to visualize, presence of shunting can be enhanced with the placement of the presaturation slab (see Fig 10.10 on p. 150) on the LA ensuring that this slab does not cover other sources of flow into the RA (ie, superior or inferior vena cava). Similarly, a saturation slab can be applied to the RA if there is a question of right-to-left shunting.[21,22] In addition, in-plane phase encoded velocity mapping can "label" blood shunting across the defect when the direction of the velocity is encoded properly (see earlier and Figs 10.2, 10.7, and 10.8); care needs to be taken with regard to thickness because of partial volume effects. Views can include off-axis sagittal and four-chamber to visualize the flow in these defects. To assess ASD rims, multiple planes are also required to decide whether it is possible to close a large defect with a device in the catheterization laboratory.

With the geometry and the thickness of the atrial septum, an "en face" view for sizing can be difficult with standard bright or dark blood techniques. The thinning at the edges of the ASD could be mistaken for part of the defect. Phase contrast velocity mapping, however, has been used to size ASDs[23] by localizing in the axial and sagittal plane and imaging in the off-axis coronal plane to demonstrate the defect, which shows the overall shape and size. That study also demonstrated that CMR can determine ASD size and rims and detect associated venous anomalies when transthoracic echocardiography results are not conclusive. Multiple other studies have also compared CMR for ASD sizing to echocardiography, cardiac catheterization, and surgery[22,24–27] and demonstrated that the combination of bright blood and phase contrast imaging methods provide accurate measurements of ASD size and rims. Measurements of the defect and the surrounding rims to adjacent structures can be performed on both the magnitude (anatomic) and phase (velocity) images. Using the prior images obtained, planning scans through the ASD to the aorta and cavae allow for more rim measurements. All

this allows the patient to be appropriately sent to the catheterization laboratory or the operating suite for defect closure.

From a function and physiology standpoint, as mentioned previously, phase contrast, velocity-encoded imaging also is used to determine the degree of intracardiac shunting by measuring Qp/Qs[29] using through-plane measurements of the main pulmonary artery and proximal ascending aorta using a velocity encoding at 150 cm/sec (Fig 10.6). This type of flow measurements has been validated against catheterization.[28–30] Through-plane measurement in the plane of the ASD, however, may not accurately quantify the shunt.[29] As a complementary technique, RV volume overload and RA size due to flow across the secundum ASDs can be evaluated with ventricular volumes by cine and diastolic flattening of the ventricular septum. Comparison of the right and left ventricular stroke volumes will also be discrepant due to the shunt volume and can be used as a comparison with velocity mapping in the absence of valve regurgitation; however, with RV dilatation, the pulmonary and tricuspid valves may also dilate and demonstrate insufficiency. These findings can all be displayed with routine CMR imaging and the different contributions to the RV volume overload (from ASD flow or valve insufficiency) can be teased out.

Sinus venosus ASD (Figs 10.4, 10.7–10.9)

This type of interatrial communication is < 10% of all ASDs and occurs as generally two types. The more common type is a deficiency of the wall between the right superior vena cava (SVC) and right upper pulmonary vein (RUPV) located in the posterior atrial septum, behind the fossa ovalis. There is a resulting significant amount of left-to-right shunting directly from the RUPV to the RA with RA and RV dilation (Figs 10.4 and 10.7). The other type is located inferiorly toward the inferior vena cava (IVC) with anomalous drainage of the right lower pulmonary vein (RLPV) (Fig 10.9). CMR is utilized to diagnose the sinus venosus ASD and to iden-

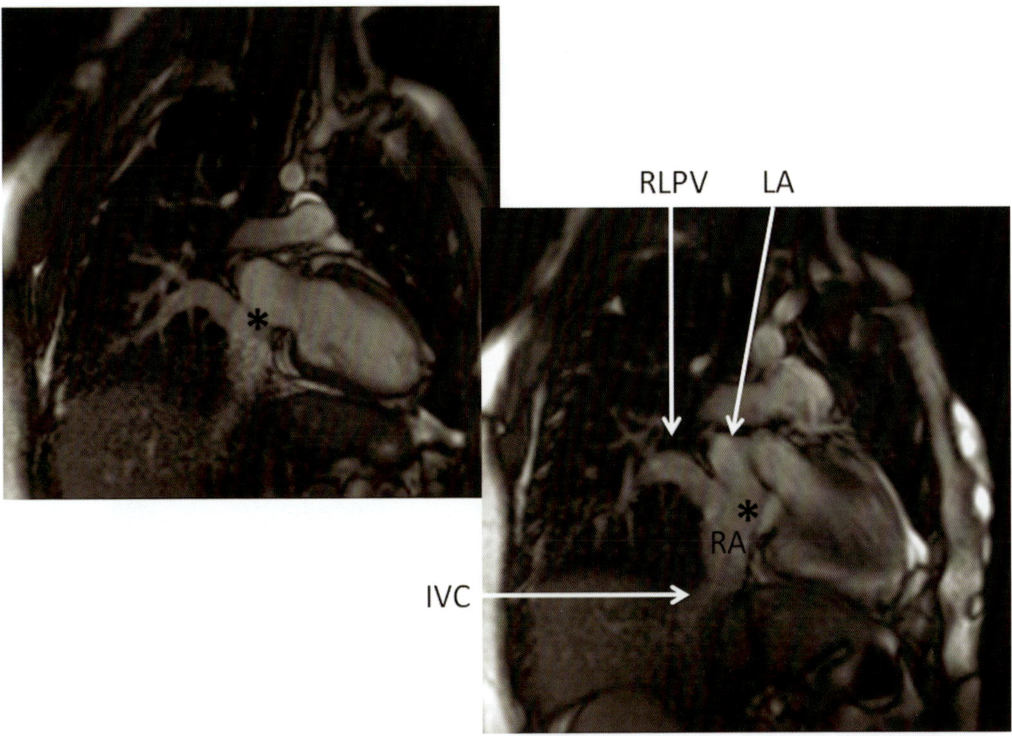

Fig 10.9—Partial anomalous pulmonary venous connection of the right lower pulmonary vein (RLPV) associated with sinus venosus atrial septal defect of the inferior vena cava type (IVC). The upper left and lower right panels are off-axis coronal images at different antero-posterior levels demonstrating the anomalous RLPV and the atrial septal defect (*). Abbreviations: RA, right atrium; LA, left atrium.

tify the pulmonary venous drainage pattern, which needs to be determined in preparation for surgical repair. One of the key advantages of CMR for sinus venosus ASDs is to identify all pulmonary veins preoperatively and to alert the surgeon to know what veins might need to be baffled and whether a Warden procedure is needed.

With standard axial bright blood or dark blood images covering the heart and great vessels, an obvious sinus venosus ASD is immediately identified (Figs 10.7 and 10.8). Anomalous pulmonary venous drainage is also easily seen (Figs 10.4, 10.7–10.9). Imaging is focused on the SVC-RA junction as well as the RUPV looking for absence of the posterior SVC wall and absence of atrial septal tissue dividing RA and LA. Similarly, IVC, RLPVs, and septal walls are also examined (Fig 10.9). Imaging planes are manipulated to identify all pulmonary venous

drainage by bright blood cine imaging. As with the secundum ASD, the hemodynamic significance of the shunting can be determined using the phase encoded velocity mapping for flow and volume analysis via cine techniques for ventricular volume overload. CMR in a recent study accurately demonstrated sinus venosus defects, anomalous pulmonary venous drainage, and additional important anomalies and was found superior to echocardiography in diagnosing these defects.[31]

Primum ASD (Fig 10.10)

A primum ASD is located inferiorly on the atrial septum near the atrioventricular valves and is a component of endocardial cushion defects which also include a common atrioventricular valve or abnormalities of the mitral valve along with a possible canal-type ventricular septal defect. These lesions are easily identified on CMR (Fig 10.10) and the effect of shunting and common atrioventricular or left atrioventricular valve insufficiency can be assessed with phase encoded velocity mapping and cine CMR for ventricular volumes. Associated defects can be delineated. CMR is an excellent tool to evaluate this type of lesion[32,33] and has proved useful in delineating the anatomy of the common atrioventricular valve, whether the common atrioventricular valve is malaligned or balanced over the ventricles, quantifying the common atrioventricular valve regurgitation and the ventricular function (using cine CMR and velocity mapping) and quantifying the pulmonary to systemic flow ratio (using velocity mapping across both the aorta and pulmonary artery). As this is treated surgically, it will not be discussed further.

Common Atrium

In this lesion, there is a lack of septal tissue and one large atrium is seen; this is often associated with heterotaxy syndromes and can be easily seen with CMR. Evaluation by CMR is

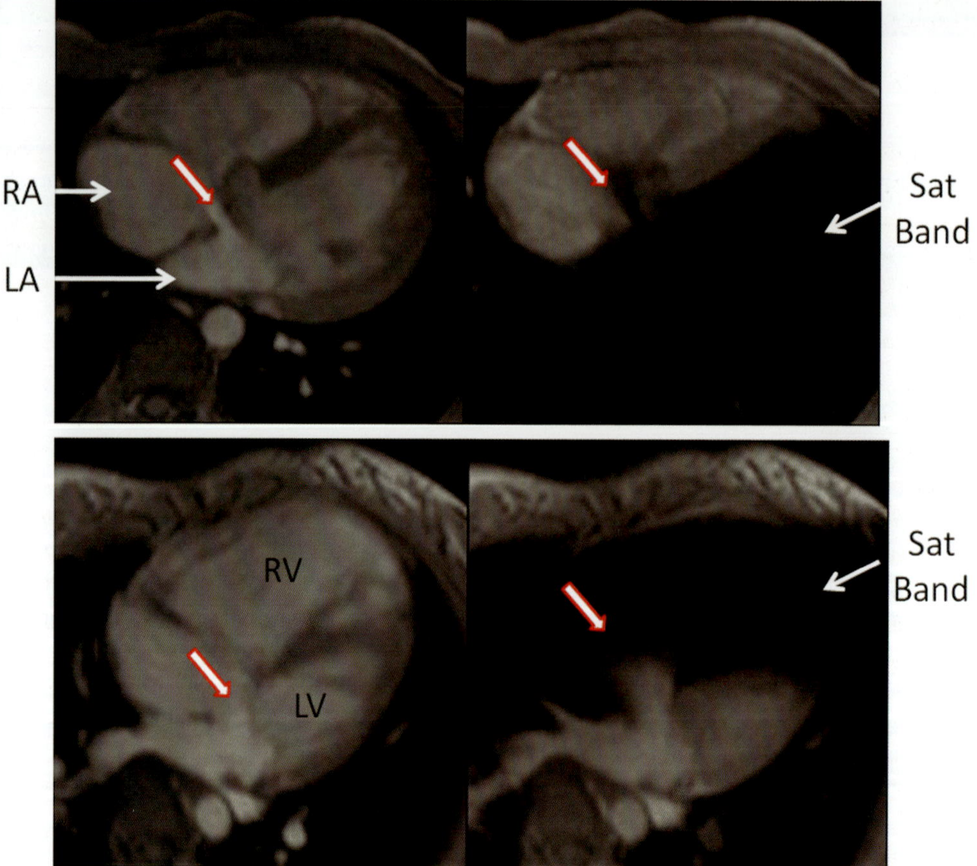

Fig 10.10—Primum atrial septal defect utilizing presaturation tagging. The upper and lower left panels are gradient echo images and the corresponding upper and lower right panels are the same images with a "presaturation tag" (Sat Band) on the left atrium (LA) (upper right) and the right atrium (RA) (lower right). The primum atrial septal defects are indicated with an arrow. Note the left-to-right flow in the upper panels with dark blood coursing into the RA with a Sat Band on the LA. With left-to-right flow in the lower panels, note the bright blood coursing into the RA with a Sat Band on the RA. Both patients have incomplete atrioventricular canal defects (note no blood crossing the ventricular septum after Sat Band placed), the child in the upper panels is 3 years old and the one in the lower panels is 2 years of age. Abbreviations: LV, left ventricle; RV, right ventricle.

especially important to clarify other associated complex anomalies as well as measuring Qp/Qs (Fig 10.6).

Patent Foramen Ovale (PFO)

When the flap of the foramen ovale fails to fully close, a PFO is present with generally a small amount of left-to-right shunting; this shunting is usually of no clinical significance. However, if right-to-left flow occurs at the PFO level, as with an ASD, individuals may be at risk for stroke or an ischemic event. This is generally evaluated using color Doppler echocardiography, contrast echocardiography ($\pm$ Valsalva maneuver), or transesophageal echocardiography, which is considered the noninvasive gold standard. There is not much data on comparing CMR and transesophageal echocardiography for PFO evaluation. As CMR is noninvasive and can image associated anomalies and transesophageal echocardiography is semi-invasive and has a smaller field of view, it may be attractive to develop for PFO evaluation, especially in adults. Dynamic contrast-enhanced CMR was studied in a small number of patients showing excellent feasibility for diagnosing both PFO and atrial septal aneurysm.[34] In a similar, larger study, CMR had a significant false negative rate.[35]

An Example of the CMR of a Lesion with an Atrial Septal Defect

Tricuspid atresia (Fig 10.3)

Tricuspid atresia (TA) is very uncommon, found in 79 of one million live births[36] and a major classification divides this lesion into three major groups: a) normally related great arteries (I) (most common), b) D-transposition of the great arteries (II), and L-transposition of the great arteries (III) (least common). The subgroups A, B, and C, categorize the presence and size of the ventricular septal defect and the presence or absence of pulmonary atresia or

stenosis.[37] With total obstruction to flow across the tricuspid valve into the RV, there is a requisite ASD (Fig 10.3) or dilated PFO (the entire cardiac output must cross the atrial septum). A persistent left superior vena cava is present in 12% to 15%, which is important surgically because of the Fontan repair.

The set of contiguous axial static SSFP images through the thorax, which begins the CMR imaging, clearly identifies not only the atretic valve but the associated anomalies as well, including the ASD. Off-axis coronal SSFP images through the long axis of the RA and RV confirms the diagnosis of TA. Cine CMR demonstrates not only a lack of flow through the tricuspid valve in the four-chamber and RV long-axis views, but is also used to assess LV function as well as flow across the ASD (Fig 10.3) and ventricular septal (if present) communications. Velocity mapping is used to assess cardiac output. Throughout staged Fontan reconstruction, CMR is used to assess the various parts of the repair, including the systemic venous pathway (Fontan baffle), the pulmonary arteries, the ASD, the reconstructed aorta (if present), ventricular function, and regional lung perfusion.[7,38–42] CMR can also be used to assess flow across the fenestration which allows communication between the systemic and pulmonary venous pathways; it allows maintenance of cardiac output at the expense of cyanosis. If a device is used to close the fenestration (ie, closing the communication between the systemic and pulmonary venous pathways similar to closing an ASD), steady-state free precession imaging can be used (see Fig 10.3 and following text).

Catheter Intervention on the Atrial Septum in the Catheterization Laboratory

(Figs 10.3, 10.11, and 10.12)

Most ASD devices used to close defects in the catheterization laboratory allow the patient to undergo CMR for other clinical cardiac or noncardiac indications. As an example, an AM-PLATZER Septal Occluder device creates only a local artifact (Fig 10.11); the remainder of the cardiovascular structures and ventricular func-

tion is easily evaluated (Figs 10.3, 10.11, and 10.12). A report of 26 pediatric patients utilizing CMR to evaluate the position of large ASD occluder devices and the impact on surround-

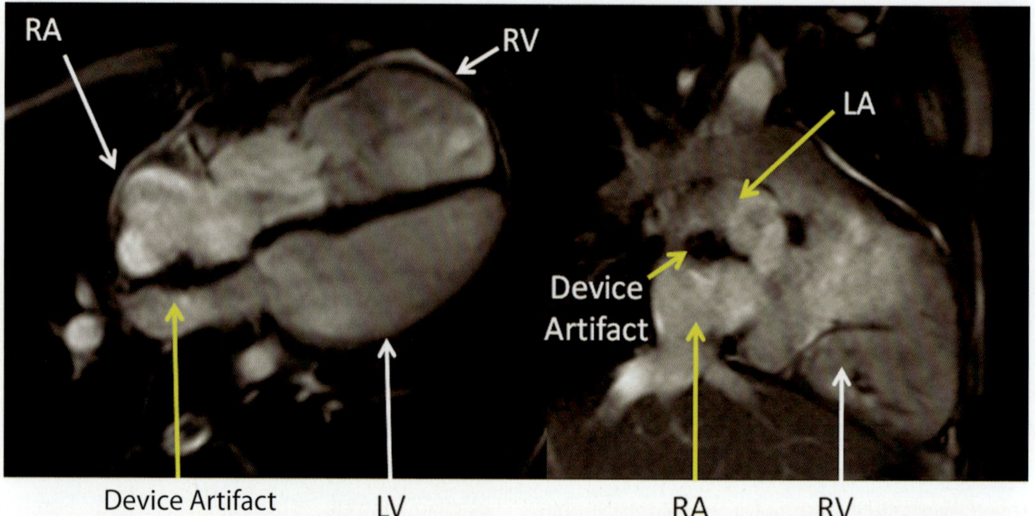

Fig 10.11—Atrial septal defect (ASD) closure by AMPLATZER device. The right image is a right ventricle (RV) long-axis view and the left image is a four-chamber view by steady-state free precession cine imaging of a 9-year-old individual with an RV cardiomyopathy and ASD after device closure. Note the rounded, black artifact created by the device as well as the finely trabeculated, thin-walled mid and apical portions of the RV. Abbreviations: LA, left atrium; LV, left ventricle; RA, right atrium; RV, right ventricle.

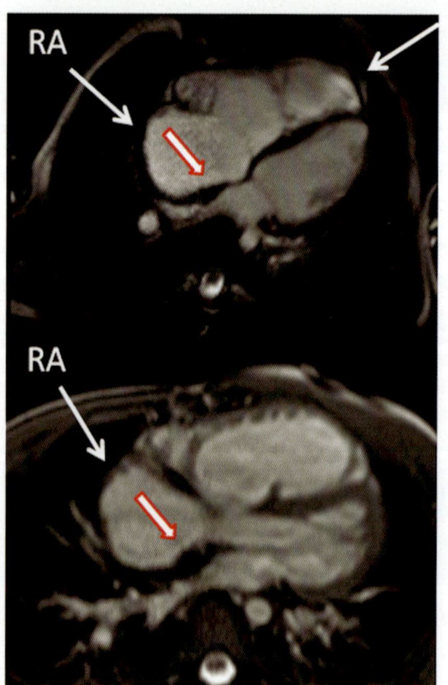

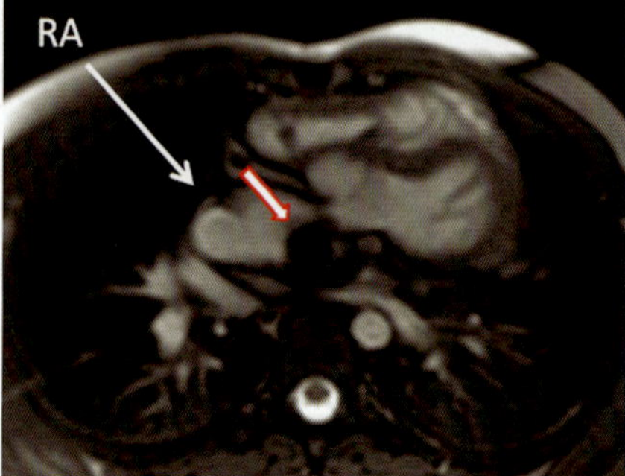

Fig 10.12—Atrial septal defect (ASD) closure by STARFlex device. The left panels are a four-chamber view (upper) and axial view (lower) by steady-state free precession of a 7-year-old with a simple ASD closed by a STARFlex device. Note the oval-shaped artifact (arrow) and a right ventricle (RV) which remains dilated. The panel above right is an axial view of a 4-year-old with transposition of the great arteries (TGA) after arterial switch operation (ASO) who is also after ASD closure with a STARFlex device as well (arrow). Again note the oval shape of the artifact.

ing structures found that a thorough evaluation was obtained.[43]

Intervention in the CMR Suite
(Fig 10.13)

ASD closure and creation

Closing an ASD in the CMR suite been successfully performed in animals using real-time CMR-sequences (obtaining images as quickly as possible in real time as a cine) with specialized interventional procedures, catheters, and equipment. [44] In addition, ASDs have been created as well in the CMR suite and have been dilated by balloon-tipped catheters (Fig 10.13).[45,46] There are still hurdles to overcome before this is practical in humans.[47] As CMR techniques improve, with better spatial and temporal resolution along with techniques to minimize artifact, CMR-guided interventions may become a reality. Radiation exposure to patient and operators could be eliminated. It has the potential to provide the interventionalist with better soft tissue representation of the atrial septum, not fully possible with catheterization or standard echocardiography.

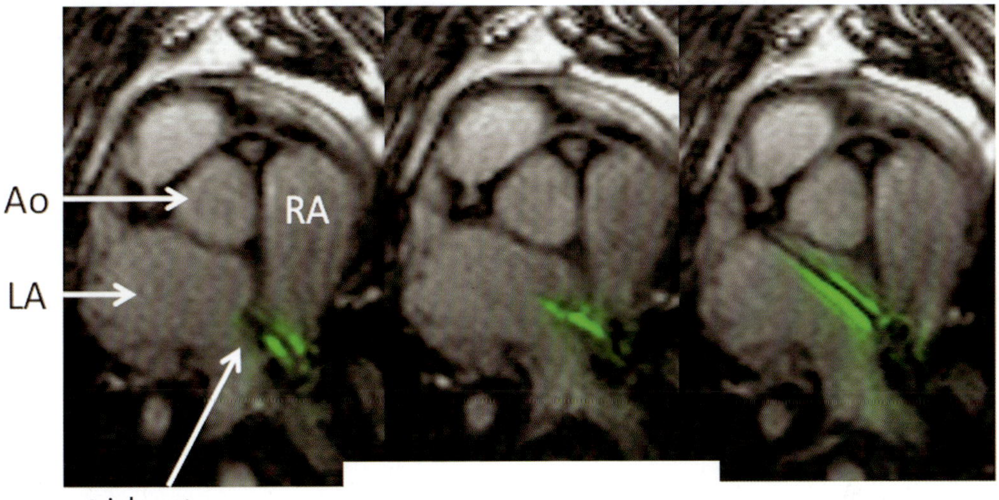

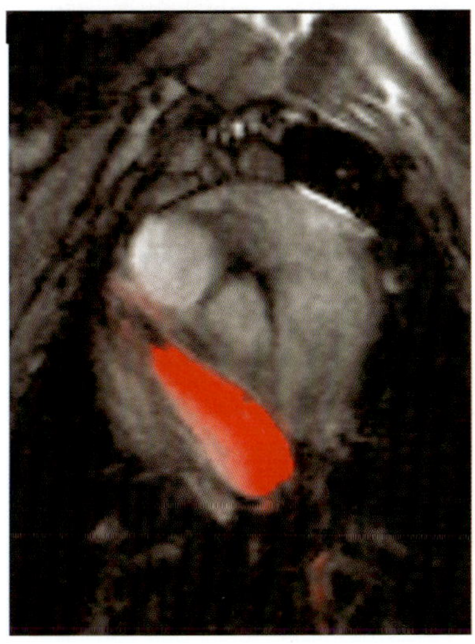

Fig 10.13—Interventional catheterization in the magnetic resonance imaging suite. The figure depicts puncture of the atrial septum by an active catheter (green tip) and balloon dilation of the created atrial septal defect (red balloon). The top three images are essentially close to the equivalent of an echocardiographic parasternal short-axis view depicting the atrial septum; the images are temporally sequential from left to right demonstrating contact with the atrial septum (left), puncture (middle), and advancing the catheter into the left atrium (LA) (right). In the lower left panel, a balloon-tipped catheter has crossed the atrial septum and the balloon has been inflated. (Images have been published previously[45] and are courtesy of Dr. Robert Lederman from the National Institutes of Health.) Abbreviations: Ao, aorta; RA, right atrium.

Conclusion

CMR of the atrial septum and ASD offers complementary imaging to echocardiography and cardiac angiography and often offers unique insights into the anatomy, physiology, and function of the various lesions that present to the clinician. Quantification of Qp/Qs, RV volume-overload, and associated anomalies such as anomalous pulmonary venous connection are just a few of the many contributions CMR can make. This added value that CMR brings to medical and surgical management along with the potential for new innovations (eg, ASD closure in the CMR suite) will ensure this modality a place in the approach to the atrial septum.

References

1. Modan L, Keinan L, Blumstein T, Sedetzki S. Cancer following cardiac catheterization in childhood. *Int J Epi.* 2000;29:424–428.

2. Brenner DJ, Elliston CD, Hall EJ, Berdon WE. Estimated risks of radiation-induced fatal cancer from pediatric CT. *AJR.* 2001;176:289–296.

3. Helbing WA, Rebergen SA, Maliepaard C, et al. Quantification of right ventricular function with magnetic resonance imaging in children with normal hearts and with congenital heart disease. *Am Heart J.* 1995;130:828–837.

4. Helbing WA, Niezen RA, Le Cessie S, van der Geest RJ, Ottenkamp J, de Roos RA. Right ventricular diastolic function in children with pulmonary regurgitation after repair of tetralogy of Fallot: volumetric evaluation by magnetic resonance velocity mapping. *J Am Coll Cardiol.* 1996;28:1827–1835.

5. Neimatallah MA, Ho VB, Dong Q, et al. Gadolinium enhanced 3D magnetic resonance angiography of the thoracic vessel. *JMRI.* 1999;10:758–770.

6. Harris MA, Ghoads G, Weinberg PM, Fogel MA. Magnetic resonance delayed enhancement for the detection of fibrous tissue in postoperative patients with various forms of congenital heart disease. *J Am Coll Cardiol.* 2005;45: (abstract).

7. Fogel MA, Weinberg PM, Chin AJ, Fellows KE, Hoffman EA. Late ventricular geometry and performance changes of functional single ventricle throughout staged Fontan reconstruction assessed by magnetic resonance imaging. *J Am Coll Cardiol.* 1996;28:212–221.

8. Papavassiliou DP, Parks, W, Hopkins K, et al. 3-D echocardiographic measurement of RV volume in children with congenital heart disease validated by MRI. *JASE.* 1998;11:770–777.

9. Nosir YF. Measurements & day-to-day variabilities of LV volumes & EF by 3-dimensional echocardiography and comparison with MRI. *Am J Cardiol.* 82:209–214.

10. Hundley WG, Li HF, Lange RA, et al. Assessment of left-to-right intracardiac shunting by velocity-encoded, phase-difference magnetic resonance imaging. A comparison with oximetric and indicator dilution techniques. *Circulation.* 1995;91:2955–2960.

11. Fogel MA. CMR in congenital heart disease. In: Lardo AC, Fayad ZA, Chronos NAF, Fuster V, eds. *Cardiovascular Magnetic Resonance. Established and Emerging Applications.* 1st ed. London: Martin Dunitz; 2003:224.

12. Boxt LM. Radiology of the right ventricle. *Rad Clin North Am.* 1999;37:379–400.

13. Boxt LM. MR imaging of pulmonary hypertension and right ventricular dysfunction. *Mag Reson Clin North Am.* 1996;4:307–325.

14. Rebergen SA, Helbing WA, van der Wall EE, Maliepaard C, Chin JG, de Roos A. MR velocity mapping of tricuspid flow in healthy children and in patients who have undergone Mustard or Senning procedure. *Radiology.* 1995;194:505–512.

15. Kim RJ, Fieno DS, Parrish TB, et al. Relationship of MRI delayed contrast enhancement to irreversible injury, infarct age, and contractile function. *Circulation.* 1999;100:1992–2002.

16. Nagel E, Klein C, Paetsch I, et al. Magnetic resonance perfusion measurements for the noninvasive detection of coronary artery disease. *Circulation.* 2003;108:432–437.

17. Nakagawa Y, Fujimoto S, Nakano H, et al. Magnetic resonance velocity mapping of transtricuspid velocity profiles in dilated cardiomyopathy. *Heart Vessels.* 1998;13:241–245.

18. Nakagawa Y, Fujimoto S, Nakano H, Hashimoto

T, Dohi K. Magnetic resonance velocity mapping of normal transtricuspid velocity profiles. *Int J Card Imaging*. 1997;13:433–436.

19. Mostbeck GH, Hartiala JJ, Foster E, Fujita N, Dulce MC, Higgins CB. Right ventricular diastolic filling: evaluation with velocity-encoded cine MRI. *J Computer Asst Tomography*. 1993;17:245–252.

20. Thomson LE, Crowley AL, Heitner JF, et al. Direct en face imaging of secundum atrial septal defects by velocity-encoded cardiovascular magnetic resonance in patients evaluated for possible transcatheter closure. *Circulation*. 2008;1(1):31–40.

21. Hartnell GG, Sassower M, Finn JP. Selective presaturation magnetic resonance angiography: new method for detecting intracardiac shunts. *Am Heart J*. 1993;126:1032–1034.

22. Holmvang G. A magnetic resonance imaging method for evaluating atrial septal defects. *J Cardiovasc Magn Reson*. 1999;1:59–64.

23. Beerbaum P, Korperich H, Esdorn H, et al. Atrial septal defects in pediatric patients: noninvasive sizing with cardiovascular MR imaging. *Radiology*. 2003;228:361–369.

24. Piaw CS, Kiam OT, Rapaee A, et al. Use of noninvasive phase contrast magnetic resonance imaging for estimation of atrial septal defect size and morphology: a comparison with transesophageal echo. *Cardiovasc Intervent Radiol*. 2006;29:230–234.

25. Lange A, Walayat M, Turnbull C, et al. Assessment of atrial septal defect morphology by transthoracic three dimensional echocardiography using standard grey scale and Doppler myocardial imaging techniques: comparison with magnetic resonance imaging and intraoperative findings. *Heart*. 1997;78:382–389.

26. Holmvang G, Palacios IF, Vlahakes GJ, et al. Imaging and sizing of atrial septal defects by magnetic resonance. *Circulation*. 1995;92:3473–3480.

27. Taylor AM, Stables RH, Poole-Wilson PA, Pennell DJ. Definitive clinical assessment of atrial septal defect by magnetic resonance imaging. *J Cardiovasc Magn Reson*. 1999;1:43–47.

28. Powell AJ, Tsai-Goodman B, Prakash A, Greil G, Geva T. Comparison between phase-velocity cine magnetic resonance imaging and invasive oximetry for quantification of atrial shunts. *Am J Cardiol*. 2003;91:1523–1525.

29. Beerbaum P, Korperich H, Barth P, Esdorn H, Gieseke J, Meyer H. Noninvasive quantification of left-to-right shunt in pediatric patients; phase-contrast cine magnetic resonance imaging compared with invasive oximetry. *Circulation*. 2001;103:2476–2482.

30. Rebergen SA, van der Wall EE, Helbing WA, de Roos A, van Voorthuisen AE. Quantification of pulmonary and systemic blood flow by magnetic resonance velocity mapping in the assessment of atrial-level shunts. *Int J Card Imaging*. 1996;12:143–152.

31. Valente AM, Sena L, Powell AJ, Del Nido PJ, Geva T. Cardiac magnetic resonance imaging evaluation of sinus venosus defects. *Pediatr Cardiol*. 2007;28:51–56.

32. Parsons JM, Baker EJ, Anderson RH, et al. Morphological evaluation of atrioventricular septal defect by magnetic resonance imaging. *Br Heart J*. 1990;64:138–145.

33. Jacobstein MD, Fletcher BD, Goldstein S, et al. Evaluation of atrioventricular septal defect by magnetic resonance imaging. *Am J Cardiol*. 1985;55:1158–1161.

34. Mohrs OK, Petersen SE, Erkapic D, et al. Diagnosis of patent foramen ovale using contrast enhanced dynamic MRI: a pilot study. *Am J Roentgenol*. 2005;184:234–240.

35. Nusser T, Hoher M, Merkle N, et al. Cardiac magnetic resonance imaging and transesophageal echocardiography in patients with transcatheter closure of patent foramen ovale. *J Am Coll Cardiol*. 2006;48:322–329.

36. Hoffman JIE, Kaplan S. The incidence of congenital heart disease. *J Am Coll Cardiol*. 200;39:1890–1900.

37. Edwards JE, Burchell HB. Congenital tricuspid atresia: a classification. *Med Clin North Am*. 1949;67:530–542.

38. Graham TP, Johns JA. Pre-operative assessment of ventricular function in patients considered for the Fontan procedure. *Herz*. 1992;17:213–219.

39. Rebergen SA, Ottinkamp J, Doornbos J, van der Wall EE, Chin JG, de Roos A. Postop-

erative pulmonary flow dynamics after Fontan surgery: assessment with nuclear magnetic resonance velocity mapping. *J Am Coll Cardiol.* 1993;21:123–131.

40. Fellows KE, Fogel MA. MR imaging and heart function in patients pre- and post-Fontan surgery, *Acta Paediatrica Suppl.* 1995;410:57–59.

41. Fogel MA, Ramaciotti C, Hubbard AM, Weinberg PW. Magnetic resonance and echocardiographic imaging of pulmonary artery size throughout stages of Fontan reconstruction. *Circulation.* 1994;90:2927–2936.

42. Fogel MA, Weinberg PM. Fellows KE, Hoffman EA. A Study in ventricular—ventricular interaction: Single right ventricles compared with systemic right ventricles in a dual chambered circulation. *Circulation.* 1995;92:219–230.

43. Lapierre C, Raboisson MJ, Miro J, Dahdah N, Guerin R. Evaluation of a large atrial septal occluder with cardiac MR imaging. *Radiographics.* 2003;23:S51–S58.

44. Rickers C, Jerosch-Herold M, Hu X, et al. Magnetic resonance image-guided transcatheter closure of atrial septal defects. *Circulation.* 2003;107:132–138.

45. Raval AN, Karmarkar PV, Guttman MA, et al. Real-time MRI guided atrial septal puncture and balloon septostomy in swine. *Cathet Cardiovasc Intervent.* 2006;67:637–643.

46. Elagha AA, Kocaturk O, Guttman MA, et al. Real-time MR imaging-guided laser atrial septal puncture in swine. *J Vasc Interv Radiol.* 2008;19:1347–1353.

47. Moore P. MRI-guided congenital cardiac catheterization and intervention: the future? *Cathet Cardiovasc Intervent.* 2005;66:1–8.

PART III

Procedure

Techniques

11

Establishing a Program in Structural Heart Disease Interventional Therapies

Ted Feldman and Ziyad M. Hijazi

> Learn from the mistakes of others. You can't live long enough to make them all yourself.
> —**Eleanor Roosevelt**

Establishing a program in structural heart disease interventional therapies requires several key components. Knowledge about the field, procedural and decision-making training, the necessary equipment, an experience base, and some form of certification represent the major components needed for programmatic development.

Knowledge Base

The knowledge base for structural intervention is broad and not well defined. The required knowledge base spans many fields, including pediatric and adult interventional cardiology, cardiovascular and cardiothoracic surgery, and vascular surgery and interventional radiology. The necessary knowledge base needed for practice is in theory and ideally the same for anyone who enters the field. In practice, instructional intervention represents a broad spectrum of practice, and the needed new knowledge base differs depending on the background and prior experience of the operator, and on the intended structural interventions the operator hopes to perform. At the entry level, for example, the adult interventional cardiologist may have substantial experience with diagnostic catheterization in aortic stenosis. In this case, the basic skills needed for balloon aortic valvuloplasty and the knowledge base for aortic valvuloplasty would be incremental and relatively easily acquired. At the same time, an adult interventional physician with no experience in transseptal catheterization would face a large hurdle in entering the wide spectrum of procedures that require left atrial access. Similarly, the management of congenital heart disease after prior surgical repair in the adult patient requires a substantial background and is often more accessible to the already-trained pediatric interventional physician.

Although no accreditation standards and no training program standards exist for a knowledge base in structural intervention, the Society for Cardiovascular Angiography and Interventions (SCAI) is developing a core curriculum for structural heart disease interventions. It will most easily apply to training programs. Some unaccredited structural heart disease training programs exist around the United States, but the infrastructure for accredited programs has yet to develop. Nonetheless, an integrated, cross-subspecialty core curriculum is a critical step in defining the knowledge base for structural intervention and is in development. The knowledge base needed for experienced practitioners entering the field will obviously depend on the individual and his or her specialty and experience, and the acquisition of this knowledge base will occur over a period of years.

Training

The traditional route or training in adult cardiac intervention has always been procedure volume based. The guidelines for training adult cardiovascular medicine, for example, recommend a minimum of 100 diagnostic cardiac catheterization procedures, an additional 200 diagnostic procedures for people who intend to practice primarily in invasive cardiology, and 250 coronary interventional procedures to develop basic competency for a dedicated interventional career.[1,2]

Structural procedures create a strong paradox for this procedure paradigm. Although coronary interventional procedures are comparatively simpler and performed in large numbers, structural procedures are relatively more complex and are performed in much smaller numbers. If one were simply to apply the logic of established training programs to structural training, many more procedures than 250 would be needed to establish basic skills in structural procedures (Fig 11.1). This is not possible, and alternative pathways to gaining training and familiarity with structural intervention are necessary as a consequence.

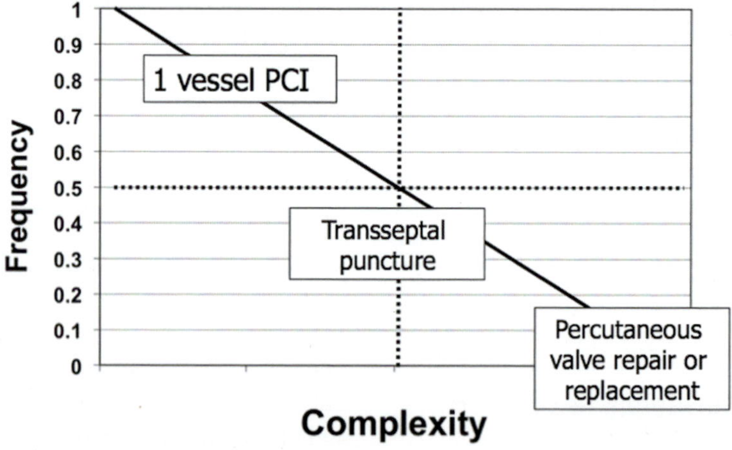

Fig 11.1—The training paradigm for invasive procedures has traditionally been to require large numbers of procedures to assure competency. The prototype is coronary intervention, whereby 250 angioplasty procedures are recommended for a single year training experience. If this principle is applied to structural intervention, the procedures are less frequent and more complex. It is not possible to require hundreds of structural interventions during the course of a single year of training, and the vast differences in types of structural interventional procedures further complicate the issue.

Imaging and diagnostics

Diagnostic methodology requires as much attention as procedural and technical training. Patient evaluation is as or more important than the performance of the interventional procedure. The interpretation of computerized tomography (CT) and magnetic resonance imaging (MRI) cardiac and vascular studies are not well studied by many interventional physicians and experience with these modalities is requisite. The interpretation of transthoracic and transesophageal echo studies is obviously important; identifying what information is missing is sometimes the hardest part of these studies. Facility with intracardiac echo is also necessary and has a substantial interpretive and technical learning curve. The emphasis in all of structural intervention in hemodynamics makes a strong background in hemodynamic and right heart catheter pressure interpretation requisite. This goes beyond the examination of waveforms and includes troubleshooting data acquisition during studies and maintaining high laboratory standards for quality in hemodynamic recording. For example, the basic methods for accurate transducer calibration have been forgotten in many catheterization laboratories (cath labs) today. Several courses exist at which detailed reviews of both didactic and case materials for hemodynamic assessments can be acquired. Visiting other laboratories as an observer is invaluable and often a way to see even more than can be shown in case transmissions from meetings.

Training methods

What training methods are available? The simpler structural procedures can be understood by attending demonstration programs. The value of both taped and live-case demonstrations for entry-level structural interventional procedures is critical. Some controversy has developed regarding the ethics and necessity of live-case demonstrations. It is our opinion that for acquiring new skills in a complex field, live demonstration courses provide an unparalleled

and irreplaceable resource. Visiting another laboratory allows you to see the more mundane but important elements, including what kind of inventory is available and the small procedural techniques that cannot be demonstrated in live-case transmissions.

Planning entry into the field using procedures that are an extension of an existing skill set is important. For operators who do not have prior transseptal catheterization skills, closure of patent foramen ovale (PFO) and simple atrial septal defects (ASDs) may represent a feasible pathway into the field. Similarly, balloon aortic valvuloplasty using the retrograde approach is an extension of skills that most adult cardiovascular interventional physicians have already achieved.

A further key route for the basic acquisition of training is via proctoring. Proctoring is device specific, and generally supported by device manufacturers. The value of having a highly experienced visitor in your laboratory to apply new technologies and learn technique is irreplaceable. At the same time, some techniques cannot be transmitted in this manner.

Transseptal puncture is among those skills that cannot be in the current circumstances brought with the proctoring approach. Septal closure devices are the paradigm for proctoring, and it is likely that in the future percutaneous left atrial appendage closure and valve interventions will follow this model.

Partnerships

Another useful way to gain training and experience is to partner with physicians from other specialties in an institution or in the community. Developing a relationship with a pediatric interventional physician, if one is an adult cardiologist, working with vascular and cardiothoracic surgeons, and any other specialists, who have an interest in complex structural heart disease, valvular heart disease, congenital heart disease, or congenital heart disease in adults is highly fruitful. The kind of amplification of knowledge and skills, which comes from working in such a partnership, especially if it can be procedural, is highly useful. Similar partnerships can be valuable in diagnostic laboratories including ultrasound vascular laboratories and radiology special procedures.

The natural evolution of the relationship among vascular surgeons, interventional radiologists, and cardiologists in the field of abdominal aortic stent grafting, is an example of partnerships, which can lead to structural partnership. Obviously, in valve interventions and the growing field of percutaneous aortic valve replacement and mitral valve repair, partnership with a cardiothoracic surgeon is essential for the interventional physician. Both parties have a great deal to learn, and generally there is a favorable transfer of skills necessary to forge a successful partnership. In some cases, these partnerships are easily forged within an institution, and also within a community. In less common cases, it is possible to develop relationships with specialists from other disciplines from other communities, cities, or states.

Simulation

Simulation is another essential element of training.[3,4] Simulators range from bench-top glass or plastic models (Fig 11.2) to the highly sophisticated and interactive mechanical and clinical simulators, which are found currently; commonly at national meetings. Simulation offers an obvious experience in practicing procedure and gaining understanding of interventional equipment. In the SimSuite simulation system, entire procedures, including clinical decision making, management of complications, pharmacologic management, and procedure flow are all incorporated.

Simulations are not available for every intervention; however, many basic skills can be learned through simulation laboratories. The value of simulation has been clearly established and should not be underestimated. Simulators have become common as part of procedure training for entry into new device trials for novel devices. The Edwards PARTNER aortic valve replacement trial uses simulators for the beginning phase of training, as does the Atritech device for left atrial appendage occlusion.

Clinical trials

Possibly, the most useful way to gain skills with new device therapy is to participate in clinical trials. Not only is training provided for a specific device but a great deal of cognitive information comes with the process. The experience gained in trial is shared, and shared learning has become a ubiquitous part of multicenter new device therapy efforts. The recently completed Evalve EVEREST trials and the Edwards PARTNER aortic valve replacement trials represent examples. Frequent conference calls, investigator meetings, critical protocol review, and special sessions at national meetings all contribute to one's knowledge and technical skill base. In some respects, it is a circular situation whereby people with skills get into trials and trials teach new skills, it remains possible to break into these trials when one's institutional and

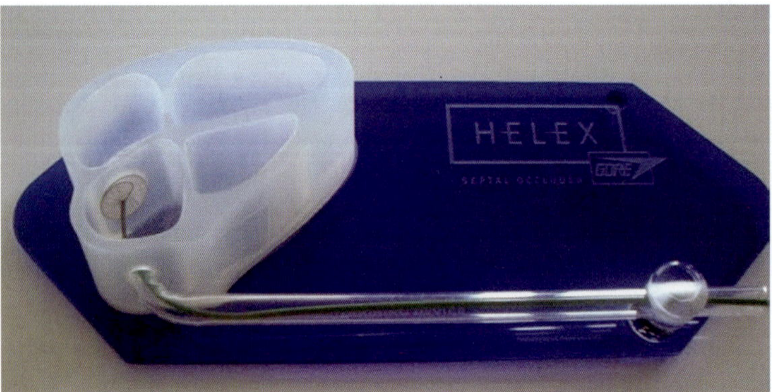

Fig 11.2—Photo of a bench-top "simulator." Simulation technology may take the form of simple bench-top models for device deployment. Here is a simple model of the aorta and an atrial septal defect, which allows practice with the deployment of atrial septal defect occluder devices. (Courtesy of W.L. Gore & Associates.)

research resources are well matched to a trial effort. This is especially true when trials expand from phase I to phase II and may need to enlist the help of 30 to 60 centers to optimize patient enrollment. Trials involving proved devices for new indications are particularly attractive as an entry point into the world of trials as a form of continued training and skill acquisition. An example, device closure for PFO in randomized trials for stroke prevention, is underway and enlists a large number of trial sites.

Training programs

Training programs unfortunately do not represent a pathway for training in structural heart interventions. There are no accredited programs, and only a few non-accredited or informal training programs around the United States. These programs are often targeted to people, who have completed all of their accredited training and thus necessitate an additional year of commitment minimum to acquire basic skills of transseptal catheterization, shunt closure, and valve intervention. This highlights the challenge in creating a new paradigm for training and the acquisition of new skills for structural heart intervention, and the curriculum being designed by the SCAI represents a key first step in this direction.

Equipment

A sizeable investment is required for basic equipment for any of the broad range of transseptal and structural interventions. Intracardiac ultrasound is requisite. Investment in a dedicated machine for the cath lab that includes the console and the disposable imaging transducers has to be committed. Although transesophageal echocardiography can be used in any situation that might require intracardiac ultrasound, TEE sometimes requires general anesthesia and thus requires more personnel and greater degrees of sedation for structural procedures. Intracardiac echocardiographic exams simplify these procedures as much as can be accomplished and provide excellent information for most septal closure procedures. The initial capital outlay may be in the range of $60,000–$100,000 depending on the equipment selected.

In addition, a wide range of disposables is necessary. A commitment from the institution is requisite and a sizeable investment is required. As an example, for ASD closure using the AGA devices, full stocking of 26 sizes of the ASO device at about $5,500 each is a substantial commitment (Fig 11.3). These have a defined shelf life so that expiration and inventory loss is an additional part of the commitment. Transseptal catheters and needles, longer guiding

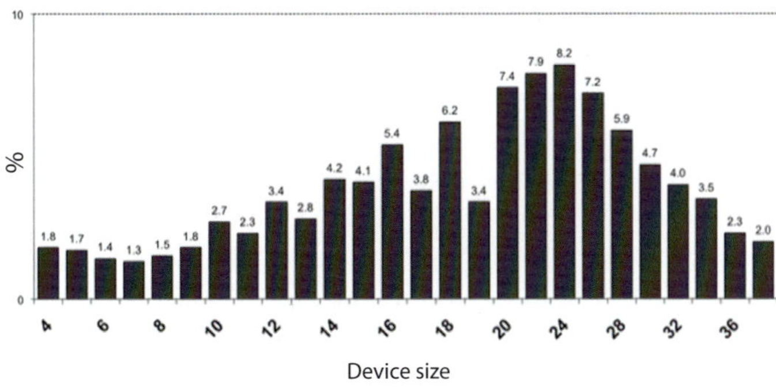

Fig 11.3—Percentages of ASO occluders shipped by size. The inventory and equipment needs for structural program can be substantial. For example, the AGA Medical AMPLATZER Septal Occluder (ASO) is manufactured in sizes ranging from 4 to 38 mm in diameter. To stock one of each of these size devices and two of the more commonly used sizes requires a substantial initial outlay.

sheaths in a wide range of diameters from 5 to 14 or 16F is necessary as are femoral sheath sizes ranging commonly in the 12 to 14F size, up to 16 or even 24F for some interventions. Large balloons, 12 to 30mm diameter, for large vessel stenting and valvuloplasty are needed. Familiarity with all of this equipment is also necessary.

The Interventional Team

Far from least among the requirements for establishing a successful program is a team approach. Interventionalists, cardiovascular surgeons, echocardiographers, noninterventional clinicians, and other specialists including anesthesiologists, interventional radiologists, pediatric cardiologists, pediatric cardiovascular surgeons, and vascular surgeons can all be team members. The concept of team is beyond the simple idea of having all of these specialties present in an institution. Real cooperation among the members of these groups is required for success, safety, and program growth. The level of cross-training and cross-teaching that occurs as a result of these partnerships cannot be overemphasized. Many of the previously discussed issues of knowledge base and training are captured by the workings of an interventional team.

In "The clinical development of percutaneous heart valve technology: a position statement of the Society of Thoracic Surgeons (STS), the American Association for Thoracic Surgery (AATS), and the SCAI," the recommendation is for a team with at least an interventionalist, cardiovascular surgeon, echocardiographer, and noninterventional clinician.[5] Experienced operators are requisite. Participation in studies in this paradigm is recommended for sites that have institutional volumes of between 100 and 150 minimum surgical valve operations per year, surgeons with 40 to 50 minimum valve operations per year, and interventionalists with at least 100 PCI procedures per year including transseptal and coronary sinus catheteriza-

tion experience. These recommendations were crafted from a multisociety interaction to characterize the elements necessary for participating in trials for new percutaneous valve therapy devices.[5]

Conclusion

Starting a program to enter the exciting and rapidly growing world of structural heart disease interventions is a long-term project that requires a substantial commitment. A large knowledge base, the acquisition of new skills, and creation of a multidisciplinary team are all essential elements. The path to developing a structural program will be different for practitioners with different backgrounds; the adult cardiologist with experience in valvular disease will not follow the same route as one with a background primarily in coronary disease, and the path for the surgeon with no catheter skills will be different as well. Because this is a young field, there are no defined training requirements or pathways. This is both a challenge and also a great opportunity.

References

1. Hirshfeld JW Jr, Banas JS Jr, Brundage BH, et al. American College of Cardiology training statement on recommendations for the structure of an optimal adult interventional cardiology training program: a report of the American College of Cardiology task force on clinical expert consensus documents. *J Am Coll Cardiol.* 1999;34(7):2141–2147.
2. Pepine CJ, Babb JD, Brinker JA, et al. Guidelines for training in adult cardiovascular medicine. Core Cardiology Training Symposium (COCATS). Task Force 3: training in cardiac catheterization and interventional cardiology. *J Am Coll Cardiol.* 1995;25(1):14–16.
3. Ahlberg G, Enochsson L, Gallagher AG, et al. Proficiency-based virtual reality training significantly reduces the error rate for residents during their first 10 laparoscopic cholecystecto-

mies. *Am J Surg.* 2007 Jun;193(6):797–804.

4. Gallagher AG, Cates CU. Virtual reality training for the operating room and cardiac catheterisation laboratory. *Lancet.* 2004 Oct 23–29;364(9444):1538–1540.

5. Vassiliades TA Jr, Block PC, Cohn LH, et al. The clinical development of percutaneous heart valve technology: a position statement of the Society of Thoracic Surgeons (STS), the American Association for Thoracic Surgery (AATS), and the Society for Cardiovascular Angiography and Interventions (SCAI). *J Thorac Cardiovasc Surg.* 2005;129(5):970-6. *J Am Coll Cardiol.* 2005;45:1554–1560. *Ann Thorac Surg.* 2005;79(5):1812–1818. *Cathet Cardiovasc Intervent.* 2005;65(1):73–79.

12

How to Close Simple ASDs

Matthew Egan and Ralf J. Holzer

Introduction

Transcatheter device closure of secundum atrial septal defects (ASDs) has replaced surgical repair as the primary method of treatment in the majority of cardiac centers, which is especially true for "simple" defects. Many devices have been developed over the years since King and Mills initially described ASD closure in the cardiac catheterization laboratory in 1976.[1] At present, the only two devices that have been granted Food and Drug Administration (FDA) post-market approval (PMA) in the United States are the AMPLATZER Septal Occluder (ASO) (AGA Medical Corporation, Plymouth, Minnesota) and the HELEX Septal Occluder (W.L. Gore & Associates, Flagstaff, Arizona). The technique to close "simple" defects utilizing these devices is described in detail in this chapter.

Simple versus Complex ASD Morphology

Whereas complex ASDs may require a variety of technical modifications to facilitate successful closure (Chapters 13 and 14), percutaneous closure of "simple" ASDs is more straightforward and usually successful, provided that operators follow some important basic guidelines. Important characteristics of complex ASDs (discussed in Chapters 8 and 9) that highlight a greater technical procedural challenge include:

- A very large ASD in excess of 30 mm (unstretched diameter)
- An ASD with more than one rim deficiency

- An ASD with a rim deficiency other than an isolated deficiency of the retro-aortic rim, which is present in 30% to 50% of patients. This applies particularly to deficiencies of the inferior caval vein rim.
- Multiple ASD and/or a multifenestrated atrial septum
- ASDs in small infants (< 5 kg)

General (Pre) Procedural Considerations

Although closure of "simple" ASD is frequently straightforward, it should only be performed in laboratories and by operators equipped to deal with complications of the procedure and unexpected technical challenges. Furthermore, a complete stock of available devices of all sizes is required, to allow the operator to choose exactly the device size most appropriate for the specific patient. Retrieval equipment, including loop snares, bailout systems, as well as surgical backup should be available in the event a device needs to be removed emergently.

The type of anesthesia used depends on institutional, operator, and patient preference. In certain adults or older children, intracardiac echocardiography (ICE) may be used to monitor device deployment, thus allowing these procedures to be performed under conscious or deep sedation (Chapter 8).[2,3] However, general anesthesia is preferable when transesophageal echocardiography (TEE) is being considered to guide device deployment, or in young and/or uncooperative patients. In elderly patients with left ventricular diastolic dysfunction, in which test occlusion of the ASD is being planned as part of the procedure, conscious sedation with ICE may be preferable, as it allows to better monitor respiratory function that could be compromised as a result of increased left atrial pressure with test occlusion.

Even though standard vascular access is usually obtained in the right femoral vein, other vascular entry sites, such as transhepatic access, will be described in Chapter 19.[4] The initial sheath size used depends on the age of the patient, and is usually 8F for adult sized patients, and 6F for most pediatric patients. A monitoring arterial line (optional) is then placed in the right femoral artery. If the procedure is going to be guided by ICE, additional venous access from the right or left femoral vein is required. Heparin is administered at a dose of 100 IU per kilogram, and the activated clotting time (ACT) is maintained above 200 seconds throughout the procedure. A dose of intravenous antibiotics, such as a cephalosporin, is administered prior to device deployment.

Hemodynamic and Angiographic Evaluation

A thorough hemodynamic evaluation should be performed prior to device deployment. This should include a complete right heart catheterization, as well as an antegrade left heart catheterization through the ASD. Particular attention should be given to pulmonary artery pressures, pulmonary vascular resistance, Qp:Qs, as well as pulmonary capillary wedge pressure (PCWP), left atrial pressure (LAP), and left ventricular end diastolic pressure (LVEDP). In elderly patients with a large left-to-right shunt, and/or evidence of left ventricular diastolic dysfunction, it may be necessary to evaluate for an exaggerated increase of PCWP, LAP, and/or LVEDP with test occlusion of the ASD (Chapter 15).[5,6]

Although angiography may not be absolutely necessary, a right upper pulmonary venous angiogram is recommended for the majority of patients. This should be obtained using a single plane in 35° left anterior oblique (LAO) and 35° cranial angulation. This angiography provides an exquisite profile of the atrial septum (Fig 12.1), which can serve as a road map when deploying the device. Further-

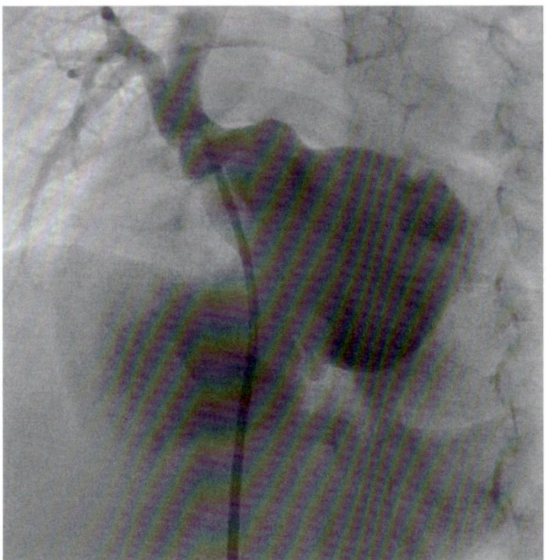

Fig 12.1—Two-year-old female with a moderate secundum ASD. Angiography taken in right upper pulmonary vein (35 RAO, 35 CR) profiles very well the atrial septum with a central secundum ASD, and facilitates measuring the total atrial septal length.

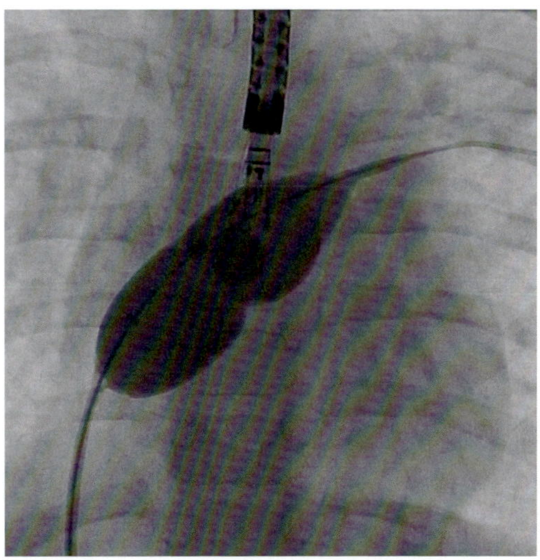

Fig 12.2—Balloon sizing of a moderate secundum ASD in a 3-year-old child. While in this patient a notable waist facilitated the use of the cine recordings, echocardiographic measurement of the sizing balloon is usually more reliable.

more, the atrial septal length can be measured very well using this angiography, which is especially important in smaller children, where the maximum device size that can be used is limited by the total atrial septal length. Even though echocardiography is essential for ASD closure, an angiographic road map allows rotating the device and aligning it with the septum, which becomes particularly useful when the TEE probe has to be pulled up during deployment, due to image blockage by the TEE probe, and/or the probe potentially interfering with device orientation during deployment.

Echocardiography and Balloon Sizing

The echocardiographic assessment by either modality includes measuring the defect in multiple planes, assessing the length of all septal rims, documenting the pulmonary venous drainage, and demonstrating the degree of AV valve regurgitation (Chapter 7). A rim is considered to be deficient if its length is < 5 mm, and absent if it is 1 mm or less.[7]

Balloon sizing of the ASD is recommended for all defects that will be closed using ASO, and it is even more important for those defects being considered for closure with the HELEX Septal Occluder. Balloon sizing is particularly helpful for irregularly shaped ASDs that have inconsistent echocardiographic dimensions on different imaging planes. The left upper pulmonary vein is entered and an exchange length, extra stiff, wire is advanced with care, which can be used for both the balloon sizing as well as for subsequently advancing the delivery sheath or delivery catheter. Typically an AGA Sizing Balloon, available at maximum diameters of 18, 24, and 34 mm (AGA Medical Corporation, Plymouth, MN), is introduced directly through the skin. Under echocardiographic guidance, the balloon is slowly inflated until no residual flow is visualized by color Doppler (Fig 12.2). It is important to stop immediately when the shunt is abolished (stop-flow diameter), to avoid oversizing the defect. Measurements are generally more reliable by echocardiography than angiography due to magnification and profiling issues.

Choosing the Appropriate Device

In general, for small defects device choice is largely based on operator preference. However, as erosions have not been reported with the HELEX Septal Occluder, this device may be preferable for patients with a small ASD. Details of the HELEX Septal Occluder are outlined in Chapter 27. Its use was originally described by Zahn and colleagues in 2001.[8] The device is available at 15, 20, 25, 30, and 35 mm total diameter. With the HELEX Septal Occluder being a non–self-centering device, the chosen device size should be at least twice the stop-flow diameter. If this diameter exceeds 18 mm, ASO may be preferable, as the 35-mm HELEX Septal Occluder is rather soft and flexible, and may not provide the overall stability required for successful closure.

ASO was first introduced in 1997, and is described in detail in Chapter 26.[9,10] It is available in the United States at sizes from 4 to 38 mm (outside the U.S., it is available up to 40 mm), with 1-mm increments up to 20 mm, and 2-mm increments thereafter. The device size specifies the diameter of the central connecting waist, with the left atrial disk exceeding the central waist circumferentially by 6 to 8 mm, depending on device size. The device size should be equal to but no larger than 1 to 2 mm above the stop-flow diameter. If balloon sizing is not used, a good estimate for device size is obtained by adding 20% to the average diameter by two-dimensional (2D) color Doppler imaging.

Closure Technique

AMPLATZER Septal Occluder

Once the device size has been selected, the appropriately sized delivery sheath is chosen, which ranges from 6 to 12F, depending on device size. In larger patients, it may be beneficial to upsize the delivery sheath by 1F, especially if the next larger device would require upsizing of the delivery sheath. That way, if the device is found to be too small during deployment, the same delivery sheath can be used for the next larger device. For simple ASD, it is recommended to initially attempt closure using the standard 45° TorqVue Delivery Sheath (AGA Medical Corporation, Plymouth, Minnesota).

To load the device, the delivery cable is passed through the loader and an attached Tuohy Borst adapter. The device is then screwed onto the delivery cable, paying meticulous attention that the cable and device interact easily. It is essential to avoid crossthreading the cable into the microscrew of the device, as this can lead to an inability to release the device, or inadvertent premature release. To enhance clotting, it may be beneficial to soak the device in blood for a few minutes prior to loading. Once the device is screwed onto the delivery cable, it is gently pulled into the loader under water seal, and subsequently the system is flushed generously through the Tuohy Borst adapter. Once the device is loaded and ready for delivery, the prepped delivery sheath including dilator is advanced over a stiff wire that has been placed within the left upper pulmonary vein. Once the dilator reaches the right atrium, the dilator is fixed and the delivery sheath advanced over the wire. This fills the distal end of the sheath with a fluid column, and reduces the risk of inadvertent air embolism. The sheath is advanced toward the mouth of the left upper pulmonary vein, and subsequently dilator and guide wire are removed slowly under water seal. This is crucial, especially in spontaneously breathing patients, as a deep inspiration or a hasty removal of dilator and cable can suck air into the sheath and result in systemic air embolism. The sheath is then flushed, using only gentle aspiration while gradually pulling back the sheath until blood can be aspirated. Subsequently the loader is attached to the delivery sheath. Under fluoroscopic guidance, the device is advanced. It is important to watch the distal end of the delivery sheath for any sign of air being pushed through the sheath by the device. Once the device is at the tip of the delivery sheath, the whole assembly is pulled back until the tip of the delivery sheath exits the mouth of the pulmonary vein and is freely within the left atrium. The following device deployment should be performed with the same fluoroscopic projection that was used during initial angiography, which serves as a road map for device deployment (Fig 12.3), as well as continuous echocardiographic guidance, preferably in short-axis view. The left atrial disk is deployed, by retracting the sheath over the delivery cable. Once the device is oriented appropriately, it is gradually pulled back toward the atrial septum. The central waist is deployed at least partially prior to the left atrial disk reaching the septum, which allows for self-centering of the device within the ASD. Occasionally, a gentle rotation of the sheath may be necessary to improve device alignment along the atrial septum. Once the left atrial disc sits in the appropriate position with the connecting waist stenting the defect itself, the right atrial disc is deployed. If the device pulls through the septum at this time, the device is recaptured, the sheath repositioned, and the deployment process repeated.

If the device cannot be aligned to the atrial septum, one should try to pull up the TEE probe during deployment and use solely the angiographic road map, as the probe can interfere with device delivery. Mild distortions of the device position during deployment can lead to the device pulling through the defect, especially in patients with a deficient retroaortic rim. If device alignment remains difficult despite pulling up the TEE probe, one should consider the use of the precurved Hausdorf sheath (Cook, Bloomington, Indiana), which allows the operator to torque the device to align it directly to the atrial septum. Other techniques for facilitating difficult device deployments, such as pulmonary vein techniques or use of a stiff second catheter/wire,[11–13] are usually only necessary in patients with significant or multiple rim deficiencies and as such are described in Chapter 13.

After deployment, the position of the ASO is carefully evaluated using echocardiography. A very gentle push-pull motion "Minnesota wiggle" on the delivery cable may facilitate

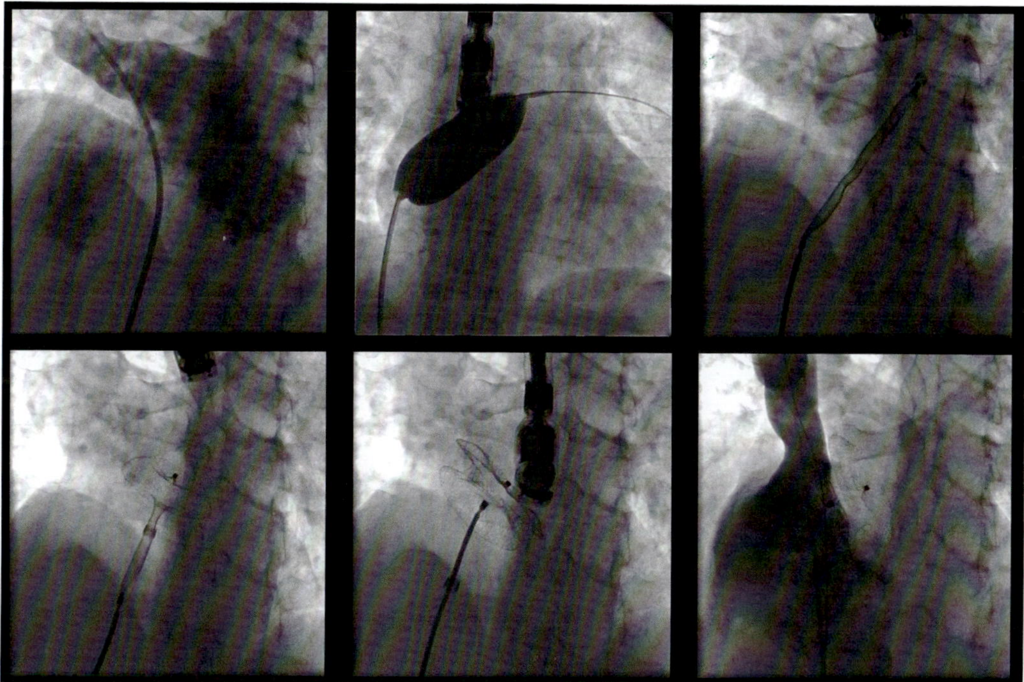

Fig 12.3—Balloon sizing of a moderate secundum ASD in a 3-year-old child. While in this patient a notable waist facilitated the use of the cine recordings, echocardiographic measurement of the sizing balloon is usually more reliable.

better disk separation and assist the echocardiographic assessment to confirm that all rims have been captured. Color Doppler flow may show some residual flow through the waist and two discs but should not show residual flow around them. The assessment should also evaluate for obstruction of adjacent structures as well as interference with the atrioventricular (AV) valves (Chapter 7). If there is residual shunting around the device or if the position is deemed unsatisfactory, the sheath is advanced while retracting the delivery cable to recapture the device. If there remain concerns about the device position, an angiography can be performed in LAO/Cranial angulation via the side arm of delivery sheath. This allows profiling the device against the atrial septum, and separating left atrial from right atrial discs. One should see the contrast capturing just the right atrial disc and part of the waist during the RA injection, while the opposite will be the case during recirculation/levophase (Fig 12.4). Once appropriate device position has been confirmed, the device is released by attaching the pin-vise to the deliv-

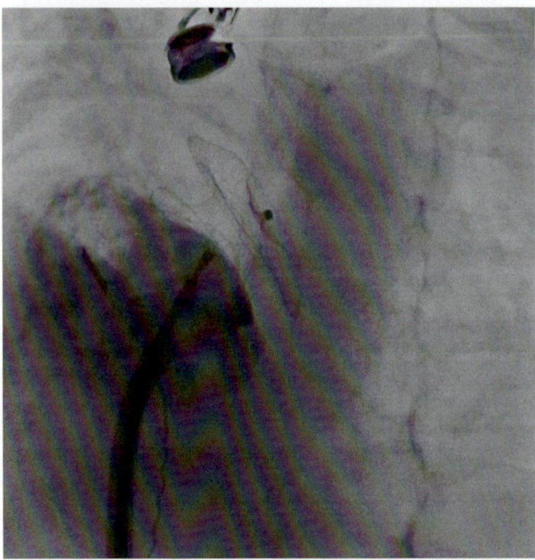

Fig 12.4—Three-year-old female with a moderate ASD. TEE was unable to confirm capture of the inferior/IVC rim, and therefore ICE imaging was obtained. Furthermore, outlined in this picture, an angiogram was performed through the delivery sheath prior to release of the device, documenting good device position and no spillover of contrast to the left atrial disc.

ery cable and rotating it counterclockwise. The delivery cable should be pulled back into the delivery sheath immediately after it detaches itself from the device, to avoid injury to the atrial wall or inadvertent device embolization. The device typically reorients itself into a more appropriate position once the tension of the delivery cable has been removed. A final echocardiographic assessment is performed after device release.

HELEX Septal Occluder

The HELEX Septal Occluder delivery system consists of three components: a 10F green delivery catheter, a gray control catheter, and a tan mandrel. The delivery catheter has a distal side-hole, which allows an "over the wire" use of this catheter, but requires upsizing the venous sheath to 12F if an 0.035" guide wire is being used. The control catheter has a retrieval cord to facilitate device retrieval if necessary. Loading is accomplished by submerging the device and delivery catheter tip in a heparinized saline bath (without removing the catheter from the plastic packing) to reduce the risk of air entrapment. A large syringe filled with heparinized saline is attached to the red retrieval cord cap and the control catheter is flushed. Subsequently the luer lock between the control catheter and green delivery catheter is loosened, and the control catheter is pulled back carefully, which pulls the device into the delivery catheter. It is essential not to engage any brute force during this process, as this may lead to a premature lock, which may only be noticed during the deployment process itself. Once all but 3 cm of the device is captured into the delivery catheter, with the mandrel starting to become slightly curved, the mandrel luer lock is loosened, which allows for pulling the remainder of the device into the green delivery catheter. The system is again flushed generously at this point, leaving a syringe attached at the end. If a guide wire is utilized (rapid-exchange), it is loaded through the distal guide wire slot at the distal end of the green delivery catheter. The delivery system is then advanced through the hemostatic sheath and across the atrial septum under fluoroscopy until the radiopaque marker at the tip of the green delivery catheter is positioned within the left atrium. Similar to deployment of an ASO, the fluoroscopic projections should mirror those used during an initial angiography, which can be used as a road map during deployment. Echocardiography verifies the location of the tip of the green delivery catheter, and if a guide wire was used it is removed at this time. The device is deployed using a "push-pinch-pull" technique. First, the gray control catheter is pushed resulting in the device leaving the sheath and entering the left atrium. Next, while holding the green delivery catheter, the gray control catheter, is pinched. Then, the tan mandrel is pulled back approximately 2 cm, thereby gradually forming the left atrial disc. This technique is repeated until the center eyelet exits the delivery catheter, which can be visualized on fluoroscopy. Figure 12.5 demonstrates various stages of the deployment process. With the left atrial disc having formed, the whole assembly is gradually pulled back against the atrial septum. However, as is the case during all stages of the deployment process, it is crucial to avoid pulling the device against any resistance, as it may

not only pull the soft device through the ASD, but may also lead to premature lock or the lock subsequently not capturing the right atrial disc. The right atrial disc is prepared for deployment by holding the gray control catheter in a fixed position while withdrawing the green delivery catheter until the mandrel luer lock stops at the Y-arm hub. The mandrel luer lock is then tightened and the right atrial disc formed by holding the green delivery catheter in a fixed position while pushing the gray control catheter until the control catheter luer lock can be tightened. The device position is then interrogated with echocardiography. Evaluation should assess for residual shunting via color Doppler flow, obstruction of adjacent structures, and interference with the AV valves. If the device position is unsatisfactory, the device is recaptured the same way as it was originally loaded. Once echocardiography confirms an appropriate device position, the red retrieval cord cap is removed. The device is locked by loosening the mandrel luer lock, fixing the green delivery catheter, and pulling sharply on the mandrel at least 2 cm to release the lock. This should be a firm and swift pull, avoiding jerkiness or a gradual pull. Sometimes the lock may not be completely freed,

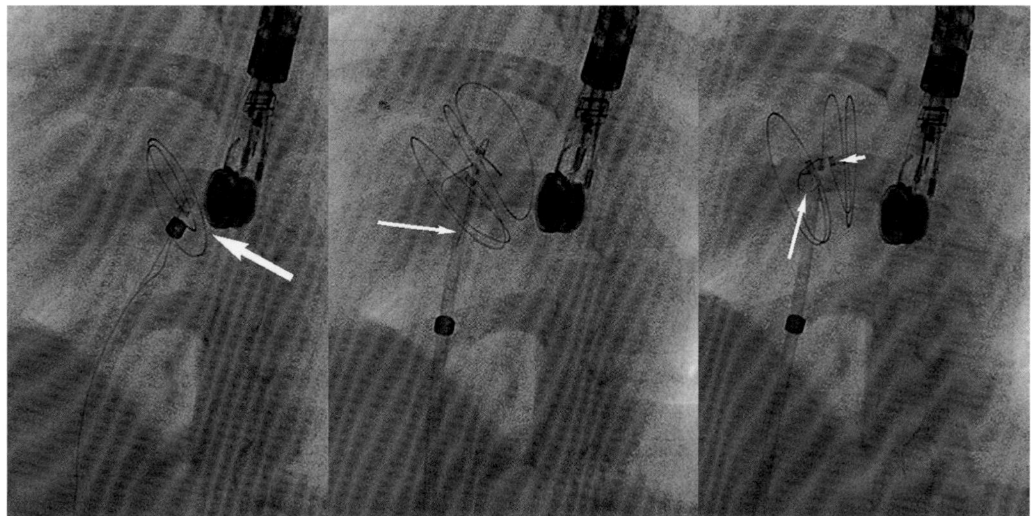

Fig 12.5—Delivery of the HELEX Septal Occluder. Left, The left atrial disc is deployed. One can see the distal eyelet just outside of the delivery catheter. Middle, Both left and right atrial disc are configured. The arrow points to the locking loop which is still sitting within the mandrel. Right, The lock has been released. Arrows pointing to the distal eyelet as well as the locking loop, which captures the proximal/RA eyelet. (Courtesy of W.L. Gore & Associates.)

in which case the catheter should be gently torqued to allow the locking loop to configure. It is crucial that the device be carefully evaluated at this stage to ensure the locking loop has captured the right atrial eyelet. At this time, the device is loosely attached to the gray control catheter by the retrieval cord. The retrieval cord can be utilized to remove the device if deemed necessary. Otherwise, the delivery system is removed as a single unit, making sure the cord moves freely without any tension on the device. A final echocardiographic evaluation should be performed at this time.

Postprocedural Care and Results

After device occlusion has occurred, the sheaths are removed and hemostasis is obtained. The patient is monitored overnight in the hospital. The next morning, a chest x-ray (CXR) is obtained to confirm device position and complemented with a transthoracic echocardiogram, which evaluates for device placement, residual shunting, and evidence of a pericardial effusion. A 12-lead electrocardiogram is obtained to evaluate for evidence of heart block or atrial arrhythmias.[14] Patients should receive aspirin therapy and require subacute bacterial endocarditis prophylaxis prior to at-risk procedures. Both can be discontinued after 6 months, provided complete closure has been confirmed.

Results are excellent with both the AMPLATZER Septal Occluder and the HELEX Septal Occluder. Closure rates with the AMPLATZER Septal Occluder are > 95% at 1-year follow-up, with few requiring repeat intervention.[10,11,15,16] The US multicenter HELEX Pivotal Study compared results of occlusion with the HELEX device compared to surgical controls. Clinical success, defined as no or insignificant residual shunting 1 year after device placement, occurred in 91.7% of patients.[17]

Summary

Transcatheter device closure of "simple ASDs" has become standard therapy. It can be performed safely with excellent results when utilizing the appropriate techniques for placement of the AMPLATZER Septal Occluder and the HELEX Septal Occluder as described in this chapter. Alterations in the technique to occlude more complex defects will be described in subsequent chapters.

References

1. King TD, Thompson SL, Steiner C, Mills NL. Secundum atrial septal defect. Nonoperative closure during cardiac catheterization. *JAMA.* 1976;235(23):2506–2509.

2. Koenig P, Cao Q-L, Heitschmidt M, Waight DJ, Hijazi ZM. Role of intracardiac echocardiographic guidance in transcatheter closure of atrial septal defects and patent foramen ovale using the AMPLATZER device. *J Interv Cardiol.* 2003;16(1):51–62.

3. Zanchetta M, Rigatelli G, Pedon L, Zennaro M, Carrozza A, Onorato E. Catheter closure of perforated secundum atrial septal defect under intracardiac echocardiographic guidance using a single AMPLATZER device: feasibility of a new method. *J Invasive Cardiol.* 2005;17(5):262–265.

4. Holzer RJ, Chisolm J, Hill S, Cheatham JP. Transhepatic cardiac catheterization in complex congenital heart disease: Where there is a will there is a way. *Congenital Cardiol Today.* 2005;3:1–7.

5. Ewert P, Berger F, Nagdyman N, et al. Masked left ventricular restriction in elderly patients with atrial septal defects: a contraindication for closure? *Cathet Cardiovasc Interv.* 2001;52(2):177–180.

6. Holzer R, Cao Q-L, Hijazi ZM. Closure of a moderately large atrial septal defect with a self-fabricated fenestrated AMPLATZER septal occluder in an 85-year-old patient with reduced diastolic elasticity of the left ventricle. *Cathet Cardiovasc Interv.* 2005;64(4):513–518.

7. Du ZD, Koenig P, Cao Q-L, Waight D,

Heitschmidt M, Hijazi ZM. Comparison of transcatheter closure of secundum atrial septal defect using the AMPLATZER septal occluder associated with deficient versus sufficient rims. *Am J Cardiol.* 2002;90(8):865–869.

8. Zahn EM, Wilson N, Cutright W, Latson LA. Development and testing of the HELEX septal occluder, a new expanded polytetrafluoroethylene atrial septal defect occlusion system. *Circulation.* 2001;104(6):711–716.

9. Sharafuddin MJ, Gu X, Titus JL, Urness M, Cervera-Ceballos JJ, Amplatz K. Transvenous closure of secundum atrial septal defects: preliminary results with a new self-expanding nitinol prosthesis in a swine model.[erratum appears in Circulation. 1998 Feb 3;97(4):413]. *Circulation.* 1997;95(8):2162–2168.

10. Masura J, Gavora P, Formanek A, Hijazi ZM. Transcatheter closure of secundum atrial septal defects using the new self-centering amplatzer septal occluder: initial human experience. *Cathet Cardiovasc Diagn.* 1997;42(4):388–393.

11. Varma C, Benson LN, Silversides C, et al. Outcomes and alternative techniques for device closure of the large secundum atrial septal defect. *Cathet Cardiovasc Interv.* 2004;61(1):131–139.

12. Wahab HA, Bairam AR, Cao Q-L, Hijazi ZM. Novel technique to prevent prolapse of the AMPLATZER septal occluder through large atrial septal defect. *Cathet Cardiovasc Interv.* 2003;60(4):543–545.

13. Berger F, Ewert P, Abdul-Khaliq H, Nurnberg JH, Lange PE. Percutaneous closure of large atrial septal defects with the AMPLATZER Septal Occluder: technical overkill or recommendable alternative treatment? *J Interv Cardiol.* 2001;14(1):63–67.

14. Hill SL, Berul CI, Patel HT, et al. Early ECG abnormalities associated with transcatheter closure of atrial septal defects using the AMPLATZER septal occluder. *J Interv Card Electrophysiol.* 2000;4(3):469–474.

15. Masura J, Gavora P, Podnar T. Long-term outcome of transcatheter secundum-type atrial septal defect closure using AMPLATZER septal occluders. *J Am Coll Cardiol.* 2005;45(4):505-507.

16. Fischer G, Stieh J, Uebing A, Hoffmann U, Morf G, Kramer HH. Experience with transcatheter closure of secundum atrial septal defects using the AMPLATZER septal occluder: a single centre study in 236 consecutive patients. *Heart (British Cardiac Society)* 2003;89(2):199–204.

17. Jones TK, Latson LA, Zahn E, et al, Multicenter Pivotal Study of the HSOI. Results of the U.S. multicenter pivotal study of the HELEX septal occluder for percutaneous closure of secundum atrial septal defects. *J Am Coll Cardiol.* 2007;49(22):2215–2221.

13

Device Closure of Difficult ASDs

Mustafa H. Abdullah Al-Qbandi and Ziyad M. Hijazi

Introduction

Secundum atrial septal defect (ASD-II) represents about 10% of congenital heart disease and beyond bicuspid aortic valve, is the most common congenital heart defect in adulthood. Transcatheter treatment of ASD-II is an alternative treatment option to traditional surgical closure both in children and adults[1-6] Indeed, in the last decade, a considerable number of patients with isolated ASD have undergone successful percutaneous closure with different devices.[5-11] However, morphologic variations of ASD-II are frequent and have important impact in determining the success of the transcatheter procedure; thus, their assessment remains crucial for the selection of the best treatment approach. Most ASDs (24%–75%) are centrally located, however, there remains a good percentage of them with deficient rims. Most of these cases are straightforward with a diagnosis made by transthoracic echocardiography; others require more detailed diagnosis and therefore decision for whether they are suitable for percutaneous closure.

ASDs termed difficult to close by percutaneous approach are frequently encountered. Some of these are large and others have deficient rims or the atrial septum is aneurysmal or fenestrated. Collectively, these difficult ASDs are better termed "Complex ASDs." In a study by Pedra et al,[14] they arbitrarily defined ASD with complex anatomy as the presence of a large (stretched diameter $\geq$ 26 mm) ASD associated with a deficient ($\leq$ 4 mm) rim located at the anterior, inferior, or posterior portion of the atrial septum; two separate ASDs within the atrial septum (distant or close to each other); and multifenetrated septum. Defects associated with a floppy, redundant, and hypermobile

Transcatheter Closure of ASDs and PFOs: A Comprehensive Assessment. © 2010 Ziyad M. Hijazi, Ted Feldman, Mustafa H. Abdullah Al-Qbandi, and Horst Sievert, editors. Cardiotext Publishing, ISBN: 978-0-9790164-9-3.

atrial septum (excursion ≥ 10 mm), considered to be aneurysmal were also regarded as ASDs with complex anatomy, irrespective of their size. Therefore, the common subtypes of secundum ASD are the following.

1. Large defects (could be centrally located or not)
2. Deficient anterosuperior rim
3. Multiple or fenestrated defects
4. Deficient posteroinferior rim
5. Aneurysmal atrial septum
6. Combination of the above (eg, large ASD with deficient rims).

In this chapter, we will define each subtype of secundum ASD and techniques used to closing each one of them. There are many devices used to close ASDs successfully. In this chapter, our main target will be focused on AMPLATZER Septal Occluder (ASO) as it is the most widely used device worldwide. Other devices that are in use include CardioSEAL/STARFlex, Occlutech-Figulla, Cardia INTRASEPT, Solysafe, and the HELEX device. The reader is encouraged to review the chapters on specific devices in Part IV.

Atrial Septal Rims

An adequate rim is 7 mm and longer. However, a minimum of a 5-mm rim of atrial septum around the defect has been suggested as a prerequisite for device closure with ASO.[15] However, due to its design, it is believed that the ASO would not require an anterior rim for anchorage and the device would wrap around the posterior wall of the aorta. A deficient or absent rim is anything < 3 mm. A questionable or inadequate rim is between 3 and 5 mm.

To close the ASD using the transcatheter technique, it is important for the interventional cardiologist to have sound knowledge of the atrial septal rims and the structures that surround the ASD (Fig 13.1). The atrial septum is surrounded by several important structures. The aortic root is located anterosuperiorly, the mitral valve and tricuspid valve anteroinferiorly,

the superior vena cava and right upper pulmonary vein posterosuperiorly, and the inferior vena cava posteroinferiorly. The simplified classification was initially proposed by Shrivastava and Radhakrishnan.[16] With minor modification to their classification, Amin[17] has suggested the following: aortic rim, the atrial septal rim that is adjacent to the aortic valve; superior vena cava (SVC) rim, the rim adjacent to the SVC; superior rim, the rim between the SVC rim and the aortic rim; posterior rim, the rim opposite to the aortic rim; inferior vena cava (IVC) rim, the rim adjacent to the IVC; atrioventricular valve (AV) rim, the rim adjacent to the AV valve rim (Fig 13.2).

Device Closure of ASD

As the AMPLATZER Septal Occluder (ASO) (AGA Medical Corporation, Plymouth, Minnesota) is the most widely used device, this review focuses on ASD closure with the ASO device. There are, however, other available devices in the market (see Part IV).[18-21] They are: GORE HELEX Septal Occluder device (W.L. Gore, Flagstaff, Arizona); Sideris Buttoned device that

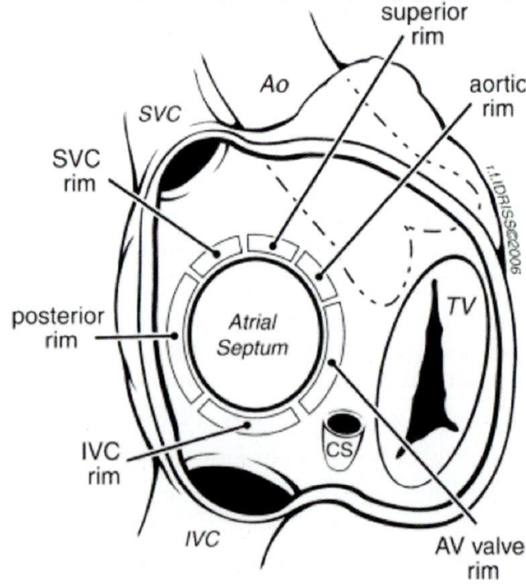

Fig 13.1—Classification of atrial septal rims. From Amin.[17] (Courtesy of Wiley-Blackwell. Used with permission.)

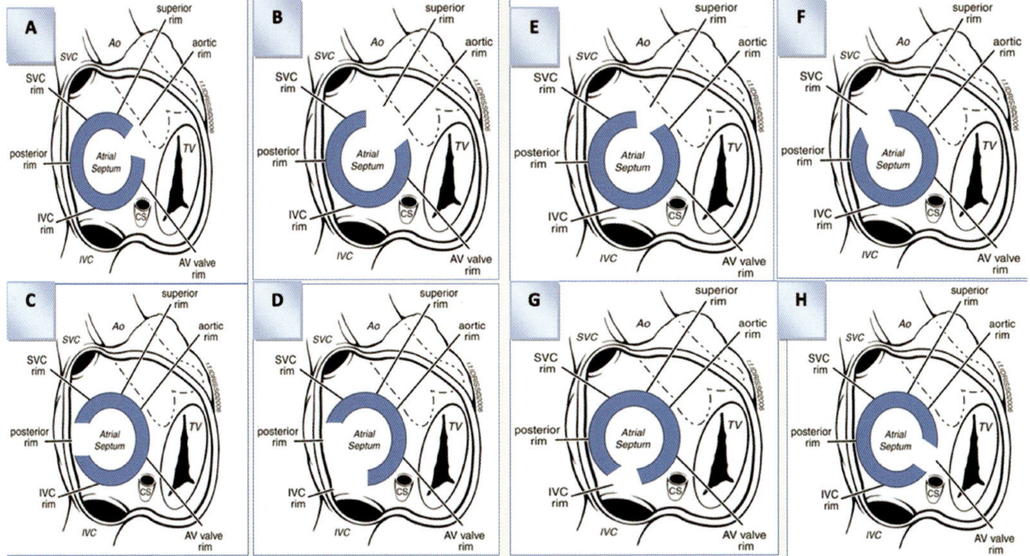

Fig 13.2—Demonstrating different scenarios for ASD-II rims. A, Anterior rim deficiency. B, Anterosuperior rim. C, Posterior rim. D, Posteroinferior rim. E, Superior rim. F, SVC rim. G, IVC rim. H, IVC rim at atrio-ventricular valves. Modified from Amin.[17] (Courtesy of Wiley-Blackwell. Used with permission.)

has undergone several modifications over the years (it is rarely being used now); STARFlex (NMT, Boston, Massachusetts) device, which is a modification of the CardioSEAL device; INTRASEPT1 PFO device that was modified for closure of ASD; and the Occlutech-Figulla device (Occlutech, Jena, Germany). Excluding the ASO and the Occlutech-Figulla, the aforementioned devices can close defects that are 20 mm or smaller in diameter. The HELEX device appears to be safe and effective in patients with small- to moderate-sized ASD.[22]

Echocardiography

The majority of ASDs are closed under either TEE guidance or ICE (see chapters 7 and 8). When performing TEE, the size of the defect should be measured in at least two orthogonal views because many of the defects are oval in shape. Complete echocardiographic examination of an ASD includes measurement in three standardized views that are utilized during the procedure: (1) the aortic short-axis view, to identify and evaluate the aortic rim and the posterior rim; (2) the bicaval view, to evaluate the SVC and IVC rims; and (3) the four-chamber view, to evaluate the AV valve rim and the superior rim. The probe is positioned in the esophagus to image the atria and the aortic valve. Small adjustments in the position of the probe in the esophagus, the degree of rotation and flexion used on the probe, and the precise angle of the plane are always necessary due to individual anatomic variability. For ICE, the readers are referred to excellent articles that address the use of ICE to guide device closure of ASDs (see chapters 7 and 8).[23–25]

Balloon sizing

Two sizing balloons are available for the stationary method of assessing the "stretched diameter or stop-flow diameter," the NuMED sizing balloon (NuMED, Hopkinton, NY) and the AGA sizing balloon (AGA Medical). Recently, a newer and improved version of the AGA sizing balloon has become available. The new AMPLATZER sizing balloon-II is available in three sizes (18, 24, and 34 mm). In contrast to the previously available AGA sizing balloons, the radiopaque marker bands are inside the balloon. Two marker bands are 0.4-mm apart for proper positioning of the catheterization laboratory camera angle. The third marker is 15 mm from the second marker for measuring the size of the defect. The balloon is made of softer and more compliant material. The distal tip is softer to prevent inadvertent injury to cardiac structures. Balloon sizing the defect is useful, as most of the defects are somewhat oval in shape and choosing a correct size device suitable for the defect may otherwise be difficult. The most important point to remember is that even these malleable balloons can stretch the ASD and falsely increase the size of the defect. Some operators do not perform balloon sizing, instead depend on the largest color Doppler flow diameter. Oversizing can be detrimental and can lead to potential complications. In a report by Amin,[17] he recommended that "stop-flow technique" be used when balloon sizing of the ASD. The stop-flow technique is described as follows: after the balloon is astride the ASD, inflate the balloon with saline or saline/contrast mixture until no shunt is seen across the ASD by color echocardiography, deflate the balloon until shunting reappears, then reinflate to eliminate the shunt (stop-flow diameter of the ASD). A device that is equal to or up to 2 mm larger than the stop-flow diameter usually works well. Oversizing should be avoided. It is not necessary to stretch the ASD diameter, and hence the term balloon-stretched diameter should be avoided. However, it is conceded that in some patients who have thin, flailing septum primum, balloon sizing may not be easy because the septum is stretched even by gentle inflation of the balloon. Despite these shortcomings that occur rarely in a few patients during balloon sizing, it is possible to measure the stop-flow diameter. Patience is a virtue. Again, it is strongly recommended to adhere to stop-flow diameter of ASD. Another area where balloon sizing can be cumbersome is in small patients with deficient rims. A good example is in a patient who weighs 15 kg and has 26-mm ASD. This patient is very likely to have deficient aortic, posterior, and/or IVC rims. Balloon sizing with long balloons in such patients may lead to obstruction of the flow from the IVC, decrease in flow of circulation from the right and left atria into the ventricles, leading to hemodynamic compromise (low cardiac output and hypotension). In addition, during balloon sizing, stop-flow diameter may not be achieved; even a minor indentation may not be seen by fluoroscopy. For such patients, balloon sizing may not be performed; instead total atrial septal length can be used to determine the size of the device. The total atrial septal length, is measured in four-chamber view by TTE and/or TEE. The AV valve rim plus the average size of the ASD (measured in at least two orthogonal views) plus the superior rim equals total atrial septal length. A device where the left atrial disc of the ASO is equal to or smaller than the total atrial septal length can be used.

Large defects

One complex anatomy of ASD is simply the defect size even with adequate rims. There is no universal definition of a large ASD. However, ASDs requiring devices > 25 mm are generally regarded as being large. In adults, ASD-II is considered too large (extra-large) for percutaneous closure if the diameter is > 38 mm. A large ASD could be defined as those with diameter range between 25 and 38 mm (stretched or unstretched). Pedra et al[14] defined a large ASD as an ASD with a stretched diameter > 26 mm. In children, the indication for percutaneous treatment is based on the defect diameter–septal length ratio with minimal differences according to the device type.

The total atrial septal length is measured in four-chamber view by TTE and/or TEE. The AV valve rim plus the average size of the ASD (measured in at least two orthogonal views) plus the superior rim equals total atrial septal length. A device where the left atrial disc of the AMPLATZER Septal Occluder is equal to or smaller than the total atrial septal length can be used.

> Left atrial disc size (for device ≤ 10 mm waist = 12 mm)
>
> Left atrial disc size (for device 11–32 mm waist = 14 mm)
>
> Left atrial disc size (for device 32–40 mm waist = 16 mm)

Total atrial septal length = measured either in, four-chamber view or using the equation:

ASD size + AVV rim + superior rim

For example, if ASD size is 20 mm, AVV rim = 5mm, Superior rim = 7 mm, stretched diameter or no flow technique ASD diameter = 25 mm

Total atrial length = 20 mm + 5 mm (AVV rim) + 7 mm (superior rim) = 32 mm
Left atrial disc size = 20 + 14 = 34 mm

In this example, ASD device > Total atrial septal length—This means higher risk for complications if device placement attempted. However, some interventional cardiologist may perform the procedure with success, as total atrial septal length may vary ± 5 mm between the four-chamber view and the calculated one and the complex nature of the three-dimensional (3D) structure of the septum allowing a large device to be seated well in the heart.

From the preceding example, using the ASO about 12 to 14 mm (12 mm in devices up to 10 mm and 14 mm in larger sizes up to 30 mm) of the rim around the central retention skirt of the device should be added to the echocardiographically measured defect diameter. When this diameter sum is larger than the maximum interatrial septal length measured in the four-chamber TTE or TEE view, device closure should not be attempted. Otherwise, if one considers using CardioSEAL/STARFlex (CS/SF; Nitinol Medical Technology, Boston, Massachusetts) or HELEX devices (W.L. Gore & Associates, Flagstaff, Arizona) in a child, a device–defect ratio of 1.8 to 2 is used as cutoff for percutaneous closure. In any case in which the diameter of device needed to close the ASD-II is equal or larger than the whole interatrial septum length, the child is referred for surgical closure.

An ASD larger than 25 mm is most likely associated with rim deficiency. Varma and colleagues[26] studied 172 patients with secundum ASD and divided them into two groups based on balloon stretched diameter: group 1, ≤ 25 mm (n=138, 80%); group 2, > 25 mm (n=34, 20%). Rim deficiency (n=62) was more frequent in group 2 compared to group 1 (50% vs. 33%; P=0.07), especially inferior rim deficiency (35% vs. 2%; P=0.005). Device deployment was successful in group 1 and group 2 (100% vs. 91%; P=0.007).

Although it seems like a simple problem, the questions would be how large a device could be used to close such a defect, whether the left atrium would accommodate such device and whether such a large device would encroach on other intracardiac structures (eg, mitral valve) or obstruct blood flow (eg, vena cavae or pulmonary veins).

Deficient anterosuperior rim

Deficient anterosuperior rim is frequently encountered with large ASDs. In a study by Podnar et al[13] among the 190 patients, 46 patients (24.2%) had centrally placed defects. In the remaining 144 patients (75.8%), various morphological variations of secundum-type ASD were found. The most frequent was a deficiency of the anterosuperior rim detected in 80 patients (42.1%).

Personal experience shows most patients the authors attempt to occlude with various devices were found to have deficient anterior superior rim. Other investigators[1,13,27] had similar experiences. In the paper reported by Varma et al[26] it was the deficient inferior rim that was found to be associated with unsuccessful AMPLATZER implantations. In contrast, with deficient anterior rim, the discs of the AMPLATZER straddle the ascending aorta. Chien-Fu Huang et al[28] found no statistical difference in closing ASDs with or without deficient anterosuperior rims. The group pointed out that in ASDs without rim deficiency, the chosen ASO size should be equal to or 1 to 2 mm larger than the measured ASD diameter. However, ASDs with deficient SA rim, the chosen ASO size should be 2 to 4 mm larger than the measured ASD diameter. Initial reports of erosion of the aortic wall by the ASO with development of aorta-to-right atrium[29] or aorta-to-left atrium[30] fistulae led to the recommendation of oversizing (ie, using a device size 4 mm larger than the measured stretched diameter) the implanted device in large defects with deficient anterior superior rim to ensure the device discs straddle and remain flared around the ascending aorta to prevent discrete areas of pressure where erosion may occur. When oversizing the device, care has to be taken not to interfere with surrounding intracardiac structures.

The difficulty in deploying the ASO in patients with deficient anterior superior rim is that the left atrial disc tends to become perpendicular to the atrial septum leading to prolapse of the left disc into the right atrium, posing a challenging difficulty. To overcome such difficulties several techniques have been proposed. Deployment of the left disc of the device in the right upper or left upper pulmonary vein followed by release of the waist and the right atrial disc while simultaneously withdrawing the deployed left atrial disc against the atrial septum[1,15,27,29,31] has been successfully used. Heat-bending the distal delivery sheath 360° plus cutting off the tip of the sheath $\geq$ 45° toward its inner circumference is another technique proposed to help overcome the prolapse of the left disc into the right atrium.[26,32,33] Another technique is the use of a specially designed sheath (Hausdorf sheath; Cook, Bloomington, Indiana) with two curves at the end to help align the left atrial disc parallel to the septum.[26,34] Supporting/holding the left atrial disc with the tip of a reinforced dilator to prevent prolapse into the right atrium is another method recently used successfully.[34]

Multiple or fenestrated defects

Multiple or fenestrated defects account for about 13% of total secundum ASDs. These represent another complex anatomy of the ASD that may be successfully closed using different techniques or devices. Of the 1013 patients studied by Butera et al,[11] multiple ASDs accounted for 46 patients (4.5%) and multifenestrated ASDs for 27 patients (2.7%). They found that in patients with multifenestrated defects, their ASDs were consistently associated with aneurysm of the interatrial septum.

Bramlet[35] studied 238 patients with secundum ASDs for device closure. In their series, 34 patients (14%) were classified as multiple ASD or cribriform type of ASD, 19 patients were closed successfully with single device. Carano et al[36] and Tchana et al[37] reported the use of balloon atrial septostomy to create a single large defect that could then be closed with a single large ASO device. The authors do not favor using such a technique. Szkutnik et al[38] reported a technique, which has been used in many institutions, and that is using a single ASO device deployed in the larger defect to occlude two or more smaller defects. In their series, a smaller defect (< 7-mm distance from the larger defect) had a 100% closure rate at 1-month follow-up. Deploying the device in the larger defect may decrease the distance between the two defects or even compress the smaller defect. They found that if the distance between the two defects is > 7 mm, a residual left-to-right shunt will persist. Other methods for closure of multiple defects with a single device include using a single CardioSEAL device[39,40,] or the new AMPLATZER Cribriform device.[42] If the smaller defect is hemodynamically significant, but is far from the other defect (> 7 mm) two devices should be used.[38] This is the approach used by Pedra et al[14] and such an approach of closure of two distant defects with two separate devices; closing the smaller defect followed by closure of larger defect is recommended. After verifying good position of both devices, release of the smaller device should precede the release of the larger device. Echocardiographic evaluation while occluding the larger defect with a balloon is helpful in deciding on the use of two devices.

Deficient posteroinferior rim

Closure of a large ASD with deficient or absent posteroinferior (PI) rim continues to be a real challenge. Insufficient number of cases with deficient PI rim reported in most series makes it even more difficult to have a solid consensus. The deficiency of the posteroinferior rim was reported by Butera et al[11] to be in the range of 33%. Those who were eligible for cardiac catheterization dropped to 10% after their exclusion criteria. All patients failed device closure. Pedra et al[14] mentioned one case with deficient anterior rim and a floppy, thin, and hypermobile posterior rim that was not a good candidate for device closure. On the other hand, Du et al[15] reported 23 patients with deficient rims, of which 3 patients had deficient inferior or posterior rims. Two patients had 2 mm of posterior rim and the third had a 4-mm posterior rim. These 3 patients were successfully closed. Hijazi and Cao[42] reported a 6.5-year-old girl, weighing 15 kg, with a 14-mm ASD with a posteriorly deficient rim that was closed successfully under ICE guidance. Certainly in the literature, there are many good success stories closing ASDs with deficient posterior or posteroinferior rims. Yet, the number of cases is too small to make a generalized conclusion. Lack of detailed anatomical description of the deficient rims and surrounding rims and defects in most reported studies adds to difficulty in drawing useful conclusions. Mathewson et al[32] defined absent PI rim as a rim < 3 mm. As the difference in radius length between right and left atrial discs of the ASO is 2 to 3 mm, a rim < 3 mm will not allow

both discs to hang on both sides of the rim. They found that defects with absent PI rim tend to be larger in diameter. They concluded that, although a stable ASO deployment is possible, these defects are more liable for complications such as pulmonary vein or IVC obstruction, encroachment onto the anterior mitral leaflet, or frank embolization.

Atrial Septal Aneurysm

The diagnostic criteria for atrial septal aneurysm (ASA) is made if a sacculation or deformity in the interatrial septum or the foramen ovale region is seen—an excursion of 10 mm into the right or left atrium or if the sum of bilateral excursions of > 10 mm.[43] Another definition of ASA (Fig 13.3) is a circumscribed bulging in the atrial septum, with a base width of at least 15 mm (or 8 mm/m^2 body surface area in children) and a depth of at least 15 mm (or 8 mm/m^2 body surface area in children), or if there is an oscillating membrane with excursions of 15 mm or more.[44] Septal aneurysms with single or multiple defects represent a different kind of complex anatomy of the ASD. Such anatomy is better dealt with

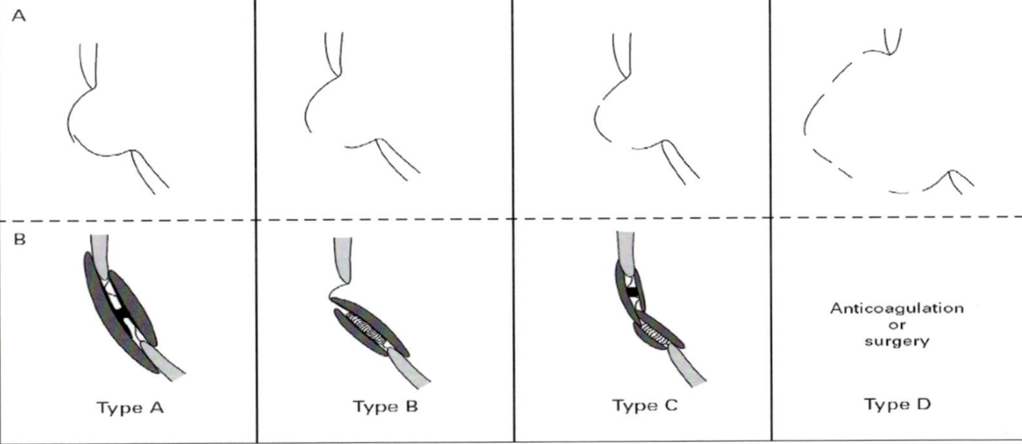

Fig 13.3—Classification of atrial septal aneurysm with respect to the interatrial communications (A) and their possible treatment (B). Type A: Persistent foramen ovale that was occluded with a large PFO device. Type B: Atrial septal defect (ASD) occluded with an AMPLATZER ASD device. Type C: Two or few perforations located in no more than two clusters and not treatable with a single device, treated with an AMPLATZER PFO and AMPLATZER septal occluders. Type D: Multiple perforations spread irregularly over aneurysm. Transcatheter treatment is currently not recommended. (Reproduced from Ewert et al.[40] with permission from BMJ Publishing Group Ltd.)

using devices that don't rely on stenting mechanism within the defect to achieve stabilization in the septum. Patch- or double disc-type devices such as the buttoned device, the HELEX, the CardioSEAL or the more recent AMPLATZER Cribriform are more appropriate choices to close such defects. Ewert et al[45] reported on 50 patients in whom closure was possible. In 9 with aneurysm and atrial septal defect (type B), 5 defects were closed and 4 required surgery. Device closure was achieved in all 10 patients with aneurysms and 2 perforations (type C), but 4 had a residual shunt. Thirteen patients with multiple perforated aneurysms (type D) underwent surgery. They concluded that classification of morphology of perforations of aneurysm is clinically useful for selecting patients for treatment by transcatheter devices.

In a study done by Numan et al,[46] 10 patients out of 16 with fenestrated ASD were diagnosed to have septal aneurysm (62%). Their use of the Cribriform AMPLATZER device proved effective in closing most ASDs (92%). A similar result was previously reported by Hijazi.[41] A large defect within an aneurysmal septum may however require a large ASO device or may not be amenable for ASO closure. Krumsdorf[47] reported that in closing two small but distant defects within an aneurysmal atrial septum may effectively close both defects, but carry a higher risk of later development of thrombus formation. Zamora et al[48] successfully closed defects associated with atrial septal aneurysms with buttoned devices by compressing the aneurysm between the occluder and the square-shaped counter-occluder.

Techniques Used to Close ASDs with Deficient Rims When Attempting AMPLATZER Occluder System

- Pulmonary vein approach
  - —Left upper pulmonary vein technique
  - —Right upper pulmonary vein technique
  - —Right lower pulmonary vein technique
- Roof of left atrium, at the entry of right upper pulmonary vein
- Hausdorf sheath technique
- Boosfeld-Spies technique
- Use of a Straight Side-Hole Delivery Sheath (SSH technique or Kutty's Method)
- Wahab technique
- Right Judkins catheter technique
- Balloon assisted technique
- Nounou technique using Agilis catheter
- The parallel wire technique

See Table 13.1

Pulmonary Vein Approach

The usual place for the ASD sheath is the left upper pulmonary vein (Fig 13.4). In most cases, this will work very well especially if the ASD is centrally placed. However, in patients with deficient aortic and/or posterior rim, device deployment is challenging.[17] In these patients, after the left disc is deployed and pulled to approximate it to the atrial septum, the superior/anterior part of the device (that is toward the aortic rim) protrudes in the right atrium. By echocardiography, the device appears perpendicular to the atrial septum. If the anterior rim is deficient, the following technique is used first. The delivery sheath is placed into the left upper pulmonary vein; the depth of the sheath should be enough to ensure that the left atrial disc will temporarily stay in the pulmonary vein when the sheath is withdrawn. The sheath is then withdrawn swiftly all the way into the right atrium so as to deploy both discs simultaneously, while the delivery cable is kept taut and stable in one location. The device resembles an American football at initial deployment. The left disc springs out of the pulmonary vein and slaps onto the atrial septum. This maneuver keeps the left disc parallel to the atrial septum, which prevents the aortic edge of the device from protruding into the right atrium. If the device does not spring out of the pulmonary vein, a gentle traction on the cable helps in withdrawing the device. Extreme care and caution should be exercised to avoid

Maneuver	Description	ASD Morphology	Reference
Pulmonary vein approach	The delivery sheath is placed in the left upper pulmonary vein or the right upper pulmonary vein and the left atrial disc is partially deployed to create an American football-like appearance. With further withdrawal of the sheath, the disc jumps parallel to the septum.	Large ASD with deficient anterior or posterior rim	Amin[17]
Left atrial roof approach	The delivery sheath is placed near the orifice of the right upper pulmonary vein (not inside the pulmonary vein). On fluoroscopy (anteroposterior view), the delivery sheath appears parallel to the spine.	Large ASD with deficient anterior or posterior rim	Amin[17]
Hausdorf sheath	The Hausdorf sheath is a specially designed long sheath with two posterior curves at its end, allowing for a better alignment of the left atrial disc parallel to the septum	Large ASD with deficient anterior rim	
Boosfeld-Spies	This is a modified Mullins sheath with a creation of a bevel at the inner curvature, also allowing a more parallel alignment of the left atrial disc to the interatrial septum.	Large ASD with deficient anterior rim	Krumsdorf[47]
SSH Kutty method	A Mullin's transseptal sheath (Cook, Bloomington, Indiana) 1–2F sizes larger than the minimum recommended sheath diameter for the intended AMPLATZER ASD occluder is cut with scissors in a direction parallel with the proximal straight length of the shaft at the base of the preexisting curve.	Large ASD with deficient anterior and/or posteroinferior rims	Remadevi[49]
Wahab technique	Following deployment of the left atrial disc, a long dilator is advanced into the left atrium, holding the superior anterior part of the left atrial disc to prevent it from prolapsing.	Large ASD with anterosuperior or posterior rim deficiency	Cooke[33]
Right Judkins catheter technique	The device (< 16 mm) is advanced via an 8F Judkins right catheter through a delivery sheath into the left atrium. Following removal of the sheath and deployment of the left disc, the assembly aligns to the septum.	Large ASD and deficient posterior rim	Hijazi[42]
Balloon-assisted technique	Similar to the dilator assisted-method, a balloon catheter is used following deployment of the left atrial disc to prevent its prolapse by holding the superior anterior part of the left atrial disc.	Large ASD and deficient posterior rim	Hijazi[42]
Nounou Agilis catheter	Agilis steerable guide catheter (St. Jude Medical) which is able to be curved by the handle on the sheath thus directing the tip of the sheath closer to the desired perpendicular plane. Can accept up to 20- to 22-mm device. Needs arterial sheath 8F to be inserted at handle.	Large ASD with deficient rims	Spies[50]
Parallel wire technique	It is not a technique to orient the device, but rather to maintain access to LA. A support 0.018" wire is used	Multiple ASD or fenestrated ASD. Large ASD with deficient rims	Kutty[52]

Table 13.1—Techniques Used to Close ASDs with Deficient Rims When Attempting AMPLATZER Occluder System

advancing the device deep into the pulmonary vein, as injury to the pulmonary vein can occur. In case the technique fails or the patient has a large ASD with deficient anterior rim, the next technique to use is deployment from the right upper pulmonary vein. In this method, after securing the sheath in the right upper pulmonary vein with the loaded device, the sheath is withdrawn partially to deploy the device from the mouth of the right upper pulmonary vein, in contact with the posterior superior septum, in an attempt to maintain the device parallel to the atrial septum as it is deployed. This maneuver can avoid rotation of the left atrial disc.[27] In case the posterior rim is deficient, the right lower pulmonary vein approach is tried.[49]

Roof of Left Atrium

This technique is also applicable in patients who have combined deficiency of aortic and poste-rior rims.[17] In this scenario, the standard device deployment technique is unsuccessful because the posterior edge of the device protrudes into the right atrium. Small patients, who have a deficient posterior rim, also have small left atrial cavity. When the left disc is deployed, it can-not expand fully in the left atrial cavity; hence, the posterior edge of the device protrudes into the right atrial cavity. To avoid this, the delivery sheath is placed near the orifice of the right upper pulmonary vein (Fig 13.5) (not inside the pulmonary vein). On fluoroscopy (anteroposte-rior view), the delivery sheath appears parallel to the spine. The device is advanced and the left disc is deployed in the atrial roof while keeping the sheath stable. The deployed left disc is per-pendicular to the spine after it is deployed in the atrial roof. The right disc is deployed by with-drawing the sheath. This maneuver keeps the posterior edge of the device inside the left atrium and away from the posterior rim of the defect, while the remainder of the device is deployed.

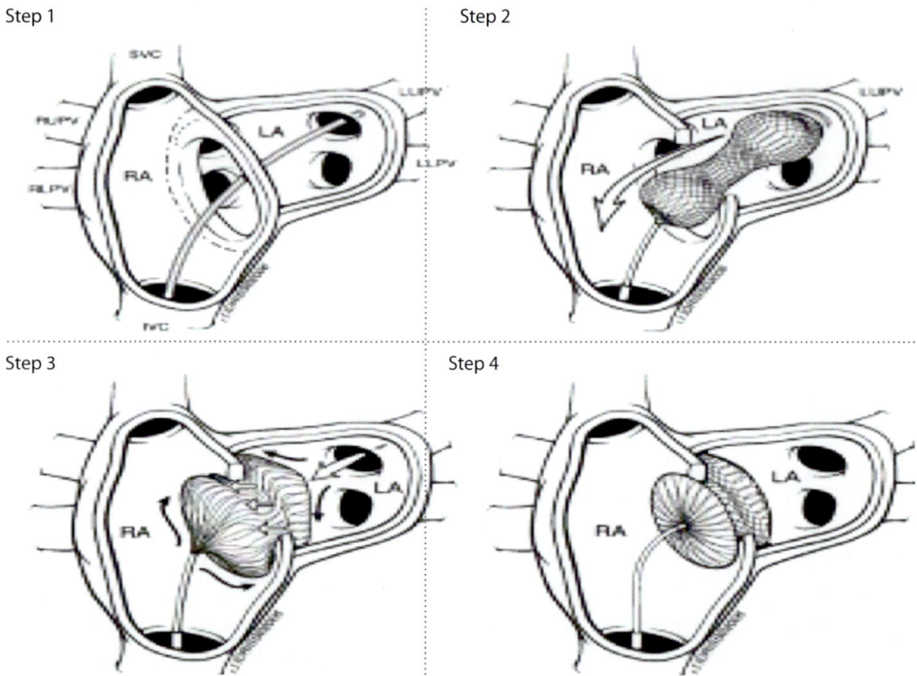

Fig 13.4—Left upper pulmonary vein approach for deployment of the AMPLATZER Septal Occluder. From Amin.[17] (Courtesy of Wiley-Blackwell. Used with permission.)

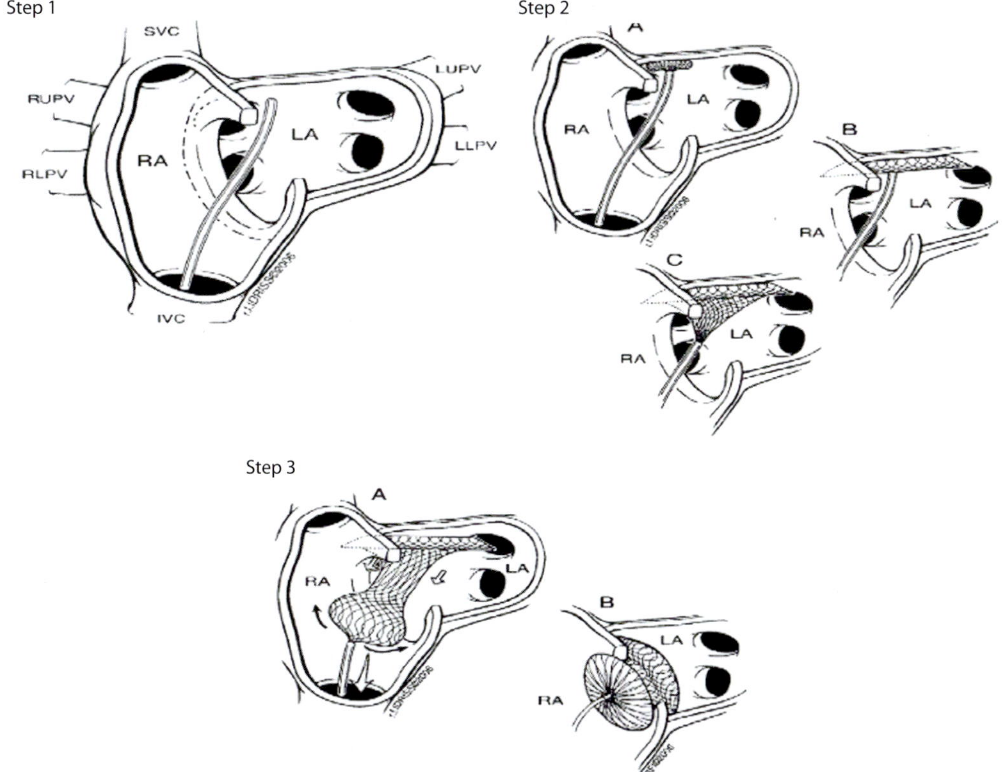

Fig 13.5—Roof of the left atrium approach for deployment of the AMPLATZER Septal Occluder. From Amin.[17] (Courtesy of Wiley-Blackwell. Used with permission.)

Hausdorf Sheath Technique

This technique is used in cases there are large ASDs with deficiency of anterior and/or anterosuperior rims. Failure to close the ASD with pulmonary venous approach may lead one to think of using this type of catheter. The late Gerd Hausdorf, MD, designed a delivery sheath (Fig 13.6) with two posterior curves and angled tip to keep the aortic edge of the disc posterior, hence parallel to the septum and away from the aortic rim. One disadvantage of the Hausdorf sheath is its bulky shape, making it difficult to maneuver through the inferior vena cava and a small right atrium. The Hausdorf sheath (Cook Medical, Bloomington, Indiana) is available in sizes 10, 11, and 12F. The sheath construction features FEP polymer which increases flexibility and maintains curve retention during pro cedural use. Radiopaque tip identifies precise location of sheath's distal tip for positioning accuracy. All the sizes come with a length of 75 cm.

The Daig sheath (St. Jude Medical, Minneapolis, Minnesota) has a somewhat similar configuration to the Hausdorf sheath and has been used by some interventionalists with good success.

Boosfeld-Spies Technique

Dr. Christoph Boosfeld and Dr. Christian Spies modified a 12F Cook Mullins-type sheath (Cook Medical) in order to close a large ASD.[50] The sheath was altered as follows (Fig 13.7). First, the entire sheath was shortened, reducing the bend of the delivery sheath. Second, the tip of the sheath was cut at the inner curvature creating a bevel reorienting the outlet of the sheath more lateral, allowing a more parallel

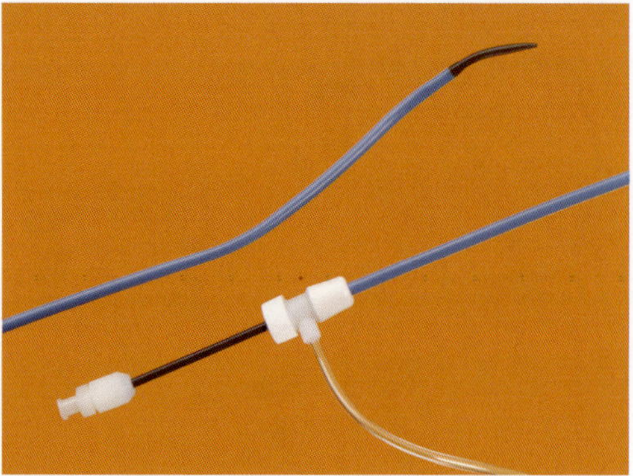

Fig 13.6—Hausdorf sheath. (Courtesy of Cook Medical. Used with permission.)

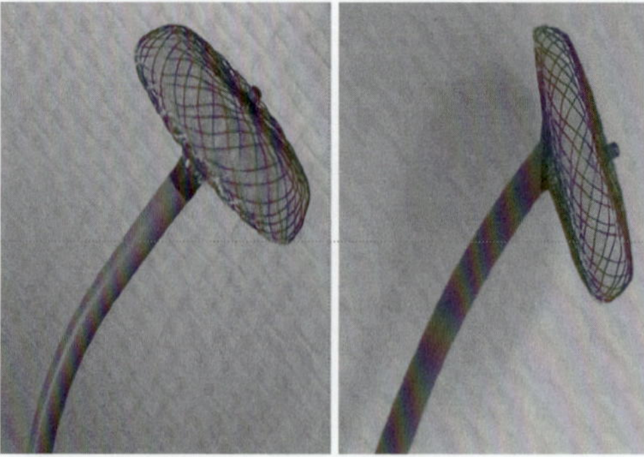

Fig 13.7—Left, regular unmodified Cook delivery sheath. Right, a bevel is placed at the inner curvature of the sheath. Note the lesser bend of the sheath and the more sideward orientation of sheath's outlet. From Spies et al.[50] (Courtesy of Wiley-Blackwell. Used with permission.)

orientation of the retention disc in relation to the interatrial septum. The patient described in their paper had 25-mm ASD with deficient inferior rim of 3 mm. A 32-mm AMPLATZER device was successfully deployed using this technique. Creation of a bevel on the inner curvature of the delivery sheath for percutaneous ASD closure devices has been described.[51] Yet a major shortcoming of this "cut tip" sheath was the occurrence of a long longitudinal split of the sheath. This complication did not allow for the retrieval of the AMPLATZER device. With the modified sheath used in the Boosfeld-Spies report, this complication did not occur.

Use of a Straight Side-Hole Delivery Sheath (SSH Technique or Kutty's Method)

This is a method whereby a Mullins transseptal sheath is modified[52] The resulting sheath is straight and has an exit orifice essentially in the side of the distal portion of the sheath—a straight, side-hole (SSH) delivery sheath. A Mullin's transseptal sheath (Cook Medical) 1 to 2F sizes larger than the minimum recommended sheath diameter for the intended AMPLATZER ASD occluder is cut with scissors in a direction parallel with the proximal straight length of the shaft at the base of the preexisting curve (Fig 13.8). This results in an elongated teardrop-shaped opening that is essentially in the side of the sheath. The distal tip of the sheath after the initial cut is sharp and is, therefore, trimmed slightly to provide a more rounded contour. The cut edges of the opening still have the potential to be relatively sharp so one must exercise caution when maneuvering this sheath in the vascular system. This modification should only be done on a sheath made from material that resists splitting longitudinally. Care must be taken as the sheath is advanced through the skin to ensure that the tip of the SSH sheath is not folded back on itself. Predilation of the entry site may be helpful. There is no radiopaque marker at the end of the modified sheath, so extra care is required to visualize and ensure the correct location of the tip of the modified sheath. Although the tip of the sheath has been blunted, there may still be relatively sharp edges. Therefore, the sheath should not be advanced unless the dilator is in place. Once the tip of the sheath is in the left atrium, wire and dilator are withdrawn and further steps follow as for ASD device closure. In this case the LA disc will be parallel to the plane of atrial septum.

The authors have used this modified delivery sheath in 140 successive patients with excel-

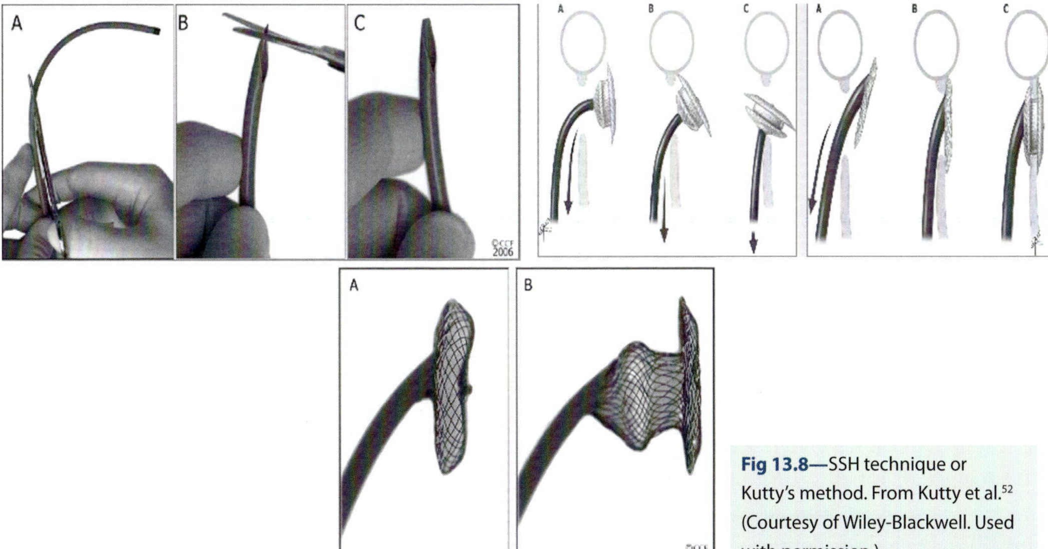

Fig 13.8—SSH technique or Kutty's method. From Kutty et al.[52] (Courtesy of Wiley-Blackwell. Used with permission.)

lent results. They reported its use in ASDs with deficient inferior rims as well anterosuperior rims.

Wahab Technique

The Wahab is another technique to help keep the left atrial disc parallel to the septum and prevent prolapse into the right atrium.[34] It could well be used for ASDs that are large with deficient anterior, anterosuperior, and/or posterior rims. In their original description of the two cases: one patient was a 4.5-year-old girl with a balloon-stretched ASD diameter of 20 mm and a 22-mm AMPLATZER device was used. The other patient was a 10-year-old girl with a balloon-stretched diameter of 23 mm and a 24-mm AMPLATZER device was used successfully. In both cases initial attempts at closure failed with the standard technique (deployment in mid left atrium) and the left upper pulmonary vein approach. Every time the device prolapsed into the right atrium or formed perpendicular angle with the atrial septum.

The technique used involves two femoral vein lines and sheaths. In their own wording "The stiff end of a 0.035" guidewire was preshaped and curved to 45°. This wire was advanced inside the dilator until it reached to the tip. The dilator was maneuvered inside the left atrium. The LA disk was deployed inside the LA. The dilator was maneuvered to hold the superior/anterior aspect of the LA disk inside the LA while deploying the waist and the right atrium disk in the defect and right atrium, respectively (Fig 13.9). The dilator was withdrawn back to the right atrium and out the patient. There are potential problems using this technique: damage to the LA disc from the stiff dilator, disturbance of the wire mesh or the fabric layers of the device. So caution should be taken in using this technique.

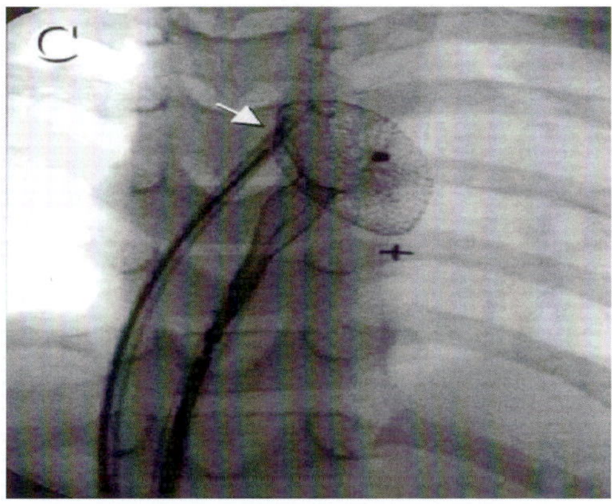

Fig 13.9—Wahab technique (dilator method). From Wahab et al.[34] (Courtesy of Wiley-Blackwell. Used with permission.)

Right Judkins Guide Catheter Technique

The right Judkins guiding catheter with an inner lumen of 0.089" (Cordis, a Johnson and Johnson Co, Miami, Florida) can accept up to 18-mm ASD AMPLATZER device (Fig 13.10). The case described by Hijazi involved a 6.5-year-old girl (weight 15.6 kg) with a posteriorly deficient rim and ASD size of 14 mm and stretched diameter of 17.5 mm. The initial attempts at closure using a 18-mm AMPLATZER device and left upper pulmonary vein approach failed due to prolapse of LA disc into the RA. ICE imaging was used. A 22-mm device was loaded into an 8F right Judkins guide coronary catheter. The guide catheter (with the device and cable) was advanced through a 9F sheath positioned in the mid left atrium until the guide catheter reached the tip of the sheath. The sheath was then retracted back into the inferior vena cava leaving the guide catheter in the middle of the left atrium. Retracting the catheter over the cable deployed the left atrial disc. The left atrial disc was parallel to the septum. Then part of the waist was deployed in the left atrium and the remainder of the waist was deployed in the defect. Further retraction of the guide catheter over the cable deployed the right atrial disc in the right atrium. This has resulted in complete occlusion of the defect. This example clearly shows that little angles are sometimes needed to deploy the device probably by making the LA disc parallel to the plane of the atrial septum.

Balloon-Assisted Technique

The balloon-assisted technique (BAT) consists of using a balloon catheter to support the left atrial disc of the AMPLATZER Septal Occluder during device deployment. This was initially reported by Dalvi et al.[53] The balloon support prevents prolapse of the LA disc into the right atrium (Fig 13.11). This technique is used mainly in cases of large ASD with deficient rims even if it is the posterior inferior rim. The procedure requires two femoral lines.

The technique is as follows: From the left femoral vein, Judkins right 4F with 3.5 curve is stationed in the left upper pulmonary vein (any other multipurpose catheter can be used). This is exchanged for the Medi-Tech sizing balloon catheter that is initially used for sizing the defect (or any sizing balloon). The left atrial (LA) disc was released well within the LA just outside the opening of the left or right superior pulmonary veins. The sizing balloon is inflated

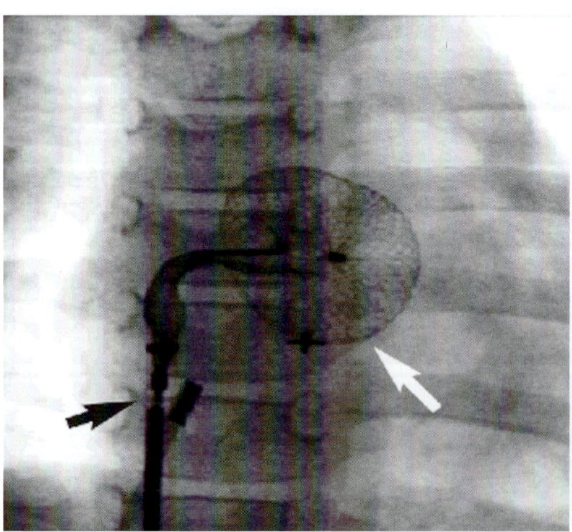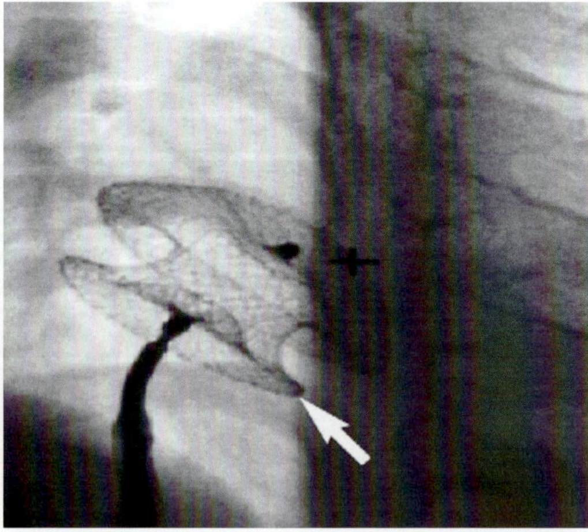

Fig 13.10—Right Judkins guide catheter technique. (Reprinted from Hijazi and Qi-Ling.[42] (Copyright 2002, with permission from Anderson Publishing Ltd.)

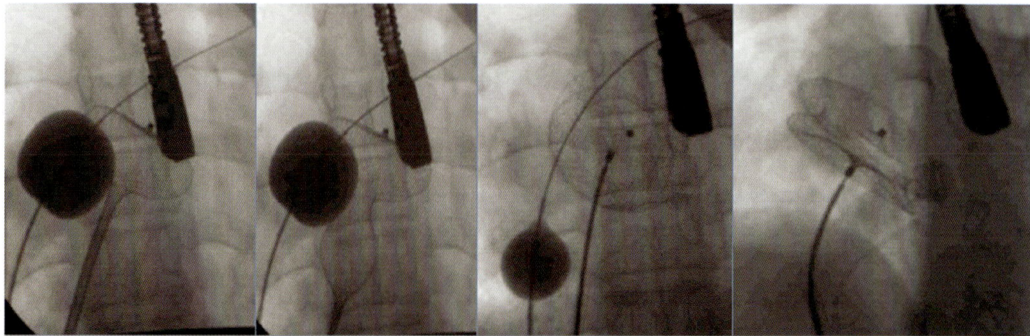

Fig 13.11—Balloon-assisted technique. From Dalvi et al.[53] (Courtesy of Wiley-Blackwell. Used with permission.)

in the right atrium (RA) and pushed over the guide wire to abut the IAS from the RA side with the assistance of another operator. The LA disc along with the delivery sheath is pulled back towards the IAS, so that the inflated balloon could support the LA disc. The waist and the RA disc are then released in succession. The LA disc that tended to prolapse through the ASD and lie horizontally across the defect when not supported is found to cuddle the aortic root with the balloon support. The balloon is gradually deflated. During the balloon deflation, the RA disc is moved toward the LA disc by pushing the loading cable. The balloon, along with the guide wire, is brought down into the inferior vena cava. The position of the device was confirmed by TEE.

Nounou Technique Using the Agilis Catheter

The Nounou is a novel technique where a steerable curved guide catheter, the Agilis catheter (Fig 13.12) (St. Jude Medical, Inc., Minneapolis, Minnesota), is used to properly position an ASO.[54] The case report describes a 29-year-old male presenting with progressive shortness of breath and found to have a moderate-sized secundum-type ASD measuring 20 mm using stop-flow technique. The anterosuperior rim was deficient. Several attempts at closure failed, including the use of a larger device at 26 mm. To properly deliver the ASO, they selected a delivery sheath with the ability to create an

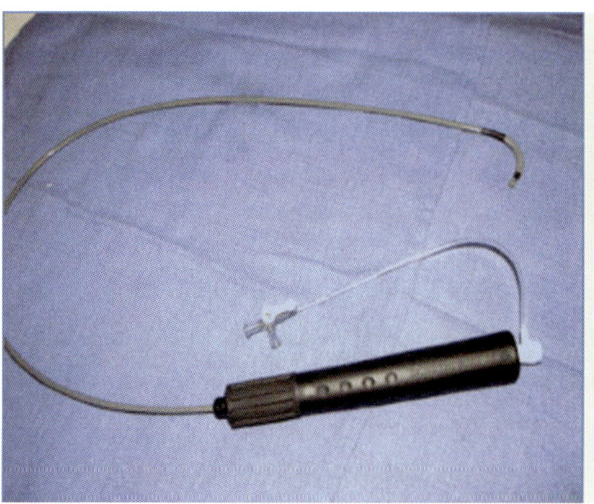
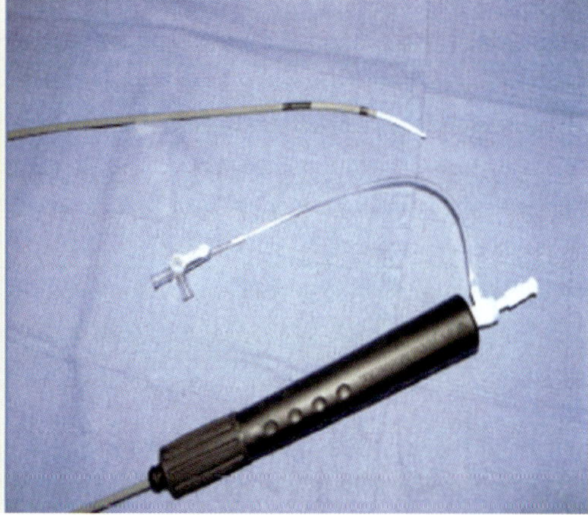

Fig 13.12—Demonstration of the curve of the Nounou technique using Agilis catheter. From Nounou et al.[54] (Courtesy of Wiley-Blackwell. Used with permission.)

acute curve to keep the introducer closer to a perpendicular axis with septal plane. They used an Agilis steerable guide catheter that was able to be curved by the handle on the sheath thus directing the tip of the sheath closer to the desired perpendicular plane. The Agilis catheter required another 8F sheath to be inserted into the handle to load the ASO device. The curved sheath was advanced and positioned in the left atrium. The ASO device was loaded into the sheath and advanced to the left atrium in standard fashion, the left atrial disc was deployed, the device assembly angled and retracted into the ASD. By doing so it was possible to place the ASO in the same plane with the atrial septum and successfully implant the closure device.

The only caveat using this catheter is the size of device that may be loaded inside can be perhaps no larger than 20 mm.

The Parallel Wire Technique for Septal Defect Closure

The Parallel Wire technique is mainly to maintain wire position in LA in case repeated attempts are anticipated.[55] Therefore, it is not a technique to position the device, but rather to maintain access to LA. The "parallel wire" technique described a novel method to maintain access to the LA until just before device release. It helps to guide device placement in fenestrated ASDs and serves as a "body wire." Similarly, in large ASDs with deficient rims, this technique could be used as a body wire for support to reduce the incidence of device prolapse. A support 0.018" wire was used, but any support 0.014" wire could also be utilized. These wires would be soft enough to allow the ASO to take its natural configuration, yet provide enough support to regain access should the need arise. Also, removing the wire after the device has been deployed but not released is easy, as wire entrapment is very unlikely to occur due to the small wire profile.

Summary

During the past decade, interventional occlusion of secundum-type ASDs has become standard treatment for most defects. As measured by the number of devices implanted worldwide and their respective results, the AMPLATZER Septal Occluder has become the first choice. In patients with appropriate anatomical dimensions of the defect, interventional closure should be favored. Adapting well-known interventional methods and developing newer techniques and device designs will also allow successful treatment of highly complicated atrial septal anatomy and atypical interatrial defects. Most complications encountered with interventional occlusion of interatrial defects are fully understood and should therefore be avoided. This technique provides equal efficacy, lower complication rates, a shorter hospitalization, and less cost than surgical closure. Surgical ASD closure should be considered only in patients with septum primum defects, sinus venosus defects, secundum defects larger than 38-mm stretched diameter, or secundum defects without sufficient rims.

References

1. Chessa M, Carminati M, Butera G, et al. Early and late complications associated with transcatheter occlusion of secundum atrial septal defect. *J Am Coll Cardiol.* 2002;39:1061–1065.

2. Berger F, Ewert P, Bjornstad PG, et al. Transcatheter closure as standard treatment for most interatrial defects: experience in 200 patients treated with the AMPLATZER Septal Occluder. *Cardiol Young.* 1999;9:468–473.

3. Du ZD, Hijazi ZM, Kleinman CS, Silverman NH, Larntz K. Comparison between transcatheter and surgical closure of secundum atrial septal defect in children and adults: results of a multicenter nonrandomized trial. *J Am Coll Cardiol.* 2002;39:1836–1844.

4. Thomson JD, Aburawi EH, Watterson KG, Van DC, Gibbs JL. Surgical and transcatheter (AMPLATZER) closure of atrial septal defects: a pro-

spective comparison of results and cost. *Heart.* 2002;87:466–469.

5. Rome JJ, Keane JF, Perry SB, Spevak PJ, Lock JE. Double-umbrella closure of atrial defects. Initial clinical applications. *Circulation.* 1990;82:751–758.

6. Sideris EB, Sideris SE, Thanopoulos BD, Ehly RL, Fowlkes JP. Transvenous atrial septal defect occlusion by the buttoned device. *Am J Cardiol.* 1990;66:1524–1526.

7. Sievert H, Babic UU, Hausdorf G, et al. Transcatheter closure of atrial septal defect and patent foramen ovale with ASDOS device (a multi-institutional European trial). *Am J Cardiol.* 1998;82:1405–1413.

8. Formigari R, Santoro G, Rossetti L, Rinelli G, Guccione P, Ballerini L. Comparison of three different atrial septal defect occlusion devices. *Am J Cardiol.* 1998;82:690–692, A9.

9. Carminati M, Giusti S, Hausdorf G, et al. A European multicentric experience using the CardioSEAL and STARFlex double umbrella devices to close interatrial communications holes within the oval fossa. *Cardiol Young.* 2000;10:519–526.

10. Dobrolet NC, Iskowitz S, Lopez L, Whalen R, Zahn EM. Sequential implantation of two HELEX septal occluder devices in a patient with complex atrial septal anatomy. *Cathet Cardiovasc Intervent.* 2001;54:242–246.

11. Butera G, Romagnoli E, Carminati M, et al. Treatment of isolated secundum atrial septal defects: impact of age and defect morphology in 1,013 consecutive patients. *Am Heart J.* 2008;156:706–712.

12. Chan KC, Godman MJ. Morphological variations of fossa ovalis atrial septal defects (secundum): feasibility for transcutaneous closure with the clam-shell device. *Br Heart J.* 1993;69:52–55.

13. Podnar T, Martanovic P, Gavora P, Masura J. Morphological variations of secundum-type atrial septal defects: feasibility for percutaneous closure using AMPLATZER septal occluders. *Cathet Cardiovasc Intervent.* 2001;53:386–391.

14. Pedra CA, Pedra SR, Esteves CA. et al. Transcatheter closure of secundum atrial septal defects with complex anatomy. *J Invas Cardiol.* 2004;16:117–122.

15. Du ZD, Koenig P, Cao Q-L, Waight D, Heitschmidt M, Hijazi ZM. Comparison of transcatheter closure of secundum atrial septal defect using the AMPLATZER septal occluder associated with deficient versus sufficient rims. *Am J Cardiol.* 2002;90:865–869.

16. Shrivastava S, Radhakrishnan S. Echocardiographic anatomy of atrial septal defect: "nomenclature of the rims." *Indian Heart J.* 2003;55:88–89.

17. Amin Z. Transcatheter closure of secundum atrial septal defects. *Cathet Cardiovasc Intervent.* 2006;68:778–787.

18. Mills NL, King TD. Nonoperative closure of left-to-right shunts. *J Thorac Cardiovasc Surg.* 1976;72:371–378.

19. King TD, Thompson SL, Steiner C, Mills NL. Secundum atrial septal defect. Nonoperative closure during cardiac catheterization. *JAMA.* 1976;235:2506–2509.

20. Rashkind WJ. Transcatheter treatment of congenital heart disease. *Circulation.* 1983;67:711–716.

21. Chopra PS, Rao PS. History of the development of atrial septal occlusion devices. *Curr Intervent Cardiol Rep.* 2000;2:63–69.

22. Jones TK, Latson LA, Zahn E, et al. Multicenter Pivotal Study of the HELEX Septal Occluder Investigators. Results of the U.S. multicenter pivotal study of the HELEX septal occluder for percutaneous closure of secundum atrial septal defects. *J Am Coll Cardiol.* 2007;49(22):2215–21.

23. Rao PS. Summary and comparison of atrial septal defect closure devices. *Curr Interv Cardiol Rep.* 2000;2:367–376.

24. Rao PS. Closure devices for atrial septal defect: which one to choose? *Indian Heart J* 1998;50:379–383.

25. Rao PS. Transcatheter closure of atrial septal defect: are we there yet? *J Am Coll Cardiol.* 1998;31:1117–1119.

26. Varma C, Benson LN, Silversides C, et al. Outcomes and alternative techniques for device closure of the large secundum atrial septal defect. *Cathet Cardiovasc Intervent.* 2004;61:131–139.

27. Berger F, Ewert P, Abdul-Khaliq H, Nurnberg JII, Lange PE. Percutaneous closure of large

atrial septal defects with the AMPLATZER Septal Occluder: technical overkill or recommendable alternative treatment? *J Intervent Cardiol.* 2001;14:63–67.

28. Huang CF, Fang CY, Ko SF, et al. Transcatheter closure of atrial septal defects with superior-anterior rim deficiency using AMPLATZER septal occluder. *J Formos Med Assoc.* 2007;106: 986–991.

29. Chun DS, Turrentine MW, Moustapha A, Hoyer MH. Development of aorta-to-right atrial fistula following closure of secundum atrial septal defect using the AMPLATZER septal occluder. *Cathet Cardiovasc Intervent.* 2003;58:246–251.

30. Aggoun Y, Gallet B, Acar P, et al. [Perforation of the aorta after percutaneous closure of an atrial septal defect with an Amplatz prosthesis, presenting with acute severe hemolysis]. *Arch Mal Coeur Vaiss.* 2002;95:479–482.

31. Harper RW, Mottram PM, McGaw DJ. Closure of secundum atrial septal defects with the AMPLATZER septal occluder device: techniques and problems. *Cathet Cardiovasc Intervent.* 2002;57:508–524.

32. Mathewson JW, Bichell D, Rothman A, Ing FF. Absent posteroinferior and anterosuperior atrial septal defect rims: Factors affecting non-surgical closure of large secundum defects using the AMPLATZER occluder. *J Am Soc Echocardiogr.* 2004;17:62–69.

33. Cooke JC, Gelman JS, Harper RW. Echocardiologists' role in the deployment of the AMPLATZER atrial septal occluder device in adults. *J Am Soc Echocardiogr.* 2001;14:588–594.

34. Wahab HA, Bairam AR, Cao Q-L, Hijazi ZM. Novel technique to prevent prolapse of the AMPLATZER septal occluder through large atrial septal defect. *Cathet Cardiovasc Interv.* 2003;60:543–545.

35. Bramlet MT, Hoyer MH. Single pediatric center experience with multiple device implantation for complex secundum atrial septal defects. *Cathet Cardiovasc Intervent.* 2008;72: 531–537.

36. Carano N, Hagler DJ, Agnetti A, Squarcia U. Device closure of fenestrated atrial septal defects: use of a single Amplatz atrial septal occluder after balloon atrial septostomy to create a single defect. *Cathet Cardiovasc Intervent.* 2001;52:203–207.

37. Tchana B, Hagler DJ, Carano N, Agnetti A, Squarcia U. Device closure of fenestrated atrial septal aneurysm: difficulties and complications with implantation of two devices. *J Invas Cardiol.* 2004;16:532–534.

38. Szkutnik M, Masura J, Bialkowski J, et al. Transcatheter closure of double atrial septal defects with a single AMPLATZER device. *Cathet Cardiovasc Intervent.* 2004;61:237–241.

39. Pedra CA, Pihkala J, Lee KJ, et al. Transcatheter closure of atrial septal defects using the CardioSeal implant. *Heart.* 2000;84:320–326.

40. Ewert P, Berger F, Kretschmar O, Abdul-Khaliq H, Stiller B, Lange PE. Feasibility of transcatheter closure of multiple defects within the oval fossa. *Cardiol Young.* 2001;11:314–319.

41. Hijazi ZM, Cao Q-L. Transcatheter closure of multi-fenestrated atrial septal defects using the new AMPLATZER cribriform device. *Ped Cardiol Today.* 2003;1–4.

42. Hijazi ZM, Qi-Ling Cao. Transcatheter Closure of Secundum Atrial Septal Defect Associated with Deficient Posterior Rim in a Child Under Intracardiac Echocardiographic Guidance. *Appl Cardiac Imaging.* 2003;7–10.

43. Olivares-Reyes A, Chan S, Lazar EJ, Bandlamudi K, Narla V, Ong K. Atrial septal aneurysm: a new classification in two hundred five adults. *J Am Soc Echocardiogr.* 1997;10:644–656.

44. Hanley PC, Tajik AJ, Hynes JK, et al. Diagnosis and classification of atrial septal aneurysm by two-dimensional echocardiography: report of 80 consecutive cases. *J Am Coll Cardiol.* 1985;6:1370–1382.

45. Ewert P, Berger F, Vogel M, Dahnert I, Alexi-Meshkishvili V, Lange PE. Morphology of perforated atrial septal aneurysm suitable for closure by transcatheter device placement. *Heart.* 2000;84:327–331.

46. Numan M, El SA, Tofeig M, Gendi S, Tohami T, El-Said HG. Cribriform AMPLATZER device closure of fenestrated atrial septal defects: feasibility and technical aspects. *Pediatr Cardiol.* 2008;29:530–535.

47. Krumsdorf U, Ostermayer S, Billinger K, et al. Incidence and clinical course of thrombus for-

mation on atrial septal defect and patient foramen ovale closure devices in 1,000 consecutive patients. *J Am Coll Cardiol.* 2004;43:302–309.

48. Zamora R, Rao PS, Sideris EB. Buttoned Device for Atrial Septal Defect Occlusion. *Curr Intervent Cardiol Rep.* 2000;2:167–176.

49. Remadevi KS, Francis E, Kumar RK. Catheter closure of atrial septal defects with deficient inferior vena cava rim under transesophageal echo guidance. *Cathet Cardiovasc Intervent.* 2009;73:90–96.

50. Spies C, Boosfeld C, Schrader R. A modified Cook sheath for closure of a large secundum atrial septal defect. *Cathet Cardiovasc Intervent.* 2007;70:286–289.

51. Hoyer MH. Delivery sheath tear after modification for ASD closure. *Cathet Cardiovasc Intervent.* 2006;68:162–164.

52. Kutty S, Asnes JD, Srinath G, Preminger TJ, Prieto LR, Latson LA. Use of a straight, sidehole delivery sheath for improved delivery of AMPLATZER ASD occluder. *Cathet Cardiovasc Intervent.* 2007;69:15–20.

53. Dalvi BV, Pinto RJ, Gupta A. New technique for device closure of large atrial septal defects. *Cathet Cardiovasc Intervent.* 2005;64:102–107.

54. Nounou M, Harrison A, Kern M. A novel technique using a steerable guide catheter to successfully deliver an AMPLATZER septal occluder to close an atrial septal defect. *Cathet Cardiovasc Intervent.* 2008;72:994–997.

55. Chiam PT, Cohen HA, Ruiz CE. The parallel wire technique for septal defect closure. *Cathet Cardiovasc Intervent.* 2008;71:564–567.

14

Device Closure of ASDs in Small Children

Mustafa H. Abdullah Al-Qbandi and Ziyad M. Hijazi

Introduction

We arbitrarily define small children undergoing percutaneous closure of secundum atrial septal defect (ASD), to be either child < 2 years of age and/or a child with weight < 15 kg. This group of children can further be divided into two subgroups. The first subgroup is patients < 1 year of age (infants) with weight < 10 kg and the other subgroup is early toddler patients with weight in the range of 10 to 15 kg. ASD is a common cardiac abnormality in up to 5% to 10% of patients with congenital heart disease. Symptoms due to ASD are uncommon during early childhood; however, on rare occasions, infants/children may present due to symptoms of failure to thrive or shortness of breath. The natural history of ASD indicates that such defects are generally benign in the first 2 to 3 decades of life (for full discussion about clinical perspectives and natural history of ASD, the reader is referred to Chapters 2 and 3). In children with no symptoms, there is a general concensus among pediatric cardiolgists to close asymptomatic ASDs prior to entering school, around 3–4 years of age (see Box 14.1). Symptomatic ASD in small children could be isolated or associated with cardiac, noncardiac, and/or genetic syndromes. Symptoms of pulmonary overcirculation, frequent respiratory infections, congestive heart failure (CHF), failure to thrive, or inability to wean from a ventilator are seen in small children.[1,2] The possible explanations of CHF in infants with ASD include[3]: (1) large left-to-right shunt; (2) presence of another left-to-right shunt; (3) earlier than usual decrease in pulmonary vascular resistance; (4) presence of a left-sided obstructive lesion; (5) abnormal ventricular compliance; or (6) abnormal atrial compliance. Those patients as well as others having associated cardiac diseases or lung diseases aggravated by the ASD may require treatment at an earlier age.[4] In a study by Hanslik et al,[5] of ASDs with a diameter of 4 to 5 mm at diagnosis, 56% showed spontaneous closure, 30% regressed to a diameter of ≤ 3 mm, and none required surgical closure. Of ASDs with a diameter of > 10 mm at diagnosis, none closed spontaneously, whereas 77% required surgical or device closure. Gender and observation time were not associated with spontaneous ASD closure or regression to ≤ 3 mm (Fig 14.1).

The incidence of symptomatic ASD in infancy as reported by Dimich and colleagues[6] varies from 5% to 10% to 13.7%; symptomatic ASD requiring surgery is even rarer (3.7%) at that age.[7]

Elective surgery is usually planned between 2 and 4 years of age. A low associated morbidity remains after surgical closure, including mainly infections, pericardial effusions, arrhythmias, and of course the scar associated with the surgery. However, there has to be a very good indication for a surgeon to close an isolated ASD in small children. Reports of percutaneous intervention for symptomatic ASD in small children are increasing.[8,9] Transcatheter device closure of an ASD in a small patient imposes certain technical challenges (Box 14.2). Dalvi[10] reported that large ASDs in small children present multiple problems for transcatheter closure. The rims are frequently deficient compared with small- and medium-sized defects. However, even with sufficient rims, there are some unique challenges in this group of patients. The small size of the left atrial cavity may not be large enough to accommodate the left atrial disc of the device. The curvature of the left atrium produced by the pulmonary veins posteriorly and the atrial appendage anteriorly causes rotation of the left atrial disc and prevents it from remaining parallel to the plane of the interatrial septum.[11] Floppiness of the inferior rim is another factor that may not offer adequate support to the device, more so if associated with deficiency of the aortic or superior vena caval rim.[12] These factors either alone or in combination lead to malalignment of the left atrial disc in relation to the plane of the interatrial septum with subsequent prolapse of the disc into the right atrium. In a study by Cardenas,[4] a total of 484 children < 18 years old underwent ASD closure over a period of 4 years. In 52/484 patients, percutaneous closure was attempted while patient weight was equal or < 15 kg. Associated lesions were frequent: cardiac in 21%, noncardiac in 32.7%, with defined genetic syndromes in 13.4%. Ten patients (19.2%) weighed < 10 kg at the time of

---

Spontaneous closure

Rare if defect > 8 mm at birth.[6,7]

Rare after age 2 years.

Very rarely an ASD can enlarge on follow-up.[6–9]

Indications for closure

ASD associated with right ventricular volume overload.

Ideal age of closure

In asymptomatic child: 2 to 4 years (in some centers closure is performed earlier by device)

Symptomatic ASD in infancy[2,10]

Congestive heart failure, severe pulmonary artery hypertension is seen in about 8% to 10% of cases.

Rule out associated lesions (eg, total anomalous pulmonary venous drainage; left ventricular inflow obstruction, or aortopulmonary window).

Box 14.1—Some Facts about Atrial Septal Defects

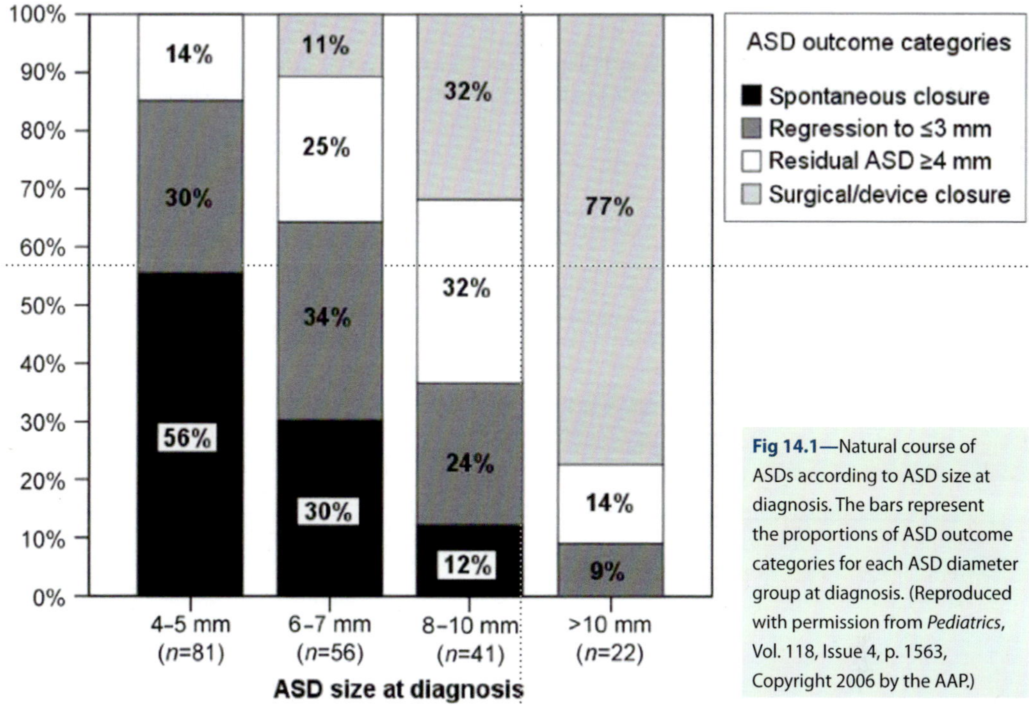

Fig 14.1—Natural course of ASDs according to ASD size at diagnosis. The bars represent the proportions of ASD outcome categories for each ASD diameter group at diagnosis. (Reproduced with permission from *Pediatrics*, Vol. 118, Issue 4, p. 1563, Copyright 2006 by the AAP.)

procedure. Associated lesions in this population group were even higher when compared with the whole cohort: 7 patients (70%) had either a cardiac or noncardiac anomaly or a genetic syndrome.

Indications and Mode of Intervention

Clearly, ASD must be closed in symptomatic patients with right ventricular volume overload, especially in small children with symptoms of pulmonary overcirculation, evidence of pulmonary hypertension, failure to thrive, or inability to wean off from the ventilator. In this group of patients, surgical closure may pose some morbidity and even mortality. Therefore, efforts should be made to close such defects either percutaneously or in a hybrid fashion (peratrial) to avoid the complications of bypass and to shorten the recovery period.

Transcatheter Approach

Imaging

Transcatheter device closure of an ASD in a small patient imposes certain technical challenges. Although the standard approach is to guide the device implantation with transesophageal echocardiography (TEE),[13] the pediatric multiplane transesophageal probe is sometimes too large as well traumatic to pass down the esophagus in small weight infants. Alternatively, transthoracic echocardiographic (TTE) imaging from the subcostal view using the ultrasound transducer in a sterile sleeve is used to guide the device delivery. Another innovative approach is the use of intracardiac echocardiography (ICE) to guide the closure procedure. The use of ICE was reported successfully to guide closure of ASDs in small children.[14–21] This technique can overcome the need for general endotracheal anesthesia and the disadvantages/risks associated with the use of TEE. The ICE catheter is inserted via a sheath into the femoral vein. The ICE catheter (AcuNav, Siemens Medical Systems) is currently available in two sizes, an 8F and a 10F. The 8F probe can be introduced in an 8F regular sheath.

Procedure

Informed consent is obtained from the parents of all patients. All procedures are conducted under general anesthesia, using fluoroscopic and echocardiographic guidance, usually transesophageal but occasionally ICE or TTE. Femoral venous access is obtained. If this is not possible due to femoral vein thrombosis/interrupted inferior vena cava, then transhepatic approach is the best approach that should be attempted. All patients must receive intravenous heparin once access is established. The largest ASD diameter, as measured by TEE at the beginning of the procedure, and the stop-flow diameter using a sizing balloon (NuMED or AGA Medical), is recorded. Some operators do not perform balloon sizing, rather they measure the largest diameter using color Doppler and choose a device approximately 25% larger than this diameter. If there is more than one defect or if the septum has multifenestrations, closure can be done using multiple devices or one single device covering the entire septum.

There are numerous devices available that can be used to close ASDs. In the United States, the only approved devices are the AMPLATZER Septal Occluder (AGA Medical Corporation, Plymouth, Minnesota) and the GORE HELEX device (W.L. Gore & Associates, Flagstaff, Arizona). Antibiotic prophylaxis is given before or during the procedure and at 8-hour intervals for a total of three doses. All patients are placed on an aspirin regimen of 5 mg/kg per day, initiated two days prior to the procedure and continued for 6 months after the procedure. All patients should have chest radiograph, electrocardiogram, and echocardiogram at 24 hours, 1 to 6 months, and 12 months after the procedure, and yearly thereafter.

If, at any time, transfemoral or transhepatic approach[22] is not possible, then the hybrid approach (surgical peratrial) is another solution that does not require cardiopulmonary bypass. The peratrial approach[23-25] is used when the size of infant is < 5 kg or has an associated cardiac defect that can also be closed/repaired without cardiopulmonary bypass (muscular VSD). This approach involves a minimal lower sternotomy that is performed after full evaluation of the ASD by TEE. The right atrial wall is then punctured with an 18-gauge needle through which a

Clinical, sedation, and intubation skills

Associated cardiac or noncardiac lesions
Syndromic or nonsyndromic
General anesthesia/sedation
Airway abnormalities

Imaging preparation in small children

Transthoracic echocardiogram
TEE: too large for small babies; near field not ideal!
ICE: some view the size of the sheath required to be large.
Epicardial echocardiogram, if peratrial approach is chosen.

Venous approach in small children

Femoral approach
Transhepatic approach
Hybrid or peratrial closure

Procedure and device data

Sheath size
ASD size
Balloon sizing
Adequacy of ASD rims
Number of ASDs
Device type and size
Size of left atrium

Box 14.2—Challenges Encountered in Percutaneous Closure of ASD in Small Children

0.035-inch wire is passed through the ASD to the left atrium. The dilator and the introducing sheath are placed in the mid left atrium. Injecting agitated saline bubbles into the left atrium confirms the position of the sheath. The device is then loaded into the sheath and the left disc is deployed first, followed by the right disc. The position of the device is then confirmed by TEE prior to its release.

Lammers et al[26] reported 24 infants with isolated secundum ASD who underwent surgical closure within the first year of life. All children were symptomatic. Signs of pulmonary hyperperfusion, such as tachydyspnea, failure to thrive, recurrent respiratory infections, or heart failure, were present. Four infants required artificial ventilation. Ten patients had additional problems, such as prematurity with chronic lung disease, hepatomphalocele and congenital diaphragmatic hernia, which were present in 1 patient each. Eleven patients had defined dysmorphic syndromes. All but 1 infant underwent preoperative invasive hemodynamic evaluation. Thirteen patients had pulmonary hypertension preoperatively. The follow-up time was 46 ± 33 months (range, 4–125 months). At follow-up, pulmonary artery pressure proved to be normal in 11 of the 13 children who had pulmonary hypertension previously. One patient died of persistent pulmonary hypertension. Clinical performance, growth, and development improved in nearly all patients. All ventilator-dependent children could be weaned shortly after ASD closure.

Similar results were reported after surgical repair of ASD in infancy.[27,28]

The smallest baby who had percutaneous closure of ASD with AMPLATZER device was reported by Lim and Matherne[29] in a patient who was 112 days old, born at 23 weeks' gestation with a birth weight of 700 g. He was referred for the inability to wean from the ventilator. At the time of the procedure, the infant's weight was 2.3 kg. The defect was successfully closed under transthoracic echocardiography guidance.

In a study conducted by Cardenas et al,[4] of 52 total cases with a weight range of 4.7 to 15 kg,

10 patients (19.2%) weighed < 10 kg at the time of procedure. Associated lesions in those < 10 kg were even higher when compared with the whole cohort. Seven patients (70%) had either a cardiac or noncardiac anomaly or a genetic syndrome (P<0.05). More than two-thirds of the population were symptomatic (36/52, 69.2%). Symptoms were respiratory in 19/52 of the patients (36.5%), failure to thrive or feeding problems in 3/52 of the patients (5.7%), and cyanosis in 2/52 (3.8%). Mean ASD diameter was 12 mm (range 5–20 mm) and mean stretched diameter was 14.2 mm (range 6–22 mm). There were two or more defects or a multifenestrated septum in 8 cases (15%). Three different devices were used, the AMPLATZER Septal Occluder, the STARFlex device (Nitinol Medical Technology, Boston, Massachusetts), and the GORE HELEX occluder. No deaths or major complications occurred. When comparing children weighing < 10 kg with the others, minor complications were not more frequent (10% vs. 16%, NS), nor was procedure failure (0% vs. 7%, NS). When comparing the group of patients with an ASD diameter ≥ 15 mm with the others, minor complications were significantly more frequent (31% vs. 3%, P = 0.015), but procedure failure was not significantly higher (9% vs. 3%, NS). The 1 patient weighing < 10 kg and with a > 15 mm ASD diameter experienced a small pericardial effusion.

Diab et al[25] in another study included 15 infants < 1 year of age with ASD. In this study, the AMPLATZER septal device was used solely. The patients ranged in age from 0.5 to 11.9 months (mean ± standard deviation; 8.2 ± 3.7 months) in the percutaneous group and from 2.2 to 3.4 months (2.9 ± 0.6 months) in the peratrial group. Their weights ranged from 3.8 to 8.3 kg (5.5 ± 1.7 kg) and from 3.0 to 4.0 kg (3.4 ± 0.6 kg) in each group, respectively. The indications for ASD closure were failure to thrive, significant chamber enlargement, hemodynamically significant shunts, and prior to liver transplantation. The size of the defect as measured by ICE (n=3) or TEE (n=12) ranged from 2.0 to 16 mm (8.0 ± 4.4 mm). The pulmonary/systemic flow ratio ranged from 1.0 to 9.0 (2.8

± 2.0). The device was successfully placed in 14 of 15 infants. The size of the AMPLATZER Septal Occluder device implanted ranged from 4 to 20 mm (10.1 ± 4.3 mm). It was percutaneously deployed in 11 of 14 patients and by the hybrid or peratrial approach (open-chest, off-pump) in 3 of 14 infants. In infants who had a successful attempt (n=14), the complete closure rates at 24 hours and 1 year were 86% and 100%, respectively. In 3 of 15 infants, minor complications occurred: transient arrhythmias (n=2) and blood transfusion (n=1). One patient had a major complication with vascular intimal injury with thrombosis of the inferior vena cava. One patient with Down syndrome died 6 weeks later of progressive pulmonary hypertension. The follow-up time ranged from 0.6 to 6.9 years (3.2 ± 1.9 years). At follow-up, clinical development and growth improved in all children with failure to thrive, and all ventilator-dependent children could be weaned shortly after closure of the ASD. In this study, in addition, they evaluated the growth of the atrial septum in some of patients as they grew. The ratio of the device to the atrial septum was calculated at the time of the procedure and then at 1-year follow-up with the four-chamber apical view by TTE. There was a trend for this ratio to decrease as these infants grew older. Thus, although the device is significantly large compared with the atrial septum at the time of closure, the septum grows significantly and the device size becomes less concerning.

Fischer et al,[30] in a retrospective study of 71 children who underwent ASD device closure before their second birthday, reported a median age and body weight of 17.2 months (range 3.9–23.8 months) and 10.0 kg (range 3.8–14.5 kg), respectively. Sixteen of their patients were in their first year of life and 18 had a body weight of 7 kg or less. Median fluoroscopy time was 13.6 minutes and median device size was 15 mm. Successful closure was achieved in 68 children (95.8%). The procedure was aborted in 3 patients: in one, the device repeatedly straddled the septum; in the other two, a small left atrium restricted the movement of the left-sided disc. One device embolized and was reimplanted

after retrieval. One infant with multiple disorders died 6 days after closure from acute sepsis probably unrelated to the procedure. No other complications occurred. The AMPLATZER Septal Occluder was used in all but two patients. These two had multifenestrated defects that were closed with the cribriform type of device. In 13 patients (18%) with a median body weight of 7.1 kg, balloon sizing was not performed. In six children, the implanted device used was 1 to 4 mm less than the balloon measurement. Both in the downsizing and the no-sizing groups they paid attention to the maximal diameter of the left-sided disc that might be accommodated on the interatrial septum. The group concluded that the results and complications of ASD closure with the AMPLATZER device in patients in their first 2 years of life compared favorably with procedures in older patients, provided that the size of the septum and the dimensions in the left atrium were taken into consideration when selecting the device size.

Few clinical studies in the literature have addressed the problem of symptomatic secundum ASD in infants. Most are publications reporting on the outcome of surgical closure in small series of patients. Results of percutaneous ASD closure are currently very similar, at least in adults and children older than 4 years old.[31,32] When comparing both techniques for smaller children, Vogel et al, reported transcatheter ASD closure in 12 symptomatic children aged < 2 years, with major complications in 2 patients due to device embolization requiring surgical retrieval.[33] Butera et al reported lower complication rates and shorter hospital stay for percutaneous closure.[34] He also reported transcatheter ASD closure in 48 children aged 5 years or less, with excellent results and low morbidity.[9] Visconti et al, related bypass surgery for ASD closure with a slightly poorer neuropsychological outcome.[35] Transcatheter ASD closure is also associated with a less negative impact on right and left ventricular function as assessed by tissue Doppler imaging.[36]

With the modern use of coronary wires for accessing the small femoral veins, skilled operators, and the use of good imaging techniques to guide closure steps either by ICE or TEE, secundum ASDs in small children can be closed safely with minimal complications.

Summary

Symptomatic ASD does occur in infancy but is uncommon. ASD should be included in the differential diagnosis of any large left-to-right shunt, especially if the systolic murmur is not harsh or loud, and the diastolic murmur is heard best at the lower left sternal border. If the condition of the patient fails to improve, intervention should be undertaken without undue delay. Percutaneous ASD closure can be performed safely and successfully in selected small children. Cardiologists and pediatricians should bear in mind that a valuable percutaneous alternative to surgery now exists for ASD closure. However, patients must be selected carefully, because the risks of the procedure, including perforation of the heart during device implantation, device erosion in the aorta, and interference with mitral and pulmonary venous flow, must be balanced against the benefits.

References

1. Bull C, Deanfield J, de LM, Stark J, Taylor JF, Macartney FJ. Correction of isolated secundum atrial septal defect in infancy. *Arch Dis Child.* 1981;56:784–786.

2. Dimich I, Steinfeld L, Park SC. Symptomatic atrial septal defect in infants. *Am Heart J.* 1973;85:601–604.

3. Hunt CE, Lucas RV Jr. Symptomatic atrial septal defect in infancy. *Circulation.* 1973;47:1042–1048.

4. Cardenas L, Panzer J, Boshoff D, Malekzadeh-Milani S, Ovaert C. Transcatheter closure of secundum atrial defect in small children. *Catheter Cardiovasc Interv.* 2007;69:447–452.

5. Hanslik A, Pospisil U, Salzer-Muhar U, Greber-Platzer S, Male C. Predictors of spontaneous closure of isolated secundum atrial septal defect in children: a longitudinal study. *Pediatrics.*

6. Dimich I, Steinfeld L, Park SC. Symptomatic atrial septal defect in infants. *Am Heart J.* 1973;85:601–604.

7. Hunt CE, Lucas RV Jr. Symptomatic atrial septal defect in infancy. *Circulation.* 1973;47:1042–1048.

8. Vogel M, Berger F, Dahnert I, Ewert P, Lange PE. Treatment of atrial septal defects in symptomatic children aged less than 2 years of age using the AMPLATZER septal occluder. *Cardiol Young.* 2000;10:534–537.

9. Butera G, De RG, Chessa M, et al. Transcatheter closure of atrial septal defect in young children: results and follow-up. *J Am Coll Cardiol.* 2003;42:241–245.

10. Dalvi B, Pinto R, Gupta A. Device closure of large atrial septal defects requiring devices > or = 20 mm in small children weighing < 20 kg. *Catheter Cardiovasc Interv.* 2008;71:679–686.

11. Varma C, Benson LN, Silversides C, et al. Outcomes and alternative techniques for device closure of the large secundum atrial septal defect. *Catheter Cardiovasc Interv.* 2004;61:131–139.

12. Nagm AM, Rao PS. Percutaneous occlusion of complex atrial septal defects. *J Invasive Cardiol.* 2004;16:123–125.

13. Kleinman CS. Echocardiographic guidance of catheter-based treatments of atrial septal defect: transesophageal echocardiography remains the gold standard. *Pediatr Cardiol.* 2005;26:128–134.

14. Hijazi Z, Wang Z, Cao Q-L, Koenig P, Waight D, Lang R. Transcatheter closure of atrial septal defects and patent foramen ovale under intracardiac echocardiographic guidance: feasibility and comparison with transesophageal echocardiography. *Catheter Cardiovasc Interv.* 2001;52:194–199.

15. Koenig P, Cao Q-L, Heitschmidt M, Waight DJ, Hijazi ZM. Role of intracardiac echocardiographic guidance in transcatheter closure of atrial septal defects and patent foramen ovale using the AMPLATZER device. *J Interv Cardiol.* 2003;16:51–62.

16. Du ZD, Hijazi ZM, Kleinman CS, Silverman NH, Larntz K. Comparison between transcatheter and surgical closure of secundum atrial

septal defect in children and adults: results of a multicenter nonrandomized trial. *J Am Coll Cardiol.* 2002;39:1836–1844.

17. Bartel T, Konorza T, Neudorf U, et al. Intracardiac echocardiography: an ideal guiding tool for device closure of interatrial communications. *Eur J Echocardiogr.* 2005;6:92–96.

18. Bartel T, Konorza T, Arjumand J, et al. Intracardiac echocardiography is superior to conventional monitoring for guiding device closure of interatrial communications. *Circulation.* 2003;107:795–797.

19. Mullen MJ, Dias BF, Walker F, Siu SC, Benson LN, McLaughlin PR. Intracardiac echocardiography guided device closure of atrial septal defects. *J Am Coll Cardiol.* 2003;41:285–292.

20. Zanchetta M, Onorato E, Rigatelli G, et al. Intracardiac echocardiography-guided transcatheter closure of secundum atrial septal defect: a new efficient device selection method. *J Am Coll Cardiol.* 2003;42:1677–1682.

21. Jan SL, Hwang B, Lee PC, Fu YC, Chiu PS, Chi CS. Intracardiac ultrasound assessment of atrial septal defect: comparison with transthoracic echocardiographic, angiocardiographic, and balloon-sizing measurements. *Cardiovasc Intervent Radiol.* 2001;24:84–89.

22. Shim D, Lloyd TR, Beekman RH III. Transhepatic therapeutic cardiac catheterization: a new option for the pediatric interventionalist. *Catheter Cardiovasc Interv.* 1999;47:41–45.

23. Zeng XJ, Chen XF, Cheng D, Ma XJ, Hu XS, Tao L. Peratrial closure of atrial septal defects without cardiopulmonary bypass. *Asian Cardiovasc Thorac Ann.* 2007;15:191–193.

24. Tao KY, An Q, Gan CP, Tang H, Feng Y, Song HB. Give the patient another chance: peratrial device closure of a secundum atrial septal defect that failed percutaneous device closure. *J Thorac Cardiovasc Surg.* 2009;137:1024–1027.

25. Diab KA, Cao Q-L, Bacha EA, Hijazi ZM. Device closure of atrial septal defects with the AMPLATZER septal occluder: safety and outcome in infants. *J Thorac Cardiovasc Surg.* 2007;134:960–966.

26. Lammers A, Hager A, Eicken A, Lange R, Hauser M, Hess J. Need for closure of secundum atrial septal defect in infancy. *J Thorac Cardiovasc Surg.* 2005;129:1353–1357.

27. Mishra S, Tomar M, Malhotra R, et al. Comparison between transcatheter closure and minimally invasive surgery for fossa ovalis atrial septal defect: a single institutional experience. *Indian Heart J.* 2008;60:125–132.

28. Parvathy U, Balakrishnan KR, Ranjith MS, Saldanha R, Vakamudi M. Surgical closure of atrial septal defect in children under two years of age. *Asian Cardiovasc Thorac Ann.* 2004;12:296–299.

29. Lim DS, Matherne GP. Percutaneous device closure of atrial septal defect in a premature infant with rapid improvement in pulmonary status. *Pediatrics.* 2007;119:398–400.

30. Fischer G, Smevik B, Kramer HH, Bjornstad PG. Catheter-based closure of atrial septal defects in the oval fossa with the AMPLATZER device in patients in their first or second year of life. *Catheter Cardiovasc Interv.* 2009;73:949–955.

31. Rome JJ, Keane JF, Perry SB, Spevak PJ, Lock JE. Double-umbrella closure of atrial defects. Initial clinical applications. *Circulation.* 1990;82:751–758.

32. Masura J, Gavora P, Formanek A, Hijazi ZM. Transcatheter closure of secundum atrial septal defects using the new self-centering amplatzer septal occluder: initial human experience. *Cathet Cardiovasc Diagn.* 1997;42:388–393.

33. Vogel M, Berger F, Dahnert I, Ewert P, Lange PE. Treatment of atrial septal defects in symptomatic children aged less than 2 years of age using the AMPLATZER septal occluder. *Cardiol Young.* 2000;10:534–537.

34. Butera G, Carminati M, Chessa M, *et al.* Percutaneous versus surgical closure of secundum atrial septal defect: comparison of early results and complications. *Am Heart J.* 2006;151:228–234.

35. Visconti KJ, Bichell DP, Jonas RA, Newburger JW, Bellinger DC. Developmental outcome after surgical versus interventional closure of secundum atrial septal defect in children. *Circulation.* 1999;100:II145–II150.

36. Di SG, Drago M, Pacileo G. et al. Comparison of strain rate imaging for quantitative evaluation of regional left and right ventricular function after surgical versus percutaneous closure of atrial septal defect. *Am J Cardiol.* 2005;96:299–302.

15

Device Closure of ASDs and PFOs in the Elderly: Hemodynamic Assessment

Mehmet Cilingiroglu and Ted Feldman

Atrial Septal Defects

Atrial septal defect (ASD) accounts for about one-third of congenital heart disease in adults.[1] It is twice as common in women as men.[2,3] Small defects, usually < 5 mm without right-sided volume overload, may have no effect on the natural history of the individual. It is well known that even large ASDs can permit survival into adulthood.[4,5] Thus, there are many patients with ASD who present as adults and even elderly adults.

Retrospective studies suggest that three-quarters of the patients with ASD become symptomatic, but symptoms may be mild to moderate and are often not progressive.[6] The most common symptom is effort dyspnea. This is usually not disabling and the majority of patients can still engage in ordinary daily activities. Unusual symptoms of orthodeoxia and platypnea can occur in the fifth to sixth decade. Clinical dis-ability increases with age, and patients over the age of 60 are usually in serious difficulties. There is no strong relationship between symptoms and shunt size, between symptoms and patients' ages, or between symptoms and pulmonary vascular resistance. Severe pulmonary hypertension is the most important single risk factor influencing the course of the ASD. Approximately 15% of patients with significant defects might develop significantly elevated pulmonary vascular resistance indicating irreversible obstructive pathology in the fourth or fifth decade of life.[6] This serious complication may be rapidly progressive, leading to shunt reversal, disability, and even death. A pulmonary vascular resistance exceeding 7 Woods Units in the presence of 100% inspired oxygen is usually considered a contraindication to ASD closure.

In older patients, progressive disability and heart failure may develop frequently with the concomitant onset of chronic atrial arrhythmias, which may lead to significant disability. Cardiac arrhythmias of atrial fibrillation or flutter can be present in as many as 52% of patients aged 60 years or older.[7] Occasionally, chronic hypoxia from shunt reversal due to pulmonary hypertension can lead to cyanosis. Paradoxical cerebral or systemic emboli rarely occur with isolated ASD, and are more prevalent with patent foramen ovale (PFO). Compared to the same age normal counterparts, older patients with ASD have a reduced life span.[3] The average age at death usually does not exceed 50 years.[2] Patients usually die from congestive cardiac failure, pulmonary arterial thrombosis or embolism, and bronchopulmonary infections.[4,8]

It is important to understand that age-related changes in cardiac chamber's compliance play a key role in natural history and progression of symptoms in adults with ASD. The atrial level shunts occur primarily in diastole and flow direction depends on the differences in the right and left atrial pressures and compliance. The compliance of the atria is determined mainly by their respective ventricular compliances. Ventricular compliance is determined by the ventricular wall thickness, fibrosis, and contractility. Ventricular wall thickness is directly proportional to the ventricular pressure needed to overcome the resistance to flow (afterload), the pulmonary vascular resistance (PVR) in the case of the right ventricle (RV) and systemic vascular resistance (SVR) for the left ventricle (LV). As RV pressure and PVR increase, the RV wall thickness increases, leading to a fall in RV and right atrial (RA) compliance. Normally, the mean left atrial pressure is 6 to 9 mm Hg and mean right atrial pressure is 1 to 4 mm Hg, favoring a left-to-right (L-R) shunt; however, this is only a real factor in small defects. In large defects with equal atrial pressures, the amount and direction of flow across the ASD is dependent on the differences in compliance of the right and left atria and ventricles. Normally, the RA and RV compliance is much higher than that of the LA and LV, resulting in a L-R shunt across the ASD and its magnitude is dependent on the relative differences between the RV and

LV compliance. LV compliance decreases with age as the systemic arteriolar elasticity decreases and SVR increases, leading to higher blood pressure and LV hypertrophy. Decreased LV compliance with a subsequent elevation in LA pressure produces an increased L-R atrial-level shunt. Thus, the magnitude and physiologic impact of L-R shunting increases with age. The L-R shunt at the atrial level results in right-sided volume overload and ultimately development and progression of symptoms. When ASD is small, and the RV is not dilated, no intervention is typically warranted except in the patient who has suffered paradoxical embolization, or in divers. However, the development of symptoms, echocardiographic signs of significant shunt volume (dilated RV or Qp:Qs > 1.5), or shunt-related pulmonary hypertension are widely accepted indications for closure of an ASD in adults.

Patients with secundum ASD have a higher incidence of associated mitral valve prolapse, partial anomalous pulmonary venous return, and complex congenital heart defects. Lutembacher was first to observe association of mitral valve stenosis with ASD,[9] possibly incidental to the frequency of rheumatic heart disease at that time, rather than representing a real association of the two conditions. Patients with Lutembacher may develop serious consequences of mitral stenosis, namely atrial fibrillation, pulmonary hypertension, and heart failure in their forties to fifties. Often, the fossa ovalis might have more than one defect in adults. Multiple ASD closure is more challenging than for a single ASD. If the septum has more than one hole, the bigger hole is usually located in the supero-anterior septum, while the smaller hole is located in the infero-posterior septum. If two defects are present and separated by > 7 mm from each other, they can be crossed separately.[10] Each one can be sized separately and then the delivery system can be left in each defect. If there are multiple fenestrations, the AMPLATZER Multi-Fenestrated Cribriform (AGA Medical, Plymouth, Minnesota) device can be used. The device should be deployed in the middle of the septum so that it can cover all fenestrations. To date, the AMPLATZER

Septal Occluder (ASO) (AGA Medical, Plymouth, Minnesota), is the only FDA-approved device suitable for the larger ASDs up to 40 mm in diameter. However, a large defect, especially associated with deficient rims, is still challenging. In such circumstances, oftentimes, when deploying the LA disc, the disc becomes perpendicular to the atrial septum, resulting in prolapse into the right atrium. There are several techniques that can be used to overcome such difficulties in aligning the LA disc parallel to the atrial septum that will result in a successful procedure.[11]

Among patients with severe pulmonary hypertension related to a larger ASD,[12] as well as in the primary pulmonary hypertension population,[13] the presence of an atrial level shunt may actually improve survival when indexed pulmonary vascular resistance exceeds 14 Woods Units. Most of these patients have some degree of right-to-left shunting at the atrial level with associated cyanosis, owing to RV dysfunction, and closing the ASD eliminates the "pop-off" route for the right heart. By closing the defect and forcing all systemic venous return through the RV and into the high-resistance pulmonary arteriolar bed, the RV may fail in more rapid

fashion than if the ASD had been left alone. Rarely, an ASD with left-to-right shunting will be newly discovered in a patient with LV myocardial dysfunction presenting with progressive congestive heart failure. It can be difficult to determine, noninvasively, whether the LV myocardial disease or the left-to-right shunt is responsible for the patient's symptoms. Similar to patients with pulmonary hypertension, the ASD in this case allows a pop-off for the left atrium and sharing of diastolic properties between right and left hearts. During ASD closure, frequently, attention is solely focused on assessing distal pulmonary artery pressures and pulmonary vascular resistance, while this protective decompressive function of an interatrial communication on the left ventricular myocardium is being ignored. Thus, in patients over the age of 60 years, it is generally recommended to balloon-test occlude their defects temporarily (15 minutes or so) using a sizing balloon to measure the left atrial pressure.

The LA pressure can be measured through the occlusion balloon lumen, with a second catheter through the defect into the LA, or with repeated measurements of the pulmonary wedge pressure. The left ventricular end-diastolic pres-

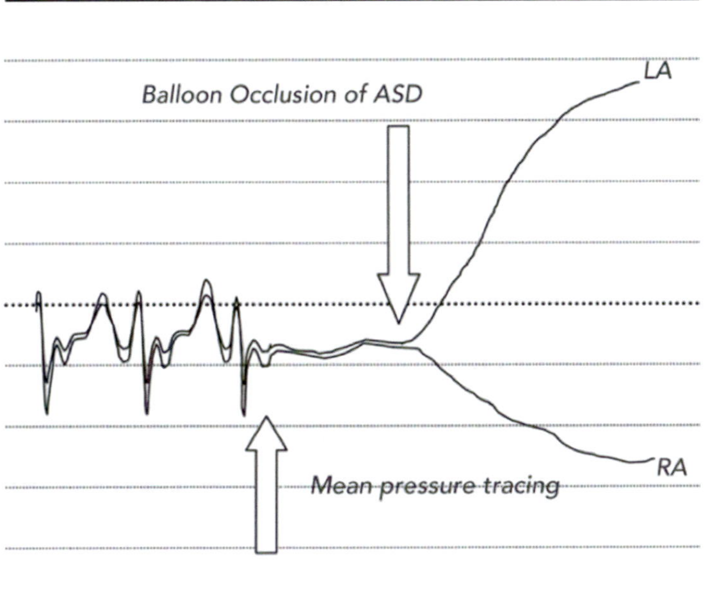

Fig 15.1—Balloon-test occlusion of ASD with sizing balloon. Simultaneous right atrial (RA) and left atrial (LA) tracings. Temporary balloon occlusion of an atrial septal defect (ASD) in a patient with left ventricular dysfunction and a large left-to-right shunt. The pressure scale (y axis) is 0 to 40 mm Hg. Mean LA pressure rises sharply, with elimination of the LA pop-off, suggesting that the LV is too sick to tolerate closure of ASD. (Reprinted from Landzberg MJ, Sommer RJ. "Profiles in congenital heart disease." In: Baim DS, Grossman W, eds. *Grossman's Cardiac Catheterization, Angiography & Intervention.* 7th ed. Philadelphia: Lippincott, Williams & Wilkins, 2005:751. Used with permission.)

sure, systemic arterial pressure, and cardiac output are monitored as well. If the LA pressure remains in a relatively physiologic range (mean < 25 mm Hg), and there are no symptoms of pulmonary edema, the defect can be closed. Typically such patients return to baseline LA pressures within a few days after closure. If mean LA pressure rises acutely with balloon occlusion to levels > 30 to 35 mm Hg, however, pulmonary venous congestion, acute pulmonary edema, and systemic desaturation may occur, indicating that the LV may be too compromised in its current state to allow ASD closure (Fig 15.1). The pathophysiologic mechanism causing this effect has been suggested to be restrictive left ventricular diastolic dysfunction or reduced diastolic elasticity, which is observed more frequently in elderly patients because of higher incidence of systemic hypertension. In these patients, interatrial communication serves as a protective pop off, thereby reducing the preload of the left ventricle. Occlusion of these defects unmasks the left ventricular diastolic dysfunction with a resulting increase in the left atrial pressures.[14] Holzer et al reported the proper technique for ASD closure in elderly patients with a large ASD and increase in left atrial pressures above physiologic range during the balloon-test occlusion.[15] Pretreatment of these patients with aggressive diuretic and afterload-reducing therapy several weeks before the procedure and use of a self-fabricated fenestrated ASO led to successful closure of ASD without adverse outcomes and long-term procedural success with improvement in left ventricular diastolic parameters. Thus, adequate preprocedural management using diuretics and afterload-reducing substances, as well as the use of a self-fabricated fenestrated ASO, may allow successful closure of large ASDs in elderly patients, in whom closure would otherwise have been prohibited by the left ventricular diastolic dysfunction and resulting increase in left atrial pressure.

ASD in elderly patients is associated with increased mortality and morbidity.[3] Initial studies produced controversial results about the effect of surgical ASD closure on mortality and morbidity. Murphy et al reported on increased mortality in patients who underwent surgical repair of ASD after the age of 25 years and compared the results with healthy controls.[16] A prospective, randomized trial by Attie et al also showed no clear survival benefit with surgical ASD closure.[17] Another retrospective study, which examined morbidity and mortality simultaneously in surgically versus medically managed ASD patients > 40 years of age, showed a survival benefit in the surgical patients.[18] Several trials have demonstrated improvement in exercise capacity in adult patients after percutaneous or surgical ASD closure, even in asymptomatic or mildly symptomatic patients.[19-22]

Elderly patients with ASDs frequently have other concomitant cardiac as well as extracardiac pathology (ischemic heart disease, diabetes, lung disease, etc). The majority of trials in the past compared surgical and conservative ASD management. Percutaneous ASD closure is a significantly less invasive procedure with a lower risk of complications compared to surgery (anesthesia, thoracotomy, heart-lung pump, etc.). Recent studies in elderly patients with percutaneous ASD closure showed uneventful recovery in majority of patients.[23-26] In one report, the mean age was 69.9 years and most of the patients were classified as NYHA I and NYHA II and a few as NYHA III functional class at their baseline. Most of these patients had class I indication for ASD closure (large shunts, right ventricular enlargement, and/or symptoms). NYHA functional class and exercise capacity significantly improved in the majority of patients. There were clear and objective signs of hemodynamic improvement in just 3 months.[24] VO2 max increased by 10% overall and the right ventricular end-diastolic diameter had significantly decreased, even normalized. Left ventricular end-diastolic diameter significantly increased while the left atrial diameter did not change. Decrease in right ventricular end-diastolic diameter significantly correlated with increase in left ventricular end-diastolic diameter after the closure. ASD closure with abolishment of left-to-right shunt leads to augmented left ventricular filling by increased left ventricular preload and therefore to improved left ventricular stroke volume.[27] The rise in left ventricular stroke volume may explain the increase in VO2 max and increase of functional capacity. Especially in this age group in which impaired diastolic function is common, this may explain the functional improvement.

In comparison to surgical ASD repair, patients' functional recovery is faster after percutaneous closure[28] because of the effects of thoracotomy and heart lung machine. The most common complication following percutaneous ASD closure immediately after and during follow-up is development of new-onset atrial fibrillation.[24–26] It is unclear whether this is part of the inflammation and healing response involved in tissue covering of the closure device or it is part of the natural history and is being detected because of close follow-up in this age group with the overall prevalence being already as high as 8% to 10%. It is also uncertain whether the atrial fibrillation is self-limiting and temporary or represents a new and persistent problem. In adults with an ASD and chronic right atrial volume overload, there may be long-term arrhythmias that are not diminished by the closure of the defect.[16] The occurrence of atrial arrhythmias could also be explained by prolonged right atrial dilatation caused by an interatrial shunt that results in structural changes in the RA that cause electrophysiological alterations that persist beyond ASD closure.[29] These studies suggest that catheter-based ASD closure in the elderly can be performed safely with minimal risk and results in improvement in symptoms as well as positive right-heart remodeling.

Surgical closure has been shown to be beneficial in patients over 60 years of age.[30,31] Average age in these retrospective studies was 65 years old. Most patients were in functional class III or VI and had moderate pulmonary hypertension and a few of them did suffer documented cerebrovascular events because of preoperative paradoxical emboli. Surgical repair was achieved either by direct suture or Dacron patch grafts depending on the size as well as associated lesions, with an operative mortality of 3% to 6%. The presence of pulmonary hypertension in the absence of a marked increase of pulmonary

vascular resistance, a large left-to-right shunt, congestive heart failure, and/or atrial fibrillation did not affect the surgical outcome and the results of surgical treatment were favorable regardless of the age. The majority of patients uniformly experienced significant improvement of at least one functional class along with a large decrease in their pulmonary artery pressures. Surgical repair was also associated with significant improvement in survival compared with that predicted for age-matched patients treated medically. These studies demonstrated that surgical closure of ASD in elderly adults could be performed successfully and safely with a low morbidity and mortality even in patients with moderate pulmonary hypertension, large left-to-right shunt, or congestive heart failure. The lower morbidity and virtual absence of mortality from ASD closure with devices compared to surgical therapy clearly speaks to the benefit of ASD closure in older patients as long as typical indications for closure are present.

Patent Foramen Ovale

Cryptogenic stroke has been highly associated with PFO and this association has been strongest in younger patients. PFO is found in over 45% of stroke patients under age 55 or 60, compared to 11% in stroke patients over age 55 years.[32] While the common view is that this is predominantly a problem in patients under age 60 years, there is evidence that older patients with PFO are also at increased risk for cryptogenic stroke.

PFO has increasingly been recognized as a potential mediator for several disease manifestations, including paradoxical embolism leading to stroke, refractory hypoxemia as a result of right-to-left shunt in a patient with right ventricular infarct, or severe pulmonary disease, orthostatic desaturation in the setting of the rare platypnea-orthodeoxia syndrome, neurological decompression illness in divers, and more recently, migraine with aura. The etiology of ischemic stroke remains unknown in up to 40% of adults, despite extensive diagnostic evaluation and is referred to as cryptogenic stroke.[33-38] Recent studies in the elderly, also suggest a strong association between the presence of PFO and/or cryptogenic stroke.[39,40]

Certain morphologic characteristics of PFO appear to predispose patients for paradoxical embolism. Both, larger PFO size, a greater degree of right-to-left shunt as assessed by crossing microbubbles, and combination of PFO with an atrial septal aneurysm constitute a higher risk situation.[41-44] Patients with both PFO and atrial septal aneurysm constitute a high-risk population with a threefold to fivefold increased risk for recurrent embolic events compared with patients with PFO alone.[45] Secondary prevention with acetylsalicylic acid has been found insufficient protection against recurrent cerebrovascular events in patients with both PFO and atrial septal aneurysm.[45,46]

Despite the growing recognition of the PFO as a risk factor for paradoxical embolism, the optimal treatment strategy for symptomatic patients remains undefined. Most patients with presumed paradoxical embolism are treated medically with antithrombotic medications, with a paucity of data concerning the efficacy of oral anticoagulation as opposed to antiplatelet therapy, or for either of these therapies alone. Surgical closure is feasible but the procedure is associated with well-known complications of cardiac surgery.[47,48] Percutaneous PFO closure using atrial septal occlusion devices can be performed with a high success and low morbidity rate even in elderly patients with presumed paradoxical embolism.[49,50] Patients with more than one cerebrovascular event at baseline may have lower risk of recurrent stroke or transient ischemic attack following percutaneous PFO closure compared with medically treated patients.[51]

The mean age of cryptogenic stroke patients is under 60 years in most reports, and this has led to uncertainty about the role of PFO in stroke in older patients. Handke et al compared patients over age 55 years with cryptogenic versus stroke of known cause. Those with cryptogenic stroke were more likely to have PFO diagnosed on TEE than were patients with stroke of known cause. The frequency of PFO was over threefold higher in the cryptogenic stroke patients, with over 40% having PFO compared to < 15% of patients with stroke of known cause. This suggests that PFO is a cause of cryptogenic stroke in older patients.[40] Another fascinating observation was made by Hagen et al. They studied the incidence and size of PFO in 965 autopsy specimens of human hearts, evenly distributed by sex and age.[33] The overall incidence of PFO was 27.3%, but it progressively declined with increasing age from 34.3% during the first three decades of life to 25.4% during the fourth through eighth decades and to 20.2% during the ninth and 10th decades. The PFO size also tended to increase with increasing age, from a mean of 3.4 mm in the first decade to 5.8 mm in the 10th decade of life. Because PFO is not known to close spontaneously, this suggests attrition in the PFO population in excess of the general or non-PFO population. The decreasing prevalence of PFO with increasing age is consistent with the concept that far more mortality risk might be associated with complications of PFO associated with other diseases of aging than we appreciate. The increased incidence of myocardial infarction and death associated with pulmonary embolism is an example. Thus, PFO closure in elderly patients should be considered similarly as in younger patients following presumed paradoxical embolism.

References

1. Marelli AJ, Mackie AS, Lonescu-lttu R, et al. Congenital heart disease in the general population: Changing prevalence and age distribution. *Circulation.* 2007;115:163–172.

2. Feldt RH, Avasthey P, Yoshimasu F, et al. Incidence of congenital heart disease in children born to residents of Olmsted County, Minnesota, 1950–1969. *Mayo Clin Proc.* 1971;46:794–799.

3. Campell M. Natural history of atrial septal defect. *Br Heart J.* 1970;32:820–826.

4. Kelly JJ Jr, Lyons HA. Atrial septal defect in the aged. *Ann Intern Med.* 1958;48:267.

5. Rodstein M, Zeman FD, Gerber IE. Atrial septal defect in the aged. *Circulation.* 1961;23:665.

6. Craig RJ, Selzer A. Natural history and prognosis of atrial septal defect. *Circulation.* 1968;37:805–815.

7. Murphy JG, Gersh BJ, McGoon MD, et al. Long-term outcome after surgical repair of isolated atrial septal defect. *N Engl J Med.* 1990;323:1645–1650.

8. Campbell M, Neill C, Suzman S. Prognosis of atrial septal defect. *Br Med J.* 1957;1:1375.

9. Lutembacher R. De la stenose mitrale avec communication interauriculaire. *Arch Mal Coeur.* 1916;9:237.

10. Cao Q-L, Radtke W, Berger F, et al. Transcatheter closure of multiple atrial septal defects. Initial results and value of two- and three-dimensional transesophageal echocardiography. *Eur Heart J.* 2000;21(11):941–947.

11. Fu YC, Cao Q-L, Hijazi ZM. Device closure of large ASDs: technical considerations. *J Cardiovasc Med (Hagerstown).* 2007;8(1):30–33.

12. Steele PM, Fuster V, Cohen M, et al. Isolated atrial septal defect with pulmonary obstructive disease long-term follow-up and prediction of outcome after surgical correction. *Circulation.* 1995;76:1037–1042.

13. Kerstein D, Levy PS, Hsu DT, et al. Blade balloon atrial septostomy in patients with severe primary pulmonary hypertension. *Circulation.* 1995;91:2028–2035.

14. Ewert P, Berger F, Daehnert I, et al. Transcatheter closure of atrial septal defects without fluoroscopy: feasibility of a new method. *Circulation.* 2000;101:847–849.

15. Holzer R, Cao Q-L, Hijazi ZM. Closure of a moderately large atrial septal defect with a self-fabricated fenestrated AMPLATZER Septal Occluder in an 85-year-old patient with reduced diastolic elasticity of the left ventricle. *Cathet Cardiovasc Interv.* 2005;64:513–518.

16. Murphy JG, Gersh BJ, McGoon MD, et al. Long-term outcome after surgical repair of isolated atrial septal defect. Follow-up at 27 to 32 years. *N Engl J Med.* 1990;323;1645–1650.

17. Attie F, Rosas M, Granados N, et al. Treatment for secundum atrial septal defects in patients >

18. Kontantinides S, Geibel A, Olschewski M, et al. A comparison of surgical and medical therapy for atrial septal defect in adults. *N Engl J Med.* 1995;333:469–473.

19. Gatzoulis MA, Redington AN, Somerville J, et al. Should atrial septal defects in adults be closed? *Ann Thorac Surg.* 1996;61:657–659.

20. Helber U, Baumann R, Seboldt H, et al. Atrial septal defect in adults: Cardiopulmonary exercise capacity before and 4 months and 10 years after defect closure. *J Am Coll Cardiol.* 1997;29:1345–1350.

21. Veldtman GR, Razack V, Siu S, et al. Right ventricular form and function after percutaneous atrial septal defect device closure. *J Am Coll Cardiol.* 2001;37:2108–2113.

22. Brochue MC, Baril JF, Dore A, et al. Improvement in exercise capacity in asymptomatic and mildly symptomatic adults after atrial septal defect percutaneous closure. *Circulation.* 2002;106:1821–1826.

23. Yalonetsky S, Lorber A. Percutaneous closure of a secundum atrial septal defect in elderly patients. *J Invasive Cardiol.* 2007;19(12):510–512.

24. Jategaonkar S, Scholtz W, Schmidt H, et al. Percutaneous closure of atrial septal defects, echocardiographic and functional results in patients older than 60 years. *Circ Cardiovasc Interv.* 2009;2:85–89.

25. Elshershari H, Cao Q-L, Hijazi ZM. Transcatheter device closure of atrial septal defect in patients older than 60 years of age: Immediate and follow-up results. *J Invasive Cardiol.* 2008;20(4):173–176.

26. Majunke N, Bialkowski J, Wilson N, et al. Closure of atrial septal defect with AMPLATZER Septal Occluder in adults. *Am J Cardiol.* 2009;103:550–554.

27. Pascoot M, Santoro G, Caso P, et al. Global and regional left ventricular function in patients undergoing transcatheter closure of secundum atrial septal defect. *Am J Cardiol.* 2005;96:439–442.

28. Thilen U, Persson S. Closure of atrial septal defect in adult. Cardiac remodeling is an early event. *Int J Cardiol.* 2006;108:370–375.

29. Morton JB, Sanders P, Vohra JK, et al. Effect of chronic right atrial stretch on atrial electrical remodeling in patients with an atrial septal defect. *Circulation.* 2003;107(13):1775–1782.

30. Nasrallah AT, Hall RJ, Garcia E, et al. Surgical repair of atrial septal defect in patients over 60 years of age. Long-term results. *Circulation.* 1976;53:329–331.

31. Sutton MGJ, Tajik AJ, McGoon DC. Atrial septal defect in patients ages 60 years or older: Operative results and long-term postoperative follow-up. *Circulation.* 1981;64;402–409.

32. Homma S, Sacco RL. Patent foramen ovale and stroke. *Circulation.* 2005;112:1063– 1072.

33. Hagen PT, Scholz DG, Edwards WD. Incidence and size of patent foramen ovale during the first 10 decades of life: an autopsy study of 965 normal hearts. *Mayo Clin Proc.* 1984;59:17–20.

34. Silver MD, Dorsey JS. Aneurysms of the septum primum in adults. *Arch Pathol Lab Med.* 1978;102:62–65.

35. Hanley PC, Tajik AJ, Hynes JK, et al. Diagnosis and classification of atrial septal aneurysm by two-dimensional echocardiography: report of 80 consecutive cases. *J Am Coll Cardiol.* 1985;6:1370–1382.

36. Agmon Y, Khandheira BK, Meisnner I, et al. Frequency of atrial septal aneurysms in patients with cerebral ischemic events. *Circulation.* 1999;99:1942–1944.

37. Hart RG, Miller VT. Cerebral infarction in young adults: a practical approach. *Stroke.* 1983;14:110–114.

38. Sacco RL, Ellenberg JH, Mohr JP, et al. Infarcts of undetermined cause: the NINCDS Stroke Data Bank. *Ann Neurol.* 1989;25:382–390.

39. Di Tullio M, Sacco RL, Gopal A, et al. Patent foramen ovale as a risk factor for cryptogenic stroke. *Ann Intern Med.* 1992;117:461–465.

40. Handke M, Harloff A, Olschewski M, et al. Patent foramen ovale and cryptogenic stroke in older patients. *N Engl J Med.* 2007;357:2262–2268.

41. Homma S, Di Tollio MR, Sacco RL, et al. Characteristics of patent foramen ovale associated with cryptogenic stroke. A biplane transesophageal echocardiographic study. *Q J Med.* 1930;23:135–150.

42. De Castro S, Cartoni D, Fiorelli M, et al. Morphological and functional characteristics of patent foramen ovale and their embolic implications. *Stroke.* 2000;31:2407–2413.

43. Schneider B, Hanrath P, Vogel P, et al. Improved morphological characterization of atrial septal aneurysm by transesophageal echocardiography: relation to cerebrovascular events. *J Am Coll Cardiol.* 1990;16:1000–1009.

44. Overell JR, Bone I, Lees KR. Interatrial septal abnormalities and stroke: a meta-analysis of case-control studies. *Neurology.* 2000;55:1172–1179.

45. Mas JL, Zuber M. Recurrent cerebrovascular events in patients with patent foramen ovale, atrial septal aneurysm, or both and cryptogenic stroke or transient ischemic attack. French Study Group on Patent Foramen Ovale and Atrial Septal Aneurysm. *Am Heart J.* 1995;130:1083–1088.

46. Mas JL, Arquizan C, Lamy C, et al. Recurrent cerebrovascular events associated with patent foramen ovale, atrial septal aneurysm, or both. *N Engl J Med.* 2001;345:1740–1746.

47. Homma S, Di Tullio MR, Sacco RL, et al. Surgical closure of patent foramen ovale in cryptogenic stroke patients. *Stroke.* 1997;28:2376–2381.

48. Dearani JA, Ugurlu BS, Danielson GK, et al. Surgical patent foramen ovale closure for prevention of paradoxical embolism-related cerebrovascular ischemic events. *Circulation.* 1999;100:II171–II175.

49. Kiblawi FM, Sommer RJ, Levchuck SG. Transcatheter closure of patent foramen ovale in older adults. *Cathet Cardiovasc Interv.* 2006;68:136–142.

50. Spies C, Khandelwal A, Timmemanns I, et al. Recurrent events following patent foramen ovale closure in patients above 55 years of age with presumed paradoxical embolism. *Cathet Cardiovasc Interv.* 2008;72(7):966–970.

51. Windecker S, Wahl A, Nedettchev K, et al. Comparison of medical treatment with percutaneous closure of patent foramen ovale in patients with cryptogenic stroke. *J Am Coll Cardiol.* 2004;44:750–758.

16

Closure of ASDs with Pulmonary Hypertension: Assessing Operability

Sara M. Trucco and William E. Hellenbrand

Introduction

Pulmonary arterial hypertension (PAH) is a rare but serious complication of unrepaired atrial septal defect (ASD), and the decision to close such defects in this patient population should be approached with caution and careful consideration. The development of advanced PAH therapies, including potent oral vasodilators, have created new hope for nonreactive patients who were previously deemed inoperable. This chapter discusses the prevalence and pathophysiology of PAH among patients with ASDs, describes catheterization techniques that are useful in assessing operability, and explores possible treatment strategies for ASD closure in patients with severely elevated pulmonary vascular resistance (PVR).

Pulmonary Arterial Hypertension Associated with Congenital Heart Disease

Definition

PAH is defined as a mean pulmonary arterial pressure (PAP) > 25 mm Hg at rest, in the setting of a normal left atrial pressure (< 15 mm Hg) and a normal resting cardiac output, thus corresponding to a resting PVR of > 3 Wood units.[1] The previously accepted definition of a mean PAP > 30 mm Hg during exercise has fallen into question after published data has shown that healthy individuals regularly achieve much higher PAP during exercise.[2,3] Eisenmenger syndrome is defined as shunt reversal that occurs after longstanding, severe

Transcatheter Closure of ASDs and PFOs: A Comprehensive Assessment. © 2010 Ziyad M. Hijazi, Ted Feldman, Mustafa H. Abdullah Al-Qbandi, and Horst Sievert, editors. Cardiotext Publishing, ISBN: 978-0-9790164-9-3.

PAH, resulting in cyanosis that in turn affects multiple organ systems.[4]

Prevalence

ASD is a common defect, encompassing approximately 7% of all forms of congenital heart disease (CHD) and affecting 1 in 1500 live births.[5,6] The development of PAH and associated pulmonary vascular disease in patients with ASD is rare in infancy and childhood, and is unusual before the age of 20 to 40 years.[7–9] In one series, only 2.2% of infants younger than 1 year of age were found to have severe PAH as a result of isolated ASD.[10] In this young age group, the frequency of PAH did not vary among different ASD subtypes. Historically, the rate of elevated PVR was reported to be approximately 5% to 10% of adult ASD patients, with females composing > 65% of those affected.[11] More recently, others have reported the prevalence of PAH in adults with unrepaired ASD to be as high as 34%.[12] In fact, histologic and structural changes of the pulmonary vasculature have been found in as many as 59% of individuals with ASD, 19% of which were graded moderate or severe.[13] These histologic changes, however, did not correlate with shunt size, degree of PAH or ASD subtype, and were not predictive of operative outcome.

It has been suggested that the variation in the prevalence of ASD-associated PAH may represent two different disease entities.[14,15] In those who develop PAH at a young age, pulmonary vascular obstructive disease may be the primary abnormality, while the ASD is an incidental and exacerbating finding.[16] Similarly, young children with CHD may have other comorbidities, such as diaphragmatic hernia, lung prematurity, or need for prolonged mechanical ventilation, which contribute to the development of PAH.[15,17] Those patients who develop PAH due to ongoing left-to-right shunt through an ASD, on the other hand, tend to do so at a much older age.

The development of Eisenmenger syndrome associated with ASD remains rare and in the majority of patients does not develop until very late in life.[18] Due to advancements in the diagnosis and treatment of PAH and CHD, the rate of Eisenmenger syndrome of all etiologies has fallen from 8% in the 1950s to its current rate of 4%.[4,19]

Pathophysiology

The development of PAH is a complex and multifactorial process that involves vasoconstriction, proliferation, and obstructive remodeling of the pulmonary vasculature, in the setting of ongoing inflammation and thrombosis[1,20] (Fig 16.1). Left-to-right shunting results in increased flow and higher pressure in the pulmonary vasculature. Over time, these shearing forces cause endothelial damage, loss of the endothelial barrier function, and endothelial dysfunction. This endothelial damage is associated with the release of fibroblast growth factor, transforming growth factor-beta (TGF-β), and the activation of endogenous vascular elastase, leading to smooth muscle cell proliferation and degradation of the extracellular matrix.[21] Furthermore, loss of the endothelial barrier leads to the adherence of platelets and the initiation of leukocytes, thus activating the immune system and coagulation pathways, resulting in inflammation and thrombosis. Finally, endothelial dysfunction alters the production of endothelin-1, thromboxane, nitric oxide, and prostaglandin I_2, thus affecting the balance of pulmonary vasoconstriction and vasodilatation.[22] Cumulatively, these endothelial changes favor vasoconstriction and ultimately lead to pulmonary vascular remodeling.[23]

Pulmonary vascular remodeling associated with CHD and PAH leads to several histologic abnormalities. Smooth muscle cells hypertrophy and proliferate, eventually extending into the peripheral pulmonary arteries.[24] An increase in connective tissue and elastic fibers contributes to the development of medial hypertrophy along with intimal and adventitial thickening.[25] It is interesting to note, however, that among ASD patients these changes are almost exclusively localized to the intima with little medial involvement, whereas in other forms of CHD, medial hypertrophy is the pre-

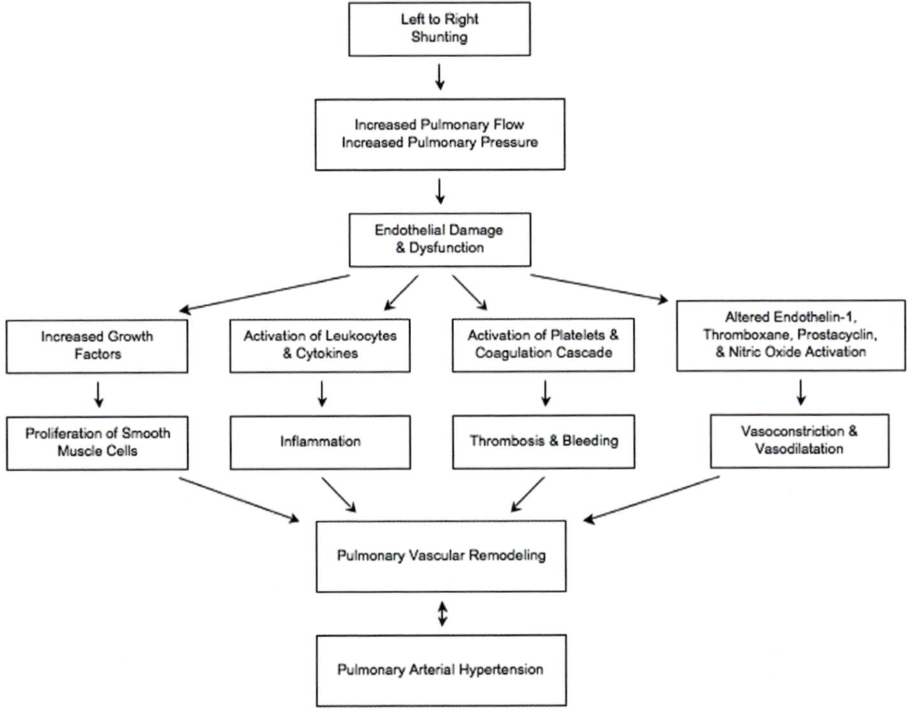

Fig 16.1—The pathophysiology of PAH and pulmonary vascular disease. Left-to-right intracardiac shunting results in increased pulmonary blood flow and pressure. This in turn, leads to endothelial damage and dysfunction. Endothelial damage activates several cellular pathways, ultimately leading to pulmonary vascular remodeling and pulmonary arterial hypertension.

dominant feature.[7] With progression, complex plexiform lesions may develop through focal proliferation of endothelial channels by myofibroblasts, smooth muscle cells, and connective tissue matrix.[26] In later stages, pruning of the pulmonary vasculature with rarification of the pulmonary arterial tree may develop, and can be observed both on lung biopsy and through pulmonary wedge angiography[23,27] (Fig 16.2). These histologic and anatomic changes are the basis for the PAH classification systems introduced by Heath and Edwards in 1958[26] and Rabinovitch in 1978,[28] both of which are still used today.

The rate of progression of CHD-induced PAH and resulting pulmonary vascular disease depends on several factors. The most important factors are the type and size of the defect, and the severity and pressure of the shunt.[29] Large ventricular septal defects (VSDs) and patent

ductus arteriosus (PDA) expose the pulmonary vasculature to higher pressures and pulmonary flows, allowing severe PAH to develop at a faster rate.[20] ASDs, on the other hand, are typically associated with normal PAP and normal PVR until 20 to 40 years of age, and when PAH develops it does so at a slower rate.[7-9] The evolution of PAH also differs among ASD subtypes: occurring in 4% of patients with secundum ASD but in 16% of those with sinus venous defects.[18] The cause of these differences remains unclear, but it has been proposed that genetic or environmental factors may be present in patients who develop PAH earlier than others. Mutations in the bone morphogenetic protein receptor type II (BMPR2), a receptor for TGF-β, have been associated with the development of familial PAH and were recently identified in 6% of patients with PAH associated with CHD.[30] The role that genetic predisposition plays in the etiology of PAH, while interacting with the hemodynamic and anatomic factors of CHD, is complex and requires further investigation.

Morbidity and Mortality

The morbidities resulting from PAH associated with CHD relate to its severity, with Eisenmenger syndrome representing the most severe form.[29] PAH patients may initially present with shortness of breath and exercise intolerance, a symptom caused by the inability to increase pulmonary blood flow during periods of increased need.[31] With Eisenmenger syndrome, right-to-left shunting leads to cyanosis and reduced arterial oxygen content, which, over time, results in hypoxic damage of multiple organ systems.[21] Chronic cyanosis leads to hepatic and renal dysfunction, in addition to thrombocytopenia, platelet dysfunction, and secondary erythrocytosis.[32,33] These hematologic changes in turn can cause hyperviscosity symptoms, bleeding,

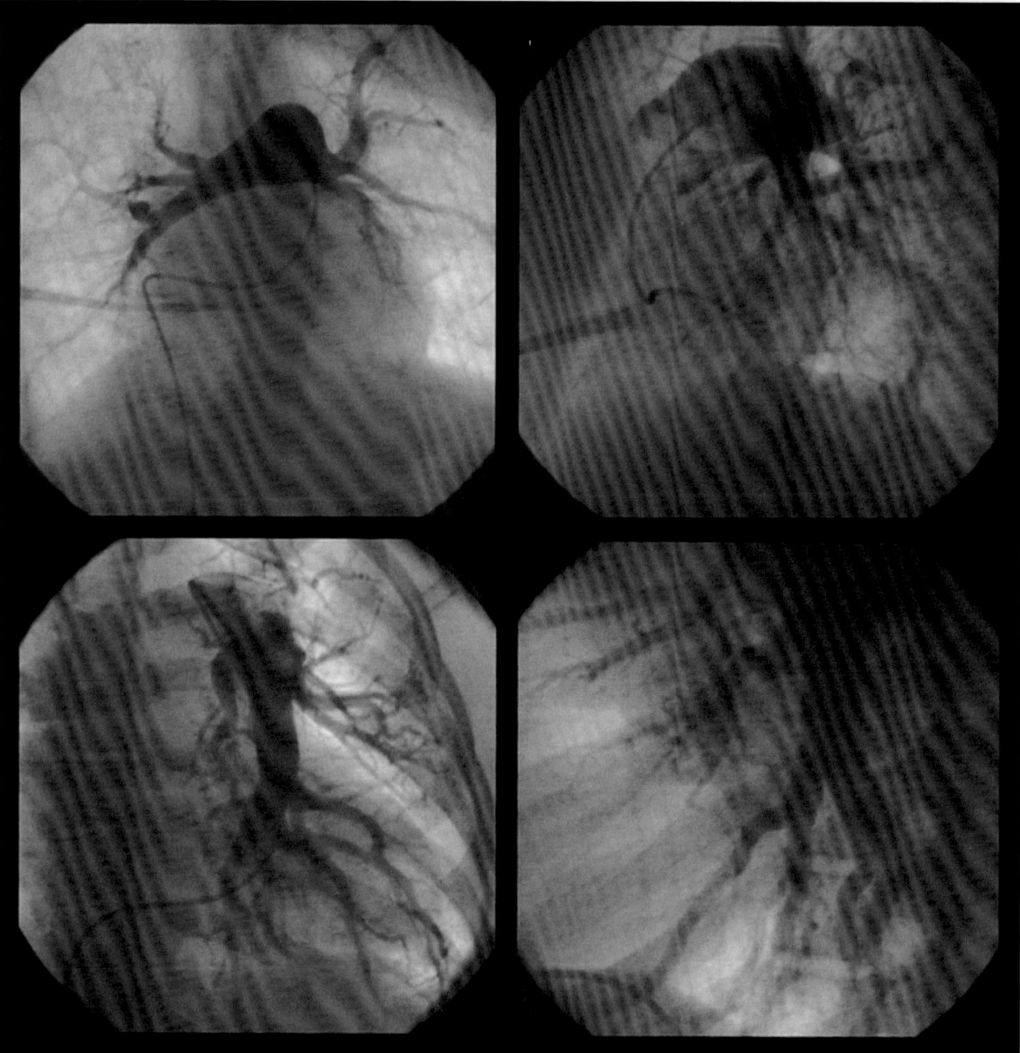

Fig 16.2—Pulmonary artery angiograms demonstrating vascular pruning and rarification of the pulmonary arterial tree. Anterior-posterior and lateral projections of pulmonary artery angiography performed in two patients with pulmonary arterial hypertension. Note that the pulmonary arteries are mildly dilated centrally, and quickly taper in size beyond the primary bifurcation. The distal arborization is pruned, and lacks normal subsegmental branching.

and thrombosis, including life-threatening pulmonary hemorrhage and paradoxical emboli. Finally, Eisenmenger patients remain at risk of cardiac complications including endocarditis, arrhythmias, right ventricular (RV) failure, and sudden cardiac death.[34]

Despite the many morbidities associated with severe PAH and Eisenmenger syndrome, mortality rates in patients with PAH associated with CHD are substantially lower than those seen in idiopathic PAH.[35] Previously, survival rates of 75%, 70%, and 55% were reported for patients aged 30, 40, and 55 years, respectively, but with the advent of new treatment options, many can reach the fifth or sixth decade of life.[36,37] In comparison, idiopathic PAH has a reported median survival of only 2.8 years after diagnosis.[38] One theory on the superior survival of PAH associated with CHD is that in this patient population, the RV is exposed to high pressures and volumes starting in infancy. Therefore, the RV may be better "trained" to support systemic PAP and less likely to develop early RV failure.[39] Secondly, patients with PAH associated with CHD are able to maintain their systemic cardiac output, despite the cost of increased cyanosis, by right-to-left shunting. In contrast, patients with idiopathic PAH have no "relief valve" and therefore have limitations to both their pulmonary and systemic cardiac outputs.[35]

Evaluation of Operability

Study modalities

Various laboratory studies and imaging modalities can help guide the diagnosis and treatment of the PAH patient with CHD. However, few of these tests have been shown to correlate with operability and outcome. Cardiac markers, coagulation studies, electrocardiograms, and pulmonary function testing can assist in determining the etiology of the PAH, but do not correlate with disease severity.[40–43] Similarly, computed tomography (CT) and ventilation perfusion (VQ) scans can help delineate anatomy and evaluate for thromboembolic disease, but cannot measure PAP.[44] Echocardiograms can assist with tracking disease progression and RV dysfunction, and can noninvasively estimate PAP with Doppler, but cannot accurately measure PVR.[45] Magnetic resonance imaging (MRI) and radionucleotide testing can calculate RV ejection fraction, which is inversely proportional to the severity of PAH,[46,47] and more recently, regression models for the accurate prediction of PVR using MRI have been developed.[48] Although this research is promising, MRI remains unable to measure PAP and left atrial pressure directly.

Lung biopsies have, in the past, been used for the evaluation of operability based on qualitative histologic changes using the Heath-Edwards classification.[25,26] The distribution of these changes, however, is not uniform and consequently, lung biopsies may underestimate or overestimate the severity of PAH. Morphometric features are distributed more uniformly within the lung, and thus Reid and colleagues developed a morphometric technique to quantify the pulmonary vascular changes associated with PAH.[28] This technique, however, has not been shown to correlate with natural history or outcome in these patients.[40] These limitations, in addition to the substantial risk such invasive testing poses to PAH patients, have limited the use of lung biopsy to cases in which tissue is required for diagnostic purposes.

Given the limitations intrinsic to other study modalities, cardiac catheterization is obligatory to accurately evaluate the operability of a patient with PAH and CHD. In addition to the direct measurement of cardiac and pulmonary pressures, cardiac catheterization allows for hemodynamic manipulations such as pulmonary vascular reactivity testing and balloon occlusion. As described later, these hemodynamic manipulations provide critical information when determining whether an ASD can be safely closed. Furthermore, cardiac catheterization also allows for pulmonary angiography. Although it should be performed with caution, pulmonary angiography is not contraindicated in this population and can be useful in ruling out other causes of PAH such as distal pulmonary artery stenosis, pulmonary venous disease, or thrombus. Finally, cardiac catheterization allows for a variety of interventions that may palliate, or even treat, the patient with CHD-associated PAH.

Calculation of PVR

PVR is a calculated value, obtained by measuring the transpulmonary gradient (the difference in mean pressure from the pulmonary arteries to the pulmonary veins) and dividing it by the pulmonary blood flow. If direct pulmonary venous pressure cannot be measured, the mean pulmonary capillary wedge pressure, or the mean left atrial pressure, can alternatively be used.

$$PVR = \frac{PAP_{mean} - PVP_{mean}}{Q_p}$$

To avoid error in calculating the PVR, several important factors need to be considered. First, oxygen consumption should be measured directly rather than assumed, and can be done with the use of respiratory mass spectrometry.[49] Oxygen consumption has been shown to change during altered physiologic states, depending on the patient's sedation level, temperature, and oxygenation status.[50,51] Therefore, oxygen consumption should be remeasured when the patient's condition changes within a catheterization, such as during pulmonary reactivity testing. Second, if using supplemental oxygen, it is imperative to incorporate dissolved oxygen into the calculation of PVR.[7] The calculated PVR will be significantly underestimated if dissolved oxygen is erroneously omitted. Therefore, the partial pressure of oxygen within the pulmonary vein should be measured, particularly in patients with intracardiac shunting.[40] Finally, polycythemia leads to increased blood viscosity, which in turn, can elevate the PVR. Lister and colleagues have reported that a drop in hema-

tocrit from 50% to 40% in children with CHD, resulted in a 30% reduction in PVR.[52] As such, the patient's oxygen consumption, oxygenation status, and hemoglobin all need to be considered to correctly calculate the PVR.

Of note, PVR cannot be accurately calculated in patients with pulmonary artery branch stenosis, or in those where a shunt is preferentially directing blood flow to one artery. Similarly, PVR cannot be calculated in patients where there are multiple sources of pulmonary blood flow, such as those with major aortopulmonary collaterals, surgically placed shunts, or other aortopulmonary connections. In these patients, pulmonary blood flow is underestimated by the Fick method, and therefore, PVR will tend to be overestimated.[7]

Pulmonary vasoreactivity testing

Pulmonary vasoreactivity testing is critical in determining the operability of a patient with CHD-induced PAH. Such testing allows one to determine whether the patient's elevation in PVR is due to reversible vasoconstriction of pulmonary artery smooth muscle cells, or if the patient suffers from irreversible fibrous changes of the pulmonary vasculature. Pulmonary vasoreactivity testing can help determine operability, but can also guide pre- and postoperative medical management and has been shown to correlate with survival.[7,40,53]

Following baseline hemodynamic testing, the patient is exposed to a short-acting vasodilatory agent and the evaluation of cardiac output and PVR is repeated. As mentioned previously, special care should be taken to measure not only the oxygen saturations, but partial pressures of dissolved oxygen as well. A positive vasoreactivity response is defined as a reduction of mean PAP of > 10 mm Hg with a resultant mean PAP of 40 mm Hg or less, without a fall in cardiac output.[36] The degree of response to pulmonary vasodilators is thought to predict the likelihood that a patient's PVR will fall once their intracardiac shunt is repaired.

Various inhaled and intravenous agents are currently available for pulmonary vasoreactivity testing. Historically, 100% oxygen was the only vasoreactive agent available and had the advantage of being easy to administer and relatively well-tolerated. Patients with decreased pulmonary venous saturation have the greatest response to oxygen. Oxygen does, however, have systemic effects including reduced systemic vascular resistance and pressure, and may increase left-to-right shunting without any change in PVR.[54] Inhaled nitric oxide (iNO) has the advantage of being a selective pulmonary vasodilator: the nitric oxide is inhaled and binds to hemoglobin, where it is quickly inactivated prior to leaving the lungs. Additionally, nitric oxide's vasodilatory effects are additive when combined with oxygen.[55,56] In past years, intravenous tolazoline hydrochloride (Priscoline) was used, but was abandoned due to undesirable systemic side effects including nausea, vomiting, and tachycardia.[57] More recently, continuous infusions of adenosine or prostacyclin have been used. Although prostacyclin does have some systemic effects, the pulmonary vasodilatory effects are greater than those on the systemic circulation, and is generally well-tolerated.[58]

Balloon occlusion testing

Temporary balloon occlusion of the ASD can provide additional information, particularly in patients who continue to have an elevated PVR despite a positive response to vasodilators and those with bidirectional shunting.[36] Two venous lines are necessary to place a balloon across the defect and measure simultaneous pressures and saturations. Echocardiography can be useful in evaluating for multiple defects. A significant increase in right ventricular filling pressures and/or a drop in cardiac output indicate a high perioperative risk, and ASD closure would therefore be contraindicated.[40]

Criteria for closure

No validated guidelines have been established regarding the closure of ASDs in patients with PAH. Some have suggested that ASD closure should only be considered when the peak PAP is < 70% of the systemic pressure, and the PVR is < 5 Wood units/m^2.[59] Others have reported that in patients with a PVR of 8 to 15 Wood units/m^2, the mortality is as high as 50% with defect closure, whereas in those with a PVR of 4 to 8 Wood units/m^2 the mortality is 10%.[7]

Several studies have been published regarding ASD closure in adult patients and those with PAH, in an attempt to retrospectively determine criteria for closure.[11,36,60–65] One series, published by Steele and colleagues, compared 40 patients with PAH who underwent either medical management or surgical closure and followed them for 4 years.[11] All those who were medically treated had progression of their disease. Among the patients who underwent closure of their ASD, those with a PVR between 7 and 9 Wood units/m^2 improved after surgery, whereas those with a PVR between 9 and 14 Wood units/m^2 had a stabilization of their disease with no progression. Those patients who underwent closure, and had a PVR of > 15 Wood units/m^2, all died. The authors concluded that ASD closure is advised in patients with a PVR < 15 Wood units/m^2. Balzer and colleagues conducted a multicenter study that evaluated preoperative hemodynamics, including pulmonary vasoreactivity testing with oxygen and nitric oxide, in 124 patients with CHD and PAH.[63] PAH was defined, in this study, as a pulmonary to systemic resistance ratio (Rp/Rs) of > 0.33. Of these 124 patients, 74 underwent surgical repair or transplantation. The authors concluded that evaluating the Rp/Rs ratio during reactivity testing with oxygen and oxygen plus nitric oxide helped to select appropriate candidates for surgical intervention. An Rp/Rs of < 0.42 with oxygen alone, and one of < 0.27 with oxygen plus nitric oxide, were associated with reduced risk of postoperative mortality and right ventricular failure and were thus identified as cut-off values for closure. More recently, percutaneous ASD closure has been reported to be safe and effective in patients with PAH, and has been shown to result in an ongoing decrease in PAP postclosure.[60,64] These studies, however, did not report specific selection criteria for closure.

Treatment Strategies for Patients with Severely Elevated Pulmonary Vascular Resistance

Classes of PAH drugs

The advent of potent oral vasodilators has expanded the options for PAH-targeted therapies, which previously were limited to inhaled or intravenous forms.[1] There are three major pathways that regulate vasoconstriction, vaso- dilatation, and cellular proliferation within the pulmonary vasculature: the endothelin pathway, the nitric oxide pathway, and the prostacyclin pathway[66] (Fig 16.3). These pathways have led to the development of three classes of PAH-targeted therapies including endothelin receptor antagonists, phosphodiesterase type-5 inhibitors, and prostacyclin analogs.[67]

Endothelin-1 is produced by endothelial cells and binds to the A and B type endothelin receptors (ET_A and ET_B) of pulmonary smooth muscle cells, resulting in powerful vasoconstriction and cell proliferation.[69] There are currently

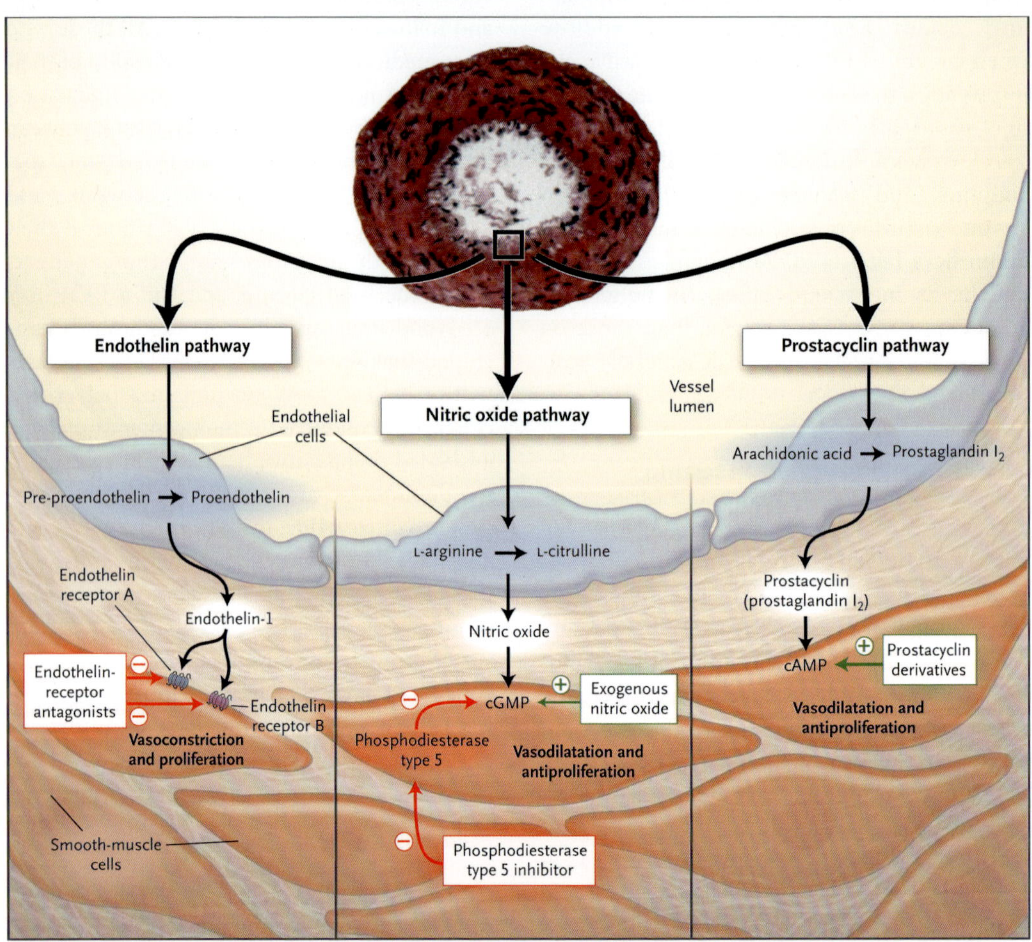

Fig 16.3—The three pathophysiological prathways in pulmonary arterial hypertension. Three major pathways involved in abnormal proliferation and contraction of the smooth muscle cells of the pulmonary artery in patients with pulmonary arterial hypertension are shown. These pathways correspond to important therapeutic targets in this condition and play a role in determining which class of drugs will be used. The classes of treatment include endothelin-receptor antagonists and nitric oxide, phosphodiesterase type 5 inhibitors, and prostacyclin derivatives. (Reproduced, with permission, from Hubert et al.[68] Copyright © 2004 Massachusetts Medical Society. All rights reserved.)

three endothelin receptor antagonists available. Bosentan is a dual endothelin receptor antagonist that acts on both ET_A and ET_B, whereas sitaxsentan and ambrisentan are ET_A selective. The benefit of selective antagonists versus dual receptor antagonists needs to be further investigated.[20] The use of bosentan in patients with Eisenmenger syndrome has been studied extensively and shown to decrease PAP, decrease PVR, and increase both exercise capacity and functional class.[70–74]

Endogenous nitric oxide produced by endothelial cells, as well as exogenous inhaled nitric oxide, cause pulmonary vasodilatation and antiproliferation by activating cyclic guanosine monophosphate (cGMP) within the smooth muscle cell. Phosphodiesterase type 5 regulates this process by breaking down cGMP. Phosphodiesterase type 5 inhibitors, such as sildenafil and tadalafil, cause vasodilatation by inhibiting the phosphodiesterase type 5 enzyme, resulting in higher levels of cGMP. Preliminary data shows that sildenafil can improve functional status, exercise capacity, and lower PAP in patients with Eisenmenger syndrome, with little associated toxicity.[75–77]

Endogenous prostacyclin and prostacyclin analogs cause vasodilatation and antiproliferation by activating cyclic adenosine monophosphate (cAMP) within the smooth muscle cell. Prostacyclin analogs are available in various forms, including intravenous epoprostenol, subcutaneous treprostinil, inhaled iloprost, and oral beraprost.[20] Intravenous epoprostenol has been reported to improve functional class, oxygen saturation, and exercise capacity, while reducing the PVR in patients with CHD-associated PAH.[78,79] Epoprostenol, however, is not without risk as it has been shown to reduce arterial oxygen, affect systemic vascular resistance, and requires long-term catheter use which is of particular risk in patients with right-to-left intracardiac shunting.[80] Inhaled iloprost, subcutaneous treprostinil, and oral beraprost are attractive alternatives due to their modes of delivery, but studies regarding their efficacy in patients with CHD-associated PAH remain limited.[81–83]

Combining medical treatment with device closure

Various potent vasodilators are available for the treatment of PAH, and preliminary research conducted in patients with Eisenmenger syndrome has demonstrated that significant improvement in hemodynamics can be achieved.[1,66,67,69,71–83] Additionally, almost one-third of patients with Eisenmenger syndrome continue to demonstrate some degree of pulmonary vasoreactivity, despite the presence of advanced pulmonary vascular disease.[36,84] Furthermore, some have proposed that endothelin-1 receptor antagonists and phosphodiesterase type 5 inhibitors have antiproliferative properties, in addition to their vasodilatory effects, that cause reverse remodeling of the pulmonary vasculature.[36,68,85] Such promising findings may allow successful defect closure in previously "inoperable" patients.[36]

The potential benefits of combining targeted PAH therapies with ASD closure are numerous. Closure of the ASD would abolish right-to-left shunting, and thereby reduce, if not eliminate, cyanosis. As previously discussed, cyanosis leads to exercise intolerance and myriad end organ dysfunctions secondary to systemic arterial desaturation and reactive erythrocytosis.[32–34] ASD closure could, therefore, result in improved exercise capacity and marked symptom relief. Elimination of the right-to-left shunt may also reduce the risk of paradoxical emboli and associated cerebrovascular events, such as stroke and abscess formation. Finally, ASD closure may protect the pulmonary circulation from further insult and progression of pulmonary vascular disease. Some have proposed that the implementation of targeted PAH therapies, without closure of the underlying defect, leads to a drop in PVR with an increase in flow and shear stress on the pulmonary vasculature.[29] Such a response would manifest itself with an initial short-term improvement followed by deterioration and further histologic changes in the lung. These adverse effects may be avoided through a staged approach that incorporates the initiation of

PAH therapies followed by partial or complete defect closure after the PVR drops.[36]

The potential risks of ASD closure in patients with severe PAH are, however, not to be understated. It has been proposed that the significant difference in long-term outcome noted between Eisenmenger patients and those with idiopathic PAH is due, in part, to the ability to unload the right ventricle through right-to-left shunting.[39] In fact, in patients with advanced idiopathic PAH, the creation of an atrial communication through atrial septostomy has been shown to decompress the right ventricle and improve cardiac output.[86,87] Thus, if an ASD is closed without significant improvement in PAP, the increased load on the heart may result in right ventricular failure, pulmonary hypertensive crisis, and death. Although percutaneous device closure eliminates the need for cardiac bypass, the sedation and airway manipulation required if anesthesia is to be employed may precipitate a pulmonary hypertensive crisis. Care should be taken to avoid hypoxia, acidosis, and airway stimulation during the procedure, all of which contribute to the high procedural risk in this patient population.[88]

Unfortunately, the literature describing successful ASD closure, in the setting of severe PAH, before or after treatment with vasodilators remains limited to small series and case reports.[89-96] Three case reports describe preclosure treatment with intravenous epoprostenol, resulting in a dramatic decrease in the PVR, and subsequent successful ASD closure.[91,92,94] Two of these patients were eventually weaned to oral vasodilators (nifedipine in one, bosentan in the other),[91,94] while the third patient continued to require epoprostenol despite an improvement in her PAP and functional class.[92] Others report the use of vasodilators as postclosure treatment in PAH patients who underwent ASD closure without preclosure therapy.[89,90,95] The largest series was reported by Yamanuchi, who utilized oral prostacyclin as postclosure treatment in four patients with ASD and associated PAH.[90] Other cases report the use of inhaled nitric oxide or bosentan in the postclosure treatment of a patient with an ASD and PDA, respec-

tively.[95,96] Although these case reports are promising, the data they offer is quite limited and long-term outcomes remain unknown. The closure of ASDs in conjunction with vasodilatory therapies cannot, therefore, be recommended as a general practice until further investigations provide strong evidence in regards to the safety and efficacy of these treatment strategies.[36]

Partial closures

Partial closure of an ASD reduces the pressure and volume load on the pulmonary vasculature, while still allowing for decompression of the right ventricle through residual right-to-left shunting. Surgical partial closures have been employed in the repair of intracardiac shunts in PAH patients and as means to decompress a stiff right ventricle in patients with right-sided obstructive lesions. Techniques include placement of a one-way flap that permits right-to-left shunting, or placement of a fenestrated interatrial patch.[97] Others have proposed the placement of pulmonary artery bands as a means of reducing pulmonary blood flow and PVR, followed by later band removal and defect closure. The morbidity and mortality associated with using this technique in patients with severe PAH, however, is high and only 50% of patients demonstrate a true benefit.[98] Percutaneous partial closures include custom-made fenestrated AMPLATZER devices or the placement of stents across such closure devices.[86,99] In patients with multiple defects, device closure of the largest defect, while leaving a smaller defect open, can achieve a similar result. With all of these techniques, residual defects may be percutaneously closed at a later time, when the PAP and PVR have dropped to safe levels.

Conclusion

The development of PAH in patients with ASDs is a complex, multifactorial process that results in serious morbidity, impaired quality of life, and reduced survival. PVR and response to vasodilators should be thoroughly evaluated prior to undertaking ASD closure in any patient with elevated PAP. In patients with mild PAH, percutaneous ASD closure can improve functional capacity and reduce PAP and PVR, without the risks associated with open-heart surgery and cardiopulmonary bypass. In patients with severe, irreversible PAH, advanced drug therapies may offer new treatment options by combining medical therapy with complete or partial defect closure. The long-term safety and efficacy of these therapies, however, are yet to be investigated. Until further data becomes available, caution and careful vigilance must be employed in the selection and follow-up of PAH patients who undergo ASD closure under this new approach.

References

1. Galie N, Hoeper MM, Humbert M, et al. Guidelines for the diagnosis and treatment of pulmonary hypertension: The Task Force for the Diagnosis and Treatment of Pulmonary Hypertension of the European Society of Cardiology (ESC) and the European Respiratory Society (ERS), endorsed by the International Society of Heart and Lung Transplantation (ISHLT). *Eur Heart J.* 2009;30(20):2493–2537.

2. Simonneau G, Robbins IM, Beghetti M, et al. Updated clinical classification of pulmonary hypertension. *J Am Coll Cardiol.* 2009;54(1, suppl):S43–S54.

3. Kovacs G, Berghold A, Scheidl S, Olschewski H. Pulmonary arterial pressure during rest and exercise in healthy subjects: a systematic review. *Eur Respir J.* 2009;34(4):888–894.

4. Wood P. The Eisenmenger syndrome or pulmonary hypertension with reversed central shunt. I. *Br Med J.* 1958;2(5098):701–709.

5. Hoffman JI. Incidence of congenital heart disease: I. Postnatal incidence. *Pediatr Cardiol.* 1995;16(3):103–113.

6. Samanek M. Children with congenital heart disease: probability of natural survival. *Pediatr Cardiol.* 1992;13(3):152–158.

7. Rudolph AM. *Congenital diseases of the heart: clinical-physiological considerations.* 3rd ed. Hoboken, NJ: Wiley-Blackwell; 2009.

8. Zaver AG, Nadas AS. Atrial septal defect—secundum type. *Circulation.* 1965;32(6, suppl):III24– III32.

9. Campbell M. Natural history of atrial septal defect. *Br Heart J.* 1970;32(6):820–826.

10. Goetschmann S, Dibernardo S, Steinmann H, Pavlovic M, Sekarski N, Pfammatter JP. Frequency of severe pulmonary hypertension complicating "isolated" atrial septal defect in infancy. *Am J Cardiol.* 2008;102(3):340–342.

11. Steele PM, Fuster V, Cohen M, Ritter DG, McGoon DC. Isolated atrial septal defect with pulmonary vascular obstructive disease—long-term follow-up and prediction of outcome after surgical correction. *Circulation.* 1987;76(5):1037–1042.

12. Engelfriet PM, Duffels MG, Moller T, et al. Pulmonary arterial hypertension in adults born with a heart septal defect: the Euro Heart Survey on adult congenital heart disease. *Heart.* 2007;93(6):682–687.

13. Sachweh JS, Daebritz SH, Hermanns B, et al. Hypertensive pulmonary vascular disease in adults with secundum or sinus venosus atrial septal defect. *Ann Thorac Surg.* 2006;81(1):207–213.

14. Andrews R, Tulloh R, Magee A, Anderson D. Atrial septal defect with failure to thrive in infancy: hidden pulmonary vascular disease? *Pediatr Cardiol.* 2002;23(5):528–530.

15. Lammers A, Hager A, Eicken A, Lange R, Hauser M, Hess J. Need for closure of secundum atrial septal defect in infancy. *J Thorac Cardiovasc Surg.* 2005;129(6):1353–1357.

16. Bull C, Deanfield J, de Leval M, Stark J, Taylor JF, Macartney FJ. Correction of isolated secundum atrial septal defect in infancy. *Arch Dis Child.* 1981;56(10):784–786.

17. Mainwaring RD, Mirali-Akbar H, Lamberti JJ, Moore JW. Secundum-type atrial septal defects with failure to thrive in the first year of life. *J Card Surg.* 1996;11(2):116–120.

18. Vogel M, Berger F, Kramer A, Alexi-Meshkishvili V, Lange PE. Incidence of secondary pulmonary hypertension in adults with atrial septal or sinus venosus defects. *Heart.* 1999;82(1):30–33.

19. Oechslin EN, Harrison DA, Connelly MS, Webb GD, Siu SC. Mode of death in adults

with congenital heart disease. *Am J Cardiol.* 2000;86(10):1111–1116.

20. Dimopoulos K, Giannakoulas G, Wort SJ, Gatzoulis MA. Pulmonary arterial hypertension in adults with congenital heart disease: distinct differences from other causes of pulmonary arterial hypertension and management implications. *Curr Opin Cardiol.* 2008;23(6):545–554.

21. Diller GP, Gatzoulis MA. Pulmonary vascular disease in adults with congenital heart disease. *Circulation.* 2007;115(8):1039–1050.

22. Haworth SG. Pulmonary hypertension in the young. *Heart.* 2002;88(6):658–664.

23. Rabinovitch M. Pulmonary hypertension: pathophysiology as a basis for clinical decision making. *J Heart Lung Transplant.* 1999;18(11):1041–1053.

24. Meyrick B, Reid L. Ultrastructural findings in lung biopsy material from children with congenital heart defects. *Am J Pathol.* 1980;101(3):527–542.

25. Heath D, Helmholz HF Jr, Burchell HB, Dushane JW, Edwards JE. Graded pulmonary vascular changes and hemodynamic findings in cases of atrial and ventricular septal defect and patent ductus arteriosus. *Circulation.* 1958;18(6):1155–1166.

26. Heath D, Edwards JE. The pathology of hypertensive pulmonary vascular disease; a description of six grades of structural changes in the pulmonary arteries with special reference to congenital cardiac septal defects. *Circulation.* 1958;18(4, pt 1):533–547.

27. Rabinovitch M, Keane JF, Norwood WI, Castaneda AR, Reid L. Vascular structure in lung tissue obtained at biopsy correlated with pulmonary hemodynamic findings after repair of congenital heart defects. *Circulation.* 1984;69(4):655–667.

28. Rabinovitch M, Haworth SG, Castaneda AR, Nadas AS, Reid LM. Lung biopsy in congenital heart disease: a morphometric approach to pulmonary vascular disease. *Circulation.* 1978;58(6):1107–1122.

29. Beghetti M. [Pulmonary hypertension associated with congenital heart disease]. *Rev Mal Respir.* 2006;23(4, suppl):13S49–13S59; quiz 13S157, 13S159.

30. Roberts KE, McElroy JJ, Wong WP, et al. BMPR2 mutations in pulmonary arterial hypertension with congenital heart disease. *Eur Respir J.* 2004;24(3):371–374.

31. Diller GP, Dimopoulos K, Okonko D, et al. Exercise intolerance in adult congenital heart disease: comparative severity, correlates, and prognostic implication. *Circulation.* 2005;112(6):828–835.

32. Spence MS, Balaratnam MS, Gatzoulis MA. Clinical update: cyanotic adult congenital heart disease. *Lancet.* 2007;370(9598):1530–1532.

33. Humbert M, Morrell NW, Archer SL, et al. Cellular and molecular pathobiology of pulmonary arterial hypertension. *J Am Coll Cardiol.* 2004;43(12, suppl S):13S–24S.

34. Daliento L, Somerville J, Presbitero P, et al. Eisenmenger syndrome. Factors relating to deterioration and death. *Eur Heart J.* 1998;19(12):1845–1855.

35. Hopkins WE, Ochoa LL, Richardson GW, Trulock EP. Comparison of the hemodynamics and survival of adults with severe primary pulmonary hypertension or Eisenmenger syndrome. *J Heart Lung Transplant.* 1996;15(1, pt 1):100–105.

36. Dimopoulos K, Peset A, Gatzoulis MA. Evaluating operability in adults with congenital heart disease and the role of pretreatment with targeted pulmonary arterial hypertension therapy. *Int J Cardiol.* 2008;129(2):163–171.

37. Cantor WJ, Harrison DA, Moussadji JS, et al. Determinants of survival and length of survival in adults with Eisenmenger syndrome. *Am J Cardiol.* 1999;84(6):677–681.

38. D'Alonzo GE, Barst RJ, Ayres SM, et al. Survival in patients with primary pulmonary hypertension. Results from a national prospective registry. *Ann Intern Med.* 1991;115(5):343–349.

39. Hopkins WE. The remarkable right ventricle of patients with Eisenmenger syndrome. *Coron Artery Dis.* 2005;16(1):19–25.

40. Moss AJ, Allen HD. *Moss and Adams' Heart Disease in Infants, Children, and Adolescents Including the Fetus and Young Adult.* 7th ed. Philadelphia: Lippincott Williams & Wilkins; 2008.

41. Kanemoto N. Electrocardiogram in primary pulmonary hypertension. *Eur J Cardiol.* 1981;12(3–4):181–193.

42. Rich S, Kieras K, Hart K, Groves BM, Stobo JD, Brundage BH. Antinuclear antibodies in primary pulmonary hypertension. *J Am Coll Cardiol.* 1986;8(6):1307–1311.

43. Karmochkine M, Cacoub P, Dorent R, et al. High prevalence of antiphospholipid antibodies in precapillary pulmonary hypertension. *J Rheumatol.* 1996;23(2):286–290.

44. Moser KM, Page GT, Ashburn WL, Fedullo PF. Perfusion lung scans provide a guide to which patients with apparent primary pulmonary hypertension merit angiography. *West J Med.* 1988;148(2):167–170.

45. Berger M, Haimowitz A, Van Tosh A, Berdoff RL, Goldberg E. Quantitative assessment of pulmonary hypertension in patients with tricuspid regurgitation using continuous wave Doppler ultrasound. *J Am Coll Cardiol.* 1985;6(2):359–365.

46. Posteraro RH, Sostman HD, Spritzer CE, Herfkens RJ. Cine-gradient-refocused MR imaging of central pulmonary emboli. *Am J Roentgenol.* 1989;152(3):465–468.

47. Debatin JF, Nadel SN, Paolini JF, et al. Cardiac ejection fraction: phantom study comparing cine MR imaging, radionuclide blood pool imaging, and ventriculography. *J Magn Reson Imaging.* 1992;2(2):135–142.

48. Bell A, Beerbaum P, Greil G, et al. Noninvasive assessment of pulmonary artery flow and resistance by cardiac magnetic resonance in congenital heart diseases with unrestricted left-to-right shunt. *JACC Cardiovasc Imaging.* 2009;2(11):1285–1291.

49. Fowler KT, Hugh-Jones P. Mass spectrometry applied to clinical practice and research. *Br Med J.* 1957;1(5029):1205–1211.

50. Li J, Stokoe J, Konstantinov IE, et al. Continuous measurement of oxygen consumption during cardiopulmonary bypass: description of the method and in vivo observations. *Ann Thorac Surg.* 2004;77(5):1671–1677.

51. Beekman RH, Rocchini AP, Rosenthal A. Cardiovascular effects of breathing 95 percent oxygen in children with congenital heart disease. *Am J Cardiol.* 1983;52(1):106–111.

52. Lister G, Hellenbrand WE, Kleinman CS, Talner NS. Physiologic effects of increasing hemoglobin concentration in left-to-right shunting in infants with ventricular septal defects. *N Engl J Med.* 1982;306(9):502–506.

53. Post MC, Janssens S, Van de Werf F, Budts W. Responsiveness to inhaled nitric oxide is a predictor for mid-term survival in adult patients with congenital heart defects and pulmonary arterial hypertension. *Eur Heart J.* 2004;25(18):1651–1656.

54. Krongrad E, Helmholz HF Jr, Ritter DG. Effect of breathing oxygen in patients with severe pulmonary vascular obstructive disease. *Circulation.* 1973;47(1):94–100.

55. Roberts JD Jr, Lang P, Bigatello LM, Vlahakes GJ, Zapol WM. Inhaled nitric oxide in congenital heart disease. *Circulation.* 1993;87(2):447–453.

56. Berner M, Beghetti M, Spahr-Schopfer I, Oberhansli I, Friedli B. Inhaled nitric oxide to test the vasodilator capacity of the pulmonary vascular bed in children with long-standing pulmonary hypertension and congenital heart disease. *Am J Cardiol.* 1996;77(7):532–535.

57. Rudolph AM, Paul MH, Sommer LS, Nadas AS. Effects of tolazoline hydrochloride (Priscoline) on circulatory dynamics of patients with pulmonary hypertension. *Am Heart J.* 1958;55:424–432.

58. Cremona G, Higenbottam T. Role of prostacyclin in the treatment of primary pulmonary hypertension. *Am J Cardiol.* 1995;75(3):67A–71A.

59. Marie Valente A, Rhodes JF. Current indications and contraindications for transcatheter atrial septal defect and patent foramen ovale device closure. *Am Heart J.* 2007;153(4, suppl):81–84.

60. de Lezo JS, Medina A, Romero M, et al. Effectiveness of percutaneous device occlusion for atrial septal defect in adult patients with pulmonary hypertension. *Am Heart J.* 2002;144(5):877–880.

61. Engelfriet P, Meijboom F, Boersma E, Tijssen J, Mulder B. Repaired and open atrial septal defects type II in adulthood: an epidemiological study of a large European cohort. *Int J Cardiol.* 2008;126(3):379–385.

62. Horer J, Muller S, Schreiber C, et al. Surgical closure of atrial septal defect in patients older

than 30 years: risk factors for late death from arrhythmia or heart failure. *Thorac Cardiovasc Surg.* 2007;55(2):79–83.

63. Balzer DT, Kort HW, Day RW, et al. Inhaled Nitric Oxide as a Preoperative Test (INOP Test I): the INOP Test Study Group. *Circulation.* 2002;106(12, suppl 1):I76– I81.

64. Balint OH, Samman A, Haberer K, et al. Outcomes in patients with pulmonary hypertension undergoing percutaneous atrial septal defect closure. *Heart.* 2008;94(9):1189–1193.

65. Suchon E, Tracz W, Podolec P, Sadowski J. Atrial septal defect in adults: the influence of age and haemodynamic parameters on the results of surgical repair. *Kardiol Pol.* 2006;64(5):470–476; discussion 477–478.

66. Beghetti M, Galie N. Eisenmenger syndrome a clinical perspective in a new therapeutic era of pulmonary arterial hypertension. *J Am Coll Cardiol.* 2009;53(9):733–740.

67. Galie N, Manes A, Palazzini M, et al. Management of pulmonary arterial hypertension associated with congenital systemic-to-pulmonary shunts and Eisenmenger's syndrome. *Drugs.* 2008;68(8):1049–1066.

68. Humbert M, Sitbon O, Simonneau G. Treatment of pulmonary arterial hypertension. *N Engl J Med.* 2004;351(14):1425–1436.

69. Galie N, Manes A, Branzi A. The endothelin system in pulmonary arterial hypertension. *Cardiovasc Res.* 2004;61(2):227–237.

70. Beghetti M, Black SM, Fineman JR. Endothelin-1 in congenital heart disease. *Pediatr Res.* 2005;57(5, pt 2):16R–20R.

71. Galie N, Beghetti M, Gatzoulis MA, et al. Bosentan therapy in patients with Eisenmenger syndrome: a multicenter, double-blind, randomized, placebo-controlled study. *Circulation.* 2006;114(1):48–54.

72. Gatzoulis MA, Beghetti M, Galie N, et al. Longer-term bosentan therapy improves functional capacity in Eisenmenger syndrome: results of the BREATHE-5 open-label extension study. *Int J Cardiol.* 2008;127(1):27–32.

73. Apostolopoulou SC, Manginas A, Cokkinos DV, Rammos S. Long-term oral bosentan treatment in patients with pulmonary arterial hypertension related to congenital heart disease: a 2-year study. *Heart.* 2007;93(3):350–354.

74. Berger RM, Beghetti M, Galiè N, et al. Atrial septal defects versus ventricular septal defects in BREATHE-5, a placebo-controlled study of pulmonary arterial hypertension related to Eisenmenger's syndrome: A subgroup analysis. *Int J Cardiol.* May 20 2009 [Epub ahead of print.]

75. Singh TP, Rohit M, Grover A, Malhotra S, Vijayvergiya R. A randomized, placebo-controlled, double-blind, crossover study to evaluate the efficacy of oral sildenafil therapy in severe pulmonary artery hypertension. *Am Heart J.* 2006;151(4):851, e851–e855.

76. Lim ZS, Salmon AP, Vettukattil JJ, Veldtman GR. Sildenafil therapy for pulmonary arterial hypertension associated with atrial septal defects. *Int J Cardiol.* 2007;118(2):178–182.

77. Mukhopadhyay S, Sharma M, Ramakrishnan S, et al. Phosphodiesterase-5 inhibitor in Eisenmenger syndrome: a preliminary observational study. *Circulation.* 2006;114(17):1807–1810.

78. Rosenzweig EB, Kerstein D, Barst RJ. Long-term prostacyclin for pulmonary hypertension with associated congenital heart defects. *Circulation.* 1999;99(14):1858–1865.

79. Fernandes SM, Newburger JW, Lang P, et al. Usefulness of epoprostenol therapy in the severely ill adolescent/adult with Eisenmenger physiology. *Am J Cardiol.* 2003;91(5):632–635.

80. Gildein HP, Wildberg A, Mocellin R. [Comparative studies of hemodynamics under prostacyclin and nifedipine in patients with Eisenmenger syndrome]. *Z Kardiol.* 1995;84(1):55–63.

81. Simonneau G, Barst RJ, Galie N, et al. Continuous subcutaneous infusion of treprostinil, a prostacyclin analogue, in patients with pulmonary arterial hypertension: a double-blind, randomized, placebo-controlled trial. *Am J Respir Crit Care Med.* 2002;165(6):800–804.

82. Galie N, Humbert M, Vachiery JL, et al. Effects of beraprost sodium, an oral prostacyclin analogue, in patients with pulmonary arterial hypertension: a randomized, double-blind, placebo-controlled trial. *J Am Coll Cardiol.* 2002;39(9):1496–1502.

83. Rimensberger PC, Spahr-Schopfer I, Berner M,

et al. Inhaled nitric oxide versus aerosolized iloprost in secondary pulmonary hypertension in children with congenital heart disease: vasodilator capacity and cellular mechanisms. *Circulation.* 2001;103(4):544–548.

84. Budts W, Van Pelt N, Gillyns H, Gewillig M, Van De Werf F, Janssens S. Residual pulmonary vasoreactivity to inhaled nitric oxide in patients with severe obstructive pulmonary hypertension and Eisenmenger syndrome. *Heart.* 2001;86(5):553–558.

85. van Wolferen SA, Boonstra A, Marcus JT, et al. Right ventricular reverse remodelling after sildenafil in pulmonary arterial hypertension. *Heart.* 2006;92(12):1860–1861.

86. Corris PA. Atrial septostomy and transplantation for patients with pulmonary arterial hypertension. *Semin Respir Crit Care Med.* 2009;30(4):493–501.

87. Kerstein D, Levy PS, Hsu DT, Hordof AJ, Gersony WM, Barst RJ. Blade balloon atrial septostomy in patients with severe primary pulmonary hypertension. *Circulation.* 1995;91(7):2028–2035.

88. Hopkins RA, Bull C, Haworth SG, de Leval MR, Stark J. Pulmonary hypertensive crises following surgery for congenital heart defects in young children. *Eur J Cardiothorac Surg.* 1991;5(12):628–634.

89. Yamauchi H, Yamaki S, Fujii M, Iwaki H, Tanaka S. Reduction in recalcitrant pulmonary hypertension after operation for atrial septal defect. *Ann Thorac Surg.* 2001;72(3):905–906, discussion 906–907.

90. Yamauchi H, Yamaki S, Fujii M, Saji Y, Ochi M, Shimizu K. Atrial septal defect with borderline pulmonary vascular disease: surgery and long-term oral prostacyclin therapy for recalcitrant pulmonary hypertension. *Jpn J Thorac Cardiovasc Surg.* 2004;52(4):213–216.

91. Schwerzmann M, Zafar M, McLaughlin PR, Chamberlain DW, Webb G, Granton J. Atrial septal defect closure in a patient with "irreversible" pulmonary hypertensive arteriopathy. *Int J Cardiol.* 2006;110(1):104–107.

92. Hirabayashi A, Miyaji K, Akagi T. Continuous epoprostenol therapy and septal defect closure in a patient with severe pulmonary hypertension. *Cathet Cardiovasc Intervent.* 2009;73(5):688–691.

93. Mizuhara A, Ino T, Adachi H, Ide H, Yamaguchi A, Kawahito K. [Surgical treatment of adult secundum ASD with severe pulmonary hypertension—two case reports]. *Nippon Kyobu Geka Gakkai Zasshi.* 1993;41(6):1089–1093.

94. Frost AE, Quinones MA, Zoghbi WA, Noon GP. Reversal of pulmonary hypertension and subsequent repair of atrial septal defect after treatment with continuous intravenous epoprostenol. *J Heart Lung Transplant.* 2005;24(4):501–503.

95. Imanaka K, Kotsuka Y, Takamoto S, Furuse A, Inoue K, Shirai T. [Atrial septal defect and severe pulmonary hypertension in an adult who needed nitric oxide inhalation after repair]. *Kyobu Geka.* 1998;51(5):403–405.

96. Eicken A, Balling G, Gildein HP, Genz T, Kaemmerer H, Hess J. Transcatheter closure of a non-restrictive patent ductus arteriosus with an AMPLATZER muscular ventricular septal defect occluder. *Int J Cardiol.* 2007;117(1):e40–42.

97. Novick WM, Sandoval N, Lazorhysynets VV, et al. Flap valve double patch closure of ventricular septal defects in children with increased pulmonary vascular resistance. *Ann Thorac Surg.* 2005;79(1):21–28; discussion 21–28.

98. Khan SA, Gelb BD, Nguyen KH. Evaluation of pulmonary artery banding in the setting of ventricular septal defects and severely elevated pulmonary vascular resistance. *Congen Heart Dis.* 2006;1(5):244–250.

99. Rothman A, Sklansky MS, Lucas VW, et al. Atrial septostomy as a bridge to lung transplantation in patients with severe pulmonary hypertension. *Am J Cardiol.* 1999;84(6):682–686.

17

Device Closure of ASDs in Patients with R-L Shunt

Anas Salkini and John W. Moore

Introduction

Interatrial communications that induce right heart volume overload by means of left-to-right shunting are usually closed to prevent late right heart failure, arrhythmias, and pulmonary hypertension.[1] Over the last two decades, the indications for transcatheter closure of communications have expanded to include patent foramen ovale (PFO) in patients after stroke or migraine,[2,3] baffle fenestrations in the Fontan circulation,[4,5] and PFOs/atrial septal defects (ASDs) in patients with bidirectional or right-to-left shunting.[6–11]

This chapter will focus on closure of the atrial level communications in patients with bidirectional or right-to-left atrial shunting. Because of the unique characteristics of patients with functional single ventricle and Fontan-type palliation, Fontan fenestration closure is discussed in the following chapter.

Pathophysiology

Right-to-left atrial shunting may be observed in patients with pulmonary hypertension and in patients with normal pulmonary pressures. Two theories have been described to explain right-to-left shunting with normal pulmonary pressure.[12] The first theory is related to the presence of a right-to-left pressure gradient which is seen in some clinical conditions such as right atrial myxoma, cardiac tamponade, right ventricular infarction, diminished right ventricular function/compliance, hypoplastic right ventricle, obstructive sleep apnea, postoperative

Transcatheter Closure of ASDs and PFOs: A Comprehensive Assessment. © 2010 Ziyad M. Hijazi, Ted Feldman, Mustafa H. Abdullah Al-Qbandi, and Horst Sievert, editors. Cardiotext Publishing, ISBN: 978-0-9790164-9-3.

respiratory distress syndrome, and in mechanical ventilation, particularly with increased pulmonary end-expiratory pressure.[13–16] In patients with repaired congenital heart defects (CHDs), a right-to-left atrial shunt through an ASD or a PFO may occur at rest or during exercise, when one or more of the following conditions are present: diminished right ventricular compliance or volume, right ventricular dysfunction, or functional or anatomical tricuspid valve restriction such as in Ebstein's anomaly. Right-to-left atrial shunting may be exacerbated by changes in posture, inspiration, Valsalva maneuvers, and during exercise[17] due to impaired right ventricular compliance when cardiac output and right ventricular end-diastolic volume are increased.

The second theory to explain right-to-left shunting with normal pulmonary pressure is related to the presence of a redundant atrial septum displaced toward the horizontal plane with atrial septal defect and the presence of a prominent Eustachian valve leading to preferential drainage of the inferior vena cava blood flow to the left atrium. A syndrome of cyanosis due to right-to-left atrial shunting with normal pulmonary pressures induced by upright posture and relieved by recumbency has been reported (the platypnea–orthodeoxia syndrome).[18–22]

Right-to-left shunting through an interatrial communication is associated with two major complications: systemic embolism and systemic desaturation. Systemic desaturation at rest or during exercise may limit physical ability and impair the quality of life of patients with repaired CHD. Cyanosis at rest is typically associated with polycythemia due to an erythropoietin-mediated response to the hypoxic environment. For that reason, such patients are at higher risk of cerebral embolism due to increased blood viscosity and clot formation.[9,23]

Agnoletti et al[9] showed that work capacity improves early after interatrial communication closure among patients with congenital heart disease and right-to-left atrial shunting. It is difficult to study right ventricular function in systole and diastole and, therefore, to evaluate right ventricular compliance with standard echocardiographic methods. Exercise testing is, however, a widely used, readily available technique that can identify patients who may benefit from closure of an interatrial communication. Indeed, if desaturation occurs only during exercise, symptoms may not be obvious. However, closure of such interatrial communications should be considered because of the risk of stroke.

Anatomical Considerations

From an embryological perspective, the inferior portion of the right venous valve develops into the valve of the inferior vena cava and valve of the coronary sinus. In the fetus, the valve of the inferior vena cava, the Eustachian valve, directs oxygen-rich blood across the foramen ovale. The remnant of this valve has no known functional significance in extrauterine life. However, maldevelopment of this valve may influence cardiac development and postnatal circulation. Complete failure of Eustachian valve regression creates an abnormal septation of the right atrium, commonly referred to as "cor triatriatum dexter." This condition has been associated with persistent cyanosis, arrhythmias, and underdevelopment of the right heart structures.[24–28]

ASDs in patients with pulmonary valve atresia and intact ventricular septum and with critical pulmonary valve stenosis differ from typical ASDs. In these lesions, the presence of elevated right atrial pressure causes right-to-left shunting, and the possible prominence of Eustachian valves or Chiari networks may divide the right atrium "cor triatriatum dexter."[29–31] Furthermore, these factors may interfere with accurate placement of ASD occluder devices. Prominence of the Eustachian valve may mimic the inferior portion of the atrial septum, potentially causing entanglement[32] and misplacement of the device if this feature is not recognized. Not surprisingly, in occasional patients undergoing surgical repair of ASDs, a prominent Eustachian valve has been mistakenly incorporated in the atrial septum during repair, resulting in postoperative obligatory right-to-left shunt and cyanosis.[33–37]

Conditions with Right-to-Left Interatrial Shunting

Pulmonary atresia with intact ventricular septum

Optimal management of infants with pulmonary atresia and intact ventricular septum has been controversial because of the anatomical heterogeneity of the hearts exhibiting this disorder.[38] The tripartite right ventricular description by Goor and Lillehei[39] and the revised classification by Bull and colleagues[40] have provided logical means for determining appropriate palliative and definitive repairs. Several studies[41–44] have demonstrated that a hypoplastic right ventricle with a patent infundibulum in pulmonary atresia or critical pulmonary stenosis with intact ventricular septum has long-term growth potential when continuity between the right ventricular cavity and pulmonary artery is established. In this subset of patients, therefore, a two-ventricle circulation is likely in the future if satisfactory palliation provides adequate pulmonary blood flow and optimizes development of the right heart.

Generally presenting as newborns, the right ventricle in such patients appears to be insufficient to maintain an adequate stroke output. As such, an aortopulmonary shunt (to support pulmonary blood flow) or a cavopulmonary connection (to unload the right ventricle) may be used as components of a management strategy. However, a coexistent atrial defect is also often present, which allows right-to-left shunting and resultant cyanosis and the potential risk of paradoxical embolization. With time, right ventricular adaptation may occur (anatomically, physiologically, or both) and closure of the atrial communication may be possible. Several factors may contribute to the increase in size of the right ventricle, including: (1) regression of

right ventricular hypertrophy after reduction in right ventricular afterload; (2) improvement of right ventricular compliance; (3) enhancement of right ventricular volumes by tricuspid valve regurgitation; (4) reduction of right-to-left shunting at the atrial level; and (5) resection of the hypertrophied muscles in the right ventricle (right ventricular overhaul).[41,45]

Ebstein's anomaly of the tricuspid valve

The right-to-left interatrial shunting in Ebstein's anomaly is the consequence of a number of factors, including functional right ventricular hypoplasia, interference of right ventricular filling by redundant tricuspid valve leaflets, and insufficiency of the tricuspid valve.

Complex congenital heart disease with 1.5 ventricle physiology

Right ventricular hypoplasia and/or dysplasia are found in association with a number of congenital anomalies. In these cardiac defects, the left ventricle is normal while the right ventricle (RV) may not be capable of completely supporting the pulmonary circulation.[46]

However, in some patients the RV pumping power may still be utilized to sustain the pulmonary circulation, provided its physiological tolerance is not exceeded.[47] Since the original report published by Billingsly et al in 1989,[48] the purpose of the so-called "one and one-half ventricle repair" has been to achieve a partial physiological correction by partially separating the pulmonary circulation from the systemic circulation while maintaining pulsatile blood flow in the pulmonary arteries. This is obtained by diverting the superior vena cava (SVC) blood to return directly into the pulmonary arteries by means of a bidirectional cavopulmonary shunt (BCPS).[49,50] In this way, the right ventricle (RV) work is reduced by about 30%[46] and the impaired ventricle may be adequate for the reduced level of function. By unloading the RV during the repair with a BCPS, a poor outcome for biventricular repair may be avoided.[46,47] In addition, by maintaining the inadequate RV as a pumping chamber for the pulmonary circulation, long-term complications of Fontan physiology such as protein-losing enteropathy may be avoided.[51] An ASD is left in place at the time of BCPS to function as a "pop-off valve." While the bidirectional cavopulmonary anastomosis reduces right ventricular workload such that the chamber may maintain a stroke volume without systemic venous congestion,[51] a residual atrial defect, while further unloading of the ventricle, may promote cyanosis. For this reason, Sano et al[45] created a restricted atrial defect in a series of 25 patients having pulmonary atresia with intact ventricular septum, who had a surgical pulmonary valvotomy. This was performed to encourage forward flow through the tricuspid valve while attempting to keep right atrial pressures < 15 mm Hg. The right atrial pressures were noted to drop in follow-up evaluations. In this situation, the defect may close spontaneously; however if it remains patent, cyanosis may persist and may be exacerbated by exercise.

Critical pulmonary valve stenosis with RV hypoplasia

Percutaneous balloon valvuloplasty has been widely used in the initial management of critical pulmonary valve stenosis in neonates and is considered to be the treatment of choice.[52,55,56] Persistent severe hypoxia following the procedure, arising from significant right ventricular hypertrophy, poor right ventricular function, and right-to-left shunting across the atrial septum, is considered an indication for a systemic-to-pulmonary shunt. Prostaglandin infusion after balloon valvuloplasty may be helpful, although there is no universal agreement on duration of therapy. Catheter closure of ASDs is technically feasible[57,58] in neonates and raises the possibility that closure of the defect will relieve the hypoxia. Success may eliminate the need for surgery with its associated complications.[53,54] The AMPLATZER occluder device has been used successfully in infants and children[57,58] and to date has been safe and effective, though long-term complications remain to be determined.

Pulmonary valve stenosis

When both pulmonic stenosis and ASD coexist, significant left-to-right shunting is prevented if right ventricular pressures increase due to the outflow obstruction caused by the pulmonic stenosis. In essence, pulmonic stenosis protects the pulmonary bed against the effects of high ASD flow. If the pulmonic stenosis is corrected initially, an increase in left-to-right shunting can occur and if not treated will lead to right ventricular volume overload and its long-term sequelae. Therefore, it is advisable to correct both lesions either simultaneously, or in a staged fashion. From a technical view, performing pulmonic balloon valvuloplasty prior to ASD occluder device deployment minimizes the risk of dislodging the ASD occluder device. On the other hand, proceeding with ASD closure prior to pulmonic balloon valvuloplasty in cases of mild-to-moderate pulmonary stenosis decreases the shunt volume into the right heart and may demonstrate that pulmonic stenosis is mild. In such cases, valvuloplasty may not be required.

Platypnea-orthodeoxia syndrome

Platypnea-orthodeoxia is a relatively uncommon but serious syndrome of arterial hypoxemia and breathlessness in the upright position caused by right-to-left interatrial shunting. Since Burchell et al[59] described this rare syndrome over half a century ago, about 50 cases have been reported.[60] The most common etiologic association is an interatrial right-to-left shunt through a PFO or an ASD.[60] Right-to-left interatrial shunting is usually associated with spontaneous or induced pulmonary hypertension. In the absence of pulmonary hypertension, a persistent Eustachian valve can cause interatrial right-to-left shunting with normal right atrial pressure.[61] Platypnea-orthodeoxia can be explained on the basis of positional modification of abnormal shunting. Standing upright may stretch the interatrial communication, whether a PFO or an ASD, thus allowing more streaming of venous blood from inferior vena cava through the defect. This redirection of flow caused by an anatomic distortion of the right atrium or the interatrial septum also may result from a loculated pericardial effusion or an aortic aneurysm. Other less common mechanisms for platypnea-orthodeoxia also exist.[60]

Right ventricular infarction

Right ventricular infarction causes reduced right ventricular myocardial compliance with increased right ventricular end diastolic and right atrial pressures. In patients with an atrial septal defect, a right-to-left shunt may develop when the right atrial pressure exceeds the left atrial pressure. The development of cyanosis and refractory hypoxemia in patients with a recent right ventricular infarction should alert the physician to the possibility of intracardiac shunting at the atrial level.

Technique of Device Closure

Atrial communication closure may be considered in the presence of mild-to-moderate desaturation at rest (O2 saturation on room air > 85%), accompanied by low flow velocity through the interatrial communication as assessed by transthoracic echocardiography (TTE) or when desaturation occurs only during exercise. Patients with increased pulmonary arterial pressure and patients with desaturation at rest < 85% may not be candidates for device closure[9] unless test occlusion of the atrial level communication proves otherwise.

The technique of device closure is the same as that used for closure of interatrial communications with left-to-right shunt; however, in patients with right-to-left shunting at rest, closure of interatrial communications should be preceded by test occlusion of the defect. Temporary test occlusion of the atrial defect should be performed with a balloon-tipped side-hole catheter or with a balloon-sizing catheter for 5 to 15 minutes. Systemic arterial and right atrial pressures and saturations should be monitored. Closure of the atrial defect may be considered

if there is not a significant drop in systemic pressures and right atrial saturation (> 10%) and there is not a significant rise in right atrial mean pressure (> 20%).[8] Test occlusion may be technically difficult if the patient has a significant bowing of the atrial septum into the left atrium caused by elevated right atrial pressure (RAP). In this case, systemic hypotension and low cardiac output may result from obstruction to pulmonary venous drainage and mitral inflow rather than from closure of the atrial level communication.

Stop-flow or stretch balloon diameter of the ASD, determined by balloon sizing at cardiac catheterization, are commonly used to select the sizes of the devices used for transcatheter closure of the secundum ASD. In the case of balloon sizing of the ASD/PFO, the stretch diameter is measured by inflating a compliant balloon through the atrial septum until the interatrial shunt is terminated and a "waist" appears on the balloon. The balloon waist is measured using both fluoroscopy and echocardiography. Stop-flow diameter is determined when interatrial shunting is terminated by the balloon, whether or not a "waist" is apparent. Using the balloon diameter, an appropriate device diameter may be chosen.

Patients with pulmonary atresia or critical pulmonary stenosis (PS) with intact ventricular septum may have prominence of Eustachian valves or Chiari network dividing the right atrium and resulting in what has been described as "cor triatriatum dexter."[29-31] Careful and thorough examination of the atrial septum and evaluation of the exact site of the drainage of the pulmonary veins allows accurate positioning of the device, excluding the Eustachian valve. In these patients, because of right atrial hypertension, there may be significant bowing of the septum into the left atrium. Echocardiography should confirm that both device discs are accurately placed across the atrial septum. Careful examination of the vital structures of the left side of the heart (including mitral valve, pulmonary vein drainage, and aortic valve flow patterns) should be performed, to confirm that the combination of leftward displacement of the atrial septum and the mass of the device does not interfere with any of these structures. The ability to test the stability of the device before release "push-pull maneuver" is an added step that should be taken to ensure stable positioning of the device, despite the increased right atrial pressure.

Literature Review

Pulmonary atresia and intact ventricular septum

Ebeid et al[6] reported the feasibility of percutaneous ASD closure in two patients (15 months and 3 years old) who underwent surgical valvotomy and Blalock/Taussig shunts as infants, with persistent significant atrial right-to-left shunt. Test occlusion of the intra-atrial communications was carried out in both patients, with evidence of satisfactory physiologic parameters. Systemic saturation increased from 75%–88% at rest to 97% after device closure. One patient had significant prominence of the Eustachian valve, mimicking a second atrial septum and producing a divided right atrium—"cor triatriatum dexter." During device placement, several imaging planes were needed to confirm satisfactory position across the true atrial septum. Imaging of the drainage site of the upper-right pulmonary veins was especially helpful in identifying the true atrial septum, allowing for accurate placement.

The results of transcatheter device closure of atrial communication in patients with pulmonary atresia and intact ventricular septum were also reported in 5 patients by Agnoletti[9] and 4 patients by Atiq et al.[8] All patients had a prior procedure to open the atretic pulmonary valve, either a surgical valvotomy or radiofrequency-assisted balloon dilation. A modified Blalock-Taussig shunt was performed in most of the patients. Children with aortopulmonary shunts underwent simultaneous temporary shunt closure and subsequent device closure if the hemodynamics were satisfactory. Atrial

communication closure was considered in the presence of mild or moderate desaturation at rest (> 84%) accompanied by low flow velocity through the interatrial communication. The age at device closure was between 4 and 15 years (median 6 years). Systemic saturation ranged 85% to 96% (median 91%) at rest, 83% to 87% at maximal exercise, and 98% to 100% after device closure. There was no significant drop in systemic pressures or right atrial saturation (> 10%) or rise in right atrial mean pressure (> 20%).

Ebstein's anomaly of the tricuspid valve

Agnoletti[9] and Atiq[8] published their experience of transcatheter device closure of atrial communication in a total of 9 patients with Ebstein's disease. The patients with unrepaired Ebstein's disease had a minor form of the disease, without major incompetence or malformation of the tricuspid valve. Surgical repair of the tricuspid valve was not indicated in this subset of patients. Before device closure, systemic saturation was between 85% and 98% at rest and between 76% and 88% on maximal exercise. After device closure, systemic saturation ranged from 94% to 100% (median 96%) and mean right atrial pressure (RAP) ranged from 6 to 12 mm Hg (median 8 mm Hg). One patient needed ablation therapy after device closure. This patient raises the consideration of whether all patients with Ebstein's anomaly should have electrophysiologic studies prior to interventional closure of their atrial communications.

Complex congenital heart disease with 1.5 ventricle physiology

Sano et al[45] created a restricted atrial defect in their series of 25 patients having pulmonary atresia with intact ventricular septum, who had a surgical pulmonary valvotomy. This was performed to encourage forward flow through the tricuspid valve while attempting to keep right atrial pressures < 15 mm Hg. In follow-up, they observed that the right atrial pressures gradually fell. In this situation, the defect may close spontaneously, but if it remains patent, then cyanosis may persist, or be exaggerated by exercise.

Atiq et al[8] reported transcatheter device closure of ASD in 5 children with pulmonary atresia with an intact ventricular septum who had undergone a bidirectional cavopulmonary connection after radiofrequency-assisted balloon dilation of the atretic pulmonary valve and a Blalock-Taussig shunt. Test occlusion of the atrial defect revealed no significant rise in right atrial or fall in systemic arterial blood pressure. Patients had mean systemic saturation of 91% at rest and 98% after device closure.

In a report published in 2005, Agnoletti et al[9] reported closure of a PFO using a 25-mm AMPLATZER PFO device in a patient with Ebstein's disease who had had a bidirectional cavopulmonary connection. In that patient, mean RAP did not change with test occlusion (8 mm Hg) and the baseline saturation was 85% at rest, 76% at maximal exercise, and 94% after device closure.

Critical pulmonary valve stenosis with RV hypoplasia

Nugent et al[7] closed an atrial defect with a device in a neonate with critical PS and hypoplastic right ventricle after initial balloon pulmonary valvoplasty. In that child, left ventricular function, cardiac output, and hypoxemia improved significantly and a systemic-to-pulmonary shunt was avoided.

This management approach in cyanotic infants with critical PS is unique. Staged palliation with a modified Blalock-Taussig shunt or PDA stent prior to ASD closure has become a more common practice.

Pulmonary valve stenosis

Agnoletti et al[9] reported closure of atrial level communication in 2 patients with pulmonary valve stenosis. The ages at device closure were 9 and 16 years. Both patients had a history of balloon pulmonary valvuloplasty. One of them had a modified BT shunt placed in the neonatal

period after balloon valvuloplasty. This patient had his shunt embolized at the time of ASD closure. Systemic saturation was 96% to 97% at rest and 78% to 94% at maximal exercise. The patient who had a higher saturation at maximal exercise had a history of migraine headache since the age of 13 years. At 16 years he had a right temporal embolism accompanied by a left facial hemiparesis and cognitive troubles. Mean RAP was 5 to 10 mm Hg at baseline and 5 to 8 mm Hg after device closure.

In managing patients with coexisting pulmonary valve stenosis and ASD, Wahl et al[62] reported balloon pulmonary valvuloplasty followed by ASD device closure in the same procedure. Performing pulmonary valvuloplasty prior to ASD occlusion probably minimizes the risk of dislodging an ASD occluder device. On the other hand, Vera et al[63] proceeded with ASD closure prior to pulmonary valvuloplasty in a patient with ASD and combined valvar and supravalvar pulmonary stenosis. After ASD closure, the shunt volume into the right heart decreased resulting in a lower gradient across the pulmonary valve (68 vs. 33 mm Hg). The gradient persisted after balloon pulmonary valvuloplasty due to supravalvar pulmonary stenosis.

Platypnea-orthodeoxia syndrome

Approximately 50 years after its first description in 1949, this syndrome has been reported in about 50 patients. In these reports, patients affected by the platypnea-orthodeoxia syndrome generally completely recovered after surgical or percutaneous closure of the interatrial communication.[11,12,22]

Right ventricular infarction

Bassi et al[64] reported the successful percutaneous closure of a right-to-left interatrial shunt in the setting of a right ventricular infarction in a 68-year-old woman who presented with right ventricular myocardial infarction complicated by refractory hypoxemia with systemic saturation down to 74%. She was found to have a significant right-to-left shunt at the atrial level through a previously undiagnosed secundum ASD. The mean right atrial pressure was 9 mm Hg, mean pulmonary artery pressure was 14 mm Hg, mean pulmonary capillary wedge pressure was 12 mm Hg, and mean left atrial pressure was 8 mm Hg. Percutaneous closure of the ASD with an AMPLATZER Septal Occluder resulted in prompt improvement in her oxygenation to 93%. Mild systemic desaturation was thought to be related to a small right-to-left shunting across a small residual PFO remote from the secundum ASD.

Repaired tetralogy of Fallot

Agnoletti et al[9] reported transcatheter closure of atrial communication in 3 patients with repaired tetralogy of Fallot. The age at device closure was 12 to 16 years old. The systemic saturation was 96% to 98% at rest, 77% to 96% at maximal exercise, and 97% to 100% after device closure. Test occlusion resulted in < 10% increase in mean RAP.

Case Examples

Case 1: Pulmonary atresia with intact ventricular septum

A 3-year-old boy with a history of pulmonary atresia, intact ventricular septum, and PDA underwent transcatheter radiofrequency perforation and then balloon dilation of the pulmonary valve. Due to significant right ventricular outflow tract (RVOT) obstruction, he underwent transcatheter RVOT stenting. At 2 years of age, patient had pulmonary valve repair (with pericardium), RVOT stent removal, RVOT muscle resection with patch augmentation, and with adjustable ASD placement. The patient had a 1-year history of progressive fatigue and a downward trend in his systemic saturation to the low 90s (%) at rest and mid 70s (%) at maximal exercise.

Right and left heart catheterization showed systemic saturation of 90% and mean right and left atrial pressure of 6 mm Hg. Indexed Qs was 3.2 L/min/m^2, Qp 1.5 L/min/m^2, and Qep 1.5 L/min/m^2. The calculated right-to-left shunting was 1.7 L/min/m^2 and Qp:Qs ratio was 0.7:1. Test occlusion was carried out for 10 minutes. This showed an increase in the systemic saturation to 100%, no change in the systemic pressure, and 1 to 2 mm Hg increase in the right atrial pressure. The ASD stretched diameter during balloon sizing was 9.6 mm. A 6F AMPLATZER delivery sheath was used to position a 10-mm AMPLATZER Septal Occluder (ASO) in the defect. TTE was used to confirm position and stability of the ASO (Fig 17.1).

Case 2: Ebstein's anomaly

A 9-year-old boy with a mild Ebstein's anomaly of the tricuspid valve has not required any intervention. He presented with systemic saturations in the low 90s at rest and in the low 80s at maximal exercise. TTE showed bidirectional shunting across secundum ASD. Because of systemic hypoxia, he was taken to the cardiac catheterization laboratory for ASD device closure. The patient had no evidence of right-to-left shunting while intubated under general anesthesia.

A 7F wedge catheter was advanced across the ASD and positioned in the left upper pulmonary vein (LUPV). A super-stiff wire was placed in the LUPV. A 24-mm AMPLATZER sizing balloon catheter was used to determine an ASD stretched diameter of 22.8 mm. A 26-mm AMPLATZER Septal Occluder was implanted using a 10F delivery sheath. TTE was used to confirm satisfactory position of the device. The stability of the device was tested, and it was released from the delivery cable (Fig 17.2).

Case 3: Critical pulmonary valve stenosis

A 3-year-old boy with history of critical pulmonary valve stenosis had balloon pulmonary valvuloplasty at 5 days of age. At 2 weeks of age, he had percutaneous PDA stenting due to low systemic desaturation caused by dynamic

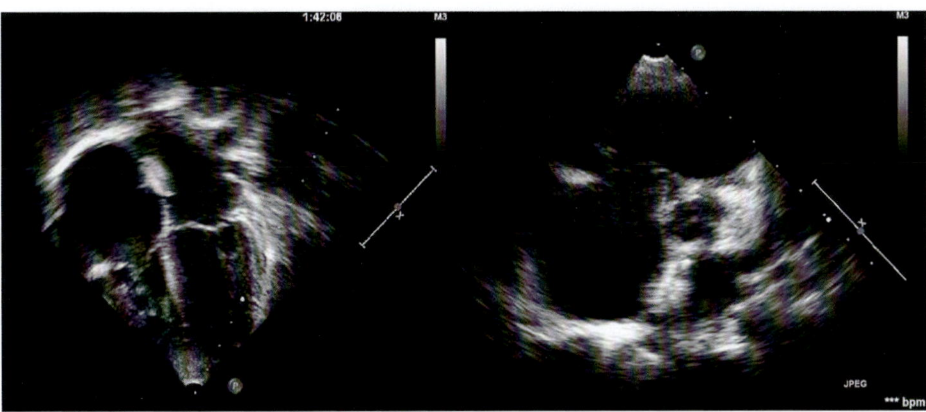

Fig 17.1—Transthoracic echocardiogram apical four-chamber and parasternal short-axis views show satisfactory AMPLATZER Septal Occluder position in a patient with pulmonary atresia and intact ventricular septum.

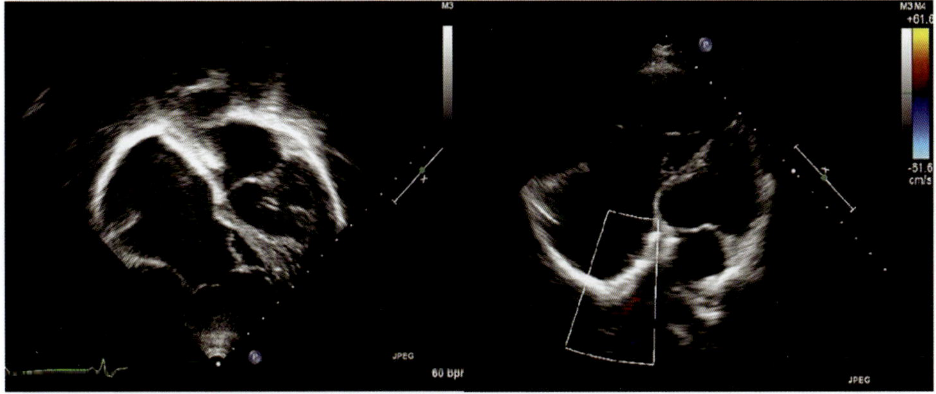

Fig 17.2—Transthoracic echocardiogram apical four-chamber and parasternal short-axis views show satisfactory AMPLATZER Septal Occluder position in a patient with Ebstein's anomaly.

right ventricular outflow tract obstruction. Due to valvar pulmonary stenosis, a repeat pulmonary valvuloplasty was done at 4 months of age. At that time, patient was also found to have coarctation of the aorta and underwent stent implantation using a Palmaz Genesis 1910B stent. Subsequently, patient has done clinically well with normal growth and development. However, patient continued to have systemic saturation in the 90% to 93% range. Most recent echocardiogram showed a small PFO with bidirectional shunting. The tricuspid valve was mildly hypoplastic with a Z-score of –1.7. The right ventricle was tripartite. Patient was referred to the cardiac catheterization to be assessed for PFO device closure.

Right and left heart catheterization showed systemic saturation of 88% and mean right and left atrial pressure of 8 mm Hg. Indexed Qs was 3.6 L/min/m^2, Qp 2.4 L/min/m^2, and Qep 2.5 L/min/m^2. The calculated right-to-left shunting was 1.1 L/min/m^2 and Qp:Qs ratio was 0.7:1. Test occlusion was carried out for 10 minutes using a Berman angiocatheter. This showed an increase in the systemic saturation to 97%, no change in the systemic pressure, and 1 to 2 mm Hg increase in the mean right atrial pressure. Right ventricular angiography showed fairly good size right ventricle. The PFO stretched diameter during balloon sizing was 8.4 mm (Fig

17.3). A 6F AMPLATZER delivery sheath was used to position a 9-mm AMPLATZER Septal Occluder in the defect. TTE was used to confirm position and stability of the ASO (Figs 17.4 and 17.5).

Conclusion

Atrial communication closure may be considered in the presence of mild or moderate desaturation at rest (> 85%) accompanied by low flow velocity through the interatrial communication

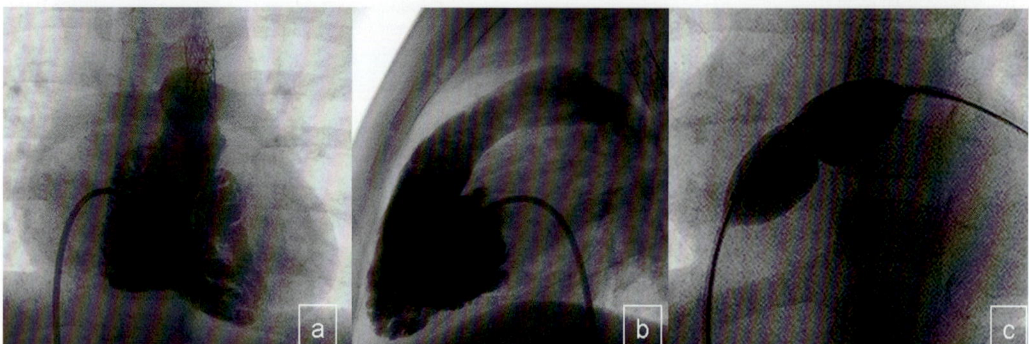

Fig 17.3—RV angiography shows a heavily trabeculated but fairly good size RV (A, B). Balloon sizing using an 18-mm balloon shows a stretched PFO diameter of 8.4 mm (C).

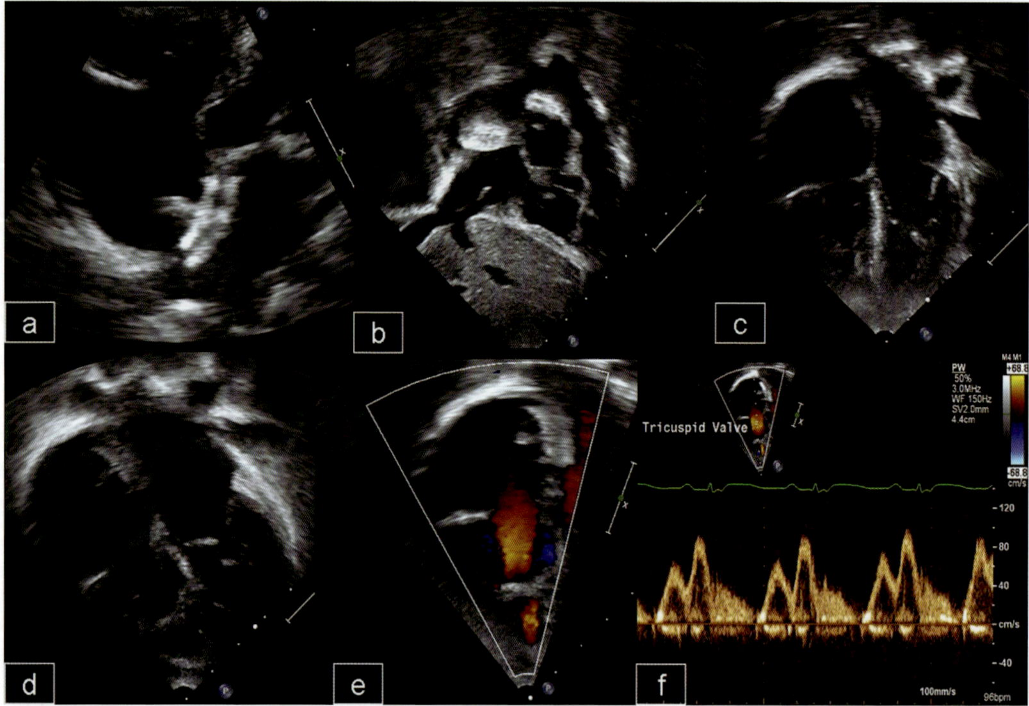

Fig 17.4—Transthoracic echocardiogram parasternal short-axis, subcostal four-chamber, and apical four-chamber views show satisfactory AMPLATZER Septal Occluder position in a patient with history of critical PS (A, C). The prominent moderator band may make the RV look small (D). However, tripartite RV is seen in other views (B, E). The tricuspid valve Z-score is –1.7. Tricuspid valve inflow Doppler after device closure shows minimal gradient across the tricuspid valve. However, the E/A reversal suggests impaired RV relaxation pattern (F).

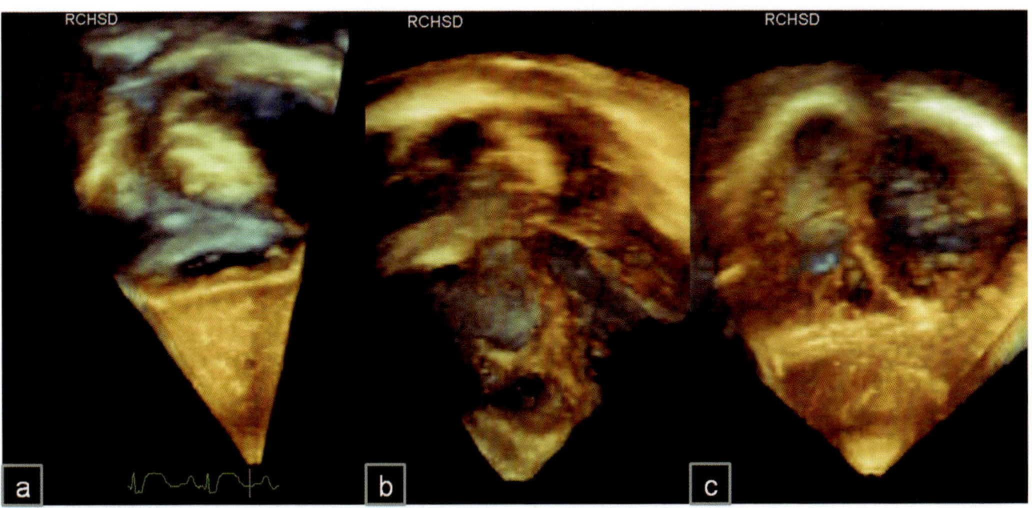

Fig 17.5—Three-dimensional (3D) transthoracic echocardiogram shows satisfactory AMPLATZER Septal Occluder position (A). B shows prominent moderator band with RV body seen below the moderator band. Widely patent RV outflow tract is seen in C.

at TTE or when desaturation occurred during exercise. Patients with increased pulmonary arterial pressure and patients with desaturation at rest < 85% may not be candidates for device closure[9] unless test occlusion of the atrial level communication proves otherwise. Percutaneous closure of interatrial communications associated with a right-to-left shunting may allow restoration of normal oxygen saturation at rest, avoidance of desaturation during exercise, and improvement of work capacity. Evaluation of oxygen consumption and more sophisticated studies of right ventricular compliance should be encouraged.

References

1. Butera G, De Rosa G, Chessa M, et al. Transcatheter closure of atrial septal defect in young children: results and follow-up. *J Am Coll Cardiol.* 2003;42:241–245.

2. Hong TC, Thaler D, Brorson J, Heitschmidt M, Hijazi ZM. Transcatheter closure of patent foramen ovale associated with paradoxical embolism using AMPLATZER PFO occluder: initial and intermediate-term results of U.S. multicenter clinical trial. *Cathet Cardiovasc Intervent.* 2003;60:524–528.

3. Sievert H, Horvath K, Zadan E, et al. Patent foramen ovale closure in patients with transient ischemic attack/stroke. *J Intervent Cardiol.* 2001;14:261–266.

4. Tofeig M, Walsh KP, Chan C, Ladusans H, Gladman G, Arnold R. Occlusion of Fontan fenestrations using the AMPLATZER septal occluder. *Heart.* 1998;79:368–370.

5. Cowley CG, Badran S, Gaffney D, Rocchini AP, Lloyd TR. Transcatheter closure of Fontan fenestrations using the AMPLATZER septal occluder: initial experience and follow up. *Catheter Cardiovasc Intervent.* 2000;51:301–304.

6. Ebeid MR, Braden DS, Gaymes CH, Heath B, Joransen JA. Post surgical use of AMPLATZER septal occluder in cyanotic patients with pulmonary atresia/intact ventricular septum: significance of cor triatriatum dexter and dilated right atrium. *Cathet Cardiovasc Intervent.* 2002;51:186–191.

7. Nugent AW, Menaham S, Goh TH, Butt W. Device closure of an atrial septal defect following successful balloon valvuloplasty in a neonate with critical pulmonary valve stenosis and persistent cyanosis. *Pediatr Cardiol.* 2000;21:170–171.

8. Atiq M, Lai L, Lee K, Benson L. Transcatheter closure of atrial septal defects in children with a hypoplastic right ventricle. *Cathet Cardiovasc Intervent.* 2005;64:112–116.

9. Agnoletti G, Boudjemline Y, Ou P, Bonnet D, Sidi D. Right to left shunt through interatrial septal defects in patients with congenital heart disease: results of interventional closure. *Heart.* 2006;92:827–831.

10. Robin E, McCauley R. An analysis of platypnea-orthodeoxia syndrome including a "new" therapeutic approach. *Chest.* 1997;112:1449–1451.

11. Kubler P, Gibbs H, Garrahy P. Platypnoea-orthodeoxia syndrome. *Heart.* 2000;83:221–223.

12. Godart F, Rey C, Prat A, et al. Atrial right-to-left shunting causing severe hypoxaemia despite normal right-sided pressures. Report of 11 consecutive cases corrected by percutaneous closure. *Eur Heart J.* 2000;21(6):483–489.

13. Tabry I, Villanueva L, Walker E. Patent foramen ovale causing refractory hypoxemia after off-pump coronary artery bypass: a case report. *Heart Surg Forum.* 2003;6:E74–E76.

14. Shah A, Tunick PA, Kronzon I. Diastolic right-to-left shunting in a patient with atrial septal defect and pericardial tamponade. *J Am Soc Echocardiogr.* 2004;17:461–463.

15. Beelke M, Angeli S, Del Sette M, et al. Obstructive sleep apnea can be provocative for right-to-left shunting through a patent foramen ovale. *Sleep.* 2002;25:856–862.

16. Cubero JM, Gallego P, Pavon M. Arrhythmogenic right ventricular cardiomyopathy and atrial right-to-left shunt. *Acta Cardiol.* 2002;57: 443–445.

17. Dubourg O, Bourdarias JP, Farcot JC, et al. Contrast echocardiographic visualization of cough-induced right to left shunt through a patent foramen ovale. *J Am Coll Cardiol.* 1984;4:587–594.

18. Gallaher ME, Sperling DR, Gwinn JL, Meyer BW, Fyler DC. Functional drainage of the inferior vena cava into the left atrium—three cases. *Am J Cardiol.* 1963;12:561–566.

19. Thomas JD, Tabakin BS, Ittleman FP. Atrial septal defect with right to left shunt despite normal pulmonary artery pressure. *J Am Coll Cardiol.* 1987;9:221–224.

20. Ciafone RA, Aroesty JM, Weintraub RM, LaRaia PJ, Paulin S. Cyanosis in uncomplicated atrial septal defect with normal cardiac and pulmonary arterial pressures. *Chest.* 1978;74:596–599.

21. Pitcher D, Fletcher P, Laszlo G, Keen G, Rees JR. Onset of right-to-left shunting through a foramen ovale in a 70-year-old woman: successful surgical treatment. *Eur Heart J.* 1986;7:541–544.

22. Bella I, Pasquino S, Da Col U, Ragni T. Cyanosis in atrial septal defect without pulmonary hypertension: a case of platypnea-orthodeoxia syndrome. *Interact Cardiovasc Thorac Surg.* 2005; 4:15–17.

23. Cottrill CM, Kaplan S. Cerebral vascular accidents in cyanotic congenital heart disease. *Am J Dis Child.* 1973;125:484–487.

24. Hansing CE, Young WP, Rowe GG. Cor triatriatum dexter. Persistent right sinus venosus valve. *Am J Cardiol.* 1972;30:559–564.

25. Morishita Y, Yamashita M, Yamada K, Arikawa K, Taira A. Cyanosis in atrial septal defect due to persistent eustachian valve. *Ann Thorac Surg.* 1985;40:614–616.

26. Raffa H, al-lbrahim K, Kaydi MT, Sorefan AA, Rustore M. Central cyanosis due to prominence of the eustachian and thebesian valves. *Ann Thorac Surg.* 1992;54:]59<50.

27. Ott DA, Cooley DA, Angelini P, Leachman RD. Successful surgical Correction of symptomatic cor triatriatum dexter. *J Thorac Cardiovasc Surg.* 1979;78:573-575.

28. Bharati S, McAllister HA Jr, Tatodes CJ, et al. Anatomic variations in underdeveloped right ventricle related to tricuspid atresia and stenosis. *J Thorac Cardiovasc Surg.* 1976;72:383–400.

29. Cooke JC, Gelman JS, Harper RW. Chiari network entanglement and herniation into the left atrium by an atrial septal defect occluder device. *J Am Soc Echocardiogr.* 1999;12:601–603.

30. Mahy IR, Anderson RH. Division of the right atrium. *Circulation.* 1998;98:2352–2353.

31. Trento A, Zuberbhler JR, Anderson RH, Park SC, Siwers RD. Divided right atrium (prominence of the eustachian and thebesian valves). *J Thorac Cardiovasc Surg.* 1998;96:457–463.

32. Douchette J, Knoblich R. Persistent right valve of the sinus venosus. *Arch Pathol.* 1963;75:105–112.

33. Becker A, Buss M, Sebening W, Meisner H, Dohlemann C. Acute inferior cardiac inflow obstruction resulting from inadvertent surgical closure of a prominent eustachian valve mistaken for an atrial septal defect. *Pediatr Cardiol.* 1999;20:155–157.

34. Staple TW, Ferguson TB, Parker BM. Diversion of the inferior vena cava into the left atrium following atrial septal defect closure. *Am J Roentgenol Radium Ther Nucl Med.* 1966;98:851–858.

35. Desnick SJ, Neal WA, Nicoloff DM, Moller JH. Residual right-to-left shunt following repair of atrial septal defect. *Ann Thorac Surg.* 1976;21:291–295.

36. Munet M, Gayet C, Buttard P, Ninet J, Chapon P, Tremeau G, Grange H, Milon H. Late discovery of inferior vena cava draining into the left atrium after surgical closure of atrial septal defect. *Arch Mal Coeur Vaiss.* 1997;90:991–994.

37. Sapin PM, Salley RK. Arterial desaturation and orthodeoxia after atrial septal defect repair: demonstration of the mechanism by transesophageal and contrast echocardiography. *J Am Soc Echocardiogr.* 1997;10:588–592.

38. Zuberbuhler JR, Anderson RH. Morphological variations in pulmonary atresia with intact ventricular septum. *Br Heart J.* 1979;41:281–288.

39. Goor DA, Lillehei CS. The anatomy of the heart. In: Goor DA, Lillehei CW, eds. *Congenital malformations of the heart.* New York, NY: Grune & Stratton; 1975:1–37.

40. Bull C, de Leval M, Mercanti C, Macartney FJ, Anderson RH. Pulmonary atresia and intact ventricular septum: a revised classification. *Circulation.* 1982;66:266–272.

41. Patel RG, Freedom RM, Moes CAF, et al. Right ventricular volume determinations in 18 patients with pulmonary atresia and intact ventricular septum: analysis of factors influencing right ventricular growth. *Circulation.* 1980;61: 428–440.

42. Lewis AB, Wells W, Lindesmith GG. Right ventricular growth potential in neonates with pulmonary atresia and intact ventricular septum. *J Thorac Cardiovasc Surg.* 1986;91:835–840.

43. Shaddy RE, Sturtevant JE, Judd VE, et al. Right ventricular growth after transventricular pulmonary valvotomy and central aortopulmonary shunt for pulmonary atresia and intact ventricular septum. *Circulation.* 1990;82(suppl IV):IV-157–IV-163.

44. Schmidt KG, Cloez J-L, Silverman NH. Changes of right ventricular size and function in neonates after valvotomy for pulmonary atresia or critical pulmonary stenosis and intact ventricular septum. *J Am Coll Cardiol.* 1992;19:1032–1037.

45. Sano S, Ishino K, Kawada M, Fujisawa E, Kamada M, and Ohtsuki S. Staged biventricular repair of pulmonary atresia or stenosis with intact ventricular septum. *Ann Thorac Surg.* 2000;70:1501–1506.

46. Arsdell GS. One and half ventricle repair. *Semin Thorac Cardiovasc Surg.* 2000;3:173–178.

47. Alvarado O, Sreeram N, McKay R, Boyd IM. Cavopulmonary connection in repair of atrioventricular septal defects with small right ventricle. *Ann Thorac Surg.* 1993;55:729–736.

48. Billingsly AM, Laks H, Boyce SW, George B, Santulli T, Williams RG. Definitive repair in patients with pulmonary atresia and intact ventricular septum. *J Thorac Cardiovasc Surg.* 1989;97:746–754.

49. Azzolina G, Eufrate S, Pensa P. Tricuspid atresia: experience in surgical management with a modified cavopulmonary anastomosis. *Thorax.* 1972;27:111–115.

50. Karl TR, Stellin G. Early Italian contribution to cavopulmonary shunt surgery. *Ann Thorac Surg.* 1999;67:1175.

51. Stellin G, Vidaa VL, Milanesib O, et al. Surgical treatment of complex cardiac anomalies: the 'one and one half ventricle repair'. *Eur J Cardiothorac Surg.* 2002;22:1043–1049

52. Colli AM, Perry SB, Lock JE, Keane JF. Balloon dilation of critical valvar pulmonary stenosis in the first month of life. *Cathet Cardiovasc Diagn.* 1995;34:23–28

53. Gladman G, McCrindle BW, Williams WG, Freedom RM, Benson LN. The modified Blalock–Taussig shunt: clinical impact and morbidity in Fallot's tetralogy in the current era. *J Thorac Cardiovasc Surg.* 1997;11:25–30.

54. Gold JP, Violaris K, Engle MA, et al. A five year clinical experience with 112 Blalock–Taussig shunts. *J Cardiol Surg.* 1993;8:9–17.

55. Rome JJ. Balloon pulmonary valvuloplasty. *Pediatr Cardiol.* 1998;19:18–24.

56. Tabatabaei H, Boutin C, Nykanen DG, Freedom RM, Benson LN. Morphologic and hemodynamic consequences after percutaneous balloon valvotomy for neonatal pulmonary stenosis:

medium term follow-up. *J Am Coll Cardiol.* 1996;27:473–478.

57. Thanopoulos BD, Laskari CV, Tsaousis GD, et al. Closure of atrial septal defects with the AMPLATZER occlusion device: preliminary results. *J Am Coll Cardiol.* 1998;31:1110–1116.

58. Wilkinson JL, Goh TH. Early clinical experience with use of the "AMPLATZER septal occluder" device for atrial septal defect. *Cardiol Young.* 1998;8:295–302.

59. Burchell HB, Helmholz HF Jr, Wood EH. Reflex orthostatic dyspnea associated with pulmonary hypertension. *Am J Physiol.* 1949;159:563–564.

60. Cheng TO. Platypnea-orthodeoxia syndrome: etiology, differential diagnosis, and management. *Cathet Cardiovasc Intervent.* 1999;47:64–66.

61. Bashour T, Kabbani S, Saalouke M, Cheng TO. Persistent Eustachian valve causing severe cyanosis in atrial septal defect with normal right atrial pressure. *Angiology.* 1983;34:79–83.

62. Wahl A, Windecker S, Misteli M, Meier B. Combined percutaneous pulmonary valvuloplasty and atrial septal defect closure for pulmonary valvular stenosis and associated secundum atrial septal defect in an adult. *Cathet Cardiovasc Intervent.* 2001;53(1):68–70.

63. Vera J, Nounou M, Kern M. Staged percutaneous atrial septal defect closure and pulmonic balloon valvuloplasty in an adult with congenital heart disease. *Cathet Cardiovasc Intervent.* 2008;72:416–423.

64. Bassi S, Amersey R, Andrews R. Right ventricular infarction complicated by right to left shunting through an atrial septal defect: successful treatment with an AMPLATZER septal occluder. *Heart.* 2005;91:e28.

18

Device Closure of Fenestrations Post Fontan Operation

Mustafa H. Abdullah Al-Qbandi and Ziyad M. Hijazi

Introduction

The Fontan operation is the definitive, conventional palliative surgical procedure for children with complex univentricular heart lesions. One of the surgical options increasingly accepted is the extracardiac Fontan,[1,2] a connection between the inferior vena cava to the pulmonary artery with a conduit placed outside the heart. It has several advantages such as absence of aortic cross-clamping, low cardiopulmonary bypass time, absence of long intra-atrial suture lines (which might decrease the risk of subsequent arrhythmias), prevention of baffle leaks, and maintenance of the laminar flow in the systemic venous return.[3,4] A modification of the Fontan operation includes creation of a fenestration between the physiologic right atrium (conduit/ lateral tunnel) and the left atrium. This persistent right-to-left shunt allows maintenance of systemic blood flow (Qs), while lowering the right atrial pressure at the expense of systemic arterial desaturation. In the extracardiac Fontan, the fenestration consists of a surgical polytetrafluoroethylene (PTFE) shunt between the extracardiac conduit and the systemic atrium (extracardiac fenestrated Fontan procedure, EFFP). This artificially induced right-to-left shunt has been invaluable in improving the condition of the patient until adaptation to the new hemodynamic situation is achieved. Subsequent to surgery, the fenestration may close spontaneously, can be closed using a snare technique, or in the catheterization laboratory utilizing a variety of devices.[5-10] Intentionally created fenestrations in patients with operated total cavopulmonary anastomosis may cause right-to-left shunt with resultant arterial hypoxemia and subsequent polycythemia.[11,12] Such defects are potential sites for paradoxical embolism leading to cerebrovascular accidents or peripheral emboli[13-17] Whereas some of these defects may close spontaneously, others do not. Due to the preceding reasons, the authors believe such fenestrations should generally be closed.[18] With the availability of a number of closure devices, such defects can be closed easily in the cardiac catheterization laboratory.

The indications for closure are:

1. Systemic arterial oxygen desaturation ≤ 90%
2. Prior cerebrovascular accidents
3. Transient ischemic attack due to paradoxical embolism
4. Peripheral emboli leading to organ infarcts/skin infarcts
5. Progressive polycythemia secondary to hypoxemia related to right-to-left shunt

Device Implantation Technique

We generally recommend performing a thorough cardiac catheterization with full hemodynamic assessment a year after the Fontan completion. Any minor hemodynamic abnormality should be addressed. Angiographic assessment of the branch pulmonary arteries is of utmost importance. Angiography in the descending aorta is also important to rule in/out presence of aortopulmonary collaterals. Finally an angiogram in the conduit (lateral tunnel or extracardiac conduit) should be done using biplane imaging. If there is a fenestration identified, the operator should cross this fenestration to the functional left atrium and assess the hemodynamics with the fenestration open and after 15 to 20 minutes of temporary balloon occlusion of the fenestration. There are double lumen catheters (5–7F) available whereby the distal lumen will measure the left atrial pressure and the proximal lumen will measure the "tunnel-RA" pressure. The operator should calculate the cardiac index and systemic oxygen transport at rest (fenestration open) and after 15

to 20 minutes of balloon occlusion of the fenestration. For full calculations of different parameters, readers are encouraged to review a paper by Hijazi et al.[19]

A significant drop in systemic arterial blood pressure and an increase in the right atrial "Fontan" pressure and heart rate would suggest that the patient does not tolerate the balloon occlusion. Occlusion of fenestration following recent surgery appears to adversely affect cardiac index and systemic oxygen delivery in a larger percentage of patients.[6,20,21] However, late occlusion (6–12 months) appears to be well tolerated in most patients.[22] Therefore, device closure of the fenestration early after surgery in high-risk Fontan patients may not be appropriate. If no significant change in the heart rate, cardiac index (no more than 15% from baseline), systemic oxygen delivery, and the Fontan pressure (no more than 5 mm Hg from baseline) occurs during the 15- to 20-minute test balloon occlusion, then device implantation is performed. One obvious benefit of fenestration closure is improvement in oxygen saturation[23] as well as exercise capacity.[24,25] Additionally, it avoids repeated activation of the inflammatory system.[26] A study by Meadows[27] found that closure of Fontan fenestrations have no acute effect on exercise capacity but improved ventilatory response to exercise. Before fenestration closure, peak oxygen consumption (VO2) was depressed and there was systemic desaturation at rest that worsened with exercise. The ventilatory response to exercise was also abnormal, characterized by elevation of the minute ventilation (VE)/CO2 elimination slope (VE/VCO2), a low end-tidal CO2, and high end-tidal O2 at the ventilatory anaerobic threshold. Although arterial saturation improved significantly after fenestration closure, there was no change in peak VO2 (70.9 ± 18.6% to 74.0 ± 18.6%, p=NS), heart rate, or O2 pulse at peak exercise. In contrast, ventilatory abnormalities (VE/VCO2) improved considerably (44.4 ± 10.9 to 33.3 ± 5.5, p≤0.001).

Various devices and techniques have been used to occlude Fontan fenestrations/baffle leaks:

Non-AMPLATZER group

Clamshell device[20]
Modified umbrella device[28]
CardioSEAL devices[10]
Buttoned device[29,30]
Modified Rashkind PDA occluder[10]
Das Angel Wing devices[31]
HELEX device[32]
BioSTAR device[33]
Modified PFO STAR device[34]

Coil group

Gianturco Coils and\or Cook detachable
coils and/or Gianturco-Grifka
vascular occlusion[7,10,35,36]

AMPLATZER group

AMPLATZER Septal Occluder[8,10,37]
AMPLATZER PFO Occluder[38,39]
AMPLATZER PDA Occluder[9,40]
AMPLATZER Vascular Plug[41]

Covered stent group

covered Cheatham-Platinum (CP) Stent[42-44]
Talent AAA Stent Graft and GORE
EXCLUDER Endoprosthesis (per-
sonal experience)

Depending on the preference of the operator and the defect nature, a device or a covered stent is chosen (Table 18.1). For some of the aforementioned devices (HELEX, CardioSEAL, etc), the reader should refer to Part IV of the book. If a coil is used, it is usually suitable for small fenestrations. The major risk using coils is embolization. A 0.038-inch Gianturco coil with a loop diameter at least twice the fenestration diameter and of sufficient length to produce four loops is to be selected for implantation. The tip of the coil delivery catheter is positioned across the fenestration into the pulmonary venous atrium and two coil loops delivered. The catheter is then gently withdrawn into the right or systemic venous atrium and the remaining two loops delivered; thus the coil straddles the fenestration. In the AMPLATZER group, one of the AMPLATZER occluder devices can be used to close the fenestration. However, these devices

are bulky and protrude into the Fontan tunnel. Their technique of deployment is the same as in the case of ASD device closure with the exception of sizing of these fenestrations. The authors tend to use a small angioplasty balloon catheter with gentle inflation. This helps determine the fenestration size as well as the shape, which is particularly helpful in extracardiac TCPC. The chosen device should be the same size as the defect. The 4-mm AMPLATZER ASD has been effective in closing fenestration baffles. For closure of many fenestrations, even the 4-mm central waist is oversized for the small opening of the fenestration, and the rigid rim of the fenestration does not allow the waist to expand, resulting in elongation "mushrooming" of the device.

The new and novel technique in closing Fontan fenestrations (especially if they are multiple, due to suture line leak) is the use of covered stents.[42-44] Many devices have been successfully used to close fenestrations. Using a device requires introduction of a guide wire and a long sheath into the pulmonary atrium. This approach can be made difficult by the fenestration's location and can be burdened by the risk of systemic embolism. The use of the covered CP stent (NuMED Inc., Hopkinton, New York) can constitute a valid tool for fenestration closure in Fontan circulation, at least in patients weighing > 15 kg. In a study by Marini,[43] six patients with fenestrated TCPC had median age and weight of 11 years and 38 kg, respectively. The femoral approach was used in all but 1 patient having bilateral thrombosis of femoral veins. The CP stent was crimped on a (NuMED, Hopkinton, New York) in 5 patients and on a regular balloon in 1 patient. The balloon's diameter was the same size or 1 to 2 mm larger than the extracardiac conduit, according to the angiographic diameter. Immediate full occlusion of fenestrations was obtained in all patients. Mean central venous pressure did not increase significantly and oxygen saturation significantly increased. No procedural or intra-hospital complications occurred. In particular, no arrhythmias, systemic embolism, or acute venous thrombosis were observed. At a median

	ASD Device	Coil	Covered Stent
Method of access	Femoral/Transhepatic	Femoral/ Transhepatic	Femoral/Jugular/ Transhepatic
Need of wire to cross fenestration	Yes	Yes	No
Balloon sizing of defect	Required	Required	Not required
Balloon occlusion testing	Required	Required	Required
Bulkiness of device	Most	Not applicable	No
Sheath size	As per device	Smallest	At least 12F
Protrusion into TCPC circuit	Yes	Yes	No
Risk of embolization into systemic circulation	Yes	Greater	No
Fenestration size and geometry	Need to know	Need to know	Not necessary
Diameter and length of extracardiac tunnel	Not necessary	Not necessary	Important to know
Anticoagulation	Needed	Needed	Needed
Residual leak	Almost none	greater	None
TCPC tunnel narrowing	Protrusion of device may make it smaller	May protrude	Fixed at the same time of fenestration closure
Multiple leaks	May need multiple device	Need multiple coils	Single stent
Cost	More expensive	Least expensive[47]	Less expensive
Postclosure access to pulmonary venous chamber if develop arrhythmia or protein losing enteropathy	Above or below the previously placed device. AMPLATZER device can be done within certain period of time, or stent placed through its disc to create fenestration[48,49]	May be difficult to retrieve. Fenestration can be created above or below the placed coil.	Can puncture through covered stent and insert a bare metal stent through struts, or go above or below the previously placed stent.

Table 18.1—Comparison of Device, Coil and Stent in Closing Total Cavopulmonary Connection (TCPC) Fenestration

follow-up of 2.8 months all patients had normal oxygen saturation and were symptom-free.

The authors' experience with the use of the Talent AAA stent graft was very encouraging. It was used in an 8-year-old patient with lateral tunnel dehiscence resulting in significant right-to-left shunt. Two grafts were deployed, one from the femoral vein and the other one overlapping the first one from the jugular vein. Oxygen saturation increased from low 80% to high 90%.

Post Fenestration Closure

Most patients post Fontan operation are placed on anticoagulation treatment such as warfarin. Some believe that such patients should receive both anticoagulation and antiplatelet therapy.

After fenestration closure, the authors believe a 6-month course of anticoagulation plus aspirin therapy is recommended. After 6 months, it is recommended to discontinue the anticoagulation and continue the aspirin therapy indefinitely.

References

1. Marcelletti C, Corno A, Giannico S, Marino B. Inferior vena cava-pulmonary artery extracardiac conduit. A new form of right heart bypass. *J Thorac Cardiovasc Surg.* 1990;100:228–232.

2. Ocello S, Salviato N, Marcelletti CF. Results of 100 consecutive extracardiac conduit Fontan operations. *Pediatr Cardiol.* 2007;28:433–437.

3. McElhinney DB, Reddy VM, Moore P, Hanley FL. Revision of previous Fontan connections to extracardiac or intraatrial conduit cavopulmonary anastomosis. *Ann Thorac Surg.* 1996;62:1276–1282.

4. Laschinger JC, Redmond JM, Cameron DE, Kan JS, Ringel RE. Intermediate results of the extracardiac Fontan procedure. *Ann Thorac Surg.* 1996;62:1261–1267.

5. Bridges ND, Lock JE, Castaneda AR. Baffle fenestration with subsequent transcatheter closure. Modification of the Fontan opera-

6. Bridges ND, Lock JE, Mayer JE Jr, Burnett J, Castaneda AR. Cardiac catheterization and test occlusion of the interatrial communication after the fenestrated Fontan operation. *J Am Coll Cardiol.* 1995;25:1712–1717.

7. Sommer RJ, Recto M, Golinko RJ, Griepp RB. Transcatheter coil occlusion of surgical fenestration after Fontan operation. *Circulation.* 1996;94:249–252.

8. Tofeig M, Walsh KP, Chan C, Ladusans E, Gladman G, Arnold R. Occlusion of Fontan fenestrations using the AMPLATZER septal occluder. *Heart.* 1998;79:368–370.

9. Rueda F, Squitieri C, Ballerini L. Closure of the fenestration in the extracardiac Fontan with the AMPLATZER duct occluder device. *Catheter Cardiovasc Intervent.* 2001;54:88–92.

10. Pihkala J, Yazaki S, Mehta R, et al. Feasibility and clinical impact of transcatheter closure of interatrial communications after a fenestrated Fontan procedure: medium-term outcomes. *Catheter Cardiovasc Intervent.* 2007;69:1007–1014.

11. Bridges ND, Mayer JE Jr, Lock JE, et al. Effect of baffle fenestration on outcome of the modified Fontan operation. *Circulation.* 1992;86:1762–1769.

12. Laks H, Pearl JM, Haas GS, et al. Partial Fontan: advantages of an adjustable interatrial communication. *Ann Thorac Surg.* 1991;52:1084–1094.

13. Wilson WR, Greer GE, Tobias JD. Cerebral venous thrombosis after the Fontan procedure. *J Thorac Cardiovasc Surg.* 1998;116:661–663.

14. Rosti L, Colli AM, Frigiola A. Stroke and the Fontan procedure. *Pediatr Cardiol* 1997;18:159.

15. Wilson DG, Wisheart JD, Stuart AG. Systemic thromboembolism leading to myocardial infarction and stroke after fenestrated total cavopulmonary connection. *Br Heart J.* 1995;73:483–485.

16. du Plessis AJ, Chang AC, Wessel DL, et al. Cerebrovascular accidents following the Fontan operation. *Pediatr Neurol.* 1995;12:230–236.

17. Hutto RL, Williams JP, Maertens P, Wilder WM, Williams RS. Cerebellar infarct: late complication of the Fontan procedure? *Pediatr Neurol.* 1991;7:293–295.

18. Hijazi ZM. Extracardiac fenestrated Fontan operation: to close or not to close the fenestration? *Cathet Cardiovasc Intervent.* 2001;54:93–94.

19. Hijazi ZM, Fahey JT, Kleinman CS, Kopf GS, Hellenbrand WE. Hemodyanmic evaluation before and after closure of fenestrated Fontan. An acute study of changes in oxygen delivery. *Circulation.* 1992;86:196–202.

20. Kopf GS, Kleinman CS, Hijazi ZM, Fahey JT, Dewar ML, Hellenbrand WE. Fenestrated Fontan operation with delayed transcatheter closure of atrial septal defect. Improved results in high-risk patients. *J Thorac Cardiovasc Surg.* 1992; 103:1039–1047.

21. Kuhn MA, Jarmakani JM, Laks H, et al. Effect of late postoperative atrial septal defect closure on hemodynamic function in patients with a Lateral tunnel Fontan procedure. *J Am Coll Cardiol.* 1995;26:259–265.

22. Goff DA, Blume ED, Gauvreau K, Mayer JE, Lock JE, Jenkins KJ. Clinical outcome of fenestrated Fontan patients after closure: the first 10 years. *Circulation.* 2000;102:2094–2099.

23. Bordacova L, Kaldararova M, Tittel P, Masura J. Experiences with fenestration closure in patients after the Fontan operation. *Bratisl Lek Listy.* 2007;108:344–347.

24. Mays WA, Border WL, Knecht SK, et al. Exercise capacity improves after transcatheter closure of the Fontan fenestration in children. *Congenit Heart Dis.* 2008;3:254–261.

25. Momenah TS, Eltayb H, Oakley RE, Qethamy HA, Faraidi YA. Effects of transcatheter closure of Fontan fenestration on exercise tolerance. *Pediatr Cardiol.* 2008;29:585–588.

26. Wessel A, Buchhorn R, Loppnow H. Interventional closure of a fenestrated Fontan avoids cytokine production. *Ann Thorac Surg.* 2000;69:1642.

27. Meadows J, Lang P, Marx G, Rhodes J. Fontan fenestration closure has no acute effect on exercise capacity but improves ventilatory response to exercise. *J Am Coll Cardiol.* 2008;52:108–113.

28. Redington AN, Rigby ML. Transcatheter closure of interatrial communications with a modified umbrella device. *Br Heart J.* 1994;72:372–377.

29. Rao PS, Chandar JS, Sideris EB. Role of inverted buttoned device in transcatheter occlusion of atrial septal defects or patent foramen ovale with right-to-left shunting associated with previously operated complex congenital cardiac anomalies. *Am J Cardiol.* 1997;80:914–921.

30. Koike K. [Transcatheter closure of the congenital cardiac defects: a review and prospect]. *Rinsho Kyobu Geka.* 1994;14:99–104.

31. Kay JD, O'Laughlin MP, Ito K, Wang A, Bashore TM, Harrison JK. Five-year clinical and echocardiographic evaluation of the Das Angel Wings atrial septal occluder. *Am Heart J.* 2004; 147:361–368.

32. Peuster M, Beerbaum P. A novel implantation technique for closure of an atypical fenestration connecting the right atrial appendage to an extracardiac conduit by use of a 15 mm HELEX device in a patient with total cavopulmonary connection. *Z Kardiol.* 2004;93:818–823.

33. Hoehn R, Hesse C, Ince H, Peuster M. First experience with the biostar-device for various applications in pediatric patients with congenital heart disease. *Cathet Cardiovasc Intervent.* 2010;75:72–77.

34. Boshoff DE, Brown SC, Degiovanni J, et al. Percutaneous management of a Fontan fenestration: in search for the ideal restriction-occlusion device. *Cathet Cardiovasc Intervent.* 2010;75:60–65.

35. Gamillscheg A, Beitzke A, Stein JI, Rupitz M, Zobel G, Rigler B. Transcatheter coil occlusion of residual interatrial communications after Fontan procedure. *Heart.* 1998;80:49–53.

36. Kim SH, Kang IS, Huh J, Lee HJ, Yang JH, Jun TG. Transcatheter closure of fenestration with detachable coils after the Fontan operation. *J Korean Med Sci.* 2006;21:859–864.

37. Cowley CG, Badran S, Gaffney D, Rocchini AP, Lloyd TR. Transcatheter closure of fontan fenestrations using the AMPLATZER septal occluder: initial experience and follow-up. *Cathet Cardiovasc Intervent.* 2000;51:301–304.

38. Bordacova L, Kaldararova M, Tittel P, Masura J. Experiences with fenestration closure in patients after the Fontan operation. *Bratisl Lek Listy.* 2007;108:344–347.

39. Masura J, Bordacova L, Tittel P, Berden P, Podnar T. Percutaneous management of cyanosis in

Fontan patients using AMPLATZER occluders. *Cathet Cardiovasc Intervent.* 2008; 71:843–849.

40. Boudjemline Y, Bonnet D, Sidi D, Agnoletti G. [Closure of extrocardiac Fontan fenestration by using the AMPLATZER duct occluder]. *Arch Mal Coeur Vaiss.* 2005;98:449–454.

41. Ebeid MR, Mehta I, Gaymes CH. Closure of external tunnel Fontan fenestration: a novel use of the AMPLATZER vascular plug. *Pediatr Cardiol.* 2009;30:15–19.

42. Boudjemline Y, Agnoletti G, Marini D, Bonnet D, Sidi D. [Use of covered stents to occlude extracardiac Fontan fenestration]. *Arch Mal Coeur Vaiss.* 2006;99:424–428.

43. Marini D, Boudjemline Y, Agnoletti G. Closure of extracardiac Fontan fenestration by using the covered Cheatham Platinum stent. *Cathet Cardiovasc Intervent.* 2007;69:1002–1006.

44. Hijazi ZM, Ruiz CE, Patel H, Cao QL, Dorros G. Catheter therapy for fontan baffle obstruction and leak, using an endovascular covered stent. *Cathet Cardiovasc Diagn.* 1998;45:158–161.

19

Unusual Vascular Access to Close ASDs and PFOs

Larry A. Latson

Introduction

The standard approach for placement of transcatheter atrial septal defect (ASD) and patent foramen ovale (PFO) closure devices is through the femoral veins. This approach is very familiar to interventionalists and provides a reasonable angle of approach to the atrial septum in the vast majority of patients. In a very small percentage of patients, the femoral approach may not be feasible. In these situations, alternative routes of vascular access are necessary to deliver a transcatheter closure device. The most commonly used alternative vascular access routes include one of the upper body veins draining to the superior vena cava (SVC) or the transhepatic route to the inferior vena cava (IVC). Minimally invasive surgical approaches are detailed elsewhere.

Primary Indications for Alternative Vascular Access

Probably the most common reason for considering alternate routes of vascular access to close an ASD or PFO is the presence of thrombi in the lower body venous system. Thrombi may have been detected in the past, or be found at the time of the contemplated procedure. The presence of an ASD or PFO in patients with venous thrombi allows for the possibility of a paradoxical embolus, which could have devastating effects. In some patients, recently discovered femoral-iliac thrombus with the potential for dislodgment makes femoral vein catheterization unattractive. In many cases, patients who have a previous history of deep vein thrombosis or pulmonary embolism have

Transcatheter Closure of ASDs and PFOs: A Comprehensive Assessment. © 2010 Ziyad M. Hijazi, Ted Feldman, Mustafa H. Abdullah Al-Qbandi, and Horst Sievert, editors. Cardiotext Publishing, ISBN: 978-0-9790164-9-3.

undergone placement of an IVC filter before discovery of the interatrial communication. In patients who have an IVC filter in place, but no evidence of persisting thrombus, it is generally possible to carefully advance one or more long sheaths from the femoral veins through the openings in the IVC filter. An ASD occlusion device may then be delivered using otherwise standard techniques (Fig 19.1).[1,2]

Patients with congenital or acquired absence of a portion of the lower body venous system also require consideration of unusual venous access routes. Acquired occlusion of the femoral-iliac system is especially common in children or adults who have required the prolonged presence of femoral venous catheters at some point in their lives. These patients often have a history of a serious medical condition necessitating a prolonged intensive care unit (ICU) stay. Less commonly, lower body acquired venous occlusions are found in patients who have required multiple cardiac catheterizations or cardiopulmonary bypass utilizing the femo-

ral vessels. It may be possible in some patients to recanalize and stent an occluded femoral-iliac venous system.[3] Other sites of vascular access however may be preferable if the only contemplated procedure is ASD closure, and the patient is otherwise asymptomatic from chronic venous occlusion.

Congenital anomalies of the venous system leading to absence of a portion of the infrahepatic IVC almost always result in a femoral venous catheter entering the atria through the azygous or hemiazygous systems, which connect to the SVC or innominate vein (Fig 19.2). Such congenitally anomalous venous pathways most commonly occur in association with complex intracardiac malformations as part of the heterotaxy syndromes. Rarely however, these venous anomalies may be seen in patients with only an ASD or PFO. In some cases, it may still be possible to deliver an ASD occlusion device through the femoral vein. The necessarily circuitous route however may make consideration of

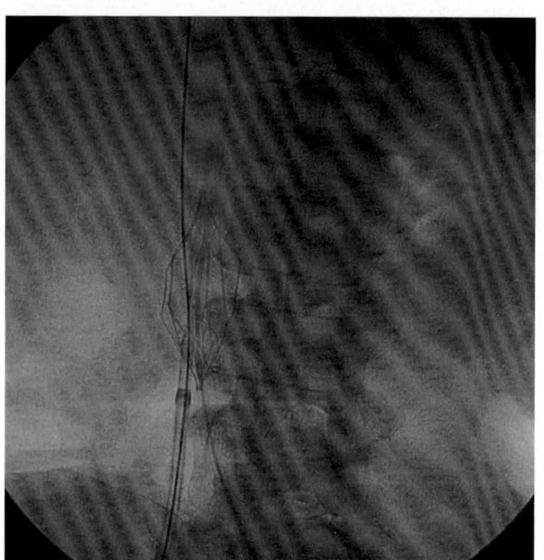

Fig 19.1—An IVC filter is in place in this patient with a history of pulmonary embolus and recently discovered PFO. Ultrasound and a preliminary angiogram demonstrated good flow through the filter with no apparent thrombus. An ICE catheter has been advanced through the filter from the left femoral vein and a long sheath is being advanced over a guide wire from the right femoral vein (marker tip visible just below the filter).

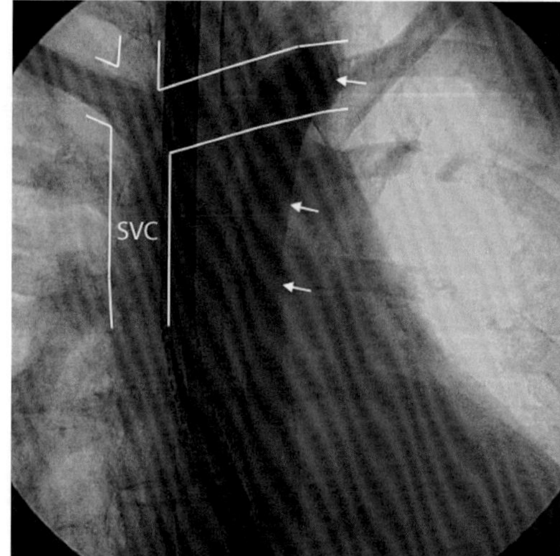

Fig 19.2—Angiogram following contrast injection in the right femoral vein in a patient with congenitally anomalous venous drainage. The infrahepatic segment of the IVC is absent. A very large hemiazygous vein (arrows) is seen to the left of the spine. This vein drains into the innominate vein and then the right-sided SVC. Another common variant is for the hemiazygous to drain into a left SVC. The PFO in this patient was closed from the right jugular venous approach.

transhepatic or upper body venous routes more attractive.

Approaches from the Upper Body Veins

The inferior portion of the atrial septum is tilted slightly away from the relatively vertical, cranial–caudal course of the superior vena cava. This orientation of the atrial septum makes it more difficult to advance a gently curved catheter across an atrial septal communication from the jugular approach than from the femoral venous approach. The difficulty is still greater if the communication is a PFO, because a PFO often has the configuration of a small channel directed cranially (Fig 19.3). In spite of this suboptimal alignment, the jugular approach has been successfully utilized in humans and in ani-mal models. In fact, the jugular approach was utilized in two of the first 12 successful placements of the original prototype AMPLATZER ASD Occluder in a swine model.[4]

To advance a catheter into the left atrium from the right superior vena cava, it is frequently necessary to utilize a relatively sharply angled catheter (such as a right coronary catheter) to first direct a guide wire across the interatrial opening. An even-more-sharply-angulated catheter, such as a left coronary catheter or an internal mammary catheter, may be especially helpful if the interatrial opening is a PFO. Although the right jugular vein is the most commonly utilized route for delivering devices from the upper venous system, the left axillary or subclavian veins can also be used.[5]

Once the jugular venous delivery sheath has been advanced across the interatrial defect to the left atrium, device deployment steps are the same as those for delivery via the femoral route. The orientation of the device relative to the septum however is different. The device

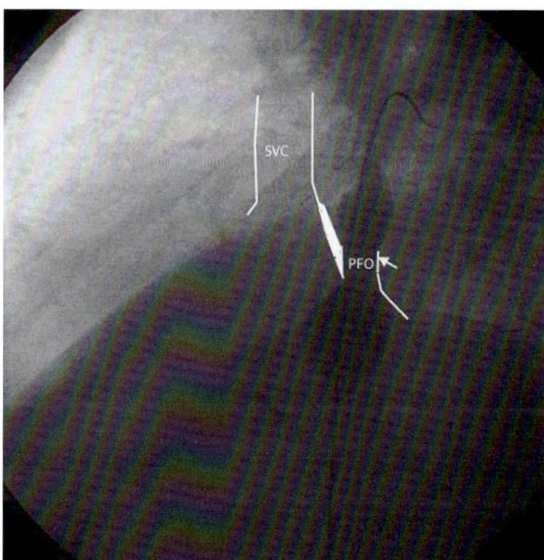

Fig 19.3—Lateral view of a partially inflated sizing balloon in a PFO. The white lines indicate the positions of the atrial septum and walls of the SVC. The arrow identifies the septum primum, which forms a flap that normally covers the opening of the foramen ovale. Notice that the inferior portion of the atrial septum angles away from the direction of the SVC and that the pathway through the PFO is oriented cephalad. The orientation of these structures makes crossing the atrial septum from the SVC more difficult than crossing from the IVC.

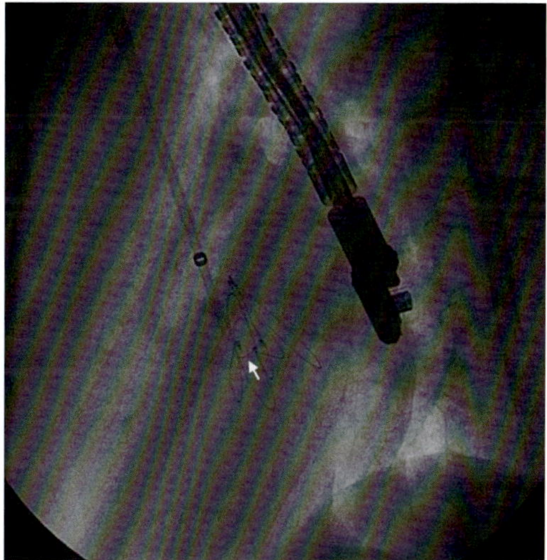

Fig 19.4—A HELEX Septal Occluder has been deployed to close an ASD from the right internal jugular vein. At this point in deployment, there is still a "safety cord" (not visible) threaded through the right atrial eyelet of the frame (opposite the arrow which points to the "locking loop" of the device). Note the device is nearly parallel to the delivery catheter from this route. TEE was used to evaluate the device placement because femoral access for an ICE probe was not possible in this patient.

must be carefully evaluated fluoroscopically and with ultrasound throughout the delivery process because the angle of approach is less than ideal. After the device has been entirely configured, the orientation may be improved by slightly advancing the delivery sheath or cable. Devices with a relatively flexible connection to the delivery catheter may be preferable to devices that more rigidly maintain a 90° angle to the tip of the delivery sheath. We and others have successfully deployed AMPLATZER and HELEX devices from the jugular venous route (Fig 19.4).[6-8]

Transhepatic Route

Transhepatic catheterization has been utilized in the pediatric cardiology community since the mid-1990s.[9-11] This approach has generally been utilized in patients with limitations to the femoral venous and jugular venous approaches. The insertion site most frequently used is between, or just below, the lowest palpable ribs near the right mid-axillary line. Different insertion sites have been used with ultrasound guidance, or if there are abnormalities of liver position as frequently seen in patients with heterotaxy syndromes.[12] Transhepatic ASD closure procedures are generally done under general anesthesia and with biplane imaging. Holding ventilation transiently at end expiration during needle insertion provides the best positioning of the liver and reduces the risk of inadvertent puncture of the diaphragm. A second sheath for an ICE probe is usually not available, so general anesthesia makes transesophageal echocardiography more tolerable. Most practitioners use fluoroscopy to advance a styleted needle cranially and slightly posteriorly from the right axillary insertion site.[13] The stylet is removed and the needle is withdrawn slightly until free flow of blood is seen and/or injection of a very small amount of contrast demonstrates the needle tip in a hepatic vein. If the needle does not enter a hepatic vein on the initial insertion, the small injections of contrast during withdrawal may

opacify a candidate vein. Recording these injections allows one to have a road map for subsequent needle insertions.

Once the needle tip is in a hepatic vein, a guide wire is advanced into the right atrium and a sheath is placed over the guide wire. It is important to use a sheath that is long enough to extend into the hepatic vein and not just into the hepatic parenchyma. We prefer not to make repeated changes in the sheath from the transhepatic approach, and usually insert a sheath large enough to accommodate the expected ASD device delivery system from the beginning. After transhepatic catheterization, we routinely place a coil or vascular occlusion device in the hepatic tract near the capsule of the liver to reduce the chance of bleeding.

The direction of approach to the atrial septum from the typical transhepatic insertion site is often even more optimal than from the femoral venous route (Fig 19.5). In most cases, the occlusion device will be nearly parallel to the plane of the atrial septum. Withdrawal movements of the delivery system from the transhepatic approach tend to move the device in a more left-to-right direction than similar movements from the femoral approach. The transhepatic approach has been utilized for ASD device placement in small infants with occluded femoral veins.[14,15] Some have recommended the transhepatic route for especially difficult ASD closures even if the femoral veins are patent.[14]

The primary concerns with the routine use of the transhepatic approach are lack of familiarity with the technique, the occasional occurrence of pain, and the possibility of significant intra-abdominal bleeding. In our experience, some older patients complain of pain that is presumably due to the small laceration and possible hematoma in the hepatic capsule caused simply by insertion of the sheath. This pain can occur even with the routine use of coils or other devices to close the intrahepatic tract. Serious bleeding into the hepatic capsule or peritoneum has been reported in up to 5% of patients.[16] Some patients with significant abdominal symptoms have undergone exploratory laparotomy. Active bleeding was no longer

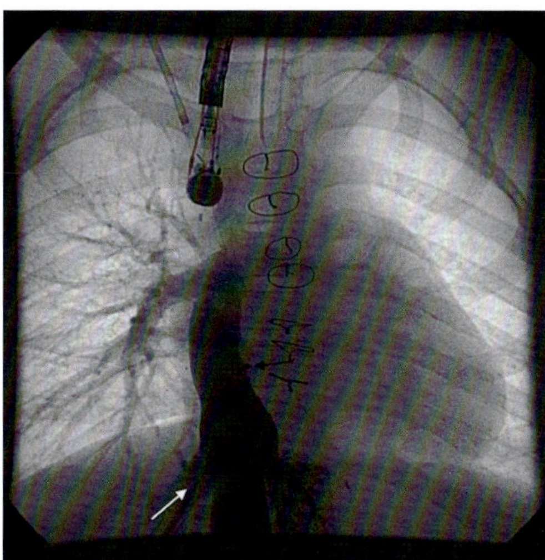

Fig 19.5—The transhepatic route was utilized to place an AMPLATZER Septal Occluder (black arrow) in the fenestration of the atrial pathway created at the time of a Fontan procedure. Note that the direction of the catheter (white arrow) allows the device to be delivered at an optimal orientation.

evident in two cases reported by Erenberg and co-workers by the time exploration could be accomplished. Conservative management with volume replacement and careful observation may be sufficient.[16] Bleeding may occur even if an occluder was placed in the insertion tract. It is important to monitor patients for development of any signs or symptoms of peritoneal irritation, drop in hemoglobin, tachycardia, or hypotension. Abdominal ultrasound should be utilized early if there are any signs of a possible complication, and some prefer to perform ultrasound imaging routinely in all patients regardless of symptoms.

Summary

The femoral venous approach is the preferred approach for ASD occlusion device delivery in nearly all patients. Alternate routes, however, may be necessary or preferable in special circumstances. Interventionalists active in transcatheter ASD closure should be familiar

with the possibility of employing these unusual routes of vascular access.

References

1. Awadalla H, Boccalandro F, Majano RA, Moustapha A, Salloum JG, Smalling RW. Percutaneous closure of patent foramen ovale guided by intracardiac echocardiography and performed through the transfemoral approach in the presence of previously placed inferior vena cava filters: a case series. *Cathet Cardiovasc Interv.* Oct 2004;63(2):242–246.

2. Rhodes JF, Miller SG, Lane GK, Latson LA. Transcatheter interventions across an inferior vena cava filter. *Cathet Cardiovasc Interv.* Jul 2003;59(3):333–337.

3. Ing FF, Fagan TE, Grifka RG, et al. Reconstruction of stenotic or occluded iliofemoral veins and inferior vena cava using intravascular stents: re-establishing access for future cardiac catheterization and cardiac surgery. *J Am Coll Cardiol.* Jan 2001;37(1):251–257.

4. Sharafuddin MJ, Gu X, Titus JL, Urness M, Cervera-Ceballos JJ, Amplatz K. Transvenous closure of secundum atrial septal defects: preliminary results with a new self-expanding nitinol prosthesis in a swine model. *Circulation.* Apr 15 1997;95(8):2162–2168.

5. Carter LI, Cavendish JJ. Percutaneous closure of a patent foramen ovale via left axillary vein approach with the AMPLATZER Cribriform septal occluder. *J Interv Cardiol.* Feb 2008;21(1):28–31.

6. Sullebarger JT, Sayad D, Gerber L, Ettedgui J, Jimmo-Waumans S, Alcebo PC. Percutaneous closure of atrial septal defect via transjugular approach with the AMPLATZER septal occluder after unsuccessful attempt using the CardioSEAL device. *Catheter Cardiovasc Interv.* Jun 2004;62(2):262–265.

7. Abdel-Massih T, Boudjemline Y, Agnoletti G, et al. [Percutaneous closure of an interatrial communication via the internal jugular route using an AMPLATZER prosthesis]. *Arch Mal Coeur Vaiss.* Oct 2002;95(10):959–961.

8. Sader MA, De Moor M, Pomerantsev E, Palacios IF. Percutaneous transcatheter patent foramen

ovale closure using the right internal jugular venous approach. *Cathet Cardiovasc Interv.* Dec 2003;60(4):536–539.

9. Sommer RJ, Golinko RJ, Mitty HA. Initial experience with percutaneous transhepatic cardiac catheterization in infants and children. *Am J Cardiol.* Jun 15 1995;75(17):1289–1291.

10. Shim D, Lloyd TR, Cho KJ, Moorehead CP, Beekman RH, 3rd. Transhepatic cardiac catheterization in children. Evaluation of efficacy and safety. *Circulation.* Sep 15 1995;92(6):1526–1530.

11. Johnson JL, Fellows KE, Murphy JD. Transhepatic central venous access for cardiac catheterization and radiologic intervention. *Cathet Cardiovasc Diagn.* Jun 1995;35(2):168–171.

12. Johnston TA, Donnelly LF, Frush DP, O'Laughlin MP. Transhepatic catheterization using ultrasound-guided access. *Pediatr Cardiol.* Jul–Aug 2003;24(4):393–396.

13. Qureshi AM, Rhodes JF, Appachi E, et al. Transhepatic Broviac catheter placement for long-term central venous access in critically ill children with complex congenital heart disease. *Pediatr Crit Care Med.* May 2007;8(3):248–253.

14. Ebeid MR, Joransen JA, Gaymes CH. Transhepatic closure of atrial septal defect and assisted closure of modified Blalock/Taussig shunt. *Catheter Cardiovasc Interv.* May 2006;67(5):674–678.

15. Javois AJ, Van Bergen AH, Husayni TS. Technical considerations for closing secundum atrial septal defect in the small child with the HELEX Septal Occluder via transhepatic access. *Catheter Cardiovasc Interv.* Jan 2006;67(1):127–131.

16. Erenberg FG, Shim D, Beekman RH, 3rd. Intraperitoneal hemorrhage associated with transhepatic cardiac catheterization: a report of two cases. *Cathet Cardiovasc Diagn.* Feb 1998;43(2):177–178.

20

Transcatheter ASD Closure without Fluoroscopy

Peter Ewert and Felix Berger

Introduction

About 80% of all septum secundum type ASD can be closed by transcatheter means. The procedure was originally introduced in clinical practice mainly under fluoroscopic guidance[1] because at that time echocardiography was less developed and available than today. With the introduction of transesophageal echocardiography its role increased considerably. Today fluoroscopy is mainly used to steer catheters, delivery systems, and occluders while echocardiography gives detailed information about the individual anatomic structure of the atrial septum and its defects. Furthermore, it reveals the relation of implanted occluders and defects, of residual shunts, and of possible interferences between occluders and adjacent anatomic structures. On the other hand, procedure and fluoroscopy times for successful interventions could

be considerably diminished, due to the easy handling of some devices in routine use and the large experience gained over the years in defects with different morphologic properties. Thus it suggests itself to systematically reduce the use of fluoroscopy further.[2] An end point of that development was the transcatheter ASD closure under echocardiography as the only imaging tool and without fluoroscopy at all.[3–5] Since then, the method has evolved to a routine procedure of first choice at our institution.

Methods

Patient selection

In all patients with an atrial septal defect (ASD) in the ovale fossa suitable for transcatheter closure on the basis of an outpatient transthoracic

---

echocardiographic study, a defect closure without fluoroscopy can be attempted. No special selection criteria are necessary in comparison to the conventional procedure. For the beginner, however, small- or medium-sized defects located centrally in the oval fossa, with sufficient margins to the atrioventricular valves and the pulmonary and caval veins are advantageous to become comfortable with the technique.

Device selection

Because two-dimensional (2D) echocardiography reveals only cross-sectional view planes, a rotational symmetry of the occluder is helpful. A good visibility of the device under echocardiography is crucial. Both are properties of the AMPLATZER Septal Occluder (AGA Medical Corporation, Plymouth, Minnesota). Thus, the procedure was developed for the implantation of AMPLATZER Septal Occluders and is performed almost exclusively with this device.

Diagnostic catheterization

The indication for defect closure of an ordinary ASD—either by surgery or by transcatheter intervention—is not dependent on a diagnostic catheterization but is derived from echocardiography. Thus, despite the possibility to perform a diagnostic catheterization under echocardiographic guidance, including pressure measurements and oximetry for shunt quantification, it is not necessary and does not belong to a routinely performed defect closure.

Catheters used to reach the left upper pulmonary vein

While by fluoroscopy the shadow of the whole catheter can be seen on the screen, echocardiographic view planes can show only small sections of the catheter whenever it is crossing the view plane. Thus, it is crucial to visualize the tip of the catheter while it is advanced through the heart. For smaller children we recommend a Berman wedge catheter with the balloon filled with a small amount of saline making it easy

to detect under echocardiography. For older children and adults an angled pigtail catheter is advantageous, because it is exactly steerable, and the tip is visible due to the double cross-section across its ring-shaped end.

How to reach the left upper pulmonary vein

Via a short sheath in the femoral vein a J-tipped guide wire is advanced into the right atrium and the superior caval vein, which can be best monitored by a bicaval transesophageal view (angulation of 90°–120°). A suitable catheter is advanced and can be seen as a thicker structure sliding over the wire. Once the catheter tip has reached the superior caval vein, the wire can be withdrawn and the catheter is visible as a double contoured tube. Now the catheter is pulled back until its tip lies directly in front of the defect. Switching to a horizontal plane (0°), the tip of the catheter and the defect can be seen simultaneously. By gently turning the catheter in a clockwise direction, it sweeps through the defect into the left atrium. A forward move of the catheter with a coordinated, simultaneous pull back and left turn of the echo probe brings the catheter under continuous vision in front of the orifice of the left upper pulmonary vein, which eventually can be entered by further advancement of the catheter.

Balloon sizing

Balloon sizing is currently under debate, and the sizing procedure can be perhaps omitted in some cases; however, we feel that it is a crucial step in transcatheter closure of ASDs revealing valuable informations about the quality of the rims of an ASD, and it helps to find the optimal occluder size avoiding oversizing and undersizing.

Exchanging the catheter against a stiff guide wire is easy, because of the different echo qualities of wire (complete extinction of ultrasound behind the metal) and catheter (inner lumen visible between double contour, no complete extinction of ultrasound). The advancement of the sizing catheter into the defect is best monitored with the balloon slightly prefilled and with a probe angle of around 70° to 80° to get a longitudinal cross-section through the balloon (Fig 20.1). The sizing itself is performed in analogy to the procedure under fluoroscopy; the balloon is filled with saline. The diameter of the sizing balloon is directly measured from the echocardiographic view plane. Care must be taken that the maximal diameter at the level of the defect is measured. Due to the accuracy of the echocardiographic measurements, the use of a sizing plate to verify the balloon diameter outside the body is not necessary in our experience.

Interventional closure

After removal of the sizing balloon, the delivery sheath is advanced over the guide wire still placed in the upper left pulmonary vein. A stiff guide wire and an angulated echocardiographic view providing the longest possible visualization of a wire section are helpful. According to the course of the wire through the atria, the angle of the transesophageal probe has to be steep (90° to 70°) to show the wire on the right atrial side and more horizontal 45° to 20° to show it on the left atrial side. The section crossing the defect is best seen in angulations in between. When the delivery sheath is advanced, it straightens the wire and consequently steeper angulations are needed, however angles larger than 90° are not helpful except in cases were the development of the device has to be performed from the right upper pulmonary vein.

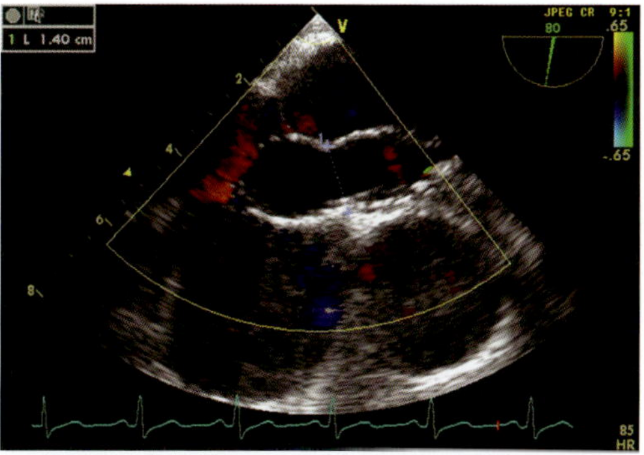

Fig 20.1—A transesophageal echocardiographic view in 80° during balloon sizing of the defect. This view outlines the entire length of the balloon.

The advancement of the sheath is seen as a thicker shadow gliding over the wire. Once the dilator is removed, the sheath can be visualized as a tube with an inner lumen. An appropriate AMPLATZER Septal Occluder is then introduced and advanced until the device is visible inside the sheath just in front of the orifice of the pulmonary vein. With the occluder held in place over the delivery system, careful retraction of the sheath deploys the distal umbrella under the roof of the left atrium. Under strict echocardiographic guidance, the occluder is pulled against the rims of the septal defect, the proximal umbrella is deployed and the correct position of the occluder is verified. During placement of the occluder, the echo view planes should show a longitudinal cross-section through the occluder and the sheath, which is the case whenever the distal wire holder and the proximal screw of the device are visible simultaneously. Due to the rigidity of the sheath and the delivery cable, relatively steep angulations (70°–90°) (Fig 20.2) are necessary. Now, with the device still on the delivery cable, a meticulous check of correct device position should be performed. This is best done in a short axis (0°–30°) scan from cranial to caudal and in a longitudinal scan (90°–120°) from left to right. Release from the delivery cable can be monitored in a longitudinal cross-sectional view across occluder and sheath. After release (Fig 20.3), correct position of the occluder should be double checked.

In selected cases of small children with small- to medium-sized defects, the procedure can be performed under transthoracic echocardiography as well. Furthermore, in cases in which balloon sizing seems not to be necessary, the procedure can be simplified by the primary introduction of the delivery sheath over the guide wire in the superior caval vein. Thereafter the occluder is loaded and advanced to the tip of the sheath pushing the device several millimeters out of the sheath forming a small, bulky "marker" at its end. The crossing of the defect from the right atrium and its placement into the defect can then be performed as described previously.

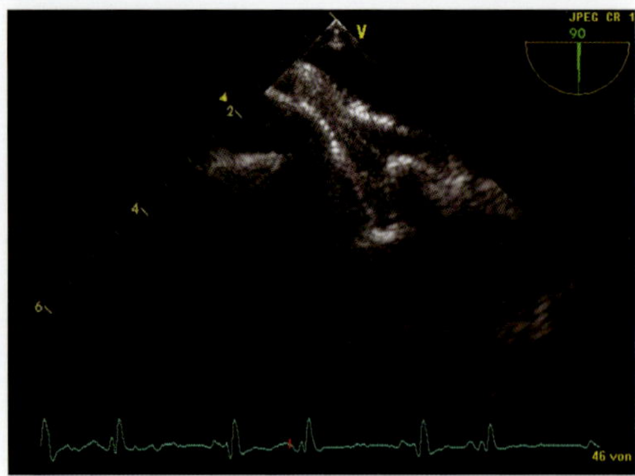

Fig 20.2—A transesophageal echocardiographic view in 90° allows visualization of the two discs of the device and the delivery cable.

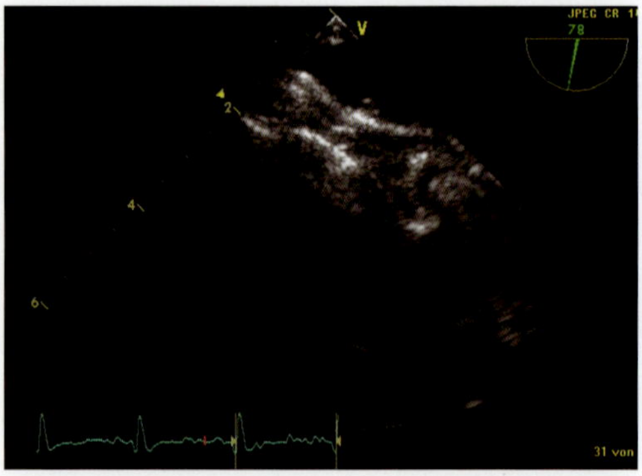

Fig 20.3—A transesophageal echocardiographic view in 78° verifies correct device position after it has been released from the cable.

Sedation

The procedure is best performed under deep conscious sedation with continuous propofol infusion. Individual tolerance of the echo probe, however, varies considerably and some adults may only need mild sedation (for example, midazolam) and a good pharyngeal anesthesia.

Results

Immediate results

From July 1998 to January 2010, successful transcatheter closures of intra-atrial communications with AMPLATZER devices were performed without fluoroscopy in 285 patients and with a Solysafe occluder in one (256 ASD and 30 PFO) (Table 20.1). One device was explanted electively, despite complete closure of the septal defect, because of a mismatch between occluder size and septum length, which had produced a serious complication in a similar case treated conventionally.

Complications

During the learning period in six additional cases, fluoroscopy was used because the opera-tor felt uncomfortable with the procedure, because of the implantation of a new device, or to verify the correct position of the occluders after successful intervention. However, there was no occasion in any of the procedures during which fluoroscopy was needed to overcome a critical or potential hazardous situation. In one patient atrial flutter occurred during the diagnostic catheterization. Sinus rhythm was established by cardioversion prior to release of the occluder.

Follow-up

Short-term follow-up was uneventful, and during a mean follow-up of 4.6 years (max. 12.3 years) no otherwise specific side effects occurred in comparison to the follow-up of conventionally treated patients with fluoroscopy.

Discussion

Transcatheter closure has become the standard technique for the treatment of ASDs. Due to increasing operator experience and the availability of easy-to-handle devices, x-ray exposure is minimized to several minutes or is not even necessary.[3,4]

The benefits of avoiding fluoroscopy to the

	Age (years)	Weight (kg)	ASO Size* (mm)	Follow-up (years)
Median	9.4	36	14	4.0
Mean	18.8	42.6	16	4.6
Minimum	0.5	8.3	6	0
Maximum	76.4	160	38	12.3

Table 20.1—Demographic Data of 286 Patients Treated with AMPLATZER and 1 Solysafe Occluders without Fluoroscopy. *ASO, AMPLATZER Septal Occluder; PFO excluded.

patient and the medical staff are obvious, as is the avoidance of iodine radiopaque contrast medium. Invasive diagnostic hemodynamic measurements such as pressure recordings and oximetric shunt estimation prior to a transcatheter closure of uncomplicated ASDs are unnecessary in the vast majority of patients. However, in order to completely avoid the use of fluoroscopy, not only must the technique of device placement itself be as safe as possible under echocardiographic guidance, but also the indispensable sizing of the defect—whether it is performed with or without balloon. If one considers the role of echocardiography in the conventional procedure, it must be acknowledged that it already plays the decisive role in many aspects. Thus, the step to abandon fluoroscopy completely is relatively small, however, it needs good communication and cooperation of echocardiographer and interventionalist which is probably ideal, if both are able to perform both, echocardiography and transcatheter defect closure. The median procedure time is comparable to the time needed for the conventional procedure and is mainly dependent on a good synchronization between echocardiographer and interventionalist. A high degree of discipline is necessary to move the catheter only if an adequate view plane is visible, then very accurate movements are possible.

For a successful intervention under echocardiographic guidance, the self-centering capabilities of the ASD devices and the rotation-symmetric shape of the AMPLATZER occluders without arms are fundamental. They have excellent occlusion rates, are easily retrievable, and have the decisive advantage to remain rotation-symmetric during the stepwise configuration. Therefore, the exact position can be reliably monitored by cross-sectional echocardiographic view planes. This is also true for the Solysafe device[6,7]; however, due to its very flat configuration in the septum it is more difficult to verify the correct occluder position. Its placement over a 0.018-inch guide wire and the advancement of the device without long sheath into the defect makes dislodgment of the guide wire more probable. As long as these difficulties are taken into account, successful implantations without fluoroscopy are possible.

With increasing experience, the successful intervention of complex defects such as atrial septal aneurysms or multiperforated defects with the need for two devices are possible accordingly.

Furthermore, the technique allows the transcatheter closure of intra-atrial communications in pregnant women[8] and, in general, outside the catheterization laboratory. This can be especially helpful in critically ill patients in the intensive care unit.

Conclusion

Transcatheter closure of ASD with AMPLATZER devices is possible in most patients under echocardiographic guidance alone and with similar results to the conventional procedure. Consequently, we perform the transcatheter closure without fluoroscopy routinely as the procedure of first choice at our institution.

References

1. Mills NL, King TD. Nonoperative closure of left-to-right shunts. *J Thorac Cardiovasc Surg.* Sep 1976;72(3):371–378.

2. Ewert P, Berger F, Daehnert I, Krings G, Dittrich S, Lange P. Diagnostic catheterization and balloon sizing of atrial septal defects by echocardiographic guidance without fluoroscopy. *Echocardiography.* 2000;17(2):159–163.

3. Ewert P, Berger F, Daehnert I, et al. Transcatheter closure of atrial septal defects without fluoroscopy—feasibility of a new method. *Circulation.* 2000;101(8):847–849.

4. Ewert P, Daehnert I, Berger F, et al. Transcatheter closure of atrial septal defects under echocardiographic guidance without X-ray: initial experiences. *Cardiol Young.* 1999;9(2):136–140.

5. Ewert P, Daehnert I, Berger F, Kaestner A, Lange PE. Closure of an atrial septal defect without surgery and without x-ray [German]. *Z Herz Thorax Gefässchirurgie.* 1998;12:221–225.

6. Ewert P, Soderberg B, Dahnert I, et al. ASD and PFO closure with the Solysafe septal occluder—results of a prospective multicenter pilot study. *Cathet Cardiovasc Interv.* 2008;71(3):398–402.

7. Kretschmar O, Sglimbea A, Daehnert I, Riede FT, Weiss M, Knirsch W. Interventional closure of atrial septal defects with the Solysafe Septal Occluder—Preliminary results in children. *Int J Cardiol.* 2009;13:13.

8. Daehnert I, Ewert P, Berger F, Lange PE. Echocardiographically guided closure of a patent foramen ovale during pregnancy after recurrent strokes. *J Interv Cardiol.* 2001;14(2):191–192.

21

New Minimally Invasive Techniques for Surgical Closure of ASDs and PFOs

Nikolay V. Vasilyev and Pedro J. del Nido

Introduction

Closure of atrial septal defects (ASD) was the world's first successful surgical open-heart procedure. The first experimental attempt of an ASD closure was performed in 1939 by Arthur Blakemore, and the first successful clinical operations were done in 1952 independently by Robert Edward Gross and F. John Lewis.[1]

For decades ASD closure has been one of the most common procedures with cardio-pulmonary bypass (CPB) performed by pediatric cardiac surgeons. More recently, since a transcatheter device technique was introduced in 1974 by King and Mills,[2] this less invasive approach gradually has become a routine procedure in most pediatric cardiology practices. However, at present transcatheter ASD closure has its limitations and occasional complications.

Poor patient selection based on inaccurate evaluation of the anatomy, presence of associated left ventricular dysfunction, inadequate device to defect ratio selection, and operator-related failures resulting from insufficient experience have been reported. These may result in late complications such as erosions of the atrial wall or the aortic root, thromboembolic episodes, and bacterial infection of these devices.[3,4] Rimless ASDs, sinus venosus type defects, and ostium primum defects are still the indication for open-heart surgical closure. More recently, a variety of minimally invasive surgical techniques for ASD closure through small incisions and later through ports with robotic assistance have been described.[5,6]

Transcatheter Closure of ASDs and PFOs: A Comprehensive Assessment. © 2010 Ziyad M. Hijazi, Ted Feldman, Mustafa H. Abdullah Al-Qbandi, and Horst Sievert, editors. Cardiotext Publishing, ISBN: 978-0-9790164-9-3.

Current Approaches for Open-Heart Closure

Most of the surgical procedures for isolated ASD closure are done via small incisions. The type of incision varies and depends on surgeon preference. In many centers a right anterolateral thoracotomy is used in adult female patients, but this approach is usually avoided in pre-pubescent females to avoid the risk of breast malformation. In small children and infants, a transxiphoid incision or ministernotomy approach provides excellent exposure for safe and complete repair of the ASD. Bichell et al. also advocated the routine creation of the peri-cardial window into the right pleural space to decrease the incidence of postoperative pericar-dial effusion and possible tamponade.[7] In adult male and elderly patients, a midline minister-notomy may also be used. Some centers advo-cate a parasternal approach with resection of one or more costochondral cartilages.[8,9] Such methods in adult patients have been proposed as resulting in less postoperative pain and improved recovery, compared to conventional sternotomy. The potential chest deformations that can occur from cartilage removal can be avoided by replacing the existing cartilage.[10]

Robotically Assisted Techniques

Telemanipulation robotic systems have been successfully used for surgical ASD closure. The advantages, as with mini-incision surgeries, include better cosmetic results, less postopera-tive pain, and shorter recovery time in com-parison with the conventional approach.[11–13] In addition, use of a robotic system may provide better ergonomic movements in the confined surgical field with 7-degrees of freedom instru-ment manipulation, high-definition stereo visu-alization optics, and tremor filtration. However, as with other robotically assisted open-heart procedures, the ischemic and CPB times are considerably longer in comparison with the conventional and mini-incision operations. In addition, robotic system set-up time is signifi-cantly longer and more cumbersome for pediat-ric patients, with the use of large diameter ports and the requirement of the peripheral vessel cannulation for CPB.

Image-Guided and Hybrid Surgical Open-Chest ASD Closure

Most of the minimally invasive surgical pro-cedures, including robotically assisted inter-ventions, have been performed on the open heart, thus requiring the use of CPB. There are widely recognized potential deleterious effects of CPB, resulting in blood coagulation abnormalities, renal and pulmonary dysfunc-tion, nonspecific inflammatory response, and neurological injury.[14] These potential compli-cations and advances in noninvasive imaging have prompted surgical investigators to explore novel techniques for ASD closure in the beat-ing heart. Given that the surgical closure does not depend on favorable anatomic features, if surgical closure can be accomplished through a smaller incision compared with conventional sternotomy, and without the use of CPB, it may become a superior alternate approach to open and transcatheter device closure for many defects.

Role of New Imaging Modalities

Reliable visualization inside the heart in the presence of blood is one of the keys for suc-cessful beating-heart surgical interventions. Fluoroscopy is still the most common imag-ing modality in most catheterization laborato-ries. The advantage of the fluoroscopy is that it provides high-resolution imaging at fast frame rates. However, it has significant limitations such as absence of three-dimensional (3D) information and lack of comprehensive representation of soft tissue. In addition, the potential harmfulness of ionizing radiation has been widely discussed.[15-17] In the past few years, the usefulness of 3D ultrasound has been demonstrated in experimental settings and in clinical practice.[18-20] The nonionizing nature of ultrasound, the ease of data acquisition, the ability to focus on a specific anatomic structure, as well as a variety of additional quantification tools have enabled virtually routine application of 3D echocardiography in the operating room and catheterization laboratory.[21] 3D echocardiography systems not only have excellent diagnostic capabilities for pre- and intraoperative assessment of intracardiac anatomy but can also serve as an imaging tool to guide instruments and devices inside the beating heart in real time. In addition to transesophageal 3D echocardiography imaging, surgeons can utilize epicardial imaging, especially in younger patients. Advances in computer graphics technology have allowed development of additional image processing tools for better comprehension of 3D visual information. For example, systems that enable stereoscopic vision display algorithms were introduced for beating-heart real-time 3D echocardiography-guided procedures (Fig 21.1). While operating inside the

beating heart, the surgeon may not always have an adequate display of intracardiac structures in 3D space and have to rely on indirect evidence for depth perception. Experimental studies have shown that use of stereoscopic displays provide significantly better spatial information and depth perception to the surgeon during beating-heart procedures, compared to conventional two-dimensional (2D) displays.[22]

One of the major disadvantages of the current 3D echocardiography systems, however, is low spatial resolution. Although it is adequate for anatomic definition and gross navigation of instruments, current 3D echocardiography systems still need to be optimized for visualization of small metal objects (staples, anchors, needles), which is especially important for safe surgical maneuvers inside the beating heart. One potential solution is to use optical imaging, such as video-assisted cardioscopy, as an adjunct to 3D echocardiography for high-resolution imaging. The authors have found that for safe navigation inside the beating heart during ASD closure, one can use combined imaging modalities.[23] 3D echocardiography gives surgeons superior large-volume spatial orientation and cardioscopy offers detailed, high-magnification imaging of the instrument tips and

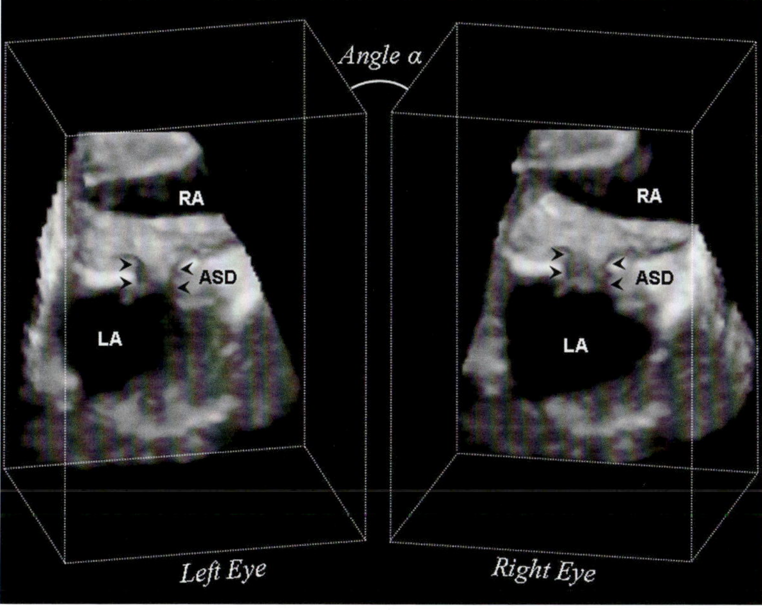

Fig 21.1—The 3D volumetric dataset of the atrial septal defect (arrowheads) is shown. Left- and right-eye views are separately generated by rendering the 3D ultrasound volume from two viewpoints skewed by angle α. By wearing the shutter-glasses the surgeon uses the real-time stereo-rendered 3D imaging for guiding a surgical procedure, as he/she controls the surgical instruments. (Reprinted from Vasilyev NV et al.[22] Copyright 2008, with permission from Elsevier.) Abbreviations: LA, left atrium; RA, right atrium.

devices, which provides surgeons with greater confidence for tissue manipulation and instrument navigation.

Novel Instruments and Devices

In conventional open-heart surgery, the techniques for ASD closure usually involve attachment and fixation of a patch to the edges of the defect using sutures. In beating-heart procedures, however, this approach is cumbersome and the need for multiple insertions of the surgical instrument into the cardiac chamber increases the risk of blood loss and introduction of air emboli. One solution is to develop alternative methods of patch placement and fixation to the tissue to perform ASD closure. This requires

use of a separate patch deployment device and a patch fixation system, which would allow the use of a single patch that can be tailored to the geometry of the defect, much the same way as in open-heart ASD closure.[22,23] This would avoid the use of a double-disc or double-umbrella device inside the atria, and also would leave a minimum amount of foreign material inside the left atrium. The authors have developed such a system, which includes the patch delivery device and the patch fixation device (Fig 21.2). The catheter-based patch delivery device consists of a self-expanding frame made of 0.25 mm × 0.75 mm Nitinol wire covered by a polyethylene tube (1.5 mm in diameter) and a grip. The polyester patch is attached to the frame by 0.1-mm Nitinol release wire. In this approach, the device is advanced through a 9F introducer sheath, and the frame with the patch is deployed through the end of the sheath and allowed to expand. The patch is then attached to the atrial septum by Nitinol-based mini-anchors deployed using a pistol-type fixation device. The mini-anchors are made of 0.31-mm Nitinol wire and have two parts, the distal arms and a proximal loop. Anchors are loaded into the fixation device, one at the time, and deployed in three steps. First, the arms of the anchor are deployed, pen-

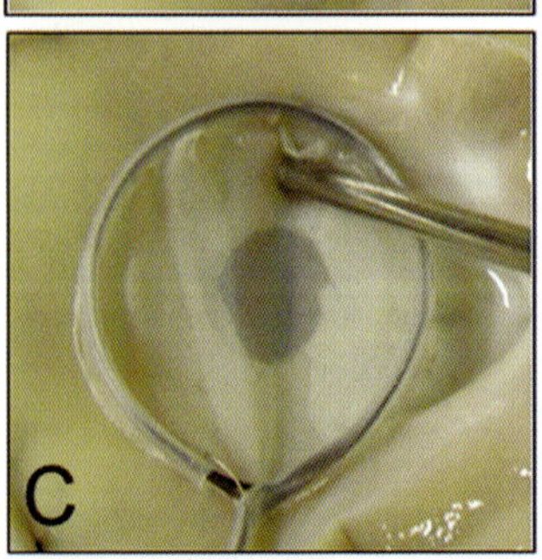
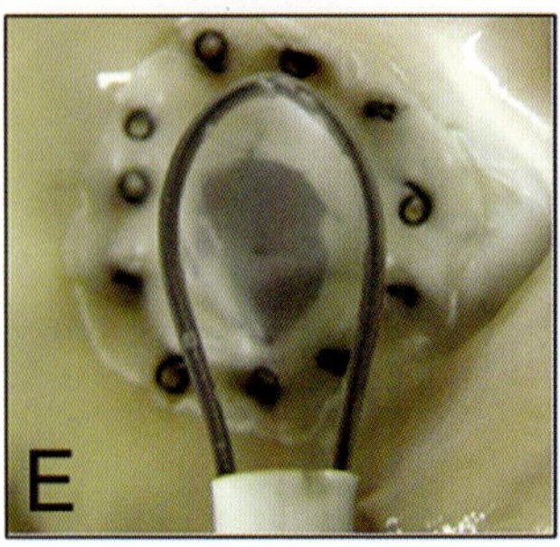
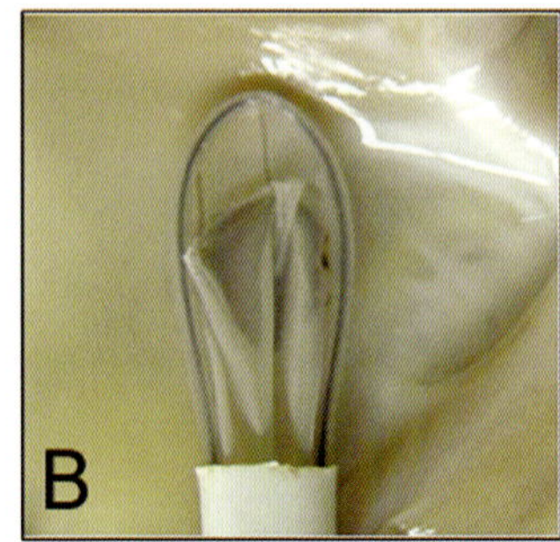
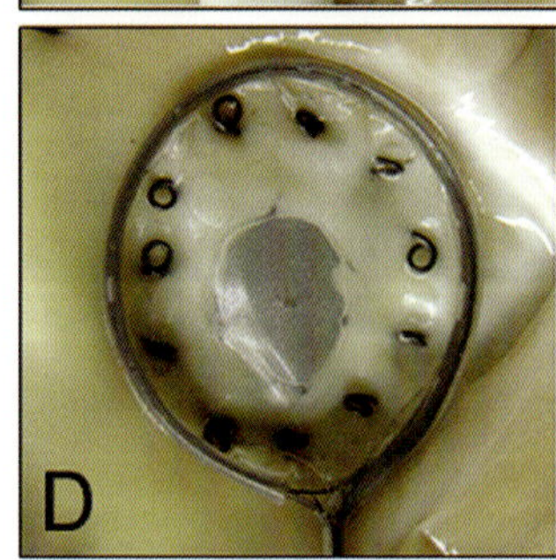
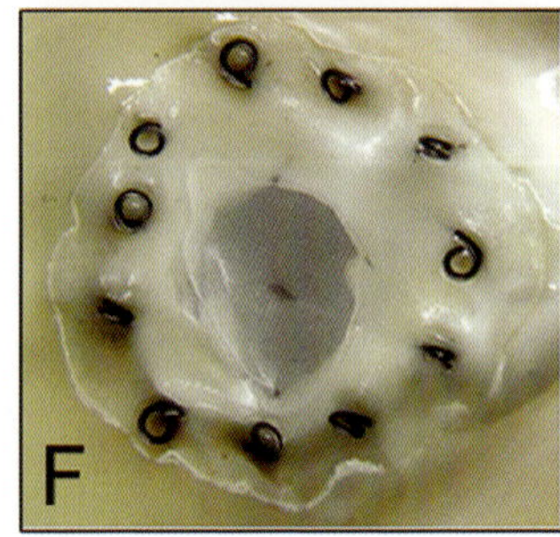

Fig 21.2—ASD patch closure system ex vivo. A and B: The patch delivery system is delivered through a 9F introducer, and the Nitinol frame expands. C and D: The polyester patch is attached to the atrial septum by Nitinol mini-anchors. E: The wire is removed, and the frame is withdrawn into the introducer. F: Final view. 2A Inset, Nitinol anchor with 2-mm loop and 10-mm arms. (Reprinted from Vasilyev NV et al.[23] Copyright 2006, with permission from Elsevier.)

etrating the patch material and the cardiac tissue with the arms expanding on the other side of the septum or within it. Before release, the operator confirms secure fixation by applying gentle tension to the anchor. Finally, the anchor is deployed completely, and the anchor loop is disconnected from the fixation device. After the patch is fixed to the septum, the release wire is removed allowing separation of the patch from the frame, and the frame is withdrawn into the sheath. This technique leaves only the polyester patch and Nitinol anchors inside the heart. During experimental animal procedures ASDs were successfully closed using such system.[22]

For image-guided interventions, novel instruments and devices have to be designed that differ from familiar surgical instruments. Because the operator uses an imaging modality such as ultrasound for guidance, the devices must be made of material that is compatible with that imaging modality. Traditional metallic surgical instruments are difficult to visualize with ultrasound imaging because sound waves bounce off metal objects creating imaging artifacts and shadows, which can confound the image of the target area. The most common artifacts seen both with 2D and 3D ultrasound are reverberations and side lobe artifacts.[24] In order to minimize these artifacts, investigators have suggested various materials to cover the metallic surface of instruments.[25] Alternatively, the surface of the metal can be roughened to minimize ultrasound reflection. In addition, the angle of incidence of the ultrasound beam with respect to the instrument is critical. The ultrasound probe position can be easily modified for epicardially guided procedures in order to visualize the atrial septum and the devices at the same time.[26,27]

Motion Compensation

Instruments that are used in image-guided surgical interventions have to be steerable in order to reach the target lesion inside the beating heart. Furthermore, in some cases, the operator is interacting with a highly mobile and very thin atrial septum. Therefore tool tip stabilization and motion compensation may be very helpful features. One option is to physically capture and stabilize the septum, and if possible, to immobilize or dampen its movements. Another alternative is to track the septal motion (image-based tracking) and mimic its motion using a robotically controlled instrument. To accomplish this, we have designed and built a one-degree-of-freedom active instrument that can easily overcome intracardiac tissue motion. The algorithm that operates this motion compensation instrument (MCI) is based on the real-time 3D echocardiography imaging. The system identifies and tracks the position of the tissue target directly in front of the instrument and a drive motor moves the instrument shaft according to the target motion. Validation animal experiments for such a system have been successfully carried out using more complex motion model of the mitral valve annulus.[28] In this study, anchors used for ASD closure were deployed into the mitral annulus using image-based motion compensation. The drawback of this image-based algorithm is that once the instruments come into contact with the annulus eliminating the gap between the tip of the instrument and the annulus, the algorithm can no longer separate tissue movement from the instrument tip and cannot control the instrument accurately. To overcome this problem a force-control tracking algorithm was developed using a force sensor on the tip of the surgical instrument.[29] It reads the force that the surgeon applies to the target tissue in real-time and actively maintains it. Further improvements are possible by using feed-forward force control to reduce vibration inherent in the system. With further development this automated motion compensation system may become a key part of other more complex image-guided intracardiac beating-heart procedures.

Another potentially beneficial feature of the instruments for intracardiac beating-heart repairs, including ASD and PFO closure, is multifunctionality. Most of the currently available devices and instruments for image-guided surgical and catheter-based interventions are designed as single-function tools and have to be continually exchanged during the procedure. Multifunctional tools may become extremely valuable for beating-heart repairs where frequent instrument exchange may lead to procedure complications such as blood loss, air embolism, and serious arrhythmias due to instrument collision with tissue. An additional feature to increase the functionality of the instrument is to incorporate an imaging modality. For example, a "cardioscope" that combines video-assisted optical cardioscopy and an instrument channel to access structures inside the beating heart may be a useful tool for beating-heart procedures. Such an instrument has been developed that incorporated both an imaging port as well as an instrument channel for safe introduction of surgical tools into the beating heart (Fig 21.3). In animal experiments, epicardial real-time 3D echocardiography was used for navigation and to image the multifunctional tool and cardiac target. The optical channel contained in the instrument was used to image the cardiac structure by pressing the

scope against the tissue, displacing the blood and permitting optical imaging of the heart surface. Beating-heart ASD patch closure without CPB was successfully achieved with combined 3D echocardiography for gross imaging and navigation and optical cardioscopy for imaging of small objects such as tissue anchors throughout the procedure.[23]

Summary

Currently, minimally invasive surgical ASD and PFO closure although performed through small incisions, still requires use of CPB. A significant number of patients are still referred for such procedures. This includes patients with rimless ASDs, primary defects, sinus venosus defects, and also patients with complex PFOs combined with other intracardiac pathology. In addition, rare but well-described complications after transcatheter device closure prompt some patients and families to choose surgery. Advancements in imaging technologies and instrument design have stimulated development of new surgical techniques that can be employed inside the beating heart. These techniques will allow surgeons not only to avoid open repair for ASDs but also develop new repairs for more complex lesions. This evolution may be seen as an intermediate step to a fully developed field of image-guided intracardiac beating-heart surgery.

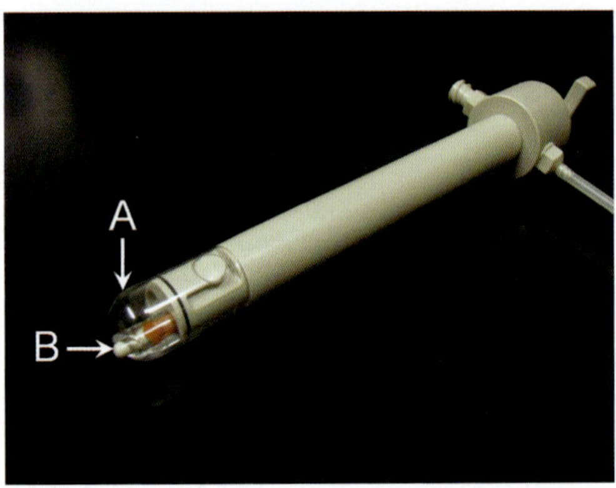

Fig 21.3— Multifunctional cardioport that combines safe instrument access inside the beating heart with cardioscopy imaging. Five-millimeter standard telescope is inserted into the optical channel (A). When the tip of the port is pressed against the tissue displacing the blood it permits optical imaging of the target inside the beating heart. The instrument is inserted into the instrument channel (B). Original valves and flush system enables safe introduction and exchange of the instruments, which prevents blood loss and air embolism throughout the procedure.

References

1. Alexi-Meskishvili VV, Konstantinov IE. Surgery for atrial septal defect: from the first experiments to clinical practice. *Ann Thorac Surg.* 2003;76(1):322–327.

2. Mills NL, King TD. Nonoperative closure of left-to-right shunts. *J Thorac Cardiovasc Surg.* 1976;72(3):371–378.

3. Knirsch W, et al. Challenges encountered during closure of atrial septal defects. *Pediatr Cardiol.* 2005;26(2):147–153.

4. DiBardino DJ, Dodge-Khatami, A, Valsangia-

como-Buechel E, et al. Analysis of the US Food and Drug Administration Manufacturer and User Facility Device Experience database for adverse events involving AMPLATZER septal occluder devices and comparison with the Society of Thoracic Surgery congenital cardiac surgery database. *J Thorac Cardiovasc Surg.* 2009;137(6):1334–1341.

5. Suematsu Y, del Nido PJ. Robotic pediatric cardiac surgery: present and future perspectives. *Am J Surg.* 2004;188(4A suppl):98S–103S.

6. Del Nido PJ, Bichell DP. Minimal-access surgery for congenital heart defects. *Semin Thorac Cardiovasc Surg Pediatr Card Surg Annu.* 1998;1:75–80.

7. Bichell DP, Geva R, Bacha E, et al. Minimal access approach for the repair of atrial septal defect: the initial 135 patients. *Ann Thorac Surg.* 2000;70(1):115–118.

8. Cosgrove DM 3rd, Sabik JF, Navia JL. Minimally invasive valve operations. *Ann Thorac Surg.* 1998;65(6):1535–1538, discussion 1538–1539.

9. Cohn LH, Adams DH, Couper GS, et al. Minimally invasive cardiac valve surgery improves patient satisfaction while reducing costs of cardiac valve replacement and repair. *Ann Surg.* 1997;226(4):421–426, discussion 427–428.

10. Lazzara RR, Kidwell FE. Right parasternal incision: a uniform minimally invasive approach for valve operations. *Ann Thorac Surg.* 1998;65(1):271–272.

11. Argenziano M, Oz MC, DeRose JJ, et al. Totally endoscopic atrial septal defect repair with robotic assistance. *Circulation.* 2003;108 (suppl 1, pt II):191–194.

12. Bacha EA, Bolotin G, Consilio K, et al. Robotically assisted repair of sinus venosus defect. *J Thorac Cardiovasc Surg.* 2005;129(2):442–443.

13. Wimmer-Greinecker G, Dogan S, Aybek T, et al. Totally endoscopic atrial septal repair in adults with computer-enhanced telemanipulation. *J Thorac Cardiovasc Surg.* 2003;126(2):465–468.

14. Menache CC, du Plessis AJ, Wessel DL, et al. Current incidence of acute neurologic complications after open-heart operations in children. *Ann Thorac Surg.* 2002;73(6):1752–1758.

15. Venneri L, Rossi F, Botto N, et al. Cancer risk from professional exposure in staff working in cardiac catheterization laboratory: insights from the National Research Council's Biological Effects of Ionizing Radiation VII Report. *Am Heart J.* 2009;157(1):118–124.

16. Clay MA, Campbell RM, Strieper M, et al. Long-term risk of fatal malignancy following pediatric radiofrequency ablation. *Am J Cardiol.* 2008;102(7): 913–915.

17. Kim KP, Miller DL, Balter S, et al. Occupational radiation doses to operators performing cardiac catheterization procedures. *Health Phys.* 2008;94(3): 211–227.

18. Suematsu Y, Martinez JF, Wolf BK, et al. Three-dimensional echo-guided beating heart surgery without cardiopulmonary bypass: atrial septal defect closure in a swine model. *J Thorac Cardiovasc Surg.* 2005;130(5): 1348–1357.

19. Marx GR, Sherwood MC, Fleishman C, et al. Three-dimensional echocardiography of the atrial septum. *Echocardiography.* 2001;18(5): 433–443.

20. Lodato JA, Cao QL, Weinert L, et al. Feasibility of real-time three-dimensional transoesophageal echocardiography for guidance of percutaneous atrial septal defect closure. *Eur J Echocardiogr.* 2009;10(4):543–548.

21. Salgo IS. 3D echocardiographic visualization for intracardiac beating heart surgery and intervention. *Semin Thorac Cardiovasc Surg.* 2007;19(4):325–329.

22. Vasilyev NV, Novotny PM, Martinez JF, et al. Stereoscopic vision display technology in real-time three-dimensional echocardiography-guided intracardiac beating-heart surgery. *J Thorac Cardiovasc Surg.* 2008;135(6):1334–1341.

23. Vasilyev NV, Martinez FJ, Freudenthal FP, et al. Three-dimensional echo and videocardioscopy-guided atrial septal defect closure. *Ann Thorac Surg.* 2006;82(4):1322–1326, discussion 1326.

24. Gottlieb RH, Robinette WB, Rubens DJ, et al. Coating agent permits improved visualization of biopsy needles during sonography. *AJR Am J Roentgenol.* 1998;171(5):1301–1302.

25. Huang J, Triedman JK, Vasilyev NK, et al. Imaging artifacts of medical instruments in ultrasound-guided interventions. *J Ultrasound Med.* 2007;26(10):1303–1322.

26. Suematsu Y, Marx GR, Stoll JA, et al. Three-

dimensional echocardiography-guided beating-heart surgery without cardiopulmonary bypass: a feasibility study. *J Thorac Cardiovasc Surg.* 2004;128(4):579–587.

27. Cannon JW, Stoll JA, Salgo IS, et al. Real-time three-dimensional ultrasound for guiding surgical tasks. *Comput Aided Surg.* 2003;8(2):82–90.

28. Yuen SG, Kesberm SB, Vasilyev NV, et al. 3D ultrasound-guided motion compensation system for beating heart mitral valve repair. *Med Image Comput Comput Assist Interv.* 2008;11(pt 1):711–719.

29. Yuen SG, Yip MC, Vasilyev NV, et al. Robotic force stabilization for beating heart intracardiac surgery. *Med Image Comput Comput Assist Interv.* 2009. In Press.

22

Complications of Device Closure of ASDs and PFOs

Zahid Amin

Introduction

Secundum atrial septal defect (ASD) and patent foramen ovale (PFO) are routinely closed in the cardiac catheterization laboratories. After the approval of AMPLATZER ASD occluder in 2001, the use of devices to close ASD increased significantly. Other devices were introduced and are under investigational protocol. For PFO, there is no device approved currently although several trials are underway and with positive results, device(s) may receive FDA approval over the next 1 to 2 years.

The technical procedure of device closure for ASD or PFO is similar, closure may lead to complications that range from minor or inconsequential to major or life threatening. The complication rate is dependent upon the experience of the operator, the type of device used, and the size of defect being closed.

This chapter will discuss all complications that have been reported in the literature, the risk of complications associated with device closure, and recommend strategies to minimize complications. The AMPLATZER (AGA Medical Corporation, Plymouth, Minnesota) devices have been used the most over the last 10 years and a significant amount of data is now available in literature for evaluation. Therefore, we will focus on AMPLATZER Septal and PFO Occluder Devices. Detailed discussion of complications encountered with the HELEX device (W.L. Gore, Flagstaff, Arizona) and CardioSEAL device (NMT Medical, Massachusetts) can be found in the following two chapters of the book.

The Devices

The following is a brief description of the available devices and is to make the reader understand the etiology of the complications that will be described in this chapter. The reader is advised to refer to part IV for more information on these devices.

Patent Foramen Ovale

A typical device that would suit the anatomy of the PFO would be a non–self-centering device with capacity to seal the septum primum and secundum and accommodate the tunnel, if present. Because of the flaplike opening, there is propensity of the right atrial disc to extrude toward the left atrial side if the limbus (septum secundum) is not sandwiched by the right atrial disc. The AMPLATZER PFO device was constructed keeping this factor in mind. The right atrial disc of two of three available sizes (25 and 35 mm) is larger than the left disc. It tends to accommodate long tunnel PFOs. For very long tunnel PFOs, there are other devices that were made to suit the length of the tunnel (such as the Premere device and Coherex FlatStent).

ASD

Two devices are currently approved for ASD closure. The AMPLATZER ASD device and the GORE HELEX Septal Occluder device. Other devices are being used but have yet to receive approval from the Food and Drug Administration (FDA). All available devices for ASD have two basic designs: self-centering (AMPLATZER) and non–self-centering (HELEX). The self-centering design of the AMPLATZER device makes it suitable for larger defects as the typical disc to defect ratio does not have to be 2:1. A defect as large as 40 mm (with adequate rims) can be closed with the AMPLATZER ASD occluder (ASO). The HELEX is a non–self-centering device and hence the largest recommended defect size to close is 18 mm (largest available device is 35 mm).

The ASD can range from a few to > 40 mm and the defects can be eccentric resulting in smaller rims than recommended by the manufacturer. Other than these minor issues, the ASDs have simpler anatomy when compared to PFOs.

As explained earlier, descriptions of other devices that are not approved are beyond the scope of this chapter. However, complications that have been published with other available devices will be mentioned.

Complications

General anesthesia

The majority of the centers perform the procedure under general anesthesia. Some centers use conscious sedation. There are potential complications related to both modalities; however, these will not be discussed further in this chapter.

Minor complications

All devices are placed during a cardiac catheterization procedure and therefore, are subject to all reported complications encountered during cardiac catheterization. These can range from minor discomfort at the catheterization site to hematoma formation, catheter-related arrhythmias, inconsequential air embolism, etc. The minor complications usually tend to resolve completely with or without any specific treatment. These complications will not be discussed further in this chapter.

Major complications

Here major complications will be defined as described by Chessa et al.[1] A complication is classified as major when (1) patient experiences a life-threatening event related to the procedure or device; (2) death occurs; (3) need arises for surgical intervention; or (4) a significant permanent anatomic or functional lesion results from catheterization procedure.

AMPLATZER Atrial Septal Occluder Device

Since its approval, the ASO device has been the most widely used device in the world. Naturally, significant numbers of publications have addressed the outcome of the device after placement. The frequent amount of publications citing results and outcome sometimes may be mistaken for higher number of complications. The risk of complications, despite significant use of ASO, remains low.[2]

Device embolization

There are various causes of device embolization.

- Large and eccentric defect
- Defect with inadequate rims
- Adequate rims without enough oomph to hold the device
- Improper sizing of the defect
- Improper placement of the device
- Absent or inadequate inferior vena caval (IVC) rim

The IVC rim, by far, is the most common cause of device embolization. The IVC is the biggest systemic vein that drains into the right atrium. The atrial septal rim, even when adequate in size, is usually paper-thin in this region. When deficient, a significant part of the atrial septal rim that corresponds to the size of the IVC is absent. When a device is placed, it appears stable as it is wedged nicely between the aortic and the posterior rims. Echocardiographically, evaluation of the IVC septal rim is usually difficult before placing the device; after device placement, it becomes even more difficult due to the difficulty in determining whether the two discs have sandwiched the thin septum.

Embolization is the most common complications reported in the literature,[1] and to the AGA Medical Corporation (personal communications) and FDA.[3] The risk has ranged from 0.5% to as high as 3%.[4] In the majority of patients, the devices can be retrieved per-

cutaneously. In some patients, surgery may be needed to retrieve the device. The defect can be closed in the same setting. The retrieval of the device is dependent upon the experience of the interventionalist primarily and location of the device secondarily.

If the device is stuck in the left ventricle or the right ventricle and entangled within the atrioventricular (AV) valve apparatus, it is strongly recommended to refer the patient for surgical retrieval of the device. Every interventionalist should be aware of his/her limitations. There are case reports of valvular injury resulting from multiple and aggressive attempts to retrieve embolized devices.[5] The most common site of embolization appears to be the left atrium, followed by right ventricle and pulmonary artery.[3] Overall, more devices embolize to the left side than the right side and commensurate with the smaller right atrial disc size. Device embolization toward the left side also suggests that the devices placed are either undersized or improperly placed.

Device embolization usually occurs during the procedure or within the first 24 hours. There are reports in the literature in which late embolization was described.[6,7] In the first report, the patient was discharged the day of the procedure without documenting whether the device was in place. In the second case report, there was documentation that the devices were stable at 18 months and embolized subsequently.

The ASO device does not hinder blood flow through the heart after embolization. Its light weight helps in making the discs parallel to the circulation and the cardiac output is maintained. Rarely there have been cases where blood flow was compromised requiring semi-urgent surgery.[8] Usually device embolization is followed by atrial or ventricular premature beats. If the device migrates further to the aorta or the pulmonary artery, the arrhythmia tends to subside.

Thrombus formation

Thrombus formation on the ASO has been described in the literature. Postprocedure, these patients are started on antiplatelet therapy (aspirin alone or aspirin with clopidogrel). The antiplatelet therapy is usually adequate for majority of patients.

If a patient suffers from systemic embolic phenomenon, thrombus formation should be one of the differential diagnoses and ruled out. A transthoracic echocardiogram may suffice in pediatric population but in adolescents and adults, transesophageal echocardiogram (TEE) is highly recommended. The management of thrombus on the device is controversial. Some physicians choose to send the patient to surgery for device removal. Some physicians start aggressive anticoagulation therapy. In general, the patient is admitted and started on intravenous heparin with serial echocardiograms. We also recommend coagulation profile in these patients to ascertain whether they are candidates for anticoagulation therapy in addition to antiplatelet therapy.

In a randomized study[9] of PFO devices, the highest risk of thrombus formation was found to be on the CardioSEAL device. In another study[10] that compared ASO, ASDOS, STARFlex, and HELEX devices, the risk of thrombus formation was the lowest on the ASO device (0.2%), followed by HELEX device (0.8%). The highest risk of thrombus formation was on the CardioSEAL device. There was no difference in thrombus formation between PFO and ASD devices. Overall risk of thrombus formation was about 1%. All thrombi were discovered at 6-month follow-up. In most cases, thrombi resolved with medical therapy (19/22), only three required surgical intervention. In another study by Krumsdorf et al[11] the incidence of thrombus on ASO device was 0%, 0.8% on HELEX device, and 7.1% on CardioSEAL device. All of these studies suggest that the risk of thrombus formation is lowest on the ASO when compared to other currently available devices.

In my own practice, I tend to continue ASA beyond 6 months in patients who required a large device for the patients' atrial septum (or if the device profile appears bulky). We consider a device large when it covers > 75% of the septum.

Arrhythmias

New-onset arrhythmias are one of the most important complications of device placement. This complication tends to be more common in adult patients as reported by Majunke et al.[12] The most common complication immediately after the procedure and during the follow-up period was new-onset atrial fibrillation (4.3%).

In the pediatric population, arrhythmias seem to be less common than adult patients. Nonetheless, arrhythmias are the second most common complication seen after ASD closure.[1] Long-term data to objectively evaluate arrhythmias is sparse at the current time. Of concern are the recent findings of progression of benign first-degree AV block to malignant arrhythmias after decades of follow-up.[13] The risk of arrhythmias after device placement may be related to marked foreign body reaction and thrombus formation may be one of the several mechanisms.[14] Anecdotally, almost every one of us has seen transient first-degree AV block after device placement. This is not limited to AMPLATZER devices though. What happens to these patients in the next 20 to 30 years remains to be seen.

Rarely, complete heart block has been reported.[15] In the majority of cases, the complication resolves after the device is removed. It is strongly recommended to electively remove the device even if intermittent complete heart block is seen. Steroids do not seem to help as the complete heart block is secondary to mechanical compression of the disc. Large device to defect ratio and in general large devices seem to increase the risk of arrhythmias. Anatomically, AV valve rim and IVC rim deficiency is common in these patients because the device has to be significantly oversized so that it will accommodate the defect.

In the AGA Medical postmarket surveillance data, a total of 698 cases have been enrolled (personal communication, Ken Lock, AGA Medical), of these 164 patients have had 5-year follow-up completed. Four patients have exhibited changes in rhythm, two had atrial flutter, one had change in P-wave axis, and one patient has unspecified arrhythmia. Overall the risk of late arrhythmias has remained low but long-term documentation is crucial.

Device-related hemodynamic compromise/ device-related cardiac injury

Injury to the atrial free wall and/or aorta has been described before ASO was introduced in the market. One of the first reports was published in 1997 where injury to the atrial wall was described by ASDOS device (not currently available in the market).[16] Subsequent to that, atrial wall injury was reported with the Angel Wing device (Microvena Corporation, Minnesota) during FDA-approved trials.

The device-related injury was most explored to investigate the cause after it occurred with the ASO device. During the FDA-approved trials in the United States, there were no cases of documented erosions seen. After premarket approval of the device, the incidence increased sharply in 2002 through 2004. A panel of physicians was convened by AGA Medical to evaluate all cases in which there was suspicion of atrial wall injury. Guidelines were established and published.[17] After the publication, the incidence decreased sharply (personal communication, AGA Medical).

There are definite device-related factors that contribute to erosion. Although erosion has been described with non–self-centering devices, I believe that self-centering device design may increase the risk of erosion. With a self-centering device, the wiggle room for the device is limited and the edges of device have constant impact on the atrial tissue if the rims are deficient or the device is oversized. When an oversized device is placed in ASD, the waist of the device tries to acquire its inherent diameter over time; the size of the discs expands as the waist expands. Sometimes a very small increase in diameter may cause the edge of the device to perforate the atrial free wall. At the same time, the size of the right atrium starts remodeling and hence decreases in size. Although the right atrial disc is smaller than the left, a significant decrease in the size of the right atrium may compromise the right atrial

disc space and cause injury to the atrial free wall.

A typical device-related atrial injury occurs at the roof of the left or the right atria, in the area separated from the aorta by the transverse sinus.[17] If the device edge protrudes into the aorta, tear in the posterior wall of the aorta may occur resulting in pericardial tamponade.

Sometimes, within 24 hours of the large ASD closure, small separation is seen between the right atrium/right ventricle and the pericardium. This separation is not due to small effusion but because of a decrease in size of the right-sided chambers resulting from acute obliteration of left-to-right atrial shunt.

Development of pericardial effusion after device closure needs to be observed closely. If the patient's ASD was a high-risk type, consideration should be given to tap the fluid. A bloody effusion is almost always diagnostic of device erosion barring catheter-related injury to the atrial appendages. Effusion in the latter tends to accumulate within the first few hours of device closure. The majority of device-related atrial perforations occur within 96 hours of the procedure.[17]

A high-risk ASD typically is a defect that is in the superior part of the atrial septum in superoinferior axis and has close proximity to the aorta with aortic rim that is either absent or negligible in size. In anterior-posterior axis (anterior wall of the chest to spine), the defect appears small but in superior-inferior axis it is large and hence an oval defect. The posterior rim,[18] which is the area between SVC and IVC rims, is either small or has thin, flailing rim. Balloon sizing of these defects is difficult as the stop-flow diameter is not achieved because of the oval shape of the defect. The device size is larger for the defect in anterior-posterior dimensions but adequate in superior-inferior dimension (oval defect). The device, therefore, is wedged in anterior-posterior dimensions.

A very small number of patients develop atrial injury where the device does not appear to be oversized. The exact mechanism of erosion in such patients remains unknown. In these patients, the edge of the atrial discs tend to wedge between the aorta and the posterior rims, with atrial systole, the disc protrudes into the atrial free wall resulting in tear.

Another rare phenomenon seen after device placement is the development of aorta-atrial fistula. This has been described with the ASO and other devices (the aorto-atrial fistula can be to either atria and has occurred with other devices as well).[19,20]

The mechanism of fistula remains the same as previously described. The location of atrial wall injury is slightly lower—not the roof of the atria but the anterior wall. This is the area where the atrial wall is adherent to the aorta. When viewed from outside, it is the area below the transverse sinus. A compromise in the integrity of the atrial wall is commensurate with compromise in the integrity of the aortic wall as well. There is no pericardial effusion because the atrial roof remains intact. The fistula tends to develop a few weeks after the procedure and generally is seen at 3- or 6-month follow-up.

Management of erosion or fistula is surgical. It is recommended that if the edge of the device is seen to compromise the atrial tissue in the operating room, the device should be removed. The device should be removed in all patients who have developed aorto-atrial fistula and the aortic wall repaired accordingly.

A careful echocardiographic evaluation of the defect, the consistency of the atrial septal rims, appropriate balloon sizing while keeping the atrial tissue redundancy and consistency in mind, avoiding device oversizing, keeping a watchful eye on the device angulation in relation to the atrial septum, and watching for change in the device size with atrial systole should decrease the risk of erosion to near 0%.

Regarding the splaying of the device discs on the aorta, there are many opinions with general consensus that splaying is better than the edge of the device pushing on the aorta.[21] In general, the discs have to splay on the aorta when aortic rim is absent. The question arises, how much splay is safe to prevent device embolization and how much splaying will result into atrial tissue injury? A gentle splay on the aorta with the edge of the device facing outward is

acceptable. If, the device edge pokes into the aorta and in atrial systole the phenomenon appears to be exaggerated, the device should be removed. In addition, if the waist touches the aorta, it is highly recommended to remove the device and exchange with a smaller device. The ASO has a significant margin of safety. When the waist touches the aorta, it means that the edges of device are 5 to 7 mm wrapped on the aorta and hence pushing on the free atrial wall. Over time, this may cause atrial wall injury.

Atrioventricular valve encroachment

In patients whose AV valve rim is not adequate, placement of a self-centering device may encroach upon the AV valves. Because the left disc is larger, the mitral valve is offset (higher than the tricuspid valve), the risk of mitral valve encroachment is higher than the tricuspid valve. As long as the left atrial disc does not touch the mitral valve, the risk of valve injury is low. There are rare reports of mitral valve injury causing significant mitral regurgitation.[22,23]

A small AV valve rim that is < 5 mm is usually not considered an absolute contraindication to device closure. It should alert the physician to evaluate the relationship of the left disc to the mitral valve. Prior to ASO release, the device is under tension because of the cable stiffness and hence the separation between the edge of the left disc to the anterior mitral valve leaflet appears more than it usually is after the release of the device. Once the device is released, the discs align the septum and the disc that initially appeared away from the hinge point of the mitral valve may sit on it. This factor should be kept in mind while closing the defect especially when the AV valve rims are small or of thin consistency.

Aortic valve distortion

Anatomically, the aortic valve and root are wedged between the left and right atrium. When a device is placed in the ASD in patients with absent aortic rim, the two discs must astride the aortic root. Because Nitinol is a shape memory alloy, the natural tendency of the two discs to approximate is inherent and hence distortion of the aortic root is conceivable. Regardless, after the publication of an article[24] in which primarily PFOs were closed in a patient population with significantly high preprocedure aortic valve insufficiency, the incidence of aortic valve insufficiency increased even further. Another study completely refuted those findings.[25] Nevertheless, the jury is still out.[26] We need to keep this potential complication in mind when choosing devices, as the risk of aortic root distortion is higher with large devices or devices that will overlap more of the aortic root than smaller devices that may just touch the aortic root.

Bacterial endocarditis

The risk of bacterial endocarditis is extremely low after ASO placement. Rarely, patients tend to develop bacterial endocarditis despite adequate prophylaxis. Although the cause remains unknown, it is conceivable that it is somehow related to incomplete endothelialization.[27]

Antibiotic prophylaxis is provided during the procedure and per protocol 6 months after the procedure for contaminated surgery. In patients with large and bulky devices, the author's policy has been to provide antibiotic prophylaxis for up to 1 year. In addition, continued antiplatelet therapy for 1 year is recommended in such patients. The author also recommends to postponing routine procedures (dental cleaning) for 6 months.

Cobra head malformation

This is a very rare complication of the ASO. It occurs when the device is being deployed inside the heart. As the left disc is extruded from the delivery sheath, it assumes the shape of cobra head. The general recommendations when this happens are to recapture the device, remove it from the delivery sheath, expand it outside the body to see if the phenomenon duplicates. If no cobra head deformity is seen, the same device can be advanced and redeployed. If the cobra head malformation persists outside the body, the device should be discarded.

The typical case in which this malformation occurs is in a patient whose procedure is complex, the size of the left atrium is small, and significant torque is applied to the delivery sheath during device deployment for proper positioning. Some devices appear to be manufactured improperly and should be returned to AGA Medical for further evaluation.

Patent Foramen Ovale

Anatomy of the PFO from the interventionalist's perspective

The author believes that PFO stands for "**p**otential **f**or **o**pening" in addition to patent foramen ovale. In the majority of the population, it is a communication that has closed completely or remains closed with the potential to open in altered physiological conditions. The communication is a flap-type opening where the septum primum (the thin septum, the frail septum, the fluttering septum, the aneurysmal septum) keeps it closed until and unless the pressure on the right atrial side increases transiently (as in straining, coughing, sneezing). If the coaptation of the septum primum to septum secundum (the thick septum, the limbus, the SVC rim, the superior rim, the aortic rim) is lost because of atrial enlargement, the communication becomes a true opening.

Although the communication is a flap-type opening, its shape is dependent upon the length of coaptation between the edge of the septum primum and secundum. Generally, the opening is small behind the ascending aorta. The opening may increase in dimension (anterior-posterior dimension) and become lacunar-type if the septum primum remains separated from the secundum. The opening will extend posteriorly toward the SVC. Hence, PFOs can come in many different sizes although they appear small if examined in one dimension only. These findings prompted physicians (including the author) to always balloon size PFO before placing a device.

The degree of overlap between the septum primum and secundum determines whether the PFO is a simple or tunnel-type. If the primum septum overlaps significantly, the PFO opening is called a tunnel-type opening and the direction of the tunnel is inferosuperior. Presence of tunnel in a PFO adds another twist, increases the complexity of the PFO, and has generated more debate than expected.

Another important consideration while evaluating PFOs is the consistency of the primum septum. If it is thin, frail, and its excursion is 15 mm or more (in some literature 10 mm or more), it is termed as aneurysmal PFO. The aneurysmal nature of the tunnel adds to PFO complexity as closure of tunnel-type PFO is difficult, and no particular device appears to be just right.

Complications of PFO Closure

Residual shunts

Because the anatomical location of the defect is somewhat similar to the ASD, the device-related complications are similar to complications related to the ASD. Some of the complications are inherent to the device itself and remains the same as described earlier, under complications of ASD closure.

Of importance are the complications related to the primary reason the patient was referred for device procedure. This is the potential for any type of shunt (right to left or vice versa) postprocedure and particularly 6 months after the procedure. These patients undergo the procedure for presumed paradoxical embolism and not for hemodynamic compromise. In an ASD patient who had significant left-to-right shunt before device procedure and had small residual shunt after device placement, the primary objective of improving the hemodynamic compromise has been achieved as opposed to a patient with PFO. The PFO patients usually

have a small shunt to begin with and if the very small shunt persists, the procedure should not be labeled as a clinical success. In a report by Taafe et al,[9] this problem persisted in all three devices that were evaluated 30 days after the procedure. The AMPLATZER device, however, had the highest closure rate when compared to HELEX or CardioSEAL group (p=0.0005 between AMPLATZER and HELEX group and p=0.0003 between HELEX and CardioSEAL group). In another study, the residual shunt rate of 34% was seen with CardioSEAL devices at 6-month follow-up.[28] Only 8% residual defect rate was seen at 6 months with the AMPLATZER PFO Occluder Device.[29]

It is the anatomical location and significant variations in the size and shape of the PFO that shunt can persist despite placement of devices that occupy the defects and cover it on both sides with discs. These subtleties have lead to increase in research for an ideal PFO device and, in the end we may discover that we need two or more types/shapes of devices that can occlude all types of PFOs.[30]

Thrombus formation

The risk of thrombus formation on these devices is similar to ASD devices. The majority of the devices used for PFO closure were originally made for ASD closure (HELEX, CardioSEAL, and ASO). Although AGA Medical has introduced a device that was designed specifically for PFO closure, the off-label use of ASD devices is rampant as the PFO device cannot be used except under FDA-approved protocol in the United States. The risk of thrombus formation on a device appears to be the highest on the CardioSEAL.[9,11]

In a review of the literature by Sherman et al[31] there were 54 cases of device thrombosis published in the literature with 9 patients who suffered from transient ischemic attack (TIA) or stroke. The mean time to diagnosis was 5 months and the majority of the thrombi were left sided.

It is strongly recommended to perform a transesophageal echocardiography (TEE) to rule out thrombus formation on the devices. The transthoracic echocardiogram may be helpful but the yield is low. In addition, the protocol for anticoagulation therapy may need to be revisited. These patients may need lifelong antiplatelet therapy or for a longer time period than 6 months. A battery of tests to rule out inherent clotting disorders is also recommended prior to device closure. These will help in sorting out patients who may be candidates for antiplatelet and/or anticoagulation therapy.

Risk of erosion or cardiac trauma

The risk of erosion with PFO devices remains low[32] but there are case reports scattered in the literature.[33] The data published from the AMPLATZER registry review[32] indicated that the risk of device-related injury was 0.018%. Cardiac catheterization-related complication (perforation of the atrial appendage) was the most common reason for cardiac trauma.

There are some rare reports of pericardial tamponade with HELEX occluder[9] requiring pericardiocentesis (according to the authors, however, it was believed to be related to a complex PFO that required multiple attempts and may not have been device related), Cardia Star[34] and CardioSEAL devices. Wire fracture resulting in mitral valve perforation has been seen with HELEX device.[35]

Conceivably, the risk of erosion or cardiac trauma with a non–self-centering device is lower when compared to a self-centering device in PFO patients. A non–self-centering device will have "wiggle room" after placement and hence can be pushed away from vital structures of the heart.

Summary

Closure of ASD and PFO using an array of devices is being performed with low risk of complications. The complications of cardiac catheterization procedure are rare. The risk of complications resulting from different devices itself is device-specific and can be lowered with mild modifications and improvements. New devices are being developed to prevent complications related to technical issues. The data on long-term complication risk will require continued follow-up especially in children. The follow-up of up to 5 years, is inadequate because children will grow up and have these devices for decades.

References

1   Chessa M, Carminati M, Butera G, et al. Early and late complications associated with transcatheter occlusion of secundum atrial septal defect. *J Am Coll Cardiol.* 2002;39:1061–1065.

2.   Masura J, Gavora P, Podnar T. Long-term outcome of transcatheter secundum atrial septal defect closure using AMPLATZER septal occluder. *J Am Coll Cardiol.* 2005;45:505–507.

3.   Dibardino DJ, McElhinney DB, Kaza AK, Mayer JE. Analysis of the IS food and drug administration manufacturer and user facility device experience database for adverse events involving AMPLATZER septal occluder devices and comparison with the society of thoracic congenital cardiac surgery database. *J Thorac Cardiovasc S.* 2009;137:1334–1341.

4.   Levi D, Moore JW. Embolization and retrieval of the AMPLATZER septal occluder. *Cathet Cardiovasc Intervent.* 2004;61:543–547.

5.   Kocyildirim E, Kanani M, Bonhoeffer P, Elliott MJ. AMPLATZER device embolization: hazards of multiple attempts at catheter retrieval. *Anadolu Kardiyol Derg.* 2007;7:329–330.

6.   Mashman WE, King SB, Jacobs C, Ballard WL. Two cases of device embolization of AMPLATZER septal occluder devices to the pulmonary artery following closure of secundum atrial septal defect. *Cathet Cardiovasc Intervent.* 2005;65:588–592.

7.   Teoh K, Wilton E, Brecker S, Jahangiri M. Simultaneous removal of an AMPLATZER device from an atrial septal defect and the descending aorta. *J Thorac Cardiovasc Surg.* 2006;131:909–910.

8.   Knott-Craig CJ, Goldberg SP. Emergent surgical retrieval of embolized atrial septal defect closure

device. *Ann Thorac Surg.* 2008;85319–85321.

9. Taafe M, Fischer E, Baronowski A, et al. Comparison of three patent foramen ovale closure devices in a randomized trial (AMPLATZER versus CardioSEAL versus HELEX Occluder). *Am J Cardiol.* 2008;101:1353–1358.

10. Baranowski A, Skowasch M, Hofmann I, et al. Thrombus formation of ASD and PFO devices: frequency and clinical importance. *Circulation.* 2006;114:785.

11. Krumsdorf U, Ostermeyer S, Billinger K, et al. Incidence and clinical course of thrombus formation on atrial septal defect and patent foramen ovale devices in 100 consecutive patients. *J Am Coll Cardiol.* 2004;43:302–309.

12. Majunke N, Bialkowski J, Szkutnik M, et al. Closure of ASD with the AMPLATZER septal occluder in adults. *Am J Cardiol.* 2009;103(4):550–554.

13. Cheng S, Keyes M, Larson MG, et al. Long-term outcomes in individuals with prolonged PR interval r first-degree atrioventricular block. *JAMA.* 2009;301(24):3571–3577.

14. Schuchlenz HW, Mannweiler S, Martin D. Marked foreign body reaction and thrombus formation after transcatheter closure of patent foramen ovale. *J Thorac Cardiovasc S.* 2005;130:591–592.

15. Al-Anani S, Weber H, Hijazi ZM. Atrioventricular block after transcatheter ASD closure using the AMPLATZER septal occluder: risk factors and recommendations. *Cathet Cardiovasc Intervent.* 2010;75:767–772.

16. Bohme J, Bettina K, Kohler F, Madman G, Concerts W. Surgical removal of ASD occlusion system. *Eur J Cardio Thorac Surg.* 1997;12(6):869–872.

17. Amin Z, Hijazi ZM, Bass JL, et al. Erosion of AMPLATZER septal occluder device after closure of secundum atrial septal defects: review of registry of complication and recommendations to minimize future risks. *Cathet Cardiovasc Intervent.* 2004;63:496–503.

18. Amin Z. Transcatheter closure of secundum atrial septal defects. *Cathet Cardiovasc Intervent.* 2006;68:778–787.

19. Chun DS, Turrentine M, Mustapha A, et al. Development of aorta to right atrial fistula following closure of secundum atrial septal defect using the AMPLATZER septal occluder. *Cathet Cardiovasc Intervent.* 2003;58:246–251.

20. Lange SA, Schoen SP, Braun MU, et al. Perforation of aortic root as a secondary complication after implantation of PFO occlusion device in a 31-year-old woman. *J Intervent Cardiol.* 2006;19:166–169.

21. El-Said H, Moore JW. Erosion by the AMPLATZER Septal Occluder: Experienced opinions at Odds with manufacturer recommendations. *CCI.* 2009;73:925–930.

22. Dialetto G, Covino F, Scognomilio G, et al. A rare complication of ASD occluder: Diagnosis by TTE. *J Am Soc Echocardiogr.* 2006;19:836, e5–e8.

23. Slesnick TC, Nugent A, Fraser C, Canno B. Incomplete endothelialization and late development of acute bacterial endocarditis after implantation of an ASO device. *Circulation.* 2008;117:e326–e327.

24. Schoen SP, Boscheri A, Lange SA, et al. Incidence of aortic valve regurgitation and outcome after percutaneous closure of atrial septal defects and patent foramen ovale. *Heart.* 2008;94:844–847.

25. Wohrle W, Kochs M, Spiess J, et al. Impact of percutaneous device implantation for closure of patent foramen ovale on valve insufficiencies. *Circulation.* 2009;119:3002–3008.

26. McElhinney DB. Patent foramen ovale closure: let's keep the heart in mind. *Circulation.* 2009;119:2967–2968.

27. Slesnick T, Nugent A, Fraser C, et al. Incomplete endothelialization and late development of acute bacterial endocarditis after implantation of an AMPLATZER septal occluder. *Circulation.* 2008;117:e326–e327.

28. Spencer MP, Mohering MA, Jesuram J, et al. Power M mode transcranial Doppler for diagnosis of PFO and assessing transcatheter closure. *J Neuroimaging.* 2004;14:342–349.

29. Anzola GP, Morandi E, Casilli F, et al. Does transcatheter closure of PFO really "shut the door?" A prospective study with transcranial Doppler. *Stroke.* 2004;35:2140–2144.

30. Sommer RJ. Patent foramen ovale: where are we in 2009? *Am J Ther.* 2009;16:562–572.

31. Sherman JM. Hagler DJ, Cetta F. Thrombosis

after septal closure device placement. A review of the current literature. *Cathet Cardiovasc Intervent.* 2004;63(4):486–489.

32. Amin, Z, Hijazi ZM, Bass JL, et al. PFO closure complications from the AGA registry. *Cathet Cardiovasc Intervent.* 2008;72:74–79.

33. Trepils T, Sievert H, Ballinger K, Troisdorf U, Sedan E. Cardiac perforation following transcatheter PFO closure. *Cathet Cardiovasc Intervent.* 2003;58:111–113.

34. Christen T, Mach F, Didier D, Kalongs A, Vermin V. Late cardiac tampon after percutaneous closure of s patent foramen ovale. *Eur J Echocardiogr.* 2005;6:465–469.

35. Qureshi A, Muta MA, Letson LA. Partial prolapsed of a HELEX device associated with early frame fracture and mistral valve perforation. *Cathet Cardiovasc Intervent.* 2009;74: 777–782.

23

Nightmare Cases in the Cardiac Catheterization Laboratory during Percutaneous Closure of ASDs

Mustafa H. Abdullah Al-Qbandi, Tarek S. Momenah, and Ziyad M. Hijazi

Introduction

This chapter presents several cases of secundum atrial septal defect (ASD) device closure that ended with a complication (erosion and device migration) despite appropriate device selection and appearance of the device after its release. Appropriate follow-up while the patient is in the hospital is of paramount importance to avoid a catastrophic outcome. In all three cases, the devices were removed surgically and the outcome was good. The major take-home message from these cases is the fact that complications do occur despite appropriate device appearance and device selection.

Case 1

ZR is a 7-year-old girl, weight 22 kg, with a diagnosis of secundum ASD and pulmonary valve stenosis. Transthoracic echocardiogram (TTE) reported volume loaded right ventricle with paradoxical septal motion. There was a moderate-size secundum ASD that measured 9 × 8 mm in size with deficient anterior rim, the other rims were adequate. There was a gradient across the pulmonary valve with a peak of 40 mm Hg. The decision was made to close the ASD percutaneously in the catheterization laboratory. Cardiac catheterization was performed under general anesthesia. Both femoral artery and vein were accessed and sheaths (5F and 6F, respectively) were introduced. Heparin at a dose of 100 units/kg was given. The right ventricular pressure was 30/3 mm Hg and the main pulmonary artery pressure was 25/10 mm Hg with a mean of 15 mm Hg. The systolic BP was 100/70 with a mean of 85 mm Hg. The calculated Qp:Qs ratio was 2:1, with low pulmonary vascular resistance. A transesophageal echocardiogram (TEE) confirmed the diagnosis. The ASD was high secundum and measured 10 × 9 mm with deficient anterior rim and adequate other rims. The total atrial septal length was 26 to 28 mm in the four-chamber view. Balloon sizing was performed using the AGA sizing balloon. The stop flow diameter was 13 mm. A 14-mm AMPLATZER Septal Occluder (ASO) (AGA Medical, Plymouth, Minnesota) device was chosen to close the defect.

Under TEE guidance, the device was easily placed at the proper position via a 9F delivery sheath. TEE and fluoroscopy confirmed good device position with no residual shunt. The device did not interfere with any structure. The procedure time was 45 minutes. Antibiotic prophylaxis was given. She was transferred to the ward in clinically good condition. Six hours later, she started to complain of nonspecific upper abdominal pain. X-ray of the abdomen and chest revealed good position of the device and abdominal gas pattern with no signs of intestinal obstruction. TTE confirmed good

position of the device with no evidence of pericardial effusion. Twelve hours later, her nonspecific abdominal pain increased in intensity, she became more restless, and pale. An emergency code was called for deteriorating clinical condition, with pulse rate at 150/min, BP = 80/60 mean at 70 mm Hg. Her hemoglobin dropped from 13g/dl to 10g/dl. The patient was intubated semi-electively to stabilize her condition. She received blood transfusion and intravenous fluids. An emergency TTE revealed a large pericardial effusion with signs of impending tamponade. This required immediate bedside pericardiocentesis. The device was in place but seen to be touching the roof of the left atrium. About a 100 ml of fresh blood was aspirated from the pericardial sac. The patient was moved back to the catheterization laboratory for angiography. Repeat TEE demonstrated good device position, however, the superior part of the left atrial disc was touching the roof of the left atrium. Left pulmonary angiogram and an ascending aortogram demonstrated no residual shunt from the left atrium or presence of connection from the ascending aorta to the pericardium. The pericardial drainage was left in the pericardial sac and she was taken to the oper-

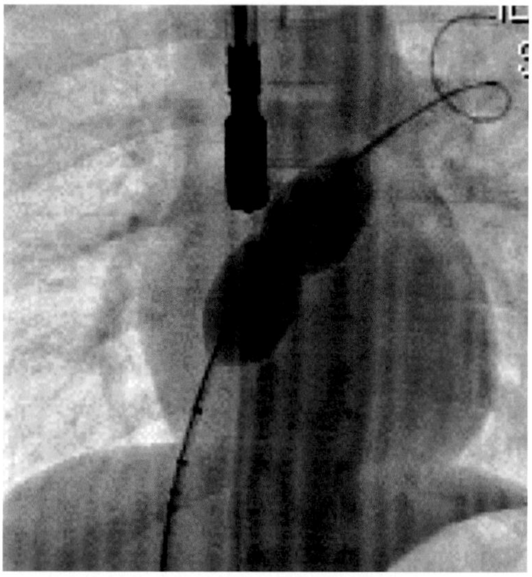

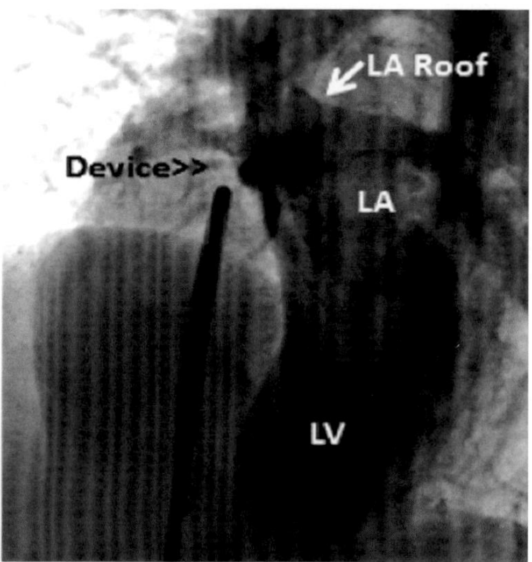

Fig 23.1—Stop-flow technique and balloon sizing of ASD. Waist can be seen clearly.

Fig 23.2—Post device closure, arrow indicates roof of LA and LA part of the device is touching the roof. Abbreviations: LA, Left atrium; LV, left ventricle.

ating room. In the operating room, the device was nicely occluding the defect but with a small hematoma around it. The device was removed. A tear on the upper part of the left atrium was found, at the entry of the right upper pulmonary vein. The ASO produced erosion into the wall of atrium. The device was also eroding the aortic wall. The ASD measured 11 mm and was closed with direct stitching. The eroded wall on both left atrial roof and aorta were also repaired with pledgeted sutures. Figures 23.1 and 23.2 demonstrate the case. The patient was discharged home a few days later in good condition and with had residual defect.

Case 2

SH is a 14-month-old toddler girl weighing 12 kg. She was diagnosed with multifenestrated atrial septal wall. A TTE showed two secundum ASDs each measuring 6 mm in size with a thin atrial septum. One of the ASDs was located at the fossa ovalis, while the other was near the inferior/posterior wall of the septum. The distance between the ASDs was 8 mm. The right ventricle was large due to the shunt, and there was paradoxical septal motion. The RV

pressure was estimated to be at half systemic pressure. There was no pulmonary valve stenosis. However, her right upper lobe branch had stenosis with peak gradient of 40 mm Hg. There was no left-sided obstruction. The case was discussed with the parents for possible ASD device closure and balloon dilatation of the stenosed right upper lobe pulmonary artery branch. Consent was given. At cardiac catheterization, the patient was intubated and mechanically ventilated. Both femoral artery and veins were accessed and sheaths (5F and 6 F, respectively) were introduced. Heparin at a dose of 100 units/kg was given. Diagnostic cardiac catheterization revealed near half systemic RV pressure (RV pressure was 40 mm Hg to systolic BP at 90 mm Hg). The calculated Qp:Qs ratio was 2:1 with low pulmonary vascular resistance. There was no RV-PA gradient and both branch PAs were of adequate size. The right upper pulmonary artery branch was narrow. No left-sided lesions. The TEE showed thin atrial septal wall with two defects each measuring 6 mm in size. One was close to the inferior vena cava and the other at the fossa ovalis area. The distance between the defects was 8 mm in length. The other rims were as follows: superior 12 mm, anterior 6 mm, posterior 8 mm, mitral 8 mm, IVC was deficient. After placing wires

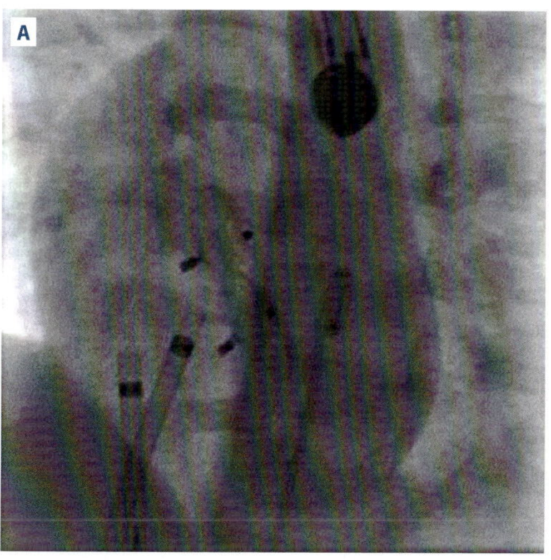

Fig 23.3 A-B—Two ASD AMPLATZER devices, 6-mm each, well-seated at AP and lateral views.

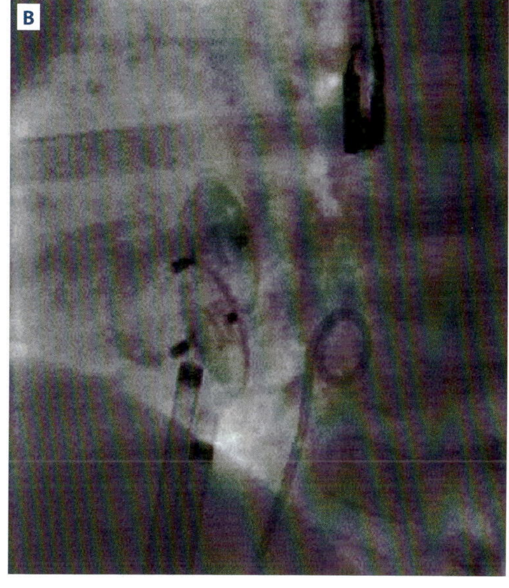

in each defect, a 24-mm AGA sizing balloon was used to measure the "stretched diameter" of each defect. Two 6-mm AMPLATZER ASD devices were chosen for the closure. After placement of sheaths (7F in each femoral vein), the central device at the fossa ovalis was deployed followed by the other one, near the IVC. Both devices looked well seated by TEE as well as by fluoroscopy (Figs 23.3). Because the RV pressure postclosure dropped to < 1/3 systemic, it was felt appropriate to defer balloon dilatation of the stenosed right upper pulmonary artery branch. There was small residual device leak. Both devices were close to each other. After a proper "Minnesota wiggle," both devices were released. Prophylactic antibiotic was given and the patient was returned to the ward.

The next day, a routine chest x-ray (CXR) (Fig 23.4) before discharge revealed one device in place, however, the other one not in the same plane. It was felt that it was sitting slightly more to the left side. The patient had no symptoms at all. A TTE showed that one of the devices (the posterior/inferior device) was in the ascending aorta at the aortic sinus at its longitudinal axis permitting flow across the aorta. The patient was taken to the operating room where both devices were removed. A longitudinal incision, 8 mm in length, was made in the ascending aorta to remove the stuck device at the aortic sinus. The atrial septum was found to be multifenestrated. The defects were closed with a GORE-TEX patch. The patient was discharged home after a few days in good condition with no residual shunt.

Case 3

Case 3 is a 7-year-old boy who was born with pulmonary atresia with intact ventricular septum. Soon after birth, he underwent cardiac catheterization where balloon atrial septostomy was performed followed by surgical placement of a modified right Blalock-Taussig (BT) shunt. Three months later, a left BT shunt was placed for a stenosed right BT shunt. At 2 years of age, repair of right ventricular outflow tract with patch enlargement was performed. The BT shunt was not taken down. It was found on serial follow-up echocardiogram that the right ventricle was growing and that the right ventricular cavity was enlarged. This was explained by either the moderate pulmonary valve regurgitation or the moderate-size secundum ASD with bidirectional flow. It was felt that cardiac catheterization was necessary to evaluate the hemodynamics and to close both the ASD and the BT shunt percutaneously. After prepara-

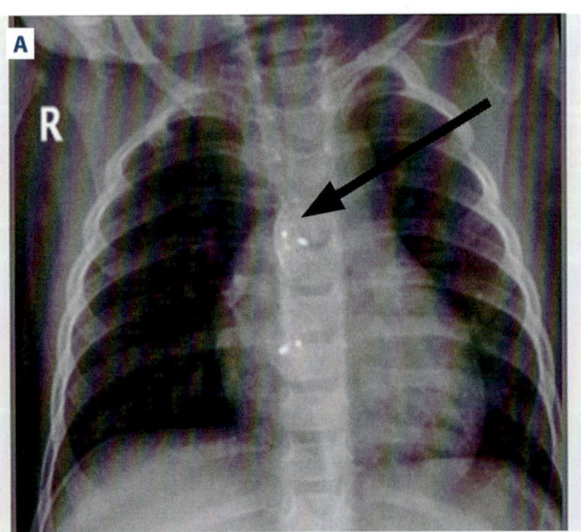

Figs 23.4 A-B—The superior device seen moved from its place and now is sitting in the ascending aorta. The other one is in place. Arrow indicates the embolized device.

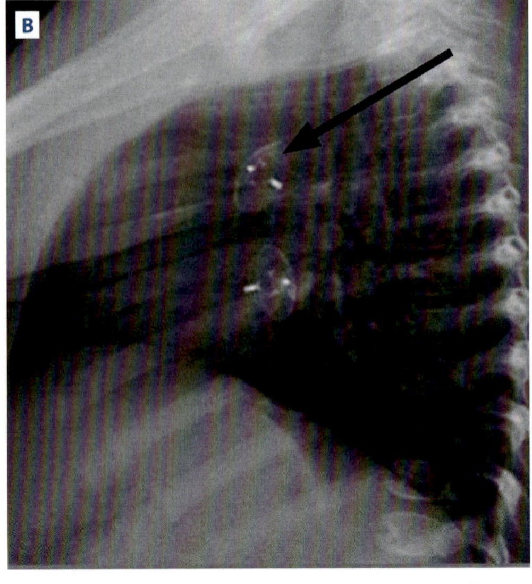

tion of the patient, both femoral artery and vein were accessed. Heparin at a dose of 100 units/kg was given. Diagnostic cardiac catheterization revealed aortic saturation of 88%, RV pressure was 40/2; LV pressure was 80/3; RA pressure was a-wave 10, V-wave 5 and mean of 5; LA pressure was a-wave 8, V-wave 7 and mean of 5; and the PA pressure was 30/11 (20). Initially, the BT shunt was coil occluded using 5 mm × 5 cm Gianturco spring coil. The next procedure was to assess possibility of ASD device closure. Balloon occlusion of ASD using 24-mm AGA sizing balloon resulted in rise of the systemic saturation to 96% with no drop in the aortic pressure or rise in RA pressure. A detailed TEE showed an ASD size of 12 mm (Fig 23.5A) with the following rim sizes: aortic 8 mm, SVC 8 mm, mitral 8 mm, and IVC 13 mm. The inferior rim was long, thin, and redundant. Balloon sizing was performed and this demonstrated a stretched diameter of 23 mm. However, slow deflation of the balloon revealed a size of about 12 mm when the flow was totally obliterated "stop-flow." The total septal atrial length was 28 to 29 mm. A bigger device was felt to be inappropriate for a small left atrium. Through a 9F long sheath, a 12-mm ASO device was deployed and released. TEE confirmed good device position (Fig 23.5B), with too much mobility during the cardiac contraction. After a few minutes the device embolized to the left ventricular cavity (Figs 23.5C, 23.6). After failed multiple attempts at retrieving the device, it was felt that surgical removal was more appropriate. At surgery, the device was removed and the ASD that measured 15 mm was closed with a GORE-TEX patch. The patient was discharged home after a

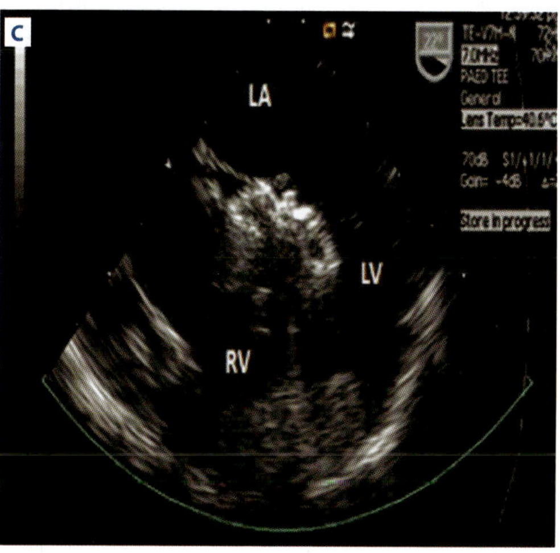

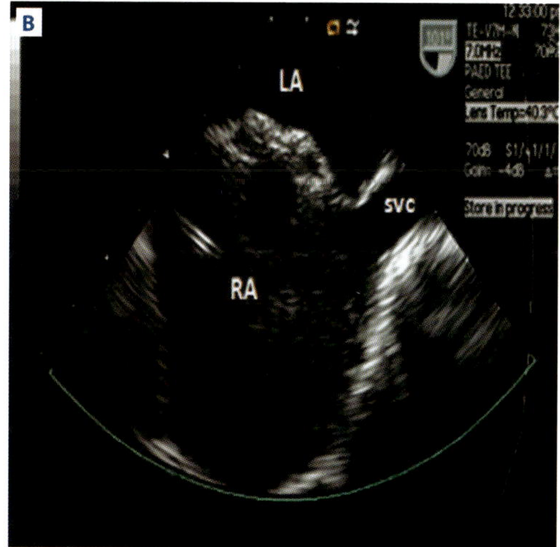

Fig 23.5 A-C—Transesophageal echocardiographic image. A: Color flow Doppler of ASD. B: Well-seated AMPLATZER device. C: The device embolized into the left ventricle just below the mitral valve. Abbreviations: Ao, Aorta; LA, Left atrium; RA, right atrium; SVC, superior vena cava; LV, left ventricle.

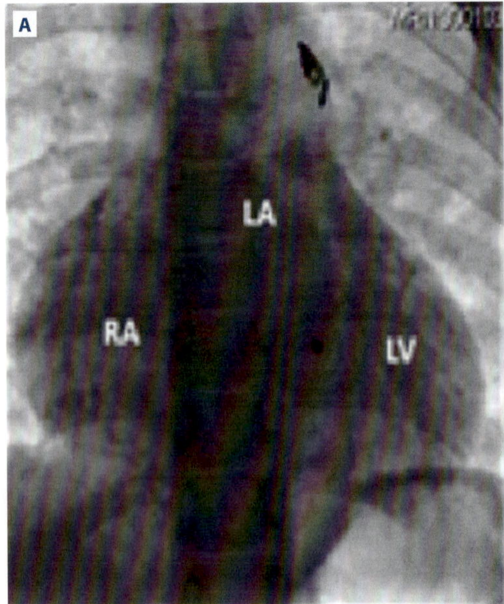

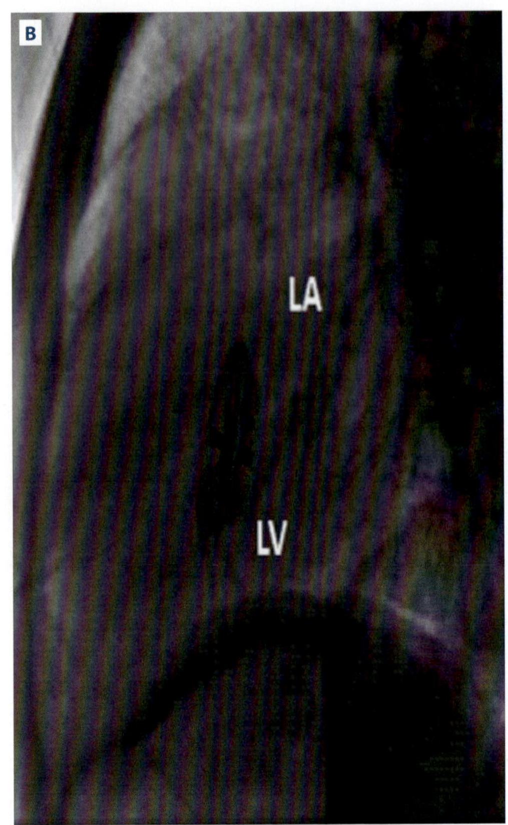

Fig 23.6 A-B Cine fluoroscopy images in frontal and lateral views post-ASD AMPLATZER device closure with the device in LV. Abbreviations: RA, Right atrium; LA, left atrium; LV, left ventricle.

few days in good condition with no residual shunt.

Discussion

The three cases represent complications following percutaneous ASD AMPLATZER device closure. Each case represents a different scenario. The first case presents acute erosion of the roof of the left atrium and the posterior part of the ascending aorta. The second case represents the risk of using multiple devices in closing multiple ASDs. The last case points to the underestimation of ASD diameter and the immediate embolization of a device into the left ventricle.

All of these cases were treated surgically. However, the authors would like to point out that successful percutaneous retrieval of an embolized device can be done. However, the laboratory should be fully equipped with all sizes and types of snares, as well as sheaths of appropriate size to remove these devices. Multiple (unsuccessful) attempts were made in the case of the embolized ASD occluder. In the first two cases, the authors believed surgical removal was more appropriate than percutaneous one.

Transcatheter ASD closure has proven to be safe and effective, and it is rapidly becoming the standard treatment for secundum-type ASDs.[1-4] When planning to discharge patients following ASD device closure, simple chest x-ray should be done to detect any change in position of the ASD.[5] This can be confirmed by echocardiography and/or chest x-ray. The authors prefer to perform an echocardiogram because it can determine shunt status as well as device position. In the event the device is not seen in its usual location, the chest x-ray can be helpful in determining the device position.

Device embolization occurs in about 0.55% of cases, regardless of ASD size, device size, or the physician's expertise.[6,7] Percutaneous retrieval of the embolized device is possible in about 50% of cases, and several techniques have been described, including the use of large sheaths,[8] gooseneck snares, or bioptomes.[4,9]

In a study by Amin et al,[10] a total of 28 cases of erosion following AMPLATZER device closure were studied (14 in the United States). All erosions occurred at the dome of the atria, near the aortic root. Deficient aortic rim was seen in 89% and the defects were described as high, suggesting deficient superior rim. The device to unstretched ASD ratio was significantly larger in the adverse event group when compared to the FDA pivotal trial group. They concluded that patients with deficient aortic rim and/or superior rim may be at higher risk for device erosion. The defect should not be overstretched during balloon sizing. Patients with small pericardial effusion at 24 hours should have closer follow-up. They further reported that 19 of the 28 patients (68%) developed symptoms within the first 72 hour of the procedure. Eight patients (29%) were diagnosed between 5 days and 8 months after the procedure, and one patient developed a pericardial effusion 3 years after the device was placed.

Awad et al[11] reported the feasibility, effectiveness, and long-term outcome of transcatheter closure of multiple ASDs using multiple ASO devices. In this study, they collected 33 patients over a period of 9 years. Sixty-seven devices were deployed in 33 patients. Immediately after the procedure 15 patients had complete closure, 8 had trivial shunt, 9 had small shunt, and 1 had large shunt. Complications included a device embolization within 24 hours and left atrial aortic wall erosion and pericardial effusion at 2 years. One patient who had large residual shunt and device embolization was a 49-year-old male patient with two defects, the larger defect measuring 24 mm with a stretched diameter of 30 mm. A 26-mm device (the largest manufactured at the time) was used to close this defect. The smaller defect measured 7 mm with a stretched diameter of 9 mm. A 9-mm device

was used to close this defect. A routine follow-up TTE at 24 hour revealed that the 26-mm device had embolized to the main pulmonary artery and the 9-mm device was in good position. The patient was completely asymptomatic. The patient underwent successful percutaneous retrieval of this device. Five months later, a 34-mm device was deployed in the larger defect with complete closure.

There are many reports in the literature about embolization of ASD AMPLATZER device.[6,11–17] Case 3 clearly emphasizes the importance of sizing the defect correctly and not undersizing the defect. If the superior rim is adequate and the aortic rim is deficient, fistulous connection between the aortic root and either atrium may occur. The exact mechanism of how the fistulous communication develops remains unknown. The device size chosen in two out of three patients who developed aorta to atrial fistula was not oversized beyond recommendation. Oversizing beyond the stretched diameter by 4 mm or more, however, is quite common in patients with deficient aortic rim to stabilize the device adequately. Although it has been recommended in the past to oversize the device by 4 mm or more, the authors recommend that oversizing beyond 2 mm should be avoided. The predominance of left atrial perforation with the ASO device may relate to the larger left atrial disc. All atrial perforations involved the roof of the atria (superior rim) and lead directly into the pericardium. When there was anterior extension, the aorta may also be involved (anterior and superior rim). This suggests that deficient superior or aortic rim may be associated with increased risk of an atrial perforation. Oversizing a device could increase this risk. Contact between the device and an atrial wall could also be related to alterations in atrial size, dimensions, and anatomy following closure of the ASD. Shrinkage of the right atrial cavity with elimination of the left-to-right atrial shunt could bring the device into contact with the atrial wall. This late hazard may be increased when the implanted device is oversized.

King et al[18] reported the first transcatheter ASD closure in 1976. Subsequently, a number of devices have been developed, with the ASO currently being the preferred implant for closure. Percutaneous transcatheter delivery of the AASO has a success rate that parallels surgery while maintaining a low complication rate.[1,19] Immediate complications include arrhythmias[1,6,20–22] transient ST-T elevation,[21] systemic and pulmonary embolization, and acute cardiac perforation.[10,20,23–25] Late complications are rare.[10] There are two published case reports of late atrial wall erosions in patients who underwent percutaneous ASD repair with the ASO. An aorta to right atrial fistula 3 months after the procedure was reported in a 10-year-old.[26] Preventza et al[27] reported a case of right atrial perforation 6 months after an uncomplicated closure of a small ASD in a 42-year-old female who presented with cardiogenic shock. A total of 29 cases of erosion of ASOs after closure of secundum ASDs have been reported in the literature.[21] Eight of the children presented in the first 72 hours postprocedure, and 2 children experienced late erosion and had a left atrium to aorta fistula with no hemodynamic compromise.[10] Possible risk factors for erosion of the ASO are deficient aortic and superior rim or oversizing of the device, which may increase the chance of contact between the device and the atrial wall. Deformations of the device at the aortic root and small pericardial effusion at 24 hours are also potential risk factors.[10] The risk factor in this case was the superior location of the defect. The balloon-stretched size of the ASD was 16 mm and the implanted device was 18 mm, as recommended.[10] Chest radiography is a rapid, noninvasive test performed at any hospital or clinic and may reveal the diagnosis in a patient who presents with cardiopulmonary symptoms. In this child, a chest x-ray showed the device, but the cardiomegaly was minimal, and migration of the device was not obvious. This case is also a clear example of the benefits of timely access to a patient's hospital records even in the initial evaluation of critically ill patients. Access to the electronic chart facilitated the diagnosis and timely management of this patient when history was not readily available and there were no obvious surgical scars to indicate previous cardiac surgical interventions.

Conclusions

In the authors' experience and the experience of others,[6] embolization/malposition is the most common serious complication of ASD device closure. Erosion must be treated with pericardial drainage and urgent surgery. Devices usually embolize into the main pulmonary artery (89%). Once a device embolizes, two different options are possible: (1) retrieve the device by a gooseneck snare or a basket catheter, or (2) refer the patient to the surgeon. The last option is indicated when the size of the device is among the largest; the surgeon will retrieve the device and close the ASD at the same time. If retrieval is attempted, an introducer of at least 2F sizes larger than the delivery sheath should be inserted to accommodate the device captured by a gooseneck snare or a basket catheter.

References

1. Du ZD, Hijazi ZM, Kleinman CS, Silverman NH, Larntz K. Comparison between transcatheter and surgical closure of secundum atrial septal defect in children and adults: results of a multicenter nonrandomized trial. *J Am Coll Cardiol.* 2002;39:1836–1844.

2. Khelashvili V, Gogorishvili I, Metreveli I, Tsintsadze A. Comparison of surgical and by transcatheter methods of closure of atrial septal defect based on the two year experience. *Georgian Med News.* 2006;17–20.

3. Berdat PA, Chatterjee T, Pfammatter JP, Windecker S, Meier B, Carrel T. Surgical management of complications after transcatheter closure of an atrial septal defect or patent foramen ovale. *J Thorac Cardiovasc Surg.* 2000;120:1034–1039.

4. Marie VA, Rhodes JF. Current indications and contraindications for transcatheter atrial septal defect and patent foramen ovale device closure. *Am Heart J.* 2007;153:81–84.

5. Lee EY, Siegel MJ, Chu CM, Gutierrez FR, Kort

HW. AMPLATZER atrial septal defect occluder for pediatric patients: radiographic appearance. *Radiology.* 2004;233:471–476.

6. Chessa M, Carminati M, Butera G, et al. Early and late complications associated with transcatheter occlusion of secundum atrial septal defect. *J Am Coll Cardiol.* 2002;39:1061–1065.

7. Tan CA, Levi DS, Moore JW. Embolization and transcatheter retrieval of coils and devices. *Pediatr Cardiol.* 2005;26:267–274.

8. Levi DS, Moore JW. Embolization and retrieval of the AMPLATZER septal occluder. *Cathet Cardiovasc Intervent.* 2004;61:543–547.

9. Berger F, Ewert P, Bjornstad PG, et al. Transcatheter closure as standard treatment for most interatrial defects: experience in 200 patients treated with the AMPLATZER Septal Occluder. *Cardiol Young.* 1999;9:468–473.

10. Amin Z, Hijazi ZM, Bass JL, Cheatham JP, Hellenbrand WE, Kleinman CS. Erosion of AMPLATZER septal occluder device after closure of secundum atrial septal defects: review of registry of complications and recommendations to minimize future risk. *Cathet Cardiovasc Intervent.* 2004;63:496–502.

11. Awad SM, Garay FF, Cao QL, Hijazi ZM. Multiple AMPLATZER septal occluder devices for multiple atrial communications: immediate and long-term follow-up results. *Cathet Cardiovasc Intervent.* 2007;70:265–273.

12. Bramlet MT, Hoyer MH. Single pediatric center experience with multiple device implantation for complex secundum atrial septal defects. *Cathet Cardiovasc Intervent.* 2008;72:531–537.

13. Saxena A, Divekar A, Soni NR. Natural history of secundum atrial septal defect revisited in the era of transcatheter closure. *Indian Heart J.* 2005;57:35–38.

14. Numan M, El SA, Tofeig M, Gendi S, Tohami T, El-Said HG. Cribriform AMPLATZER device closure of fenestrated atrial septal defects: feasibility and technical aspects. *Pediatr Cardiol.* 2008;29:530–535.

15. Balbi M, Casalino L, Gnecco G, et al. Percutaneous closure of patent foramen ovale in patients with presumed paradoxical embolism: periprocedural results and midterm risk of recurrent neurologic events. *Am Heart J.* 2008;156:356–360.

16. El-Said HG, Moore JW. Erosion by the AMPLATZER septal occluder: experienced operator opinions at odds with manufacturer recommendations? *Cathet Cardiovasc Intervent.* 2009;73:925–930.

17. Truong QA, Gupta V, Bezerra HG, et al. Images in cardiovascular medicine. The traveling AMPLATZER: rare complication of percutaneous atrial septal occluder device embolism. *Circulation.* 2008;118:e93–e96.

18. King TD, Thompson SL, Steiner C, Mills NL. Secundum atrial septal defect. Nonoperative closure during cardiac catheterization. *JAMA.* 1976;235:2506–2509.

19. Podnar T, Martanovic P, Gavora P, Masura J. Morphological variations of secundum-type atrial septal defects: feasibility for percutaneous closure using AMPLATZER septal occluders. *Cathet Cardiovasc Intervent.* 2001;53:386–391.

20. Wang JK, Tsai SK, Wu MH, Lin MT, Lue HC. Short- and intermediate-term results of transcatheter closure of atrial septal defect with the AMPLATZER Septal Occluder. *Am Heart J.* 2004;148:511–517.

21. Berger F, Vogel M, Alexi-Meskishvili V, Lange PE. Comparison of results and complications of surgical and AMPLATZER device closure of atrial septal defects. *J Thorac Cardiovasc Surg.* 1999;118:674–678.

22. Vogel M, Berger F, Dahnert I, Ewert P, Lange PE. Treatment of atrial septal defects in symptomatic children aged less than 2 years of age using the AMPLATZER septal occluder. *Cardiol Young.* 2000;10:534–537.

23. Maimon MS, Ratnapalan S, Do A, Kirsh JA, Wilson GJ, Benson LN. Cardiac perforation 6 weeks after percutaneous atrial septal defect repair using an AMPLATZER septal occluder. *Pediatrics.* 2006;118:e1572–e1575.

24. Thanopoulos BD, Laskari CV, Tsaousis GS, Zarayelyan A, Vekiou A, Papadopoulos GS. Closure of atrial septal defects with the AMPLATZER occlusion device: preliminary results. *J Am Coll Cardiol.* 1998;31:1110–1116.

25. Perry YY, Triedman JK, Gauvreau K, Lock JE, Jenkins KJ. Sudden death in patients after transcatheter device implantation for congeni-

tal heart disease. *Am J Cardiol.* 2000;85:992–995.

26. Chun DS, Turrentine MW, Moustapha A, Hoyer MH. Development of aorta-to-right atrial fistula following closure of secundum atrial septal defect using the AMPLATZER septal occluder. *Cathet Cardiovasc Intervent.* 2003; 58:246–251.

27. Preventza O, Sampath-Kumar S, Wasnick J, Gold JP. Late cardiac perforation following transcatheter atrial septal defect closure. *Ann Thorac Surg.* 2004;77:1435–1437.

24

My Worst Nightmare Cases of PFO Closure

Tina Lehr, Sonya Joy, Kristina Renkhoff,

Nina Wunderlich, and Horst Sievert

Introduction

Catheter closure of patent foramen ovale (PFO) is performed worldwide in many centers with excellent results. In most cases it is a very safe and straightforward procedure. Nevertheless technical problems and complications can occur.

Case 1

Due to a sudden aphasia, a 43-year-old man was admitted to the neurological department of his local hospital. The patient had no cardiovascular risk factors. The cranial computer tomography (CCT) scans, as well as the magnetic resonance imaging (MRI) scans detected multiple ischemic cerebral lesions. Further diagnostics including color-coded duplex scan of the brain-supplying neck vessels, a Holter electrocardiogram (ECG) as well as a thrombophilia lab testing showed normal findings. Transesophageal echocardiography (TEE) however revealed a typical PFO with an atrial septal aneurysm, and a large right-to-left shunt during the contrast study at rest and under Valsalva maneuver. By reason that no other causes for the ischemic stroke could come into consideration, and a PFO was diagnosed, it was assumed that the patient had suffered from paradoxical embolisms. He was referred for PFO closure.

Prior to the intervention the patient was administered cefuroxime for subacute bacterial endocarditis prophylaxis, as well as aspirin and clopidogrel. During intervention 10.000 units of heparin were given. We performed a TEE under deep sedation, which confirmed the diagnosis of a PFO, with a highly mobile atrial

Transcatheter Closure of ASDs and PFOs: A Comprehensive Assessment. © 2010 Ziyad M. Hijazi, Ted Feldman, Mustafa H. Abdullah Al-Qbandi, and Horst Sievert, editors. Cardiotext Publishing, ISBN: 978-0-9790164-9-3.

septum. This was followed by catheterization using a 9F sheath via the right femoral vein. The left atrium was probed with a multipurpose catheter, and subsequent balloon sizing measured a PFO of 10-mm diameter. We selected a 20-mm HELEX Septal Occluder and implanted it according to the standard technique. Postclosure fluoroscopy and TEE confirmed the correct and stable position of the device (Fig 24.1). The contrast study under Valsalva maneuver showed a mild residual shunt. Aspirin and clopidogrel were prescribed for 6 months to prevent thrombus formation on the device and to bridge the period while residual shunting might still be present. He was discharged the day after the procedure without any complications.

One-month follow-up TEE disclosed that there was no occluder visible in the PFO. There

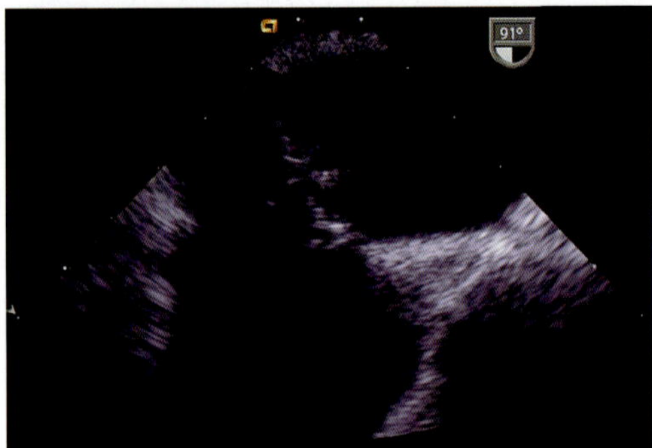

Fig 24.1—20-mm HELEX occluder in 90° TEE view.

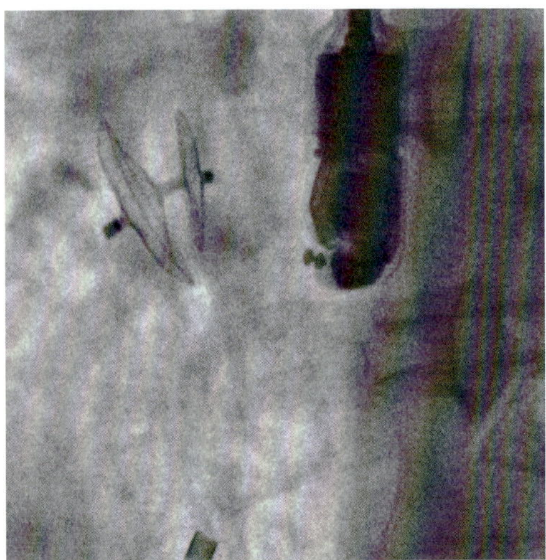

Fig 24.2—25-mm AMPLATZER occluder.

was a right-to-left shunt of contrast agent at rest and under Valsalva maneuver, as it had been before the procedure. Neither transthoracic echocardiography (TTE) nor TEE could determine the location of the device.

Fluoroscopy disclosed that the 20-mm HELEX device had embolized into the abdominal aorta.

A 9F sheath was introduced into the right femoral vein, and subsequently the left atrium was probed with a multipurpose catheter. This time we selected a 25-mm AMPLATZER PFO occluder for implantation. Correct and stable device position was confirmed by TEE and fluoroscopy (Fig 24.2). The contrast study under Valsalva maneuver showed a mild residual shunt.

In the same session we obtained arterial access with a 6F sheath via the right femoral artery. The embolized device caused a hemodynamically relevant obstruction with a pressure gradient of 55 mm Hg between the aorta and the right femoral artery (Fig 24.3). To mobilize and retrieve the device, we used various catheters and snares (Fig 24.4). But because the device was already covered by endothelial tissue, neither of them could mobilize it, in spite of very laborious efforts. The 6F sheath in the right

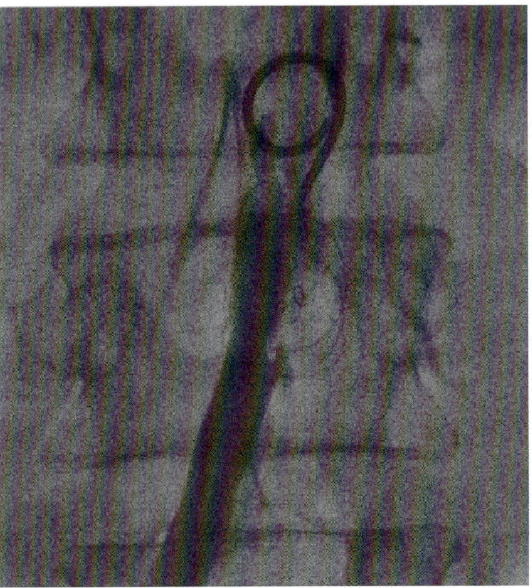

Fig 24.3—HELEX occluder in the aortic bifurcation. Obstruction of the right common iliac artery.

femoral artery was replaced with a 9F sheath. Additionally we introduced a 6F sheath via the left femoral artery to access the aortic bifurcation. Having access via both groins, we were finally able to separate an anterior located adhesion between the device and the vessel wall (Fig 24.5). The partial mobilization of the device reduced the pressure gradient between the aorta and the right femoral artery significantly from previously 55 mm Hg to 5 mm Hg (Fig 24.6). The patient was discharged one day after the procedure without further complications.

In the course of the follow-up investigations up to 1 year, the patient remained asymptomatic regarding both the embolized device as well as the PFO.

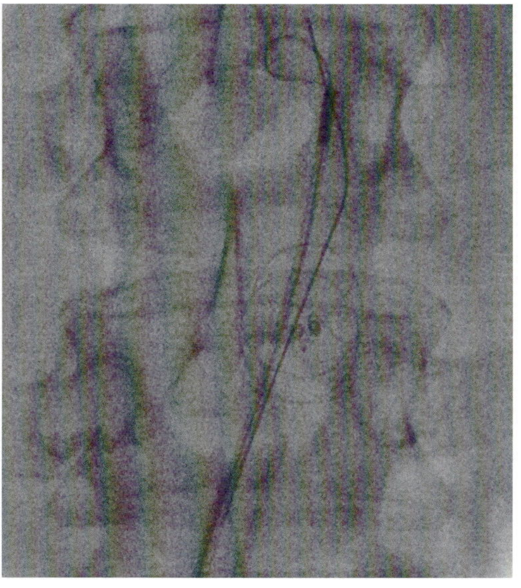

Fig 24.4—Attempted device retrieval with snare catheter and guide wire.

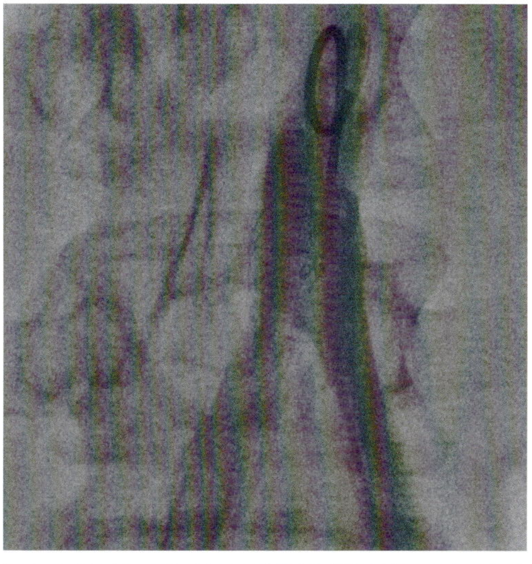

Fig 24.6—Simultaneously filling of the iliac arteries after the device had been mobilized.

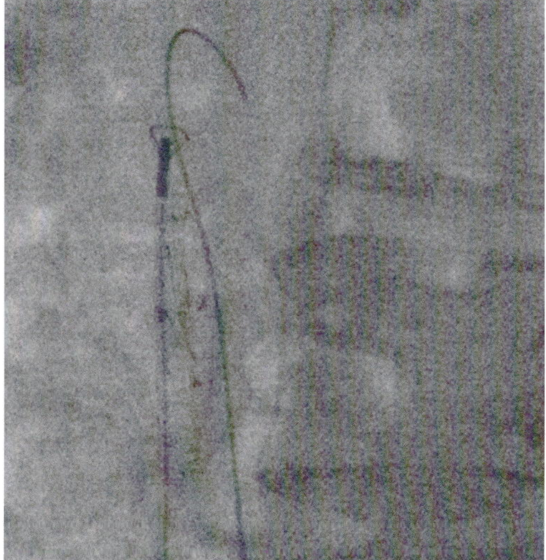

Fig 24.5—Bilateral access finally succeeded in mobilizing the device.

Case 2

A 50-year-old male patient was admitted with acute hemiparesis. MRI revealed an ischemic infarction of the right middle cerebral artery. A duplex scan of the carotid arteries and a 24-hour ECG showed normal findings. He had a history of recurrent migraine attacks. TTE showed normal findings. TEE revealed a PFO with an atrial septal aneurysm. Contrast study showed a large right-to-left shunt. Complete regression of the paresis could be observed within several days. After 11 days, the patient was discharged with phenprocoumon therapy based on International Normalization Ratio (INR). It was assumed that the PFO was the cause of the stroke.

The procedure was performed under deep sedation and the patient was administered

10.000 units of heparin. The TEE confirmed a typical PFO and a large atrial septal aneurysm (Fig 24.7). The right femoral vein was punctured and a 9F sheath inserted. Balloon sizing of the PFO measured 13.5 mm. Initially, a 25-mm Occlutech PFO occluder was implanted. Correct position was confirmed by TEE, fluoroscopy, and by performing a tug test (Figs 24.8 and 24.9). The release of the delivery cable proved to be difficult. The device rotated and the right atrial disc dislocated into the PFO tunnel (Fig 24.10).

The occluder was caught with a snare (Fig 24.11) and successfully repositioned (Fig 24.12). A few seconds later, the left atrial disc slipped into the tunnel (Fig 24.13). Once more, the device was caught with a snare and we chose to remove it completely. Thereafter, a 30-mm Occlutech PFO occluder was introduced. The device was in good position and remained so during the removal of the delivery cable (Fig 24.14). When we were about to remove the TEE probe, this device also dislocated into the PFO tunnel, this time with the right atrial disc (Fig 24.15). Repeated attempts to catch the occluder with a snare failed. The device slipped into the left atrium (Fig 24.16) and finally embolized into the descending aorta (Figs 24.17 A–C).

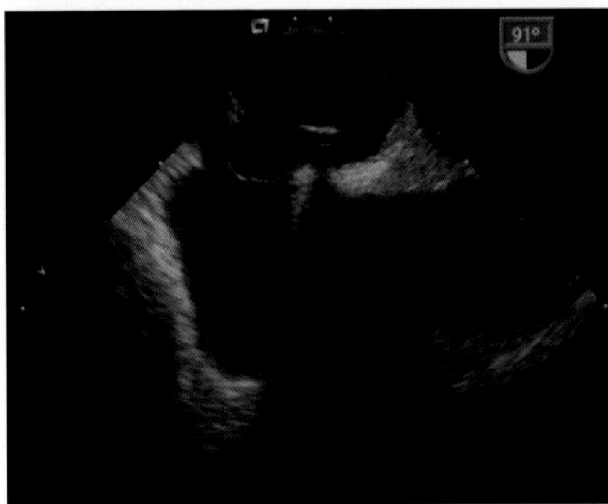

Fig 24.7—Long axis view of patent foramen oval with atrial septal aneurysm and transseptal sheath.

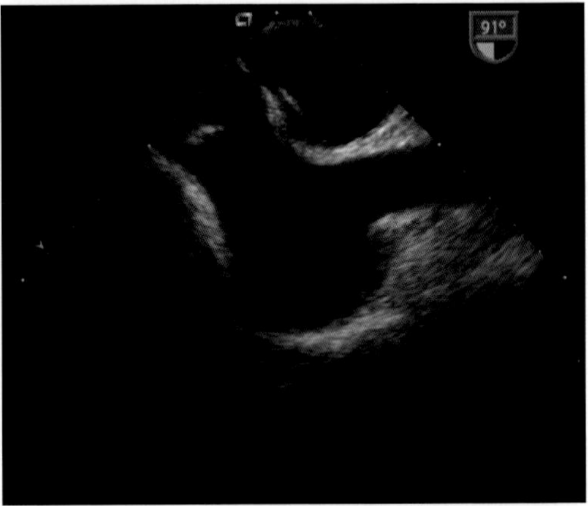

Fig 24.8—Long-axis view of PFO with 25-mm Occlutech occluder.

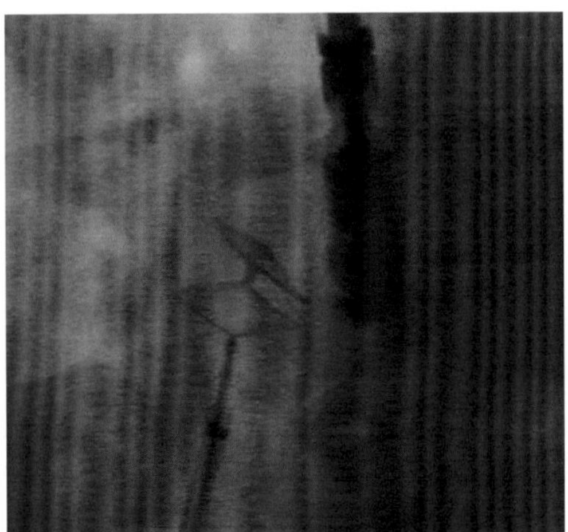

Fig 24.9—25-mm Occlutech occluder. Tug test under fluoroscopic control.

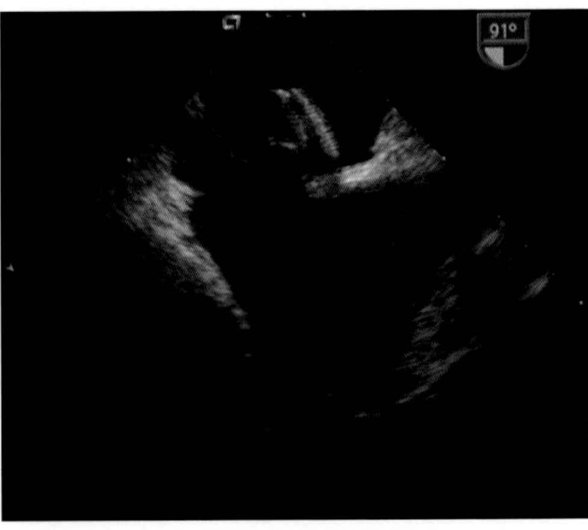

Fig 24.10—Long-axis view: Right atrial disc of 25-mm Occlutech dislocated into PFO tunnel.

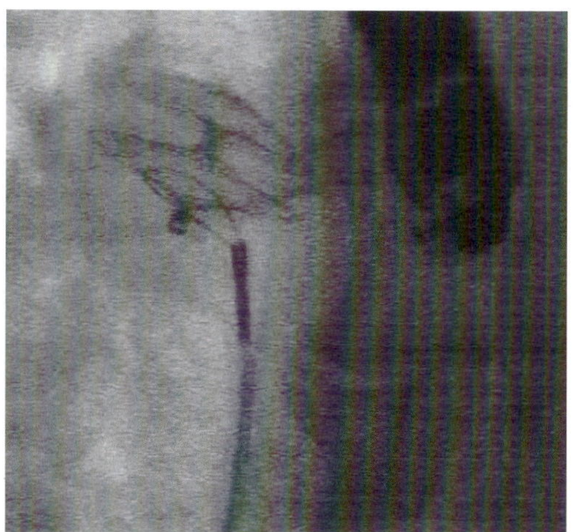

Fig 24.11—Snare catheter gripping 25-mm Occlutech occluder.

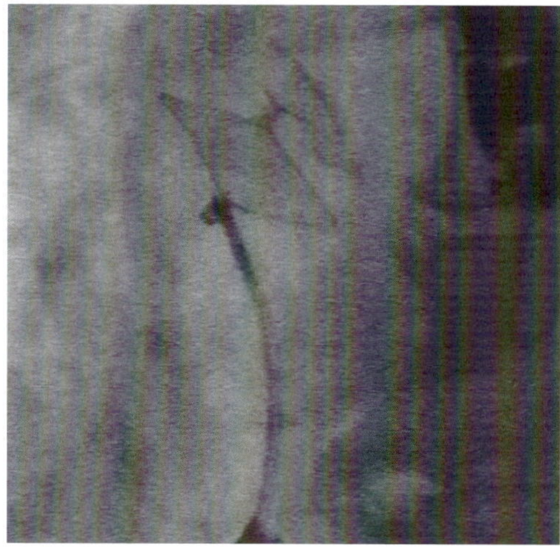

Fig 24.12—Repositioning of 25-mm Occlutech occluder attached to snare catheter under fluoroscopy guidance.

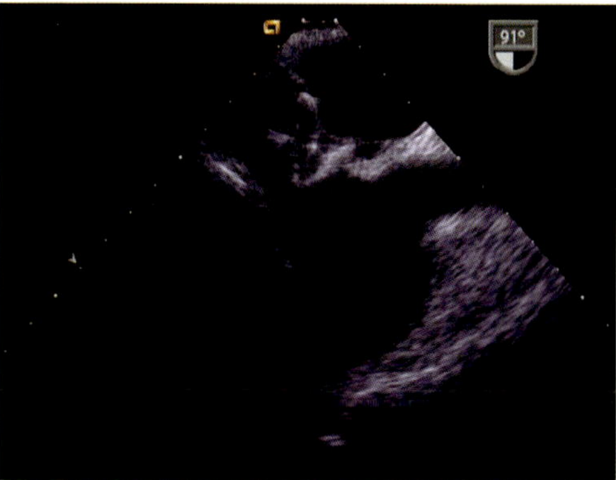

Fig 24.13—Left atrial disc of 25-mm Occlutech occluder dislocated into PFO tunnel.

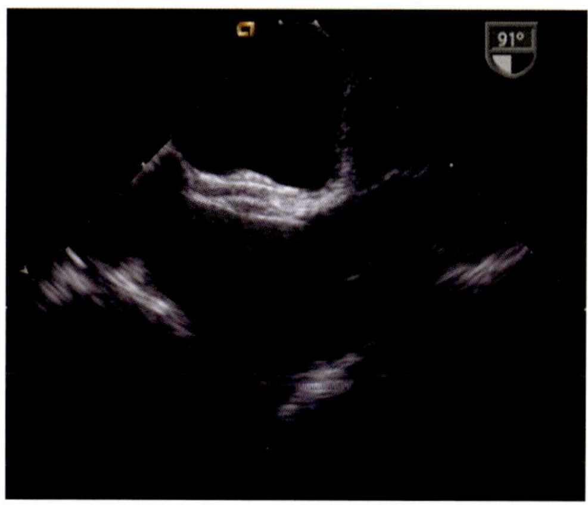

Fig 24.14—30-mm Occlutech occluder in correct position.

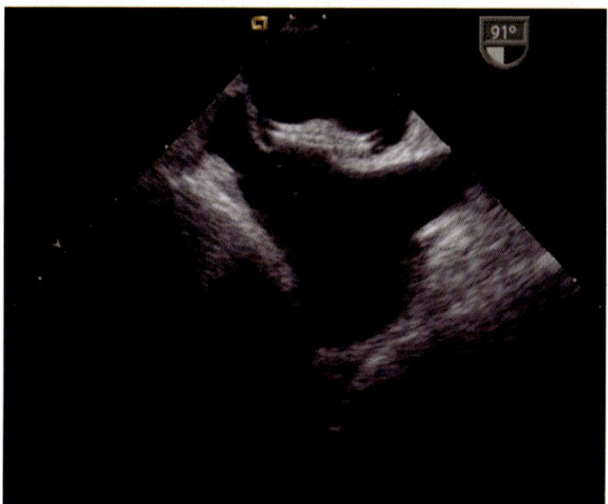

Fig 24.15—30-mm Occlutech device dislocated into PFO tunnel.

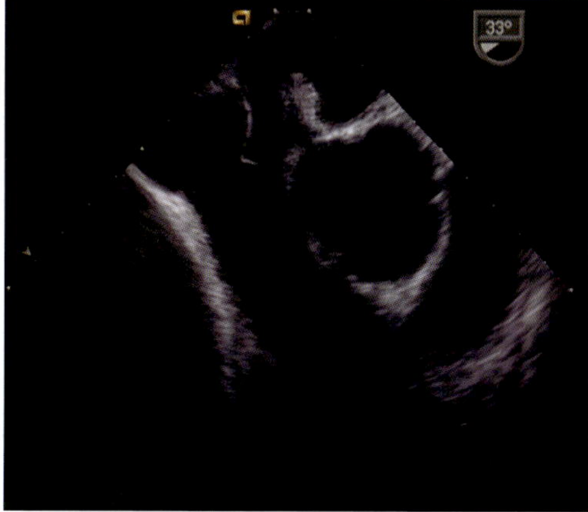

Fig 24.16—30-mm Occlutech occluder embolizing into the left atrium.

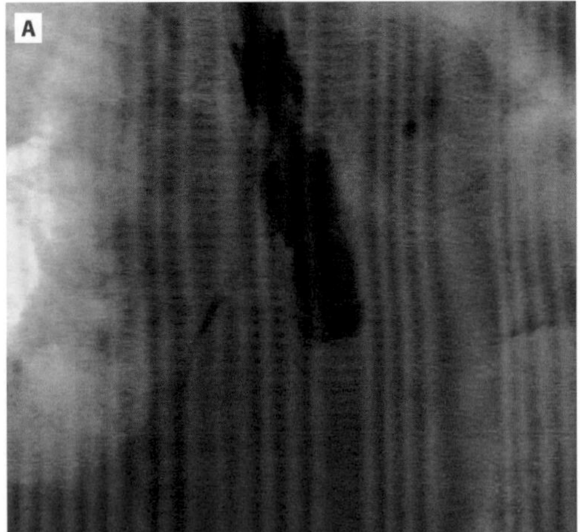

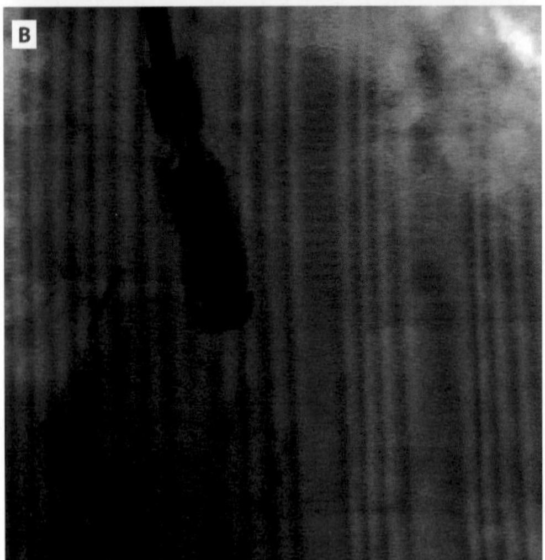

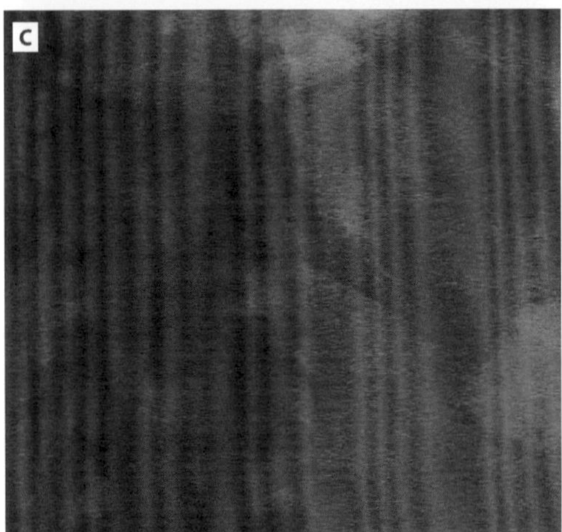

Fig 24.17 (A–C)—30-mm Occlutech occluder embolizing via left atrium and ventricle into ascending and descending aorta.

The right femoral artery was then punctured and an 11F sheath was inserted. The device was caught with a snare (Fig 24.18), but it could not be pulled back into the sheath. Therefore we extended the skin incision and widened it with a forceps, to withdraw sheath and occluder as a whole.

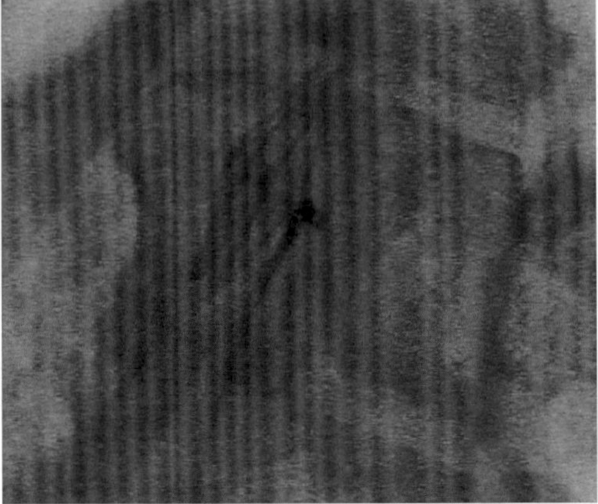

Fig 24.18—Embolized 30-mm Occlutech occluder caught with snare catheter in descending aorta.

Finally, we chose a 35-mm Occlutech PFO occluder and inserted it via a 12F sheath in the right femoral vein. This time the delivery catheter could be removed without further complications. We observed the device for another 10 minutes with fluoroscopy and TEE and confirmed correct position (Figs 24.19 and 24.20).

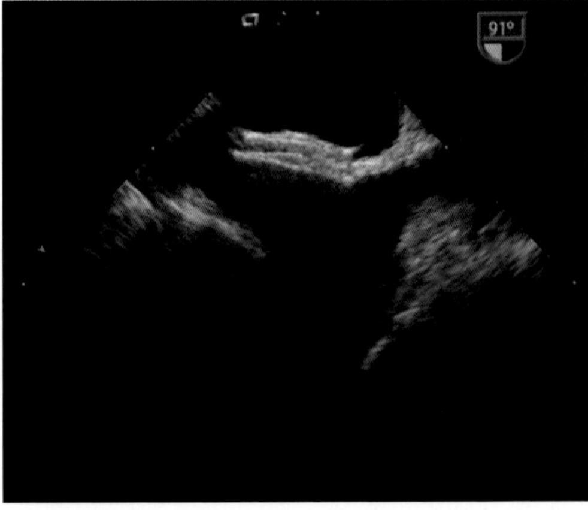

Fig 24.19—90° TEE long-axis view of 35-mm Occlutech occluder in correct position.

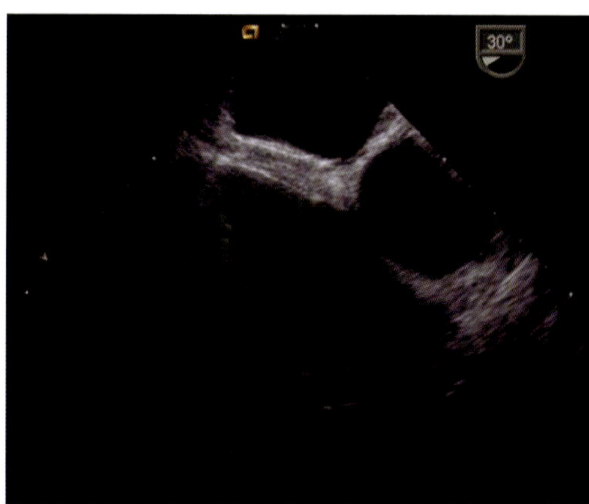

Fig 24.20—Short-axis view of 35-mm Occlutech device in correct position.

Follow-up TEE confirmed the occluder to be in good position, there were no thrombi, and in contrast study there was no residual shunt at rest or under Valsalva maneuver.

Case 3

A 58-year-old female patient was admitted to the hospital because of a stroke. CCT showed no pathological findings. MRI detected an infarction of the thalamus. Several additional diagnostic examinations, including a duplex scan of the carotid arteries, Holter ECG, 24-hour blood pressure monitoring, and an electroencephalogram (EEG) were performed, but no pathologic findings could be revealed. In TEE a PFO with a right-to-left shunt and an atrial septal aneurysm was found. All other cardiovascular risk factors were excluded. The patient fully recovered from the stroke without any persistent neurological dysfunctions. She was initially started on ticlopidine. Four months later, the patient experienced a second stroke. From then on she was treated with phenprocoumon.

Nearly 12 years later, she suffered from persisting severe back pain, hepatomegaly, and elevated liver enzymes. It was assumed that this was caused by the concurrent use of phenprocoumon and nonsteroidal anti-inflammatory drugs (NSAIDs). Not only on account of the liver damage, but also because the combined use of phenprocoumon and NSAIDs produces a dangerously high bleeding risk, the therapy was changed. Catheter PFO closure was recommended to replace phenprocoumon therapy.

The procedure was performed under deep sedation. Additionally the patient was administered 10.000 units of heparin. The right femoral vein was punctured and a 9F sheath inserted. The left atrium was probed with a multipurpose catheter and balloon sizing of the PFO measured 14 mm. The TEE showed a large PFO with a large atrial septal aneurysm. The implantation of a 23-mm BioSTAR occluder was performed without complications. Correct position was confirmed by fluoroscopy and TEE (Fig 24.21). After the device was released from the delivery cable, the device slid into the PFO tunnel. The device was caught with a snare, but during retrieval the occluder slipped off the catheter and remained in the external iliac vein (Figs 24.22–24.24). There it was caught again with a snare and finally removed (Fig 24.25). We then chose a 33-mm STARFlex occluder, which was implanted via an 11F sheath without any further complications. After a stable position was confirmed with fluoroscopy and TEE while performing a tug test, the occluder was released (Figs 24.26 and 24.27). The procedure was successfully completed after a total duration of 85 minutes.

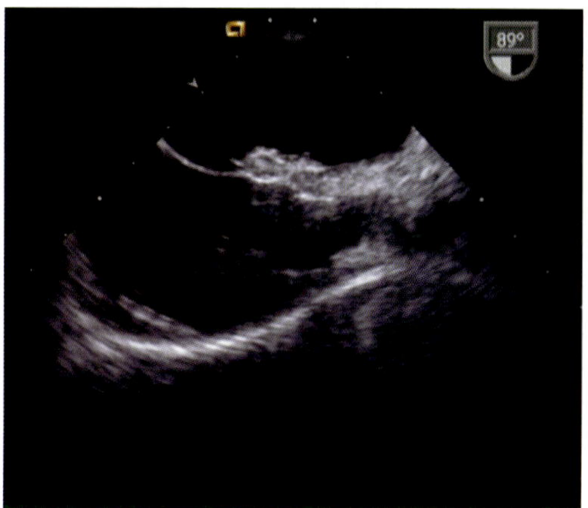

Fig 24.21—23-mm BioSTAR occluder in TEE long-axis view.

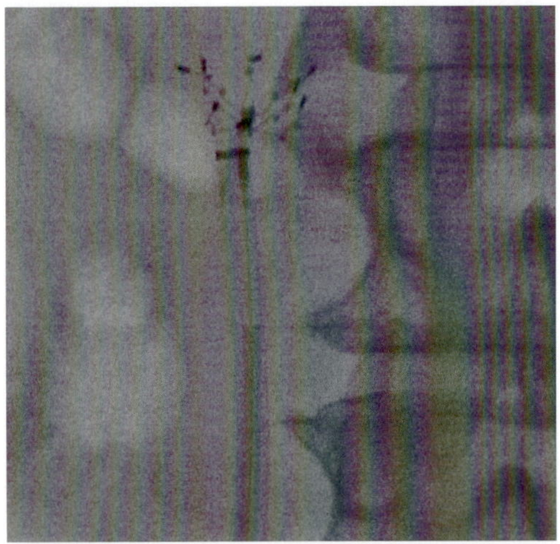

Fig 24.22—Retrieval of 23-mm BioSTAR occluder with snare catheter.

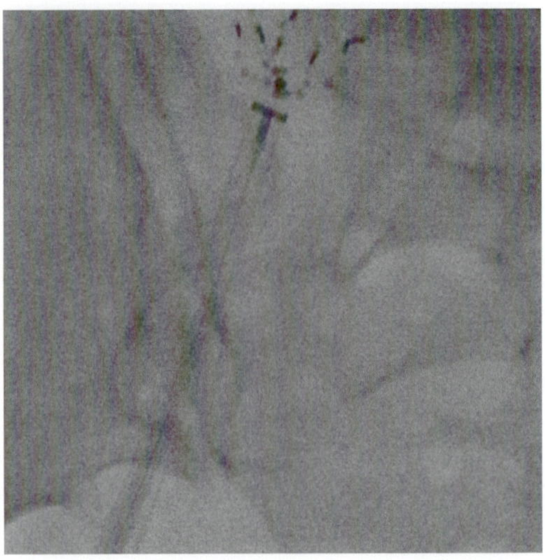

Fig 24.23—Retrieval continuing of 23-mm BioSTAR occluder with snare catheter.

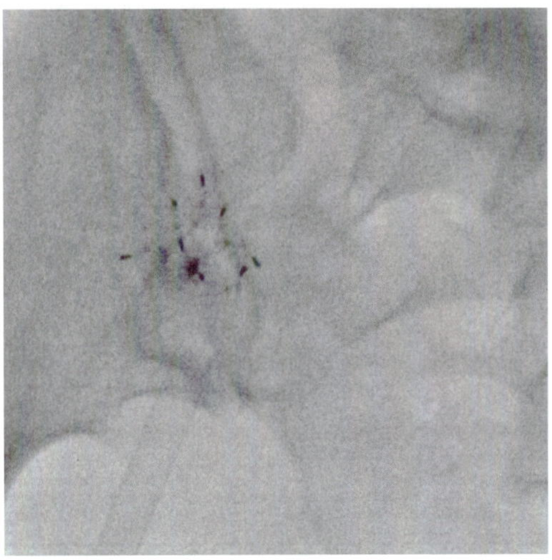

Fig 24.24—23-mm BioSTAR occluder in right femoral vein.

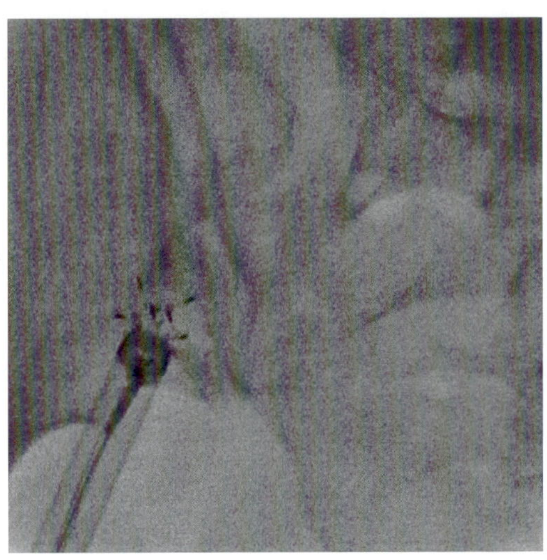

Fig 24.25—Final retrieval of 23-mm BioSTAR occluder.

During the observatory stay in the hospital, no complications occurred. The patient was discharged two days later. She was prescribed aspirin and clopidogrel. Later on, she experienced several episodes of atrial fibrillation without further consequences.

Discussion and Conclusion

Procedural complications in PFO closure are very rare. Nevertheless "easy" cases can still pose the potential of serious complications. Therefore one should be attentive to potential complications and be prepared to intervene and solve the tasks—at best via catheter in the same session.

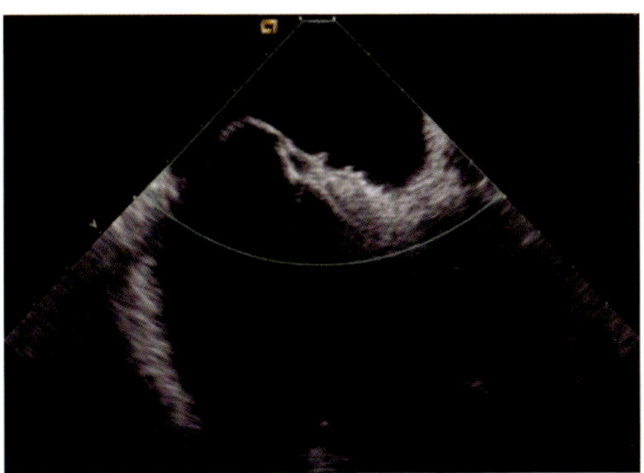

Fig 24.26—33-mm STARFlex occluder in TEE short-axis view.

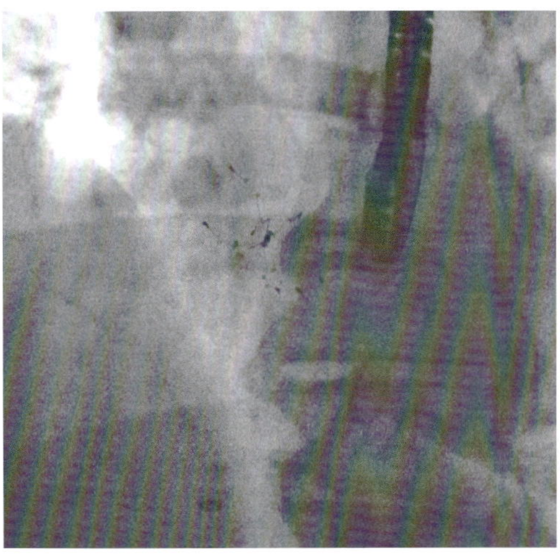

Fig 24.27—33-mm STARFlex occluder in projection onto the atrial septum.

One of the trickiest complications that can occur during PFO closure is embolization of the device. TEE is a very good imaging modality to confirm correct position of the device and to monitor even very minor changes. Screening the septum and the occluder carefully in multiple planes will reveal whether the device encompasses the septum correctly. Color Doppler may provide additional information about flow around the edge of the device as a hint of an unstable position.

In fluoroscopy one can verify whether the occluder grasps the septum correctly when contrast agent is injected via the delivery sheath.

It is important to screen and observe the occluder after the intervention is finished, because sometimes even perfectly deployed devices may slip and embolize as seen in Case 2.

When talking about imaging, it is worth mentioning that intracardiac echo (ICE) has very good abilities in monitoring these complications and is better tolerated by the patient. On the other hand it is often—depending upon the local situation and logistics—more expensive than TEE.

Case 1 shows an occluder that has embolized into the descending aorta and been covered with endothelium. If we had not succeeded in resolving the adhesion, the next step would have been to stent the obstruction caused by the device. If doing so, one has to keep in mind that the occluder underneath the stent means stress to the vessel at that particular point and may function as predetermined breaking point.

A very effective tool we used in all of the presented cases is a snare catheter. It is one of the tools one should have available in the catheterization laboratory (cath lab).

There are no predictors of embolization per se, but we have to point out that all of the patients presented had an atrial septal aneurysm in addition to the PFO. The occluders embolized were all of different designs. Therefore we cannot advise one particular occluder that should or should not be used in atrial septal aneurysms but rather motivate to evaluate every individual patient before, during, and after the procedure using appropriate imaging, especially when an atrial septal aneurysm is present.

PART IV

Devices

25

Engineering Aspects of Metallic and Bioabsorbable Devices

Carol A. Devellian, Stephanie M. Kladakis,

Steven W. Opolski, and John A. Wright Jr.

Introduction

The majority of septal occluders in use today are fabricated from a metallic framework and a polymeric tissue scaffold. Such devices have been shown to be quite effective at closing a variety of structural heart defects including atrial septal defect (ASD), ventricular septal defect (VSD), fenestrated fontan (FF), and patent foramen ovale (PFO).[1-8] Limitations include the development of allergic reactions,[9,10] arrhythmias,[6,11-13] embolizations,[14,15] erosions/perforations,[16-19] metal arm fractures,[20-22] residual leaks,[2,3,23,24] and thrombus.[25-27] Because the device remains in the patient forever, late complications (> 1 year) can occur.[22,28-40]

Several new technologies developed specifically for PFO closure have attempted to circumvent these potential complications by avoiding or limiting the amount of foreign material left in the heart. Such attempts include radiofrequency (RF) to weld the PFO flaps shut,[41-43] percutaneous suturing,[44,45] and in-the-tunnel designs,[46] which limit the exposure of foreign material to blood flow.

Recently, hybrid devices that combine a metal frame with a bioabsorbable tissue scaffold have been introduced. The objective is to minimize the amount of permanent foreign material and promote tissue remodeling and regeneration at the defect site.[47-53] Materials that promote tissue regeneration may be preferable alternatives over currently utilized permanent textiles which have been documented to elicit fibrous capsule formation and stimulate a chronic foreign body reaction when used for septal closure.[54] Bioabsorbable materials have the potential to avoid a chronic inflamma-

Transcatheter Closure of ASDs and PFOs: A Comprehensive Assessment. © 2010 Ziyad M. Hijazi, Ted Feldman, Mustafa H. Abdullah Al-Qbandi, and Horst Sievert, editors. Cardiotext Publishing, ISBN: 978-0-9790164-9-3.

tory response and promote the formation of a native-like septum.[50] Such native tissue may prove simpler to recross later in a patient's life if transseptal access to the left atrium is required for a procedure such as atrial ablation, left atrial appendage obliteration, or percutaneous mitral valve repair or replacement.[55]

Ideally, in the future, fully bioabsorbable septal occluders will be able to maintain the simple deliverability and functionality of the currently available permanent devices, but be designed to regenerate healthy native tissue and then go away completely, exhibiting no toxic behavior in the process.

The goal of this chapter is to review the design considerations and available materials for both metallic and bioabsorbable septal occluders.

Background

Understanding the history of septal occluder device design is extremely important prior to designing a new device. Design tends to be evolutionary in nature and changes are typically made to avoid functional limitations. It is important to learn from past experience including an understanding of the different designs, materials, and tissue scaffolds that have been utilized and their respective successes and failures.

Transcatheter closure of intracardiac defects was first described by King and Mills in 1976.[56] This device, comprised of two separate, rigid, stainless steel arm discs covered with polyester fabric and a locking catheter,[57] was used in only a few patients. In the late 1970s/early 1980s, William Rashkind, MD, developed the Rashkind PDA and ASD Umbrellas, both comprising stainless steel frames with polyurethane foam. The Rashkind PDA Umbrella (CR Bard, Billerica, Massachusetts) was the first double umbrella approach to defect closure and was utilized successfully in a large number of patients.[58] The Rashkind ASD device then evolved which was a six-arm, single disc

device that included hooks on alternating arms to anchor it on the septum and required a 16F sheath. Due to the hooks on the device, a centrally located ASD was required and there was no tolerance for misplacement. As a result, it was only used in a few patients. The Clamshell Septal Occluder (CR Bard, Billerica, Massachusetts), specifically designed for the cardiac septa, was subsequently developed by James Lock, MD.[21,59,60] The Clamshell was composed of a stainless steel frame and polyester fabric. Over the course of 4 years (1987–1991) approximately 1000 septal defects, primarily ASD and PFO, were treated until clinical trials were halted due to fracture of the metal arms.[21] This device eventually went through an extensive engineering redesign to reduce arm fractures and improve closure rates[61] and evolved into the CardioSEAL device (NMT Medical, Boston, Massachusetts), which became commercially available in late 1996.

Other devices emerged in the early 1990s that are also no longer on the market.[62] This includes the Das Angel Wings[63] (Microvena, Vadnais Heights, Minnesota), a Nitinol frame and polyester tissue scaffold; the ASDOS device[64] (Osypka, Grenzach-Wyhlen, Germany), a Nitinol frame and polyurethane film tissue scaffold; and the button device[65,66] (Custom Medical Devices, Amarillo, Texas), a stainless steel frame and a polyurethane foam tissue scaffold. Each of these devices was used in clinical trials, principally for ASD, with moderate success in terms of closure rates; however, they are no longer available due to complexity of use and a host of complications.[63,66-7]

Starting in the mid- to late-1990s, several new devices were introduced, most of which are still on the market today. Those commercially available via CE Mark at the time of writing are described in Table 25.1. Other devices in development include SeptRx (SeptRx), an in-the-tunnel device composed of Nitinol and polyester and BioTREK (NMT Medical, Boston, Massachusetts), a fully bioabsorbable device fabricated from a polymer, poly-4-hydroxybutyrate (P4HB).

Trade name	Manufacturer	Frame	Tissue Scaffold
AMPLATZER	AGA Medical (Plymouth, MN)	Nitinol	Polyester**
ATRIASEPT	Cardia (Eagan, MN)	Nitinol	Polyvinyl alcohol foam
BioSTAR	NMT Medical (Boston, MA)	MP35N*	Collagen
Figulla Occluder	Occlutech (Helsingborg, Sweden)	Nitinol	Polyester**
FlatStent	Coherex (Salt Lake City, Utah)	Nitinol	Polyurethane foam
HELEX	W.L. Gore (Flagstaff, AZ)	Nitinol	Expanded PTFE
Premere	St. Jude Medical (St. Paul, MN)	Nitinol	Polyester**
Solysafe	Swissimplant (Solothum, Switzerland)	Phynox	Polyester**
STARFlex	NMT Medical (Boston, MA)	MP35N*	Polyester**

Table 25.1—Currently Available Devices. *STARFlex and BioSTAR also incorporate a Nitinol centering spring. **Polyester refers to knits and other textiles made from polyethylene terephthalate (PET).

All of these implants (excluding BioTREK) are very similar in basic construction in that they contain a metallic framework—stainless steel, Nitinol, MP35N, or Phynox—and are covered with a tissue scaffold—polyester, expanded polytetrafluoroethylene (ePTFE), polyurethane or polyvinyl alcohol foam, or collagen. The metallic frame must be capable of being collapsed to travel through the femoral vein then re-expand within the heart, positioning the tissue scaffold across the defect. The tissue scaffold then promotes defect closure via tissue encapsulation (fibrous capsule) and endothelialization. In the case of BioSTAR, the tissue scaffold is bioabsorbable and promotes tissue remodeling and regeneration as opposed to the formation of a fibrous capsule.[50]

General Design Considerations

There are certain general considerations when designing a permanent cardiovascular implant. Specific to a septal occluder, the device is going to need to travel through a relatively small sheath, easily deploy within the cardiac chambers, close the hole, be durable enough to withstand stresses during the cardiac cycle for the patient's lifetime, and result in minimal adverse effects. It needs to be stiff enough to clamp onto the septum with adequate force to prevent leakage and embolization yet not so stiff as to result in erosion. It should be biologically active enough to promote quick and thorough tissue coverage and encapsulation yet not so thrombogenic or flow disruptive as to result in pathogenic thrombus formation.

The entire implantation procedure, including retrieval of the device, should be intuitive to avoid device damage and minimize patient risk. The implant and catheter system should be compatible with imaging systems to be used during the implantation procedure (ie, fluoroscopy and echocardiography). The implant should also be MR (magnetic resonance) safe. Other considerations include "designing in" competitive advantages, patent protection, freedom to operate without infringing existing intellectual property, development costs and timing, and manufacturability. And, of course, they need to be biocompatible, defined by Williams as "the ability of a material to perform with an appropriate response in a specific application."[72]

It is also important early in the design process to decide what type of septal defects will be the target of a new design. The device requirements to close atrial and/or ventricular septal defects can differ quite remarkably from the requirements for closure of a PFO, although in an ideal world one device can cover a wide range of defect morphologies. This is preferred to maximize the potential within the marketplace, to justify the development costs, to simplify life within the cardiac catheterization laboratory by limiting the number of device types and sizes that must be stocked, and to accelerate enroll-

ment in clinical trials by increasing the pool of patients eligible for the device and, therefore, the trial.

Because ASDs and VSDs are truly a "hole" and a PFO is usually a "flap" or tunnel, a one-device-fits-all approach is often not technically feasible. As outlined in Table 25.2, PFOs come in a wide range of shapes and sizes beyond the "simple" PFO (Fig 25.1) including long tunnels, thick or hypertrophic septum secundum, hypermobile or aneurysmal, and fenestrated variations.[48] Although centering mechanisms are typically desired for most ASD occluders,

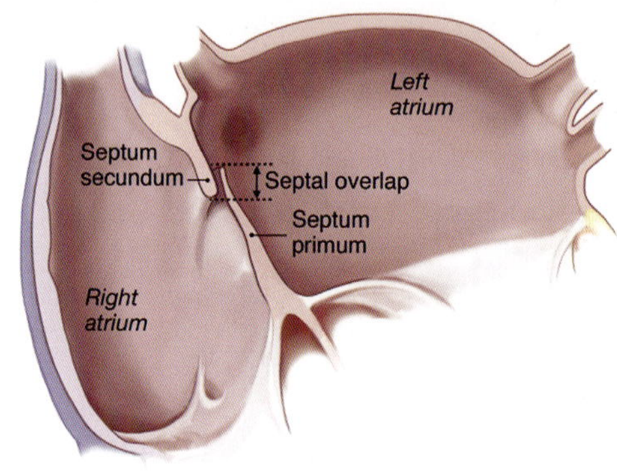

Fig 25.1—Diagram of a PFO. Reproduced from Expert Rev Med Devices. 2007;4(6):781–791 with permission of Expert Reviews Ltd.

Class	Characteristics
Simple PFO	Normal septum secundum (< 5 mm); septum primum overlap < 10 mm
Long tunnel PFO	Septum primum overlap ≥ 10 mm
PFO with thick or hypertrophic septum secundum	Thick septum secundum ≥ 6 mm Hypertrophic septum secundum ≥ 15 mm
PFO with hypermobile (floppy) septum primum/atrial septal aneurysm (ASA)	Total excursion of septum primum into left atrium and/or right atrium ≥ 10 mm
PFO associated with fenestrated septum primum	PFO combined with one or more tiny "pin-hole" shunts or small ASDs (defects of septum primum)

Table 25.2—PFO Morphological Classifications. Reproduced from *Expert Rev Med Devices*. 2007;4(6):781–791 with permission of Expert Reviews Ltd.

depending upon the type of centering mechanism, they may be beneficial or detrimental to safe and effective PFO closure.

Design Goals for the Ideal Septal Occluder

Although there may never be a septal occluder that meets all the criteria for an "ideal" device, all new designs should start with a lofty list of goals and objectives. Compromises are then inevitably made during the design process when certain objectives have an adverse relationship with a higher priority design objective, become overly technically challenging, too time consuming, cost prohibitive, or violate the laws of physics. Presented in Box 25.1 is a comprehensive list of objectives that most likely will

Immediate complete closure
Low complication rate
No permanent foreign material
Intuitive delivery
Easily retrievable and repositionable
No change to current procedure
Radiopaque and echogenic
Conformable and atraumatic
Low thrombogenicity
Minimizes size of insertion site
Minimizes risk of air introduction during all steps of procedure
Effective in most shapes and sizes of septal defects (ie, PFO, ASD, VSD, FF)
Does not require postimplant antiplatelet medications
Cost effective to manufacture
Infinite shelf life

Box 25.1—Characteristics of the Ideal Septal Occluder

never be met by a single device but provides a good starting point.

Traditional Approach: Permanent Metal Frames

The design goals for an ideal septal occluder are written after decades of design and clinical experience. In the infancy of septal repair, the concept of creating an "ideal" device was easily supplanted with creating a "workable" device. Now, after significant clinical experience demonstrating both robust safety and effectiveness, the workable device has begun to be replaced by more ideal devices and methods. Furthermore, one device design may be more appropriate for a specific anatomy than another.

It is common in new product development that engineers often iterate and expand based on prior experience. Twenty-five years ago when septal occluders were in their design infancy, a typical medical device engineer would have experience with common interventional devices and techniques of that era. Earlier work with metal guide wires afforded a familiarity and availability of fine wire, which lead to many early designs based on a wire framework. Vascular graft material became tissue scaffolds because of availability and knowledge that they worked clinically in the vascular environment. Sheaths, balloons, and catheters, which were typical tools of the interventionalist, were also incorporated based on availability and familiarity.

While familiarity with common materials and equipment of the era was advantageous for both engineers and interventionalists, it was also an advantage in the regulatory environment. Regulatory bodies are often learning about new materials, products, and techniques along with industry and physicians. The more a product is similar to existing clinically successful products, the easier the regulatory path. The more innovative a product, the higher and more numerous the regulatory hurdles. Sometimes revolutionary products are introduced after significant effort. More often though, products are evolutionary due to the less significant regulatory hurdles and decreased cost of development in both time and money.

Design considerations

Many septal occluders attempt to mimic what has been done for years by cardiac surgeons. It is known that when a patch of material is sutured on the septum, the body's natural healing response encourages tissue to grow into the material and permanently occlude the defect. Therefore, many designs use the approach of delivering a patch of material to the septum and holding it in place with a metal framework. Three examples of FDA-approved devices that use this approach are the AMPLATZER, HELEX, and STARFlex septal occluders. There are also numerous other devices with CE Mark available in Europe and other parts of the world as listed in Table 25.1.

There are several requirements for the material and the chosen design for which metals are a common and natural choice. The framework needs to have the flexibility to compress into a small delivery system and yet expand and hold a patch of scaffold material against the septum to promote healing. Typically there is a marriage of the design and the chosen material to achieve this objective. Rarely can the material be changed in a design without profound effects on the device performance. For example, the Nitinol framework material used in the AMP-LATZER could not be switched for the MP35N frame material used in the STARFlex. Neither the AMPLATZER nor the STARFlex would then perform properly. An AMPLATZER made from MP35N would not have the familiar self-expanding characteristic. Similarly, a STARFlex would expand but lack the stiffness to stay on the septum and resist dislodgment or embolization. Therefore, the material chosen is an integral part of the design for a properly functioning occluder and substitutions, even among metals, is often not possible.

Once the device is compressed and delivered to the targeted site, the metal framework needs to survive and cause no clinical sequelae. The components of the device must be biocompatible. Being biocompatible encompasses many issues over acute and chronic time frames for the life of the patient which could be many decades. There is a standard battery of tests that device materials are subjected to, which can demonstrate both short- and long-term biocompatibility.[73] Common materials that have demonstrated proven biocompatibility often require less testing and risk, whereas more novel or innovative materials with limited human use can require significantly more testing (and risk).

The framework also must hold the patch material against the septum long enough for the body to grow into the scaffold and heal the defect. After healing has occurred, the metal framework no longer provides a necessary function. However, the framework needs to cause no chronic clinical issues.

One requirement that is related to biocompatibility and is often discussed is corrosion resistance. A metal framework that corrodes in vivo can cause numerous problems. Device corrosion can cause a local adverse tissue response[9] as well as a variety of systemic responses.[10,74–79] Another possible effect of corrosion is loss of structural integrity or fracture of the metal framework. Fractures can also occur due to damage during implantation or due to cyclic fatigue following days, months, or years of in vivo stresses. Fracture occurring before tissue encapsulation may lead to device instability[20,80] or perforation/damage of surrounding cardiac structures.[81,82] Late fracture associated with thrombus has been reported.[22] Fractures occurring after complete tissue encapsulation often have no long-term clinical sequelae[21,83–86] although such occurrences should certainly be minimized. Therefore, fatigue and corrosion resistance are very important factors and both must be carefully assessed.

Earlier devices were designed when fluoroscopy was the primary means of imaging in the cardiac catheterization laboratory. This allowed for good device imaging but poor visualization of cardiac structures. Since the inception of transesophageal echocardiography (TEE) and intracardiac echocardiography (ICE), current and future devices must also be echogenic. Fortunately, the metal frameworks of current devices are all radiopaque to some degree. Marker bands of a higher radiopacity material are often used to augment the natural radiopacity in key locations. Most polished metal is not particularly echogenic but can be treated or coated to increase its echogenicity. All tissue scaffolds are not radiopaque but are often echogenic. Therefore, between fluoroscopy and TEE/ICE, most of the device and surrounding heart tissue can be imaged effectively.

MRI is becoming an increasingly important imaging modality. Although some experimental work has been conducted using MR-guided placement of septal occluders,[87–89] the most common concern is patient safety if an MRI is conducted after placement of a metal implant. At the very least, septal occluders should ideally be nonferromagnetic which means they should not be attracted to a magnet. However, even a device that is nonferromagnetic may distort or disrupt the magnetic field and affect the resulting image in the immediate vicinity of the device. With the increasing use of MRI for cardiac imaging, the concept of MR safety for septal occluders is taking on new and more restrictive meaning so as to not compromise the quality of future MR imaging scans. Based upon FDA guidelines introduced in 2008, labeling going forth will state a product is "MR Conditional," as opposed to "MR Safe," meaning it is safe only at the conditions under which it was tested.[90,91]

There are a series of other design requirements that must also be addressed. The device needs to be manufacturable in a reasonable amount of time and with an acceptable cost of goods. While manufacturability is not often discussed, it is essential for a viable, commercial product. Similarly, some level of patent protection is often needed. Very large investments are typically required to produce a regulatory-approved product, especially if a clinical trial is warranted. Patent protection helps protect the ability to recoup prior investment costs and also fund future investments in next-generation products.

Available materials

Stainless steel alloys

There are > 100 types of stainless steel alloys. These are defined as iron-based metals that contain at least 10.5% chromium.[92] Although no currently available septal occluders use stainless steel as the main framework material, it was used in some early generation devices such as the Clamshell and the Sideris Button device. Stainless steel types 304 and 316 have a long history of use outside septal repair and have been applied to both temporary and permanent implants such as devices for orthopedic fracture fixation,[93] stents,[94] embolic coils,[95] and aneurysm clips.[96] As shown in Table 25.3, the major constitutive elements of 316 stainless are chromium, nickel, iron, and molybdenum. The purpose of adding molybdenum to 316 (when compared to 304) is to increase the corrosion resistance through modification of the surface passive film. 316 stainless is considered a standard for comparison when performing evaluations for implantation biocompatibility and corrosion resistance. Stainless steels are low cost, have good strength and ductility, and come in an array of stock configurations. They can be processed by a variety of fabrication techniques, such as wire and tube drawing, laser cutting and machining, and are amenable to surface enhancement technologies. One disadvantage is that they contain iron and are therefore ferromagnetic, which may generate artifacts during MR imaging.[97] They are also susceptible to certain types of localized corrosive attack, especially when comparing 304 to 316. A typical reference for implant grade stainless steel is ASTM F138.[98]

Cobalt-based alloys

MP35N (Multiphase 35% Nickel) is a cobalt-based alloy utilized for the framework in the CardioSEAL, STARFlex, and BioSTAR septal occluders. MP35N comprises cobalt, chromium, molybdenum, and nickel as outlined in Table 25.3. MP35N has good ductility and formability, high strength, excellent corrosion resistance under stress, high fatigue strength in corrosive media, and is nonferromagnetic.[99,100] If the alloy is subjected to cold work, a heat treatment process will further increase strength and a combination of the two may be used as part of device fabrication to generate the desired mechanical properties. MP35N has been utilized in stents,[101] pacemaker leads,[102] aneurysm clips,[96,103] and reconstructive orthopedic applications.[104] A typical reference for the use of MP35N in implant applications is ASTM F562.[105]

Phynox, also known as Elgiloy, is another cobalt-based alloy used in septal repair, specifically in the Solysafe Septal Occluder. As defined in Table 25.3, the major elements are cobalt, chromium, iron, nickel, and molybdenum. This material provides a combination of high strength, ductility, and good mechanical properties. The presence of iron means that Phynox is ferromagnetic and may cause interference during MR imaging, especially at high field strengths.[103] However, in certain applications it has demonstrated acceptable MR safety.[96,106] Similar to MP35N, this alloy is age hardenable for additional strength after cold working, has excellent fatigue life, and good corrosion resistance.[106,107] A typical reference for the use of Phynox in implant applications is ASTM F1058.[108]

Nitinol alloys

An array of nickel and titanium alloys with unique properties were developed at the U.S. Naval Ordinance Laboratory (NOL) in 1959 and named Nitinol to reflect the main constitutive elements (nickel and titanium) and this location (NOL).[109,110] As shown in Table 25.3, this alloy is generally composed of 55/45 weight percent nickel/titanium. Small variances in this balance can lead to dramatic changes in transition temperature and hence the properties and performance of the material. Subsequent processing of Nitinol can also modify the transformation temperatures, mechanical properties,

and surface conditions, all of which the designer needs to define. Nitinol has excellent flexibility and kink resistance, good corrosion resistance, and is nonferromagnetic.[111] It is a unique material due to its shape memory properties in that it can withstand large deformations (strain) with minimal permanent shape change and elicit a high recovery force. The shape modification, dependent upon a phase change from martensite to austenite, results from an atomic rearrangement within the material and can be either driven by stress or temperature. With superelastic memory, the transformation is controlled mechanically by stress and the material exhibits springy, almost "rubberlike" deformation behavior. The superelastic form has been used extensively in medical device development such as guide wires. In thermal shape memory, a desired transition temperature can be preprogrammed and the desired shape set at a high temperature, resulting in a shape change at a lower temperature, such as body temperature. Nitinol, in both the thermal shape memory and superelastic embodiments, is utilized in many septal occluders, including the AMPLATZER, HELEX, and Occlutech devices, to name a few. Refer to Table 25.1 for a comprehensive list. It is the alloy also used as the centering spring component in the STARFlex and BioSTAR septal occluders and has a history of use for stents,[112] vena cava filters,[113,114] bone anchors,[115] and staples.[116] Its extensive use within the medical device industry has helped precipitate the formation of standards which are also referenced within FDA guidance documents pertaining to its chemistry[117] and transition temperature determination.[118,119]

Radiopaque alloys

To aid fluoroscopic visualization during implantation, several septal occluders include radiopaque markers. The radiopacity level is based on the material alloy or compound type, its inherent density, mass absorption coefficient, and thickness.[120] The importance of radiopaque markers has become less of an issue due to the advancements in fluoroscopic imaging equipment resolution as well as the introduction of

	316 Stainless Steel	MP35N	Phynox	Nitinol
Cobalt (Co)	—	35	40	—
Chromium (Cr)	18	20	20	—
Iron (Fe)	65	—	17	—
Molybdenum (Mo)	3	10	7	—
Nickel (Ni)	14	35	16	55
Titanium (Ti)	—	—	—	45

Table 25.3—Primary Element Compositions (Approximate Weight %)

ICE and TEE imaging during the implantation procedure. Radiopaque markers on septal occluders are commonly a platinum-based alloy (eg, 90 weight %, 10% Iridium). Adding platinum increases the product cost as well as the complexity of preclinical testing due to the possible need to conduct galvanic corrosion studies. The inherent properties of platinum allow very thin (< 0.004" thick) markers to be easily fabricated and provide adequate radiopacity while not significantly adding to the implant's delivery profile. Other alloys and elements including gold[121] and tantulum[122] have been utilized although almost any metal/alloy can be viewed fluoroscopically (ie, stainless steel, MP35N, and Nitinol) if there is enough material thickness. Platinum-based alloy markers are incorporated in the AMPLATZER (distal tip) and on the tip of each arm of the STARFlex and BioSTAR. The Nitinol frames of the Premere and Coherex FlatStent are enhanced by the addition of radiopaque markers located at the tip of each arm. The Solysafe frame, composed of Phynox, also employs radiopaque markers to achieve adequate fluoroscopic visualization.

Durability/fatigue

Durability evaluation of a septal occluder is a major hurdle during the design process. While the term *durability* often implies a long time period and is often associated with fatigue, in reality, durability testing encompasses both short and long time periods. This includes the ability of the device to withstand the stresses imparted during the implantation procedure as well as longer term in vivo.

Fatigue is a common potential failure mode for many metal objects. Fatigue implies a *repeated cycling* of a force or motion on an object. To illustrate, think of a basic metal paper clip. One can grasp the paper clip and open it 180° so the two ends will be facing away from each other. The clip will stay in that new configuration because of the significant amount of deformation to the metal in the hinged region. For most paper clips, they will not break into two parts and the clip can be folded back to its original position and still perform as a paper clip. If this process is repeated, many paper clips will fail before ten repetitions are finished. In this instance, the paper clip has failed due to fatigue but more specifically, high stress/low cycle fatigue. High stress because of the significant deformation or stress in the hinge region and low cycle because of a low number of repetitive cycles.

This analogy can be used to help explain septal occluder durability. Most septal occluders are compressed into a small catheter and then allowed to expand in the body at the intended location during delivery. This is analogous to the single back-and-forth bend of the paper clip. Most septal occluders also have some ability to be retrieved and reused if malpositioned initially. As the occluder is retrieved back into its sheath or delivery system before being expanded again, this is analogous to the repeated back-and-forth motion imparted on the paper clip. Like the paper clip, the occluder is often subjected to its highest stress or deformation during the delivery and retrieval cycle for only a small number of cycles. Unlike the paper clip, the occluder must not fracture or become weakened after this small number of cycles.

Therefore, part of the durability evaluation consists of directly subjecting devices to multiple simulated delivery and retrieval cycles. This is one way occluders are tested for high stress/low cycle fatigue. One outcome from this testing is a recommended maximum number of delivery and retrieval cycles that a particular device can be subjected to and still perform properly.

Thinking about the paper clip again, the deflection imparted in the initial example was fairly extreme and was roughly 180° in one direction and then 180° back in the opposite direction. If the deflection imparted is less, for example 90°, the number of cycles the paper clip will survive before fracture would be larger, such as 50. Reduce the deflection even more and the paper clip may survive for thousands of cycles. This scenario is commonly referred to as a low stress/high cycle fatigue. While the deflection, deformation, or stress is significantly reduced from previous values, the number of repeating cycles has also significantly increased. Finally, reducing the deflection more will allow the paper clip to survive for millions of cycles and often for an infinite number of cycles. Therefore, the fatigue limit for the paper clip may be described as being the deflection level (and below) that will never break the part even after millions of repeated cycles.

Figure 25.2 illustrates a typical fatigue response curve for an object such as a paper clip or a septal occluder. The left axis displays the amount of repeated stress (or deformation)

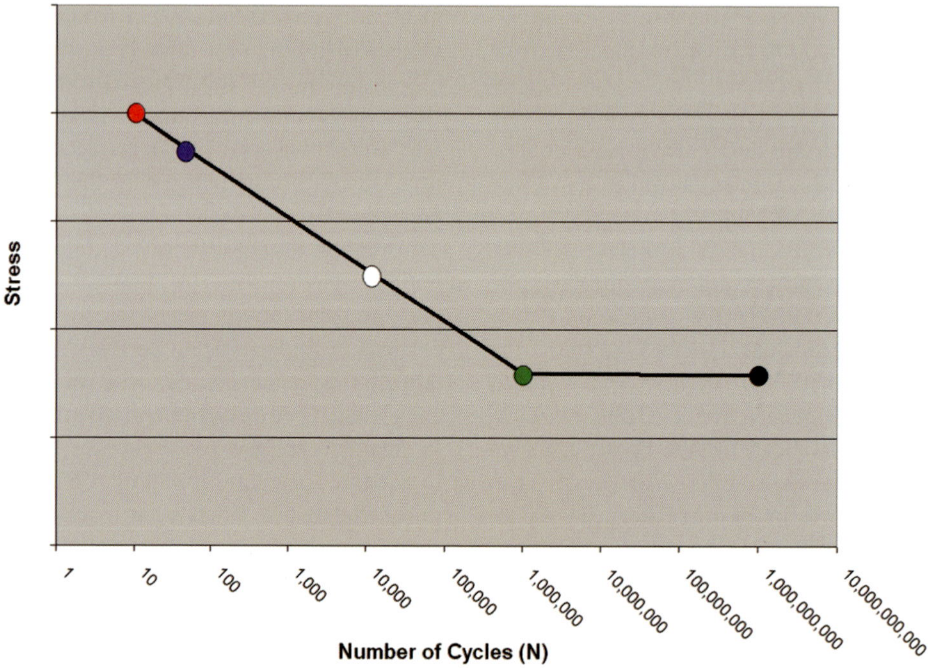

Fig 25.2—Typical metal fatigue graph

imparted to the test object. The bottom axis displays the number of cycles a given stress (or deformation) is imparted to the test object. One should note that the bottom axis is typically a log scale.

To illustrate by example, the paper clip could be characterized with a graph as shown in Fig 25.2. The red point near the top left is a high stress with low cycle fatigue fracture point. This point is the case in which the paper clip is bent back and forth nearly 180° repeatedly to fracture. The graph shows a fracture after 10 cycles at a high stress level. The blue point is for a lower stress value but a much higher number of cycles such as 50. The green point is for an even lower stress level with an even higher number of cycles. Lastly, the black point is for a stress level that is very close to the green level but with a huge number of cycles and the paper clip in this case did not fracture. Essentially, this is the fatigue limit (also called endurance limit) for the paper clip and is the stress point where the part will not fracture, even after an infinite number of repeated cycles.

Many metallic objects have been tested to millions of cycles with no failures. Typically, once a metal object can withstand one million repeated cycles without a fatigue fracture, the device will not fracture after an infinite number of fatigue cycles.[123] Because septal occluders are permanent implants and experience low stress/high cycle fatigue because of their placement in a beating heart, they are typically designed for infinite fatigue life. They are usually tested for 400 million cycles representing 10 years of real life, similar to cardiac stents. Although the testing is typically accelerated, it can still take many months to complete.

In addition to direct fatigue testing, devices are typically analyzed using computer-modeling techniques. Finite element analysis (FEA) is used to not only model the geometry and materials but also the forces or deflections applied to the device during the manufacturing process, delivery process, and a lifetime in vivo. Over the last 2 decades, computer modeling has made enormous strides in capabilities. Early modeling was limited often to small sec-

tions of devices even with powerful computers of the day. Today, modeling of entire devices simulating the interaction with common heart structures is quite common. Typically, the biggest unknowns for computer modeling are the many and varied in vivo conditions.

FEA is often first used in the design phase to screen possible designs before making a time-consuming and costly prototype. The screening may be used to select the best design based on certain performance criteria. The modeling may also look at the deformations or stresses within the structure to address common questions. For example, to determine the smallest possible sheath size a septal occluder can be compressed into for delivery, FEA can be used to determine whether it will recoil fully once released. It can also be used to determine whether the device has the strength to remain on the septum when subjected to the various forces and pressures common to the in vivo environment as well as to determine whether the motion of the heart will cause the structure to fatigue and break.

Computer modeling and direct testing often complement each other during the product development cycle. Computer modeling continues to get better and more capable but cannot replace all direct testing. Although direct testing often remains the gold standard, it is costly, time consuming, and often provides only a fail/no fail result. While valuable, a "failure" often will not indicate why the part failed and a "no failure" often will not indicate how close the part came to failing. Therefore, computer modeling and direct testing continue to both be used and complement each other.

One part of a durability assessment that can be challenging is how to deal with wear between various parts of the device. Metal devices, or components of devices, that contact or cross over one another can and do rub on each other due to the cyclic motion of the heart. This rubbing can cause damage to the surface oxide and release of metal ions/particles. This can affect the corrosion rate and the effective fatigue life of the device. Typically, a device is assessed for this type of durability as part of in vitro fatigue testing in a simulated heart environment.

Corrosion

As part of the design process for any metallic implant, the in vivo electrochemical response, also referred to as corrosion susceptibility, must be evaluated. Corrosion can be defined as the interaction of a material with an aqueous environment generating a deleterious affect on that material. "Uncontrolled" corrosion can lead to premature device failure due to a structural breakdown. Corrosion can also affect the biocompatibility of an implant due to release of metal ions/particles. The use of traditional metallic materials focuses on inhibiting the corrosion process and trying to make a device resistant to breaking down in the body's saltwaterlike environment. Future metallic devices, applying designer corrosion profiles, such as with the Biotronik (Berlin, Germany) magnesium alloy stent, apply the corrosive mechanism as a positive design attribute. This concept of "biocorrosion" was also studied by Peuster and colleagues in evaluating a stent fabricated from pure iron that demonstrated no evidence of systemic or local toxicity due to corrosion products in minipig descending aorta for up to 12 months.[124] Biocorrosion was also observed, albeit unexpectedly, when tungsten alloy-based embolization coils were found to corrode and reallow vessel patency as well as produce elevated tungsten serum levels.[125-128] Fortunately, no toxicity was noted. Bioabsorbable polymers, discussed later in the chapter, could also be argued to incorporate a potentially more elegant biocompatible version of corrosion.

Corrosion is constantly occurring. Some corrosion is desired, such as in the protection of a domestic hot water tank through use of a magnesium rod which, until the rod is consumed, corrodes preferentially by galvanic corrosion to protect the steel water holding tank.[129] On a very macroscopic scale, everyone recognizes that painting the metal surface of a ship or bridge prolongs service life by providing a barrier to corrosive attack. For a metallic cardiovascular implant, designed to last a lifetime, repairing or replacing components of the structure with a maintenance schedule obviously is not practical. A desirable material property for longer in vivo stability is to produce a material that corrodes via "passive" dissolution. The *ASM Handbook* (Volume 13) defines *passivation/passivity* as "changing of a chemically active surface of a metal to a much less reactive state/a condition in which a piece of metal, because of an impervious covering of oxide or other compound, has a potential much more positive than that of the metal in the active state."[130] Simply, the presence of a passive film provides a barrier to corrosive attack. When this passive layer is damaged, the metal can be susceptible to an increase in the rate of corrosion/metal ion dissolution.

To promote a desirable metal surface that has a stable and defined passive dissolution response with minimal ion release, engineering design and evaluation is focused on promoting the growth of a specific oxide on the metal, introducing a mechanical or electrochemical polishing technique to the raw material or device, or applying a coating to the final device. One example of surface oxide differences can be seen by the visual appearance of some common but similar septal occluders. It's interesting to compare an AMPLATZER, with its grayish color, to a Figulla occluder, with its shiny gold color. Both devices use Nitinol woven basket frameworks but with very different appearances due to the difference in surface oxide.

Depending on the design of a specific implant and the material(s) used, there are many different types of corrosion that must be considered in the design process. One needs to first look at the types that will potentially accelerate a local area attack on the structure and compromise functionality.[131] One type of localized corrosion is pitting corrosion, which can be initiated at surface imperfections or localized breakdown of the passive layer and, as the name implies, creates a deep pit (Fig 25.3). Crevice corrosion can be caused by a space created due to overlap of two materials (a narrow crack or opening), which then alters the environment in that confined area. Fretting corrosion can be caused by dynamic metal-to-metal contact resulting in surface wear that damages the pas-

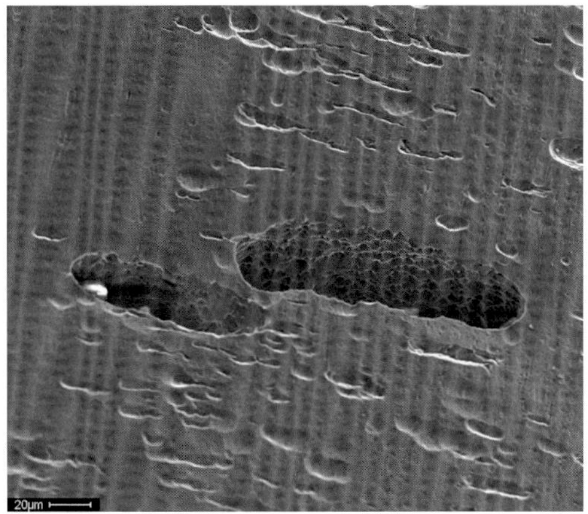

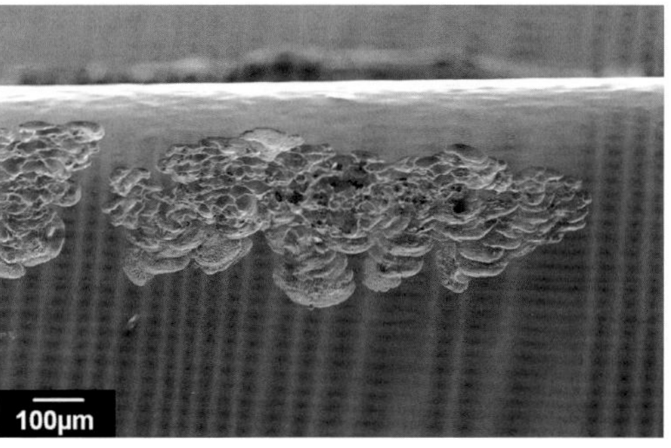

Fig 25.3—Pitting in CP4 titanium (Left) and Nitinol (Right, above). (Nitinol image courtesy of Exponent, Inc., Natick, Massachusetts.)

sive layer and may also create particles. And, lastly, galvanic corrosion can be caused by dissimilar metals in contact. Examples of this are radiopaque markers of one material attached to a metal framework of a different material or two different metal devices implanted in contact or close proximity. For example, Kong et al reported on an AMPLATZER device that showed pitting of the titanium oxide layer when examined after it had been in contact with a platinum pacemaker electrode, presumably due to a galvanic interaction.[132] Fortunately, there was no structural or clinical significance.

In addition to localized forms of corrosion, material corrosion susceptibility must also be studied. To aid in the material selection as well as to assess the impact of manufacturing processes, test methods have been defined and also recommended within FDA guidance documents to characterize corrosion susceptibility of devices and help define the metal/device passive region, where applicable.[133,134] Ideally, knowledge of the in vivo loading conditions must also be leveraged because a corrosive mechanism in combination with an applied load typically will cause greater structural degradation and less service life than if these factors were tested independently. Figure 25.4 is a fatigue response curve that demonstrates how a material that shows the presence of an endurance limit in an air environment can fail in a corrosive environment, such as the body.[135] The lower curve represents the combined effects

of corrosion and fatigue. Testing can be done to help mitigate and understand this failure mechanism. The implant design can be challenged for corrosion fatigue (CF) susceptibility, as it is now common place for engineers to test final implants (eg, stents, septal occluders) in phosphate-buffered saline solution at 37°C with anatomical location specific loads/deflections being applied. Alternatively, if the load is statically applied and the structure is placed within a corrosive environment, the potential for stress corrosion cracking (SCC) could occur. CF and SCC failure mechanisms are complex and surprisingly can occur at relatively low stresses, typically within the materials' elastic range. When the crack propagates through the structure due to the local environment combined with the load, final failure will occur when the cross-sectional area has been sufficiently reduced such that the material no longer has the strength to maintain the load. Both of these failure concepts, if and when they do occur, are implant-specific and based on electrochemical, mechanical loading, and metallurgical and microstructural specifics.

The alloys used today in septal occluders have the inherent properties to provide acceptable corrosion resistance in the blood environment. However, this corrosion resistance can be enhanced or adversely influenced by any number of factors such as the design, materials selected and their oxides, surface areas and finish, and the processes subjected to during

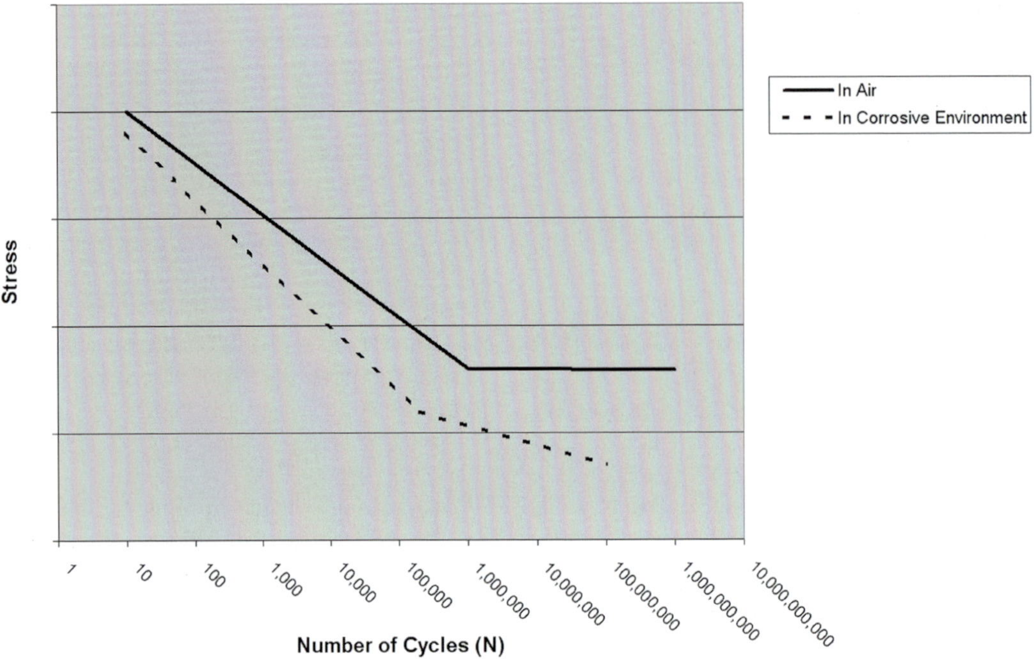

Fig 25.4—Typical S-N curve including corrosion fatigue.

manufacturing. Corrosion enhancement features, such as the surface finish or oxide, can be interrelated with biocompatibility by inhibiting the release of metal ions and by promoting a cell-friendly surface.[136,137]

Metal ion release

Due to corrosion mechanisms, all metallic implants release metal ions at some rate and will therefore be a source of both local and systemic trace metals. The dose/response relationship is unknown and most likely site-specific. Individual responses may vary dramatically. In conjunction with the corrosion evaluation, the toxicity of metal ion leaching should be part of the analysis to specifically address questions regarding what ions can leach into the body and at what rate, the form of these corrosion products, and the potential clinical implications. Controlling the type and rate of corrosion is critical for any implant as degradation can lead to device failure prior to appropriate healing and/or local or systemic toxicity can occur depending on metal ion type and particle size. Preclinical in

vivo engineering studies can be conducted to assess metal ion presence in blood, urine, and tissue. Microscopic evaluation, via scanning electron techniques or others, of a device post in vitro testing or explantation to inspect the device for structural integrity/corrosion degradation can provide invaluable data. In theory, until proven otherwise, engineers should consider all metal ions to be of concern and work to produce designs that minimize their release. The challenge becomes that the constitutive elements of the most commonly used framework materials have the potential for toxic behavior[137-148]—chromium, cobalt, molybdenum, and most notably, nickel—as discussed in the next section.

Nickel allergy

Nickel hypersensitivity is quite common, occurring in 10% to 15% of the population[149-152] and the incidence appears to be increasing.[153] Because it is well known that all metals in contact with biological systems will corrode[143] and that nickel ions leached in sufficient quantities from nickel-containing alloys may induce nickel sensitization,[147] it is important in the design process to choose materials, create designs, and develop processes that will minimize the amount of metal ions released from an implant. An important point to remember when designing is that it is not the alloy itself that causes such reactions but rather the nature of the alloy.[146] The nature of the alloy and how it is used in a device will affect the release rates under normal use. As discussed previously, these rates should be kept to a minimum under conditions of passive dissolution and avoid localized types of corrosion mechanisms such as pitting corrosion (initiated at surface imperfections or localized breakdown of the passive layer), galvanic corrosion (due to material mismatch), fretting corrosion (due to rubbing of two metals), or crevice corrosion (due to crevices where physiological fluid can be stagnant).[131] Although nickel is the allergen that is the most often discussed, this is true for other metal ions, such as cobalt, chromium, and molybdenum.[138–146] In a study conducted by Koster and colleagues, patients with allergic patch-test reactions to nickel and molybdenum had a higher frequency of in-stent restenosis within stainless steel stents than did patients without hypersensitivity.[142]

These basic guidelines for minimizing metal ion release from implants are of particular importance for devices in direct blood contact. Blood contacting metallic implants can induce a systemic response and there have been numerous publications on the topic of nickel allergy and septal occluders.[9,10,74–79,132,154–158] Increased nickel levels have been observed in both serum and urine samples from patients[154,156] and systemic allergic reactions have been observed.[10,74–79] These reactions have been associated with a wide range of symptoms including rash, chest discomfort or pain, palpitations, dyspnea, high-grade fever, edema, and migraine headache. In one case, a localized pericardial reaction resulting in pericarditis, atrial fibrillation, and migraine headache was observed.[9] Symptoms can sometimes be treated medically, using corticosteroids such as prednisone, with or without additional antiplatelet medication,[9,10,77,79] although severe cases have required surgical explantation.[74,76,78] If the desire is to eventually design septal occluders that are virtually complication-free, then sensitivity reactions are a problem as they are hard to diagnose and in the worst cases, can require the surgical procedure they have been developed to avoid. Fortunately, the incidence appears to be fairly low and by choosing the proper device for high-risk patients, physicians can avoid this type of complication. There have been several publications demonstrating the successful use of septal occluders in patients with known nickel sensitivity.[52,157–159]

Going forth, there are new technologies to treat the surface of nickel-containing alloys with a variety of coatings. While the objective would be to minimize dissolution rates, this needs to be done with great caution to avoid creating areas where corrosion can initiate (ie, a crevice) if the coating integrity is breached. Fully polymeric devices, by their nature "metal free," may also be advantageous as a means of treating nickel-sensitive patients.

Future Approach: Bioabsorbable Frames

Much has been written about the long-term goal of fully bioabsorbable implants for cardiovascular applications and in recent years, bioabsorbable stents have made significant progress.[160–163] The desire for bioabsorbable septal occluders has also been discussed although until recently, with the commercial introduction of BioSTAR and the development of BioTREK, minimal progress had been made. Septal closure devices with bioabsorbable tissue scaffolds have the potential to regenerate functional tissue as opposed to scar tissue, avoid the presence of a chronic foreign body reaction,[50,164] and allow simpler transseptal access to the left atrium for future interventions.[55] *Fully* bioabsorbable septal occluders, which contain no permanent components, should provide these benefits as well as a decreased risk of long-term complications when compared to their metallic counterparts (ie, late erosion), potential improvements in MR safety (heating and artifact), and no risk of nickel allergy.

Design considerations

Bioabsorbable materials, in general, have several key limitations for use as replacement materials for metals in existing designs. They tend to be lower in strength, lack inherent radiopacity, have been known to elicit a rather robust foreign body reaction,[165,166] and come with a risk of embolization of the fragments and particulate that will inevitably develop as part of the absorption process. This lack of inher-

ent strength, when compared to metals, makes simply switching a polymer for a metal—in the same design—impossible. Completely new designs, which take into account the strength and elasticity properties of the polymer, need to be developed. That being said, by using creativity in the design process and incorporating novel technologies and materials, a safe and effective, totally absorbable septal occluder is most likely achievable.

The critical design considerations for a bioabsorbable septal occluder are outlined in Table 25.4. These include mechanical properties as required for implant deliverability, functionality, and durability; bulk and surface biocompatibility including acceptable metabolism and clearance of degradation by-products; bioacceptability which encompasses a con-

Property	Requirements
Mechanical properties	Implant deliverability, functionality, and durability
Bulk biocompatibility	Low inflammatory response Metabolism and clearance of degradation by-products
Surface biocompatibility	Acceptable thrombogenicity Quick rate of encapsulation and endothelialization
Bioacceptability	Conformance to septal anatomy Low potential to cause trauma (erosion/perforation) Minimize flow disturbance within cardiac chambers
Deliverability/ergonomics	Ease of use/intuitiveness Retrievability and repositionability
Resorption profile	Acceptable time to strength and mass loss No potential to embolize fragments
Imaging	Radiopacity/echogenicity/MR safety
Manufacturability	Reproducible and cost effective Minimal damage due to sterility process Package protects device from moisture

Table 25.4—Design Considerations for Bioabsorbable Septal Occluders.

formable and atraumatic design; ease of use; resorption profile; imaging compatibility; and manufacturability. The objectives are, in general, similar to those of any septal occluder although the challenges are often greater (eg, radiopacity, inherent for many metals, requires additional creativity with bioabsorbable materials). In designing a bioabsorbable implant, it is important to also consider the added hurdle of strength loss with time due to the resorption process and safe elimination of degradation by-products. Also, significant effort should be focused on promoting thromboresistance and quick endothelialization, which can depend upon the tissue scaffold architecture and may require the use of biological response modifiers.

Challenges faced when "replacing" metals with bioabsorbable materials

Three properties need to be understood when deciding to design a new device and, in particular, when trying to understand the challenges that will be encountered when trying to "replace" metals with polymers. These properties are stiffness, strength, and elasticity.

Stiffness is essentially the amount of resistance to deformation. It is related to both the material as well as the shape of the part. Some materials are inherently stiffer than other materials. For example, most metals are much stiffer than most plastics. But, by changing the shape and size, even a plastic part can have as high or even higher stiffness than a metal part. Therefore, a plastic part consequently often needs to be thicker to have the same stiffness as a metal part. Stiffness is important with many septal occluders because resistance to embolization is directly related to device stiffness. Devices that exhibit a less stiff response tend not to squeeze the septum as much and are more likely to be dislodged due to various forces applied in vivo. They may also be prone to residual leaks.

The second key property is strength, which can be thought of as resistance to breakage. While stiffness is resistance to deformation, strength has to do with failure but nothing directly to do with stiffness. Strength is related

to both the type of material and also the amount. To make a septal occluder stronger, one would tend to use metals with thicker metals being stronger. However, like many things, there are limits and trade-offs. Making a device stronger may also sacrifice other important properties or features it needs to possess such as being atraumatic to the heart tissue.

The third key property is elasticity, which can be defined as resistance to permanent deformation. Something that is elastic can deform and recoil back to its original shape without taking a different shape such as becoming bent and distorted. Septal occluders are typically required to respond elastically within a significant range of motion. They need to fold or compress into relatively small catheters and then expand onto the septum. Therefore, a common feature to current septal occluders is that they are relatively elastic and they properly function due to high elasticity.

Working knowledge of stiffness, strength, and elasticity, is useful to understand existing septal occluder designs. For example, the STARFlex device has a framework made from MP35N, which is a high strength cobalt-based alloy. The stiffness (resistance to deformation) of the material is also quite high. This is apparent in Fig 25.5 because it takes a high force to create only a small amount of deformation. MP35N breaks at a high force so it has high strength. Lastly, the elastic deformation (resistance to permanent deformation) extends to about 1.5% before eventually breaking at about 2% deformation. As the material for the STARFlex has a limited amount of elastic deformation capacity, the design of the device must use a series of coil springs along the length to accommodate the required elastic deformation required by the device to compress into a delivery sheath and expand fully in vivo. So, while the material by itself is not very elastic, the design of the device (coil springs) allows the overall device to respond elastically over a considerable range.

A stainless steel balloon-expandable stent is a common cardiovascular device. Although each design differs, the basic annealed stainless steel material is quite similar. As illustrated in Fig 25.5, the stiffness at small deformations is very similar to MP35N as it follows that same curve up to almost 5 on the force scale. This initial stiff region also defines the elastic region. Up to approximately 0.2%, the annealed stainless steel responds elastically but after that point, the material permanently deforms to a level that is off the displayed graph. The strength (resistance to breakage) of this material is at a fairly low force but also after a significant amount of deformation. This is a very good material choice for a balloon expandable stent because it allows expansion with relatively low force and the stent deforms without elastically recoiling a significant amount. If the MP35N illustrated was used for a balloon expandable stent, it would require much higher pressures to expand and then once expanded, the stent would tend to elastically recoil much more. This recoil would leave a stent that is likely smaller in diameter than desired.

The third material is Nitinol, which is a nickel-titanium alloy commonly used in self-expanding stents and several septal occluders such as the AMPLATZER and HELEX devices. As previously discussed in this chapter, Nitinol can be configured to respond as either a thermal shape memory or super elastic alloy. However, once above a particular temperature, the two different Nitinol types essentially respond in a similar manner. Figure 25.5 shows this unusual, general characteristic of Nitinol, specifically its extended elastic response compared with most other metals. Initially, Nitinol is only about one-third as stiff as MP35N or stainless steel. Then, over an extended range, Nitinol deforms with little increase in force. After this extended region, Nitinol deforms like many other metals and eventually breaks.

There is one stent using a magnesium material that is both a metal and bioabsorbable. The force deformation curve for magnesium is also shown in Figure 25.5. The initial stiffness is similar to Nitinol but magnesium has a much more limited elastic region before fracturing at approximately 3% deformation. In some ways this material is similar to annealed stainless steel but it is less stiff, less elastic, and less strong, which can make designing with this material a challenge.

The last two materials shown in Figure 25.5 are poly-L-lactide (PLLA) and poly-4-hydroxybutyrate (P4HB), both bioabsorbable polymers. Their curves are typical of many polymers and

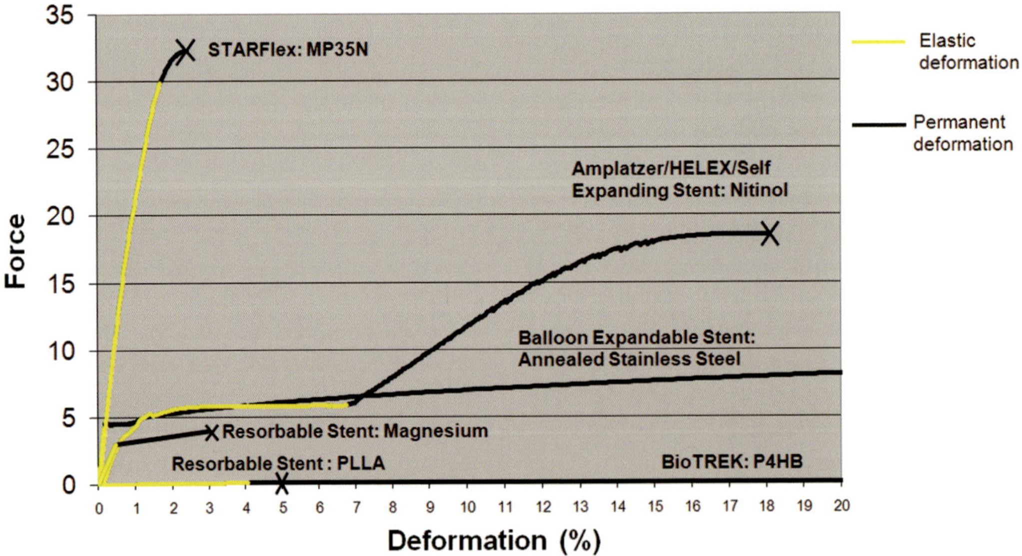

Fig 25.5—Material properties comparison

compared with metals, respond very similarly. The stiffness of these materials is a small fraction compared with most metals. A significant permanent deformation can be imparted into these polymers (either elongation or fracture) while that same force would produce very little deformation for a metal. Similarly, these polymers possess only a small fraction of the strength of metals. For the same device made of a polymer compared with a metal, the polymer device will have only a small percentage of the strength. Lastly, the elasticity of these polymers is similar to many metals. Therefore, the typical material properties of bioabsorbable polymers create a challenge of how to use these materials effectively for stents and septal occluders.

As already mentioned, there is a close synergy between a product's design and the material chosen for the design. Changing the material can create a much different and often unworkable product. Bioabsorbable polymers present a particularly challenging situation for the design of any septal occluder. The combination of low stiffness, low strength, and only moderate elasticity makes designing with these materials difficult. The concept of making just a material change and using an existing design is out of the question. The new device would not perform adequately. The concept of making a material change and some dimensional changes but keeping the product concept may be possible for some designs, but the resulting product might lack the required strength or stiffness or the device might be too bulky to be delivered percutaneously. This leaves designing a new product from scratch with the constraint of picking from the limited number of available bioabsorbable materials. Although this route is not impossible, it is a significant effort and it is not evolutionary but rather revolutionary, which is why the currently available devices all use metal frames.

Biologics are another family of materials starting to be utilized in septal occluders. While useful for a tissue scaffold to promote tissue regeneration and defect closure, they do not have the strength for use as a frame material and as such will not be covered in this section. They are discussed in the section on Tissue Scaffolds.

Available materials: absorbable polymers

One major challenge of designing a new bioabsorbable implant is the lack of available materials. Five common families of bioabsorbable

Polymer Family	Examples
Poly(α-hydroxy acids)	Polylactic acid (PLA)
	Poly-L-lactide (PLLA)
	Polyglycolic acid (PGA)
	Various copolymers and blends
Polyanhydrides	Poly(anhydride-ester)
Polyhydroxyalkanoates (PHA)	Poly-4-hydroxybutyrate (P4HB)
Tyrosine-derived polycarbonates	Poly(12DTE-12DT carbonate)
Polyether-esters	Polydioxanone (PDO)

Table 25.5—Bioabsorbable Polymers

polymers are outlined in Table 25.5 with more detail on each material included next.

Poly(α-hydroxy acids)

The most common family of bioabsorbable polymers is the poly(α-hydroxy acids), linear aliphatic polyesters that have a long history of use in medical implants dating back to the 1960s.[167] They are the first choice for a bioabsorbable polymer as they are readily available at a reasonable cost from multiple suppliers. With known biocompatibility, the development costs and time to market for a new implant can be shortened by choosing a known material over a novel one. The poly(α-hydroxy acids) includes polyglycolic acid (PGA), polylactic acid (PLA), poly-L-lactide (PLLA), and all the various copolymers and blends. PGA and PLA are often co-polymerized with polycaprolactone (PCL), another linear polyester, which degrades too slowly on its own to be of much use.

PGA is highly crystalline. Lactic acid is a chiral molecule that exists in two stereoisomeric forms giving rise to four morphologically distinct polymers of which three are commonly used: D-PLA and L-PLA (also known as PLLA), both semi-crystalline, and the racemic form D,L-PLA, which is always amorphous and therefore popular for drug-delivery.[168] L-PLA (PLLA) is used when high strength is required such as in sutures, orthopedic applications, and in the development of cardiac stents.[160–163] PGA sutures have been used commercially since 1970 under the trade name Dexon. One limitation is rapid strength loss in vivo, on the order of 2 to 4 weeks. Copolymers of PGA with PLA can slow the degradation process as PLA is more hydrophobic, although 50:50 copolymers degrade quicker than either PLA or PGA.[168] Vicryl and Polyglactin 910 sutures are copolymers of PLA and PGA.

Absorption of poly(α-hydroxy acids) is primarily via hydrolysis and the duration can be tailored from weeks to years depending upon the polymer composition, molecular weight, and crystallinity. They tend to be very stiff and rigid materials, probably not ideal for use in a septal occluder, and the degradation products, while natural metabolites, tend to

be highly acidic and can illicit a fairly intense foreign body reaction both acutely and as the implant starts to lose integrity and form particulate.[165,166,169,170] It appears that high-molecular-weight PLLA may be better tolerated[171–173] and incorporation of pharmacologic agents (eg, Paclitaxel [rapamycin] or sirolimus), as are used in drug-eluting stents, may help to suppress the inflammatory response.[174,175]

Polyanhydrides

Polyanhydrides are well suited for drug delivery.[176] Aliphatic polyanhydrides degrade quickly (days), whereas aromatic versions can take years, so copolymers are typically utilized.[168] Good biocompatibility has been demonstrated.[177,178] The first FDA-approved product was in the mid-1990s[179] and a salicylate-based poly(anhydride-ester) has been evaluated in development of a coronary stent.[180] In this application, as the polymer degrades, salicylic acid is released and taken up by the artery wall to reduce inflammation and restenosis.

Polyhydroxyalkanoates (PHA)

Polyhydroxyalkanoates (PHA) are a family of biologically produced polyesters isolated from

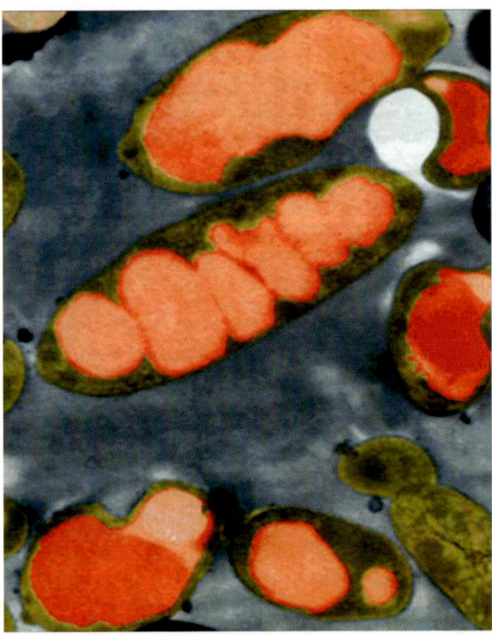

Fig 25.6—P4HB in recombinant bacteria. (Photo courtesy of Tepha, Inc., Lexington, Massachusetts.)

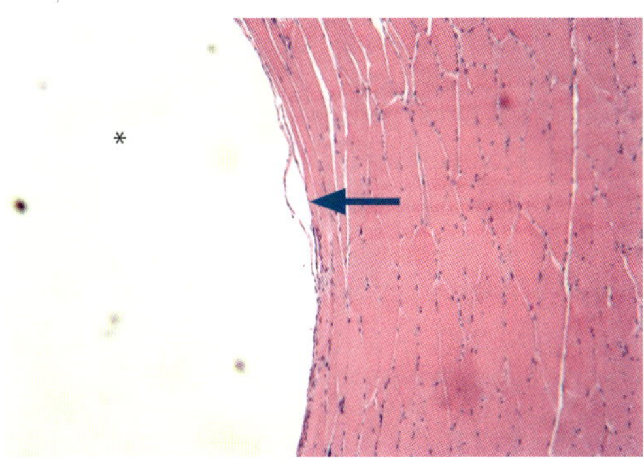

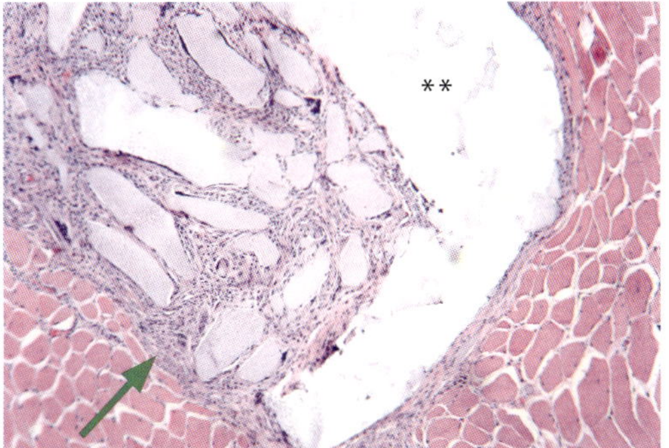

Fig 25.7—Inflammatory response of P4HB (upper figure) and PGA/PLA (lower figure) tubes at 4 weeks in vivo. One asterisk (*) denotes P4HB location. Two asterisks (**) denotes PGA/PLA location. Blue arrow points to minimal foreign body reaction with few cells and little collagen deposition. Green arrow points to giant cells, macrophages, and lymphocytes recruited as PGA/PLA tube degrades.

bacteria. They offer a unique set of physical properties not previously available to designers. PHAs are linear aliphatic polyesters, similar to the poly(α-hydroxy acids), however, the monomers are less acidic. PHAs are naturally produced (as opposed to synthetic materials) using technology common to the pharmaceutical industry. *Escherichia coli* bacteria, modified by recombinant DNA technology (Fig 25.6), is utilized to produce polymer for medical applications. Production using fermentation is advantageous in that the end polymer contains no residual metal catalysts that can potentially cause inflammation.[181,182] A poly-4-hydroxybutyrate (P4HB) with the trade name TephaFLEX (Tepha, Lexington, Massachusetts) was first FDA cleared in 2007 for use in bioabsorbable sutures and absorbable surgical meshes. This is the first commercially available medical-grade PHA

material. P4HB exhibits significant strength and flexibility and absorbs as a noninflammatory natural metabolite (4-hydroxybutyric acid) which is well tolerated and has a short half-life (35 minutes).[183] The 4-hydroxybutyric acid is ultimately broken down via the Krebs cycle to carbon dioxide and water and excreted. Bioabsorption occurs both via hydrolysis and enzymatic degradation.[182] TephaFLEX is currently being used in the development of the BioTREK septal occluder, the Tepha stent[184,185] (Tepha, Lexington, Massachusetts), and a tissue-engineered heart valve for pediatric applications[186,187] (Children's Hospital, Boston, Massachusetts). The noninflammatory nature of P4HB is shown in Fig 25.7. As can be seen, the PGA/PLA tube elicited significantly more giant cells, macrophages, and lymphocytes than the P4HB after 4 weeks of implantation in rabbit muscles.

Tyrosine-derived polycarbonates

Tyrosine-derived polycarbonates are based on the natural amino acid L-tyrosine, a major nutrient.[188] They have high strength and good biocompatibility.[189-191] Poly(12DTE-12DT carbonate) is the material furthest along in development and has been evaluated in patients in the RESORB Trial in the ReZolve stent (REVA Medical, San Diego, CA).[192] In this application, polyethylene glycol (PEG) is added for enhanced blood compatibility and the polymer has been rendered radiopaque by the iodination of tyrosine units in the copolymer backbone.[188,193] Although in vitro studies demonstrated that the incorporation of iodine may counteract the effect of PEG, differences in protein absorption have not been observed in porcine coronary arteries with iodine- and non–iodine-containing polymer stents.[194] The ability to bind iodine to the backbone to produce a radiopaque material has obvious advantages for percutaneous cardiovascular implants. The material absorbs slowly (years) and in vivo studies confirmed water uptake (hydrolysis) is the primary catalyst for the polymer degradation and at later stages there is enzymatic involvement.[166,191,195] The material breaks down to form the amino acid L-tyrosine, material monomers, ethanol, carbon dioxide, and PEG.

Polydioxanone

Polydioxanone is a polyether-ester that resulted in the first clinically tested monofilament synthetic suture.[179] It has comparatively long suture retention strength making it ideal for slow-healing wounds. It has also been used in the development of a biodegradable annuloplasty ring for mitral and tricuspid valvuloplasty in adults and children (Bioring, Lonay, Switzerland).[196–199] Polydioxanone has good flexibility and strength. Its modulus, and therefore stiffness, is lower than PLA.[168] It elicits minimal tissue response and is absorbed by hydrolysis.[200]

Absorption mechanisms: absorbable polymers

Most absorbable polymers absorb principally by hydrolysis although some are susceptible to surface erosions via enzymatic degradation. Chain scission degrades the polymer to small particles that undergo phagocytosis and are, in most cases, metabolized into carbon dioxide and water via the Krebs cycle. While most degrade to form naturally occurring metabolites, the by-products of some are highly acidic and can illicit a fairly intense foreign body reaction.[165,166]

The absorption time is a function of many factors including the chemical structure, molecular weight, crystallinity, and geometry of the device with thicker parts lasting longer than thin ones. Although clinicians would probably prefer that a bioabsorbable septal occluder maintain its strength and integrity for 6 months to allow for complete encapsulation and closure of the defect, then magically disappear overnight. This scenario (Fig 25.8) is not realistic. A more realistic example is depicted in Fig 25.9, which shows complete endothelialization occurring early and structural integrity maintained to the 3- to 6-month time point. From the start of implantation, molecular weight is starting to drop so to maintain structural integrity for 3 to 6 months, a fairly high starting point will be necessary. Therefore, complete loss of molecular weight may then take 12 months or longer with full mass loss taking as long as 2 or more years.

Available materials: absorbable metals

In addition to absorbable polymers, there are also absorbable or corrodible metals that have been used in the development of stents. The most progress to date has been with magnesium alloys, which were first introduced as orthopedic biomaterials,[201] although some limited studies have been conducted on corrodible iron stents with promising results.[124,202,203]

Magnesium has potential advantages over alternatives such as PLA and PGA, as they can be less inflammatory while absorbing quickly. In its purest form, magnesium degraded too fast and released large amounts of hydrogen gas.[204] The development focus then changed to alloys of magnesium in an attempt to slow the degradation process. The Magic stent (Biotronik, Berlin, Germany) is constructed from a magnesium alloy (WE43) containing also zirconium (< 5%), yttrium (< 5%), and rare earths (< 5%).[205,206] Magnesium (Mg) alloys degrade principally by oxidation with the Mg component corroding to form soluble Mg hydroxide, Mg chloride, and hydrogen gas.[207] The space left behind when the implant absorbs is eventually replaced by calcium, accompanied by a phosphorous compound.[208,209] Side effects of degradation products are expected to be unlikely given that magnesium is an important nutrient.[205] Limitations of these materials are that they are fairly low in strength, absorb quickly, and are radiolucent.[208]

Major challenges

There are several major challenges in designing a bioabsorbable septal occluder including the lack of inherent radiopacity of available materials; stiffness, strength, and elasticity limitations requiring thicker, bulkier designs complicating delivery; the phenomenon where strength is changing with time postimplantation; challenges to utilizing computer modeling/finite element analysis during the design process; and temperature and moisture sensitivity of the materials. Each of these is briefly discussed.

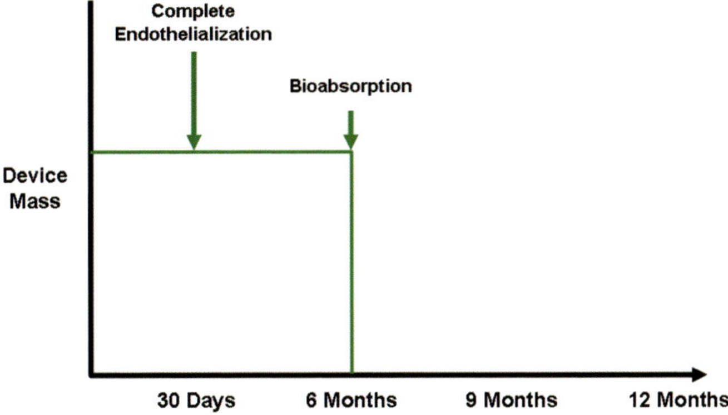

Fig 25.8—Bioabsorption rate: What the cardiologist would like.

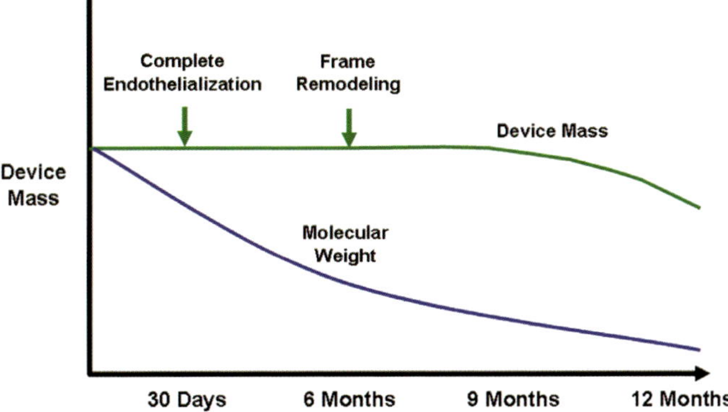

Fig 25.9—Bioabsorption rate: Reality.

Radiopacity

Polymers by nature are radiolucent. This is also the case with the one commonly utilized bioabsorbable metal—magnesium. Therefore, a significant engineering challenge that is being confronted is making a truly 100% bioresorbable implant that will provide radiopaque features.

There are several approaches to this problem. One is to hope that the characteristic of bioabsorption will be attractive enough to make up for the shortcomings of a radiolucent device. The other is to impart some level of radiopacity through the use of marker bands, fillers, or other creative methods of imparting radiopacity to inherently radiolucent materials. The use of metal markers can be seen in one of the bioabsorbable stents (Abbott Laboratories, Abbott Park, Illinois). As previously mentioned, the ReZolve stent utilizes a novel polymer with iodine bound to the backbone to impart radiopacity.

Stiffness, strength, and elasticity limitations

As illustrated in Figure 25.5, bioabsorbable materials have many significant limitations compared with commonly used metals. The stiffness of bioabsorbable materials is considerably lower. This can impact the ability of the device to clamp onto the septum to resist dislodgment and prevent leaks. To address this, thicker components and therefore bulkier designs, may be necessary. Strength can be low with some bioabsorbable materials, causing fractures. Some materials will not break but their elasticity is so low that it is difficult to design a workable product that can be percutaneously delivered and retrieved.

Strength changes with time

Durability testing of a new septal occluder can be a challenge as it is difficult to predict the in vivo loading conditions. This can be even more daunting for a device whose strength/stiffness/elasticity are also changing with time due to degradation. One way to address this issue is to design the device to maintain its strength above a minimum required level during the healing process and then design the tissue scaffold to accelerate the healing response, minimizing the healing period.

Finite Element Analysis (FEA)

Computer modeling or FEA is a commonly used mathematical tool to determine performance and longevity of septal occluders. Modeling of bioabsorbable devices is challenging because of the material properties of the polymers. Not only do bioabsorbable polymers erode over time physically, they also change significantly regarding stiffness, strength, and elasticity due to heat and moisture when implanted in the body. So, during the manufacturing process, the device will exhibit a particular response. After packaging and sterilization, the response of the material typically is different. When subjected to the temperature and moisture of the body, the material and thus device response will again be different. Then, over the course of months, the material properties will continue to change as the device absorbs in the body. Although FEA can take into consideration many of these changes, understanding the material property changes is a very significant challenge.

Temperature and moisture sensitivity

Bioabsorbable materials can, by nature, be sensitive to temperature and moisture. This requires bench testing to be conducted in a body temperature bath environment and can cause packaging challenges. Ethylene oxide sterilization subjects devices to a very moist environment and requires packaging that allows vapor transmission. As long-term packaging should ideally inhibit vapor transmission to prevent degradation due to moisture, poststerilization processing is often required to remove moisture from the package and securely seal the device in a moisture barrier material while not compromising sterility. Gamma sterilization can simplify this process by allowing sterilization through a moisture barrier, such as a foil pouch, however many polymers are mechanically degraded by radiation. Occasionally, medical device engineers develop ingenious packaging schemes that inadvertently involve refrigeration. This results in much unhappiness amongst manufacturing personnel, sales representatives, and hospital personnel and should be avoided at all costs.

Unique regulatory requirements

Bioabsorbable implants can have unique regulatory requirements, in particular if they incorporate a biologic or a pharmacologic agent, resulting in a combination product. The review process then involves multiple agencies and can require added time to commercialization. Testing will be required to demonstrate absence of adverse reactions due to the resorption process and show that the body can safely eliminate the by-products. When new materials are utilized in a cardiovascular implant, toxicity, immunogenicity, and carcinogenicity testing will need to be conducted. Another unique characteristic of such devices—and a challenge during durability testing—is that they have mechanical properties that are changing with time. The loss in strength due to degradation will affect device function and durability and testing will be necessary to show there is no risk of device or particulate embolization. To avoid this risk, high-molecular-weight materials with long absorption times will most likely be chosen, which can mean increased follow-up time for preclinical and clinical trials. Another challenge will be imaging of these devices using clinically available technologies. In some cases, the device may not show up on standard imaging technologies such as fluoroscopy and echocardiography. Even if they do, the ability to see them will most likely decrease over time following implantation, as the material resorbs.

New patient risks

Currently available permanent septal occluders have a known list of potential complications, as previously mentioned. While bioabsorbable devices may potentially eliminate some of these complications, they also may inherently create new potential complications. It will be important to design new devices to avoid these pitfalls including using appropriate safety factors to prevent an incompatibility between the healing profile and resorption profile to avoid an embolic risk, to conduct appropriate immunological screening tests on all new materials, and to monitor the immune response in preclinical and clinical trials.

Tissue Scaffolds

The tissue scaffold not only serves as a blood barrier immediately after defect closure but also as a scaffold to promote tissue in-growth for safe and effective long-term closure. Due to the inherent high surface area of tissue scaffolds, the choice of tissue scaffold will be one of the key design factors for determining the overall device–blood compatibility and healing response.

Traditional tissue scaffolds have consisted of synthetic, permanent materials previously used in other cardiovascular applications, such as polyester. The BioSTAR porcine intestinal collagen layer (ICL) scaffold is the first bioabsorbable scaffold to be clinically used in a septal occluder. Other xenograft, allograft, and bioabsorbable, synthetic materials are available as potential tissue scaffolds for the next generation of devices. Generally, tissue scaffolds are not fabricated from metals.

Design considerations

As with all medical device materials, tissue scaffolds must be biocompatible. In the case of a septal occluder, the requirements are most stringent because it is a permanent (> 30 days) implantable device with blood contact. Therefore, the International Organization for Standardization (ISO) 10993 standard[73] requires cytotoxicity, sensitization, irritation/intracutancous, acute systemic toxicity, subchronic toxicity, genotox-

icity, implantation, hemocompatibility, chronic toxicity, carcinogenicity, and reproductive/developmental testing. In addition to these standard biocompatibility tests, the tissue scaffold must also be blood compatible in the blood flow conditions at the septal wall. Although in vivo testing in the heart septal wall in a large animal model is the gold standard to determining blood compatibility, specialized in vitro testing[210] can be conducted to screen various materials, implant designs, or scaffold architectures.

Another key design consideration in choosing a tissue scaffold is the host healing response such as rapid encapsulation, complete endothelialization, and minimal scar formation (fibrosis). The polyester fabric in both the AMPLATZER and CardioSEAL/STARFlex septal occluders shows plasma protein deposition at 1 week after implantation in humans.[54] By 1 month, an endothelial cell layer covers a majority of the occluder surface.[54] When the polyester was replaced with ICL on the STARFlex framework to create the BioSTAR, the resulting occluder showed accelerated endothelialization with endothelial cell coverage beginning at 1 week and completed by 1 month postimplantation in an ovine model.[50] At later time points, a quiescent fibrous capsule forms around the polyester materials.[164] In opposition, native-like tissue forms around the BioSTAR ICL material as the materials absorbs near the two year time point.[211] These examples show that using the same material with different frameworks may result in similar host healing responses. Alternatively, changing the tissue scaffold material and using the same framework has the potential to elicit a clinically significant difference in host healing response.

The mechanical properties of the tissue scaffold are also a key design consideration. The scaffold must be flexible enough to conform to both the deployed and delivery configurations, have sufficient tear strength to withstand the forces created during tracking through a long sheath, and be strong enough to withstand the fluid flow conditions within the heart. Depending on the attachment method to the frame, the tissue scaffold may also need to have a sufficiently high suture pullout strength.

Less obvious but equally important design considerations when choosing a tissue scaffold are ease of attachment to the implant frame and implant profile in the delivery configuration. Scaffold attachment, thickness, and construction can affect the delivery profile such that the delivery sheath size must be increased to accommodate the chosen scaffold.

Available materials

Polyester

Polyesters are a category of polymers that contain an ester functional group. Although there are many different polymers with ester functional groups, polyester frequently refers to polyethylene terephthalate (PET). A common trade name for PET is Dacron by Dupont. The Clamshell device used polyester as the tissue scaffold as early as 1989. Several currently available septal occluders utilize polyester as the tissue scaffold. The STARFlex Septal Occluder utilizes a knitted polyester fabric as the tissue scaffold. The AMPLATZER Septal Occluder also utilizes a polyester fabric as its tissue scaffold. In both cases, the polyester fabric is sewn to the frame with polyester thread. In addition, the Premere, Figulla, and Solysafe septal occluders all use polyester fabric as their tissue scaffolds. Polyester knits have been widely used as vascular graft materials.[212,213]

Polyester is considered to be very biocompatible in the variety of medical applications for which it is used. In 10 of 12 cases, Clamshell explants from time points ranging from 2.7 months to 3.6 years showed mild focal foreign body reaction without inflammation near the polyester fabric.[214] One short-term (3.4 month) and one long-term (37 months) explant showed intense foreign body reaction without inflammation.[214] Histopathology conducted after a single AMPLATZER device was explanted 15 months postimplantation showed a mild inflammatory response with few lymphocytes and foreign bodies cells near the polyester fibers.[215] A more detailed histopathology study of both animal and human septal occluder explants with polyester tissue scaffold was conducted by Sigler and Jux.[164] At the 4 to 7 day time points, the polyes-

ter in the AMPLATZER and STARFlex devices induced a covering of fibrin, plasma proteins, and blood cells. At longer time points, multinucleated foreign body cells neighbored the polyester fabric. A mild lymphocytic infiltration also surrounded the polyester fibers. This mild lymphocytic and foreign body reaction continued at the longest time point of 4 years.

Expanded PTFE (ePTFE)

The HELEX Septal Occluder tissue scaffold is a hydrophilically coated, expanded polytetrafluoroethylene (ePTFE) fabric. The hydrophilic coating is to improve echocardiographic imaging of the HELEX occluder. Expanded PTFE has been widely used as a cardiovascular implant material.[212,216,217] Like polyester, ePFTE is considered a very biocompatible medical device material. ePTFE is very hydrophobic and lubricious making it thromboresistant. In a canine study in which 24 HELEX devices were implanted for 1, 3, 6, and 12 months, a thin layer of fibrous tissue infiltrated the interstices of the ePTFE with no evidence of inflammation by the 1-month time point.[218] By 12 months, vascularized connective tissue (fibrous capsule) with a covering of neoendothelial cells surrounded the ePTFE.

Polyvinyl alcohol

Ivalon is the trade name for a polyvinyl alcohol sponge. Ivalon is created by foaming polyvinyl alcohol (PVA) to create a spongelike architecture then fixing this architecture with formaldehyde. Because of PVA's high compressibility and hydrophilicity, PVA sponges are commonly used for household cleaning. Ivalon is used by Cardia (Eagan, Minnesota) as the tissue scaffold in their ATRIASEPT products. Ivalon sponges were used for the surgical repair of septal defects decades prior to the development of percutaneous septal occluders. Although very biocompatible, Ivalon was abandoned for this use after late sponge dissolution occurred.[219] Late failure of Ivalon sponge material also occurred when used for aortic grafts.[220] Porstmann et al[221] used Ivalon for catheter closure of patent ductus arteriosus (PDA). As a PDA closure device, Ivalon had excellent clinical success (94.7%).[222]

Polyurethane foam

Polyurethanes are copolymers with both soft and hard segments. By choosing the correct copolymers, the material properties can be tailored to meet the mechanical and biostability requirements of a given application. Examples of hard segment polymers are 2,4-toluene diisocyanate (TDI) and methylene di(4-phenyl isocyanate) (MDI). Polyethers or polyester polyols are examples of soft segment polymers. Despite good biocompatibility and excellent mechanical properties such as compressibility, fatigue strength, and flexibility, the safety of polyurethanes has been extensively studied due to their inherent susceptibility to biodegradation.[223–229]

The FlatStent Septal Occluder utilizes polyurethane foam as its scaffold for promoting healing from within the PFO tunnel. Although no reports on the biocompatibility or healing of the FlatStent have been published, polyurethane has been used for decades in the cardiovascular system. First developed in 1976, the Rashkind PDA Umbrella utilized two open pore polyurethane discs in a double umbrella configuration in its percutaneous implant.[58] Three months after implantation in a calf ductus, heavy tissue in-growth covered the foam and incorporated it within the endothelium.[58] In the patient population followed in Rashkind's early study, no clinical adverse events were reported with respect to the polyurethane foam.[58] Polyurethane foam patches were also used in both the original Sideris Button device[65] and the Sideris Patch device. For the patch, a preclotted fibrin matrix was applied to the polyurethane patch prior to implantation to accelerate integration with the host tissue.[230] In a piglet study using one variation of the Sideris Button device, a severe granulomatous inflammatory nodule was observed on the right atrial portion 2 months after implantation.[231] At the same time, endothelial cell coverage was observed.

Bioabsorbable polymers

Although no currently available septal occluders utilize a bioabsorbable polymer tissue scaffold, several bioabsorbable scaffolds are already in clinical use for other applications such as

reinforcement of soft tissues,[232] hernia repair,[233] and reconstruction of the pelvic floor.[234] Materials such as polylactides, polyglycolides, and poly-ε-caprolactones have been used. More recently, poly-4-hydroxybutyrate (P4HB) has been cleared by the FDA for clinical use. As previously mentioned, P4HB is sold by Tepha with the trade name TephaFLEX. The BioTREK Septal Occluder, currently in preclinical studies, utilizes P4HB as its tissue scaffold in addition to the frame. The properties of these bioabsorbable polymers are discussed in greater detail in the section, Available Materials: Absorbable Polymers.

Biologics

Using extracellular matrix (ECM) as a scaffold presents to the host a native collagen network as the framework for cellular growth and healing. The ECM scaffold may include collagen as well as growth factors, fibronectin, laminin, and other bioactive molecules that can direct the healing response. By tailoring the ECM source and manufacturing processes, a biologic scaffold can provide both a mechanical support and the correct signaling for regenerating native-like tissue at the implantation site.

Biologics can be xenografts, autografts, or allografts. Xenografts have been widely used in medical applications other than septal repair. Porcine valve replacements and catgut suture are two examples. Sources for xenograft tissue are nearly infinite but there is a risk of zoonotic infections. Allograft tissue is more limited in quantity than xenograft materials and risk of disease transmission from donor to recipient remains. Autologous tissue removes the disease transition risk but autologous tissue sources are quite limited. The possibility of abundant autologous tissue sources relies on in vitro tissue culture technology evolving to include native-like tissue formation and large-scale manufacturability.

Harvesting and processing techniques can alter the strength, growth factor concentration, immune response, degradation time, sterility, and bioburden of the final biologic product. The tissues must first be harvested in a manner to minimize microbial contamination. After har vest, the tissues are chemically and mechanically cleaned to remove tissue debris, lysed cells, and unbound proteins. While cleaning minimizes host response to the tissue, excessive cleaning may remove growth factors and other ECM constituents that promote cellular infiltration and proliferation. Once cleaned, the biologic material can be crosslinked. Crosslinking increases the resorption time but may also reduce cellular infiltration. Therefore, the crosslinking process must be tuned to provide the correct balance between degradation and cellular infiltration. The final processing step is sterilization. Gamma irradiation is the most commonly used method for biologic materials due to potential toxic residuals from ethylene oxide sterilization. Gamma irradiation may affect the collagen crosslinking leading to reduced mechanical properties. Table 25.6 summarizes the effect of processing on the biologic scaffold. The arrows represent an increase or decrease with respect to unextracted or noncrosslinked scaffolds.

Intestinal collagen layer (ICL) (Organogenesis, Canton, Massachusetts) is the one biologic currently utilized in a septal occluder, the BioSTAR. ICL is derived from the tunica submucosa of the porcine small intestine, which is then purified to form a sheet of acellular Type 1 collagen. ICL is a well-characterized material that is very pure and reproducible with undetectable amounts of porcine DNA.[235] Materials derived from small intestinal submucosa have been shown to remodel into functional native-like tissue, promoting site-specific tissue regeneration[236–239] as opposed to scar tissue formation. It also has the flexibility and strength required for suture attachment and catheter delivery. In the BioSTAR preclinical studies, ICL was shown to promote tissue regeneration with no fibrous capsule observed at 2-years postimplantation in the ovine model.[50] ICL is actively remodeled by native cells and its degradation by-products are peptides. As the matrix disintegrates, it is infiltrated by cells and undergoes phagocytosis. In preclinical studies of the BioSTAR device, ICL was shown to be approximately 90% resorbed at 2 years and replaced by autologous tissue with no fibrous capsule.[50]

Processing Step	Bioscaffold Property				
	Inflammatory cell response	Strength	Humoral immune response	Resorption time	Cellular infiltration
Cellular extraction			↓258		
Glutaraldehyde crosslinking	↓259	↑259	↓258	↑↑258,259	↓↓258,259
Epoxy crosslinking	↓259	↑259	↓↓258	↑258,259	↓↓258,259
Carbodiimide crosslinking			↓↓258	↑258	↓258
Gamma irradiation	↑260	↓260			↑260
Ethylene oxide		↔261,262			

Table 25.6—Implications of Different Chemical Processing Steps on Bioscaffolds.
Reprinted from De Deyne PG, Kladakis SM. Bioscaffolds in tissue engineering: a rationale for use in the reconstruction of musculoskeletal soft tissues. *Clin Podiatr Med Surg.* 2005;22(4);521–32. Copyright 2005, with permission from Elsevier.

Scaffold architecture

When designing a tissue scaffold, fabrication method is as critical as material choice. Mesh scaffolds can be made by knitting or weaving. Nonwoven scaffolds can be made through mechanical entanglement, melt blown, dry spun, wet spun, or electrospun processes. Foams are also frequently used as tissue scaffolds. The best fabrication method is determined by polymer processing characteristics, blood interaction, tissue in-growth, porosity, thickness, fiber size, and mechanical strength. The fabrication method can also be influenced by the desired attachment process. For example, a foam scaffold can be formed directly onto a frame foregoing a secondary attachment step. Exemplary

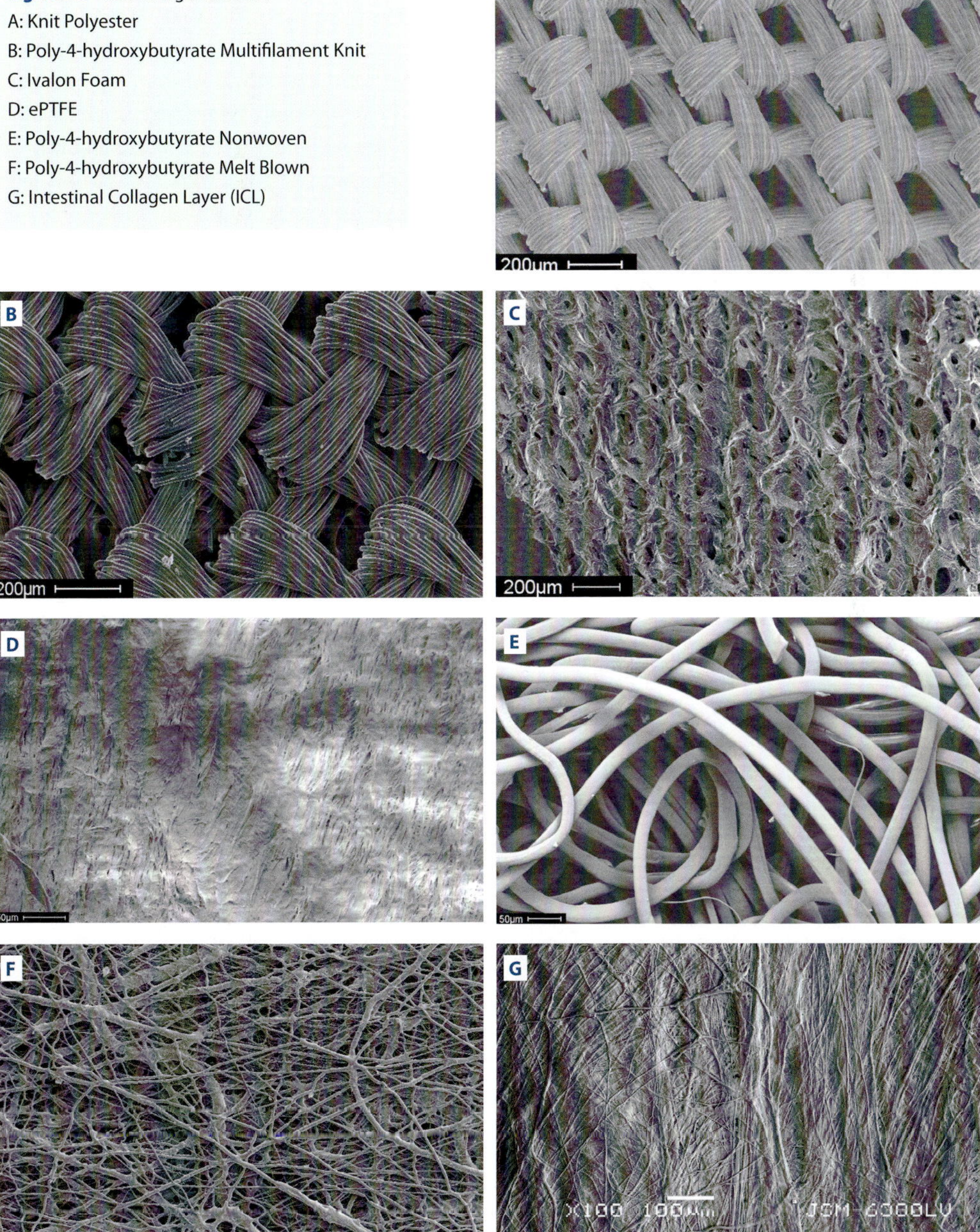

Fig 25.10—Scaffold geometries.
A: Knit Polyester
B: Poly-4-hydroxybutyrate Multifilament Knit
C: Ivalon Foam
D: ePTFE
E: Poly-4-hydroxybutyrate Nonwoven
F: Poly-4-hydroxybutyrate Melt Blown
G: Intestinal Collagen Layer (ICL)

scaffold images can be seen in Fig 25.10. The knit structures have uniform repeating patterns with large pores. The foam has various pore sizes forming an interconnected pore structure. Expanded PTFE has small, irregular-shaped pores. The nonwoven has uniform filament size arranged in a random entanglement. The melt blown has variable filament size randomly oriented with adhered joints between fibers. The ICL scaffold has dense collagen fibers arranged in an anisotropic pattern with few pores.

Cells interact differently with the tissue scaffold based on the scaffold architecture. For example, the BioTREK occluder made with a nonwoven tissue scaffold induced greater tissue coverage at 1-month postimplantation in an ovine model than when a film tissue scaffold was used. The occluder with the film tissue scaffold (Fig 25.11) is only partially covered with a glistening neoendothelial layer. Significant portions of the surface remain covered with unorganized plasma protein deposition. By comparison, the occluder with the nonwoven tissue scaffold (Fig 25.11) is almost completely covered with a glistening neoendothelial layer with a minimal amount of residual protein deposition. In the previous example, the architecture varied widely between the two tissue scaffolds of the same material, but subtle differences can also influence healing potential. In a rat in vivo study using polyurethane foam, vascular grafts with an external pore size of 30 µm induced faster neoendothelial layer coverage than grafts with 20, 10, or 5 µm.[240] Similarly, increasing the ePTFE pore size from 30 µm to 90 µm significantly increased the endothelialization rate of vascular grafts in an in vivo canine study.[241]

Biological response modifiers (drugs, proteins, genes, cells)

In certain designs, it may make sense to incorporate biological response modifiers to regulate endothelialization and/or thrombo-resistance. Biological response modifiers can include growth factors, ECM molecules, peptide sequences, or other bioactive molecule that provide a biological stimulus. With nonabsorbable devices, surface modifications are most frequently employed to achieve the desired biological response. With the development of absorbable devices, modifiers can be incorporated within the frame and/or tissue scaffold materials to provide a controlled release to extend the bioactive period.

An increased rate of healing can be induced either by preseeding the occluder with cells or by attracting cells once implanted. Preseeding the occluder would allow for immediate cell coverage but issues such as cell source, cell culture conditions, and time delay between

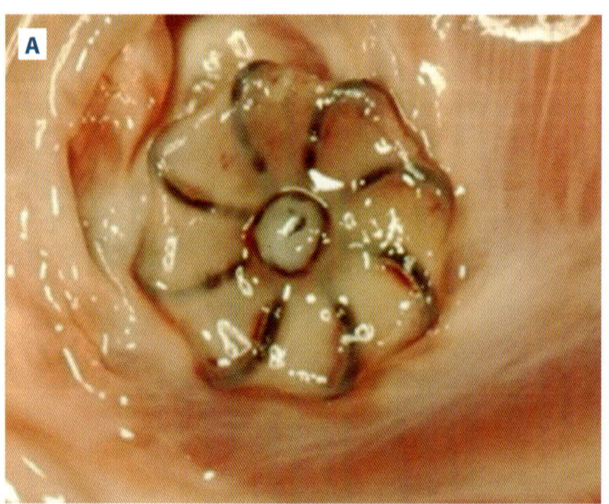 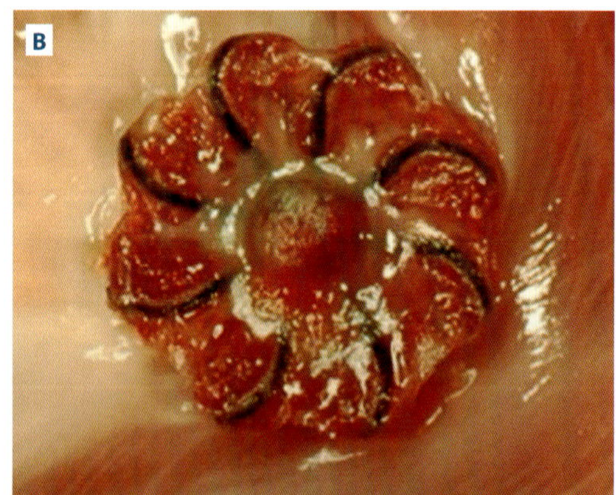

Fig 25.11—BioTREK Occluder with nonwoven (A) and film tissue (B) scaffolds at 1 month. In panel A, > 95% of the implant surface is covered with a glistening neointima. In panel B, < 20% of the implant surface is covered with neointima. The remainder is covered with plasma proteins.

occluder preparation and implantation must be resolved. Like bioscaffolds, cells can be autologous, allogeneic, and xenogeneic. In a sheep in vivo study, autologous fibroblasts were preseeded on STARFlex occluders and implanted for 30 days.[242] A thicker and more complete cell layer was apparent on the preseeded occluders in comparison to unseeded occluders. However, the preseeded occluders also demonstrated greater thrombogenicity. Preseeding an endothelial cell layer on top of the fibroblast surface might minimize the thrombogenicity but a clinically feasible source of autologous endothelial cells has yet to be identified. As tissue-engineering technology matures, living tissue grown in vitro could also be used with septal occluders. For example, the technology developed by Hoerstrup et al to grow trileaflet heart valves from myofibroblasts and endothelial cells seeded on PGA nonwoven scaffolds coated with P4HB[186] could be modified to develop septal occluder tissue.

As an alternative strategy to preseeding or tissue engineering, specific and nonspecific cell recruitment can increase early tissue encapsulation of septal occluders. Nonspecific cell recruitment can be induced by making surfaces more cell friendly through plasma treament,[243–245] collagen or other protein coating,[246–248] or peptide coating.[249, 250] Nonspecific cell recruitment can increase healing by allowing for cells to more easily attach, migrate, and proliferate on the tissue scaffold. For septal occluders, the nonspecific cell types could include endothelial cells, fibroblasts, and cardiac smooth muscle cells. Many surfaces that are nonspecific for cell recruitment may also recruit platelets or plasma proteins. Therefore, when designing septal occluder surface treatments, testing should be completed to determine both cell recruitment and thrombus formation potential. By designing tissue scaffolds to recruit a specific cell type, the risk of thrombus formation is minimized. For example, a murine monoclonal anti-human CD34 antibody has been used to cover a stainless steel stent.[251] CD34 antibody is specific to attract endothelial progenitor cells (EPC) from the circulating blood. A CD34 coating on a septal occluder could then accelerate neointimal formation via EPC recruitment without increasing thrombus formation. Short, high affinity peptides can also be used to modify substrates for recruiting and retaining specific cell types. For example, a collagen sponge modified with a mesenchymal stem cell (MSC) binding peptide (Affinergy, Durham, North Carolina) and then incubated in the presence of MSCs retained many more cells compared to the unmodified sponge (Fig 25.12).

Biological response modifiers can also be used to serve a temporary function prior to tissue encapsulation. For septal occluders, minimization of thrombus formation prior to neointimal formation is a requirement. The BioSTAR occluder accomplishes this by the application of heparin-benzalkonium chloride (HBAC) to the ICL scaffold. After 7 days post-implantation in a sheep model, uncoated ICL induced greater thrombus formation than ICL coated with HBAC.[50] The ionically bound HBAC coating elutes from the surface as the neointima is formed. Although BioSTAR is the first septal occluder to use heparin, heparin is commonly used on the surface of vascular grafts. For example, the GORE PROPATEN Vascular Graft uses covalent bonding to permanently bind heparin molecules to the luminal surface through a proprietary end-point attachment mechanism. Although few biological response modifiers beyond heparin are commonly used on cardiovascular implants, many modifiers, such as nitric

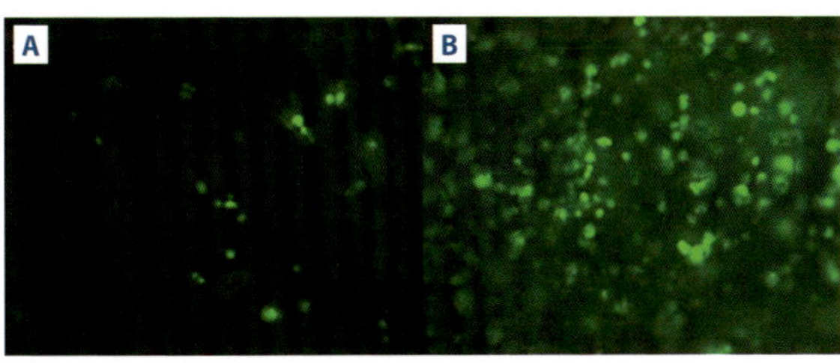

Fig 25.12—High-affinity peptides promote specific cell binding on collagen sponge. The application of peptides to a collagen sponge showed increased specific cell adhesion (panel B) in comparison to an uncoated collagen sponge (panel A). (Photo courtesy of Affinergy, Inc. (Durham, North Carolina.)

oxide, glycoprotein VI, CD39, hepatocyte growth factor, insulinlike growth factor, vascular endothelial growth factor, fibroblast growth factor-2, and transforming growth factor-beta, have been studied. As research continues and manufacturing techniques to create clinically viable products advance, a greater variety of modifiers will be available.

Preclinical Testing

Significant preclinical testing should be conducted on any cardiovascular implant prior to human testing. If significant design, material, and/or process changes are made subsequent to

Raw material analyses (chemical composition, tensile strength, etc.)
Biocompatibility/toxicity
Corrosion/resorption
Stress analysis
Integrity and durability (fatigue)
Joint integrity
Simulated end use (loading, flushing, tracking, deployment, retrieval)
Characterization of biological response modifiers (ie, drug release rates, if applicable)
Dislodgement resistance
Septal clamping force
Radial stiffness
Imaging (MR safety)
Packaging, sterility, shelf life, transport
Host response (animal testing)
Human clinical trials

Box 25.2—Typical Tests for a Septal Occluder

this testing, relevant re-testing must be considered. A list of typical tests for a septal occluder are outlined in Box 25.2. This includes dimensional, physical, mechanical, chemical, biological and electrochemical analyses, hemocompatibility and testing for equipment interfaces.

Some testing is quite basic such as raw material analyses, joint integrity, and simulated end-use. Some require significant development effort such as stress analysis and integrity and durability, which usually involves fatigue testing of complete devices in physiological buffered saline at body temperature. The most difficult aspect of this test is predicting the stresses that will be imparted to a given device in vivo followed by determining the best method to duplicate this on the bench. Certain tests, such as biocompatibility,[73] MR safety,[90] and packaging integrity, have fairly standard protocols and are more straightforward. Some tests relate to septal occluder *relative* performance, such as septal clamping force and radial stiffness and are typically done as part of the design process using available devices as controls. These tests usually don't result in quantitative performance specifications but are rather done as a screening tool to be sure a design is in the "ballpark" of existing devices relative to ability to close the defect, resist embolization, and avoid perforation. Corrosion resistance and metal ion release/toxicity is usually done in conjunction with both fatigue and biocompatibility. Fortunately, guidelines have been introduced to help guide the corrosion testing portion of this effort.[133] For bioabsorbable polymers, resorption studies can be more complex, especially if the material is susceptible to both hydrolytic and enzymatic degradation.

Host response evaluation in a large animal model is the gold standard for deliverability and healing response including toxicity. While much has been written on this subject, it is still useful to either include a few controls (an existing commercially available device) or have that data available for comparative purposes. While the porcine model has been shown to have naturally occurring PFOs of similar characteristics to human PFOs[252] and some testing of septal closure has been conducted in this model,[253,254] most long-term healing data has been done in created septal defects in the canine or ovine models.[50,51,59,218,242,255–257] These models are more manageable for long-term (> 1 year) studies and have the most historical use.

After completion of design validation testing, including a pivotal animal study, the next step is usually human clinical trials. Adequate up-front design work should be conducted to avoid significant design iteration during the human-testing phase, for obvious reasons.

The Future

The future will likely bring the development and commercialization of more hybrid-type designs that utilize bioabsorbable scaffolds combined with metallic frames, followed eventually by completely absorbable tissue regeneration devices. The availability of new materials and technologies will allow design engineers the flexibility to create fully absorbable devices that will match or surpass the performance characteristics of metallic ones. Through the use of novel materials and biological response modifiers, devices will be designed that promote immediate closure of the defect and that can be tolerated with minimal postimplant pharmacologic treatment. The risk of long-term complications for such devices should be low due to the lack of permanent foreign material, although initially acute and short-term (2-year) follow-up should be scrupulous. As with all devices, long-term follow-up in patients, including a thorough analysis of explanted devices, will be the only way to truly understand the safety and efficacy of a new implant.

References

1. Nugent AW, Britt A, Gauvreau K, Piercey GE, Lock JE, Jenkins KJ. Device closure rates of simple atrial septal defects optimized by the STARFlex device. *J Am Coll Cardiol.* 2006;48(3):538–544.

2. Billinger K, Ostermayer SH, Carminati M, et al. HELEX Septal Occluder for transcatheter closure of patent foramen ovale: multicentre experience. *EuroIntervention.* 2006;1(4):465–471.

3. Buscheck F, Sievert H, Kleber F, et al. Patent foramen ovale using the Premere device: the results of the CLOSEUP trial. *J Intervent Cardiol.* 2006;19(4):328–333.

4. Everett AD, Jennings J, Sibinga E, et al. Community use of the AMPLATZER atrial septal defect occluder: results of the multicenter MAGIC atrial septal defect study. *Pediatr Cardiol.* 2009;30(3):240–247.

5. Taaffe M, Fischer E, Baranowski A, et al. Comparison of three patent foramen ovale closure devices in a randomized trial (AMPLATZER versus CardioSEAL-STARFlex versus HELEX occluder). *Am J Cardiol.* 2008;101(9):1353–1358.

6. Kiblawi FM, Sommer RJ, Levchuck SG. Transcatheter closure of patent foramen ovale in older adults. *Cathet Cardiovasc Intervent.* 2006;68(1):136–142; discussion 143–134.

7. Arora R, Trehan V, Thakur AK, Mehta V, Sengupta PP, Nigam M. Transcatheter closure of congenital muscular ventricular septal defect. *J Intervent Cardiol.* 2004;17(2):109–115.

8. Goff DA, Blume ED, Gauvreau K, Mayer JE, Lock JE, Jenkins KJ. Clinical outcome of fenestrated Fontan patients after closure: the first 10 years. *Circulation.* 2000;102(17):2094–2099.

9. Lai DW, Saver JL, Araujo JA, Reidl M, Tobis J. Pericarditis associated with nickel hypersensitivity to the AMPLATZER occluder device: a case report. *Cathet Cardiovasc Intervent.* 2005;66(3):424–426.

10. Wertman B, Azarbal B, Riedl M, Tobis J. Adverse events associated with nickel allergy in patients undergoing percutaneous atrial septal defect or patent foramen ovale closure. *J Am Coll Cardiol.* 2006;47(6):1226–1227.

11. Alaeddini J, Feghali G, Jenkins S, Ramee S, White C, Abi-Samra F. Frequency of atrial tachyarrhythmias following transcatheter closure of patent foramen ovale. *J Invasive Cardiol.* 2006;18(8):365–368.

12. Hill SL, Berul CI, Patel HT, et al. Early ECG

abnormalities associated with transcatheter closure of atrial septal defects using the AMPLATZER septal occluder. *J Intervent Card Electrophysiol.* 2000;4(3):469–474.

13. Post MC, Van Deyk K, Budts W. Percutaneous closure of a patent foramen ovale: single-centre experience using different types of devices and mid-term outcome. *Acta Cardiol.* 2005;60(5):515–519.

14. Gadhinglajkar S, Unnikrishnan KP, Sreedhar R, Kapoor MC, Neema PK. Surgical retrieval of embolised atrial septal occluder device from pulmonary artery: pathophysiology and role of the intraoperative transoesophageal echocardiography. *Ann Card Anaesth.* 2009;12(1):40–48.

15. Peuster M, Reckers J, Fink C. Secondary embolization of a HELEX occluder implanted into a secundum atrial septal defect. *Cathet Cardiovasc Intervent.* 2003;59(1):77–82.

16. Amin Z, Hijazi ZM, Bass JL, Cheatham JP, Hellenbrand WE, Kleinman CS. Erosion of AMPLATZER septal occluder device after closure of secundum atrial septal defects: review of registry of complications and recommendations to minimize future risk. *Cathet Cardiovasc Intervent.* 2004;63(4):496–502.

17. Divekar A, Gaamangwe T, Shaikh N, Raabe M, Ducas J. Cardiac perforation after device closure of atrial septal defects with the AMPLATZER septal occluder. *J Am Coll Cardiol.* 2005;45(8):1213–1218.

18. Preventza O, Sampath-Kumar S, Wasnick J, Gold JP. Late cardiac perforation following transcatheter atrial septal defect closure. *Ann Thorac Surg.* 2004;77(4):1435–1437.

19. Pinto FF, Sousa L, Fragata J. Late cardiac tamponade after transcatheter closure of atrial septal defect with CardioSEAL device. *Cardiol Young.* 2001;11(2):233–235.

20. Fagan T, Dreher D, Cutright W, Jacobson J, Latson L. Fracture of the GORE HELEX septal occluder: associated factors and clinical outcomes. *Cathet Cardiovasc Intervent.* 2009;73(7):941–948.

21. Prieto LR, Foreman CK, Cheatham JP, Latson LA. Intermediate-term outcome of transcatheter secundum atrial septal defect closure using the Bard Clamshell Septal Umbrella. *Am J Cardiol.* 1996;78(11):1310–1312.

22. Narayan V, Puri P, Mehra AO. Late presentation of CardioSEAL PFO closure device fracture and thrombus formation three years after device implantation. *J Invasive Cardiol.* 2008;20(8):E247–249.

23. Meier JM, Berger A, Delabays A, et al. Percutaneous closure of patent foramen ovale: head-to-head comparison of two different devices. *EuroIntervention.* 2005;1(1):48–52.

24. Donti A, Giardini A, Salomone L, Formigari R, Picchio FM. Transcatheter patent foramen ovale closure using the Premere PFO occlusion system. *Cathet Cardiovasc Intervent.* 2006;68(5):736–740.

25. Sherman JM, Hagler DJ, Cetta F. Thrombosis after septal closure device placement: a review of the current literature. *Cathet Cardiovasc Intervent.* 2004;63(4):486–489.

26. Anzai H, Child J, Natterson B, et al. Incidence of thrombus formation on the CardioSEAL and the AMPLATZER interatrial closure devices. *Am J Cardiol.* 2004;93(4):426–431.

27. Krumsdorf U, Ostermayer S, Billinger K, et al. Incidence and clinical course of thrombus formation on atrial septal defect and patient foramen ovale closure devices in 1,000 consecutive patients. *J Am Coll Cardiol.* 2004;43(2):302–309.

28. Cecconi M, Quarti A, Bianchini F, et al. Late cardiac perforation after transcatheter closure of patent foramen ovale. *Ann Thorac Surg.* 2006;81(6):e29–30.

29. Celiker A, Bilgic A, Ozkutlu S, Demircin M, Karagoz T, Ayabakan C. A late complication with the CardioSEAL ASD occluder device and need for surgical revision. *Cathet Cardiovasc Intervent.* 2001;54(3):335–338.

30. Chessa M, Carminati M, Butera G, et al. Early and late complications associated with transcatheter occlusion of secundum atrial septal defect. *J Am Coll Cardiol.* 2002;39(6):1061–1065.

31. Christen T, Mach F, Didier D, Kalangos A, Verin V, Trindade PT. Late cardiac tamponade after percutaneous closure of a patent foramen ovale. *Eur J Echocardiogr.* 2005;6(6):465–469.

32. Cotts T, Strouse PJ, Graziano JN. Late migration of a Sideris buttoned device for occlusion of atrial septal defect. *Cathet Cardiovasc Intervent.*

2006;68(5):754–757.

33. Egred M, Morrison L. A late complication of a patent foramen ovale amplatzer occluder device. *Eur Heart J.* 2006;27(13):1604.

34. Hsiao JF, Hsu LA, Chang CJ, et al. Late migration of a Sideris septal occluder device for closure of atrial septal defect into the left atrium with mitral valve obstruction. *Am J Cardiol.* 2007;99(10):1479–1480.

35. Lysitsas DN, Wrigley B, Banerjee P, et al. Presentation of an embolised AMPLATZER septal occluder to the main pulmonary artery 2 years after implantation. *Int J Cardiol.* 2009;131(3):e106–107.

36. Palma G, Rosapepe F, Vicchio M, Russolillo V, Cioffi S, Vosa C. Late perforation of right atrium and aortic root after percutaneous closure of patent foramen ovale. *J Thorac Cardiovasc Surg.* 2007;134(4):1054–1055.

37. Raghu A, Kawalsky D, Feldman M. Embolic stroke due to a left atrial thrombus two years after placement of an atrial septal defect closure device. *Am J Cardiol.* 2006;98(9):1294–1296.

38. Ruge H, Wildhirt SM, Libera P, Vogt M, Holper K, Lange R. Images in cardiovascular medicine. Left atrial thrombus on atrial septal defect closure device as a source of cerebral emboli 3 years after implantation. *Circulation.* 2005;112(10):e130–131.

39. Stollberger C, Finsterer J, Krexner E, Schneider B. Stroke and peripheral embolism from an AMPLATZER septal occluder 5 years after implantation. *J Neurol.* 2008;255(8):1270–1271.

40. Teoh K, Wilton E, Brecker S, Jahangiri M. Simultaneous removal of an AMPLATZER device from an atrial septal defect and the descending aorta. *J Thorac Cardiovasc Surg.* 2006;131(4):909–910.

41. Sievert H, Ruygrok P, Salkeld M, et al. Transcatheter closure of patent foramen ovale with radiofrequency: acute and intermediate term results in 144 patients. *Cathet Cardiovasc Intervent.* 2009;73(3):368–373.

42. Sievert H, Fischer E, Heinisch C, Majunke N, Roemer A, Wunderlich N. Transcatheter closure of patent foramen ovale without an implant: initial clinical experience. *Circulation.*

2007;116(15):1701–1706.

43. Walpoth NB, Habermacher K, Moarof I, et al. Device-less patent foramen ovale closure by radiofrequency thermal energy. *Swiss Med Wkly.* 2008;138(7–8):108–113.

44. Majunke N, Baranowski A, Zimmermann W, et al. A suture not always the ideal solution: problems encountered in developing a suture-based PFO closure technique. *Cathet Cardiovasc Intervent.* 2009;73(3):376–382.

45. Ruiz CE, Kipshidze N, Chiam PT, Gogorishvili I. Feasibility of patent foramen ovale closure with no-device left behind: first-in-man percutaneous suture closure. *Cathet Cardiovasc Intervent.* 2008;71(7):921–926.

46. Reiffenstein I, Majunke N, Wunderlich N, Carter P, Jones R, Sievert H. Percutaneous closure of patent foramen ovale with a novel Flat-Stent. *Expert Rev Med Dev.* 2008;5(4):419–425.

47. Mullen MJ, Hildick-Smith D, De Giovanni JV, et al. BioSTAR Evaluation STudy (BEST): a prospective, multicenter, phase I clinical trial to evaluate the feasibility, efficacy, and safety of the BioSTAR bioabsorbable septal repair implant for the closure of atrial-level shunts. *Circulation.* 2006;114(18):1962–1967.

48. Mullen MJ, Devellian CA, Jux C. BioSTAR bioabsorbable septal repair implant. *Expert Rev Med Dev.* 2007;4(6):781–792.

49. Hoehn R, Hesse C, Ince H, Peuster M. First experience With the biostar-device for various applications in pediatric patients with congenital heart disease. *Cathet Cardiovasc Intervent.* 2009;75(1):72-77.

50. Jux C, Bertram H, Wohlsein P, Bruegmann M, Paul T. Interventional atrial septal defect closure using a totally bioresorbable occluder matrix: development and preclinical evaluation of the BioSTAR device. *J Am Coll Cardiol.* 2006;48(1):161–169.

51. Jux C, Wohlsein P, Bruegmann M, Zutz M, Franzbach B, Bertram H. A new biological matrix for septal occlusion. *J Intervent Cardiol.* 2003;16(2):149–152.

52. Ussia GP, Cammalleri V, Mule M, et al. Percutaneous closure of patent foramen ovale with a bioabsorbable occluder device: single–centre experience. *Cathet Cardiovasc Intervent.*

2009;74(4):607–614.

53. Van den Branden BJ, Post MC, Jaarsma W, ten Berg JM, Suttorp MJ. New bioabsorbable septal repair implant for percutaneous closure of a patent foramen ovale: short–term results of a single-centre experience. *Cathet Cardiovasc Intervent.* 2009;74(2):286–290.

54. Sigler M, Jux C. Biocompatibility of septal defect closure devices. *Heart (Br Card Soc).* 2007;93(4):444–449.

55. Solomon SB. The future of interventional cardiology lies in the left atrium. *Int J Cardiovasc Intervent.* 2004;6(3–4):101–106.

56. King TD, Thompson SL, Steiner C, Mills NL. Secundum atrial septal defect. Nonoperative closure during cardiac catheterization. *JAMA.* 1976;235(23):2506–2509.

57. King TD, Mills NL. Nonoperative closure of atrial septal defects. *Surgery.* 1974;75(3):383–388.

58. Rashkind WJ, Mullins CE, Hellenbrand WE, Tait MA. Nonsurgical closure of patent ductus arteriosus: clinical application of the Rashkind PDA Occluder System. *Circulation.* 1987;75(3):583–592.

59. Lock JE, Rome JJ, Davis R, et al. Transcatheter closure of atrial septal defects. Experimental studies. *Circulation.* 1989;79(5):1091–1099.

60. Rome JJ, Keane JF, Perry SB, Spevak PJ, Lock JE. Double-umbrella closure of atrial defects. Initial clinical applications. *Circulation.* 1990;82(3):751–758.

61. Ryan C, Opolski S, Wright J, et al. Structural Considerations in the Development of the CardioSEAL Septal Occluder. *Proceedings of the 2nd World Congress of Pediatric Cardiology and Cardiac Surgery,* Futura Publishing Co. 1998:191–193.

62. Latson LA. Per-catheter ASD closure. *Pediatr Cardiol.* 1998;19(1):86–93; discussion 94.

63. O'Laughlin MP. Microvena atrial septal defect occlusion device—update 2000. *J Intervent Cardiol.* 2001;14(1):77–80.

64. Babic UU. Experience with ASDOS for Transcatheter Closure of Atrial Septal Defect and Patent Foramen Ovale. *Curr Intervent Cardiol Rep.* 2000;2(2):177–183.

65. Hung J, Landzberg MJ, Jenkins KJ, et al. Closure of patent foramen ovale for paradoxical emboli: intermediate-term risk of recurrent neurological events following transcatheter device placement. *J Am Coll Cardiol.* 2000;35(5):1311–1316.

66. Lloyd TR, Rao PS, Beekman RH 3rd, Mendelsohn AM, Sideris EB. Atrial septal defect occlusion with the buttoned device (a multi-institutional U.S. trial). *Am J Cardiol.* 1994;73(4):286–291.

67. Rao PS. Summary and Comparison of Atrial Septal Defect Closure Devices. *Curr Intervent Cardiol Rep.* 2000;2(4):367–376.

68. Agarwal SK, Ghosh PK, Mittal PK. Failure of devices used for closure of atrial septal defects: mechanisms and management. *J Thorac Cardiovasc Surg.* 1996;112(1):21–26.

69. Ten Freyhaus H, Rosenkranz S, Sudkamp M, Hopp HW. Dysfunction of an atrial septal defect occluder 8 years after implantation. *J Intervent Cardiol.* 2006;19(2):163–165.

70. Bohm J, Bittigau K, Kohler F, Baumann G, Konertz W. Surgical removal of atrial septal defect occlusion system-devices. *Eur J Cardiothorac Surg.* 1997;12(6):869–872.

71. Khatchatourov G, Kalangos A, Anwar A, et al. Massive thromboembolism due to transcatheter ASD closure with ASDOS device. *J Invasive Cardiol.* 1999;11(12):743–745.

72. Williams DF. *The Williams' Dictionary of Biomaterials.* UK. Liverpool University Press; 1999.

73. ANSI/AAMI/ISO 10993-1:2003: Biological evaluation of medical devices—Evaluation and testing in order to assess the potential biological effects post implantation.

74. Vincent RN, Raviele AA, Diehl HJ. Single-center experience with the HELEX septal occluder for closure of atrial septal defects in children. *J Intervent Cardiol.* 2003;16(1):79–82.

75. Slavin L, Tobis JM, Rangarajan K, Dao C, Krivokapich J, Liebeskind DS. Five-year experience with percutaneous closure of patent foramen ovale. *Am J Cardiol.* 2007;99(9):1316–1320.

76. Fukahara K, Minami K, Reiss N, Fassbender D, Koerfer R. Systemic allergic reaction to the percutaneous patent foramen ovale occluder. *J Thorac Cardiovasc Surg.* 2003;125(1):213–214.

77. Kim KH, Park JC, Yoon NS, et al. A case of allergic contact dermatitis following transcath-

eter closure of patent ductus arteriosus using AMPLATZER ductal occluder. *Int J Cardiol.* 2008;127(2):e98–99.

78. Rabkin DG, Whitehead KJ, Michaels AD, Powell DL, Karwande SV. Unusual presentation of nickel allergy requiring explantation of an AMPLATZER atrial septal occluder device. *Clin Cardiol.* 2009;32(8):E55–57.

79. Rigatelli G, Cardaioli P, Giordan M, et al. Nickel allergy in interatrial shunt device-based closure patients. *Congenit Heart Dis.* 2007;2(6):416–420.

80. Ahmad Z, Wilson N, Veldtman G. Percutaneous stabilization of a HELEX device following locking-loop fracture: a case report. *J Invasive Cardiol.* 2009;21(11):E213–215.

81. Qureshi AM, Mumtaz MA, Latson LA. Partial prolapse of a HELEX device associated with early frame fracture and mitral valve perforation. *Cathet Cardiovasc Intervent.* 2009;74(5):777–782.

82. Mertens L, Meyns B, Gewillig M. Device fracture and severe tricuspid regurgitation after percutaneous closure of perimembranous ventricular septal defect: a case report. *Cathet Cardiovasc Intervent.* 2007;70(5):749–753.

83. Latson LA, Jones TK, Jacobson J, Zahn E, Rhodes JF. Analysis of factors related to successful transcatheter closure of secundum atrial septal defects using the HELEX septal occluder. *Am Heart J.* 2006;151(5):1129 e1127–1111.

84. Scott P, Wilson N, Veldtman G. Fracture of a GORE HELEX septal occluder following PFO closure in a diver. *Cathet Cardiovasc Intervent.* 2009;73(6):828–831.

85. Kaulitz R, Peuster M, Jux C, Paul T, Hausdorf G. Transcatheter closure of various types of defects within the oval fossa using the double umbrella device (CardioSEAL)—feasibility and echocardiographic follow-up. *Cardiol Young.* 2001;11(2):214–222.

86. Sievert H, Horvath K, Zadan E, et al. Patent foramen ovale closure in patients with transient ischemia attack/stroke. *J Intervent Cardiol.* 2001;14(2):261–266.

87. Buecker A, Spuentrup E, Grabitz R, et al. Magnetic resonance-guided placement of atrial septal closure device in animal model of patent foramen ovale. *Circulation.* 2002;106(4):511–515.

88. Buecker A, Spuentrup E, Grabitz R, et al. Real-time-MR guidance for placement of a self-made fully MR-compatible atrial septal occluder: in vitro test. *Rofo.* 2002;174(3):283–285.

89. Rickers C, Jerosch-Herold M, Hu X, et al. Magnetic resonance image-guided transcatheter closure of atrial septal defects. *Circulation.* 2003;107(1):132–138.

90. *Guidance for Industry and FDA Staff, Establishing Safety and Compatibility of Passive Implants in the Magnetic Resonance (MR) Environment;* Document issued on: August 21, 2008.

91. Shellock FG, Woods TO, Crues JV 3rd. MR labeling information for implants and devices: explanation of terminology. *Radiology.* 2009; 253(1):26–30.

92. *ASM Handbook Volume 1 Properties and Selection: Irons, Steels, and High Performance Alloys.* Materials Park, Ohio: ASM International; 1990;841–901.

93. Disegi JA, Eschbach L. Stainless steel in bone surgery. *Injury.* 2000;31 Suppl 4:2–6.

94. Ellis SG, Savage M, Fischman D, , et al. Restenosis after placement of Palmaz-Schatz stents in native coronary arteries. Initial results of a multicenter experience. *Circulation.* 1992;86(6): 1836–1844.

95. Prasad V, Chan RP, Faughnan ME. Embolotherapy of pulmonary arteriovenous malformations: efficacy of platinum versus stainless steel coils. *J Vasc Intervent Radiol.* 2004;15(2 Pt 1):153–160.

96. Becker RL, Norfray JF, Teitelbaum GP, et al. MR imaging in patients with intracranial aneurysm clips. *AJNR.* 1988;9(5):885–889.

97. Holton A, Walsh E, Anayiotos A, Pohost G, Venugopalan R. Comparative MRI compatibility of 316 L stainless steel alloy and nickel-titanium alloy stents. *J Cardiovasc Magn Reson.* 2002;4(4):423–430.

98. ASTM F138 - 08 Standard Specification for Wrought 18Chromium-14Nickel-2.5Molybdenum Stainless Steel Bar and Wire for Surgical Implants (UNS S31673). West Conshohocken, PA: ASTM International; 2008.

99. Younkin CN. Multiphase MP35N alloy for medical implants. *J Biomed Mater Res.* 1974;8

(3):219–226.

100. Escalas F, Galante J, Rostoker W, Coogan PH. MP35N: a corrosion resistant, high strength alloy for orthopedic surgical implants: bio-assay results. *J Biomed Mater research.* 1975;9(3):303–313.

101. Borin JF, Melamud O, Clayman RV. Initial experience with full-length metal stent to relieve malignant ureteral obstruction. *J Endourol/ Endourol Soc.* 2006;20(5):300–304.

102. Altman PA, Meagher JM, Walsh DW, Hoffmann DA. Rotary bending fatigue of coils and wires used in cardiac lead design. *J Biomed Mater Res.* 1998;43(1):21–37.

103. Kangarlu A, Shellock FG. Aneurysm clips: evaluation of magnetic field interactions with an 8.0 T MR system. *J Magn Reson Imaging.* 2000;12(1):107–111.

104. Weiler PJ, Medley JB, McNeice GM. Numerical [corrected] analysis of the load capacity of the human spine fitted with L-rod instrumentation. *Spine.* 1990;15(12):1285–1293.

105. ASTM F562 Standard Specification for Wrought 35Cobalt-35Nickel-20Chromium-10Molybdenum Alloy for Surgical Implant Applications (UNS R30035).West Conshohocken, PA: ASTM International; 2007.

106. Clerc CO, Jedwab MR, Mayer DW, Thompson PJ, Stinson JS. Assessment of wrought ASTM F1058 cobalt alloy properties for permanent surgical implants. *J Biomed Mater Res.* 1997; 38(3):229–234.

107. Es-Souni M, Fischer-Brandies H, Es-Souni M. On the in vitro biocompatibility of Elgiloy, a co-based alloy, compared to two titanium alloys. *J Orofac Orthop.* 2003;64(1):16–26.

108. ASTM F1058-08 Standard Specification for Wrought 40Cobalt-20Chromium-16Iron-15Nickel-7Molybdenum Alloy Wire and Strip for Surgical Implant Applications (UNS R30003 and UNS R30008). West Conshohocken, PA: ASTM International; 2008.

109. Buehler WJ, Gilfrich JV, Wiley RC. Effect of Low-Temperature Phase Changes on the Mechanical Properties of Alloys near Composition TiNi. *J Appl Phys.* 1963;34(5):1475.

110. Kauffman GB, Mayo I. The Story of Nitinol: The Serendipitous Discovery of the Memory Metal and Its Applications. *Chem Educator.*

111. Duerig TW, Pelton AR, Stockel D. The utility of superelasticity in medicine. *Biomed Mater Eng.* 1996;6(4):255–266.

112. Doi H, Maehara A, Mintz GS, Dani L, Leon MB, Grube E. Serial intravascular ultrasound analysis of bifurcation lesions treated using the novel self-expanding sideguard side branch stent. *Am J Cardiol.* 2009;104(9):1216–1221.

113. Simon M, Kaplow R, Salzman E, Freiman D. A vena cava filter using thermal shape memory alloy. Experimental aspects. *Radiology.* 1977;125(1):87–94.

114. Hull JE, Robertson SW. Bard Recovery filter: evaluation and management of vena cava limb perforation, fracture, and migration. *J Vasc Intervent Radiol.* 2009;20(1):52–60.

115. Saweeres ES, Thomas AP. Modified technique for arthroscopic Bankart repair using anchor sutures. *Arthroscopy.* 2004;20 Suppl 2:121–124.

116. Russell SM. Design Considerations for Nitinol Bone Staples. *J Mater Eng Perform.* 2009;18(5/6):831–835.

117. ASTM F2063 "Standard Specification for Wrought Nickel-Titanium Shape Memory Alloys for Medical Devices and Surgical Implants. West Conshohocken, PA: ASTM International; 2005.

118. ASTM F2004-05 "Standard Test Method for Transformation Temperature of Nickel-Titanium Alloys by Thermal Analysis". West Conshohocken, PA: ASTM International; 2005.

119. ASTM F2082 Standard Test Method for the Determination of Transformation Temperature of Nickel-Titanium Shape Memory Alloys by Bend and Free Recovery. West Conshohocken, PA: ASTM International; 2006.

120. Cullity BD. *Elements of X-Ray Diffraction.* 2nd ed. Addison-Wesley Publishing Company; 1978:13.

121. Nolan BW, Schermerhorn ML, Powell RJ, et al. Restenosis in gold-coated renal artery stents. *J Vasc Surg.* 2005;42(1):40–46.

122. Ribeiro PA, Gallo R, Antonius J, et al. A new expandable intracoronary tantalum (Strecker) stent: early experimental results and follow-up to twelve months. *Am Heart J.* 1993;125(2 Pt 1):501–510.

123. Budynas RG, Nisbett JK. *Shigley's Mechanical*

Engineering Design. McGraw Hill; 2008.

124. Peuster M, Hesse C, Schloo T, Fink C, Beerbaum P, von Schnakenburg C. Long-term biocompatibility of a corrodible peripheral iron stent in the porcine descending aorta. *Biomaterials.* 2006;27(28):4955–4962.

125. Bachthaler M, Lenhart M, Paetzel C, Feuerbach S, Link J, Manke C. Corrosion of tungsten coils after peripheral vascular embolization therapy: influence on outcome and tungsten load. *Cathet Cardiovasc Intervent.* 2004;62(3):380–384.

126. Peuster M, Fink C, Wohlsein P, et al. Degradation of tungsten coils implanted into the subclavian artery of New Zealand white rabbits is not associated with local or systemic toxicity. *Biomaterials.* 2003;24(3):393–399.

127. Peuster M, Kaese V, Wuensch G, et al. Composition and in vitro biocompatibility of corroding tungsten coils. *J Biomed Mater Res B Appl Biomater.* 2003;65(1):211–216.

128. Peuster M, Kaese V, Wuensch G, et al. Dissolution of tungsten coils leads to device failure after transcatheter embolisation of pathologic vessels. *Heart (Br Card Soc).* 2001;85(6):703–704.

129. Fontana MG. *Corrosion Engineering,* New York, NY: McGraw-Hill Book Company; 1986;295.

130. *ASM Handbook, Volume 13 Corrosion.* ASM International; 1987:10.

131. Virtanen S, Milosev I, Gomez-Barrena E, Trebse R, Salo J, Konttinen YT. Special modes of corrosion under physiological and simulated physiological conditions. *Acta Biomater.* 2008;4(3):468–476.

132. Kong H, Wilkinson JL, Coe JY, et al. Corrosive behaviour of AMPLATZER devices in experimental and biological environments. *Cardiol Young.* 2002;12(3):260–265.

133. ASTM F2129 Standard Test Method for Conducting Cyclic Potentiodynamic Polarization Measurements to Determine the Corrosion Susceptibility of Small Implant Devices. West Conshohocken, PA: ASTM International; 2008.

134. ASTM G71-81 Standard Guide for Conducting and Evaluating Galvanic Corrosion Tests in Electrolytes. West Conshohocken, PA: ASTM International; 2008.

135. Uhlig RH, Revie RW. *Corrosion and Corrosion Control.* New York. Wiley; 1985:149.

136. Palmaz JC, Benson A, Sprague EA. Influence of surface topography on endothelialization of intravascular metallic material. *J Vasc Intervent Radiol.* 1999;10(4):439–444.

137. Shabalovskaya SA. Surface, corrosion and biocompatibility aspects of Nitinol as an implant material. *Biomed Mater Eng.* 2002;12(1):69–109.

138. Eiselstein LE, Proctor DM, Flowers TC. Trivalent and hexavalent chromium issues in medical implants. *Mater Sci Forum.* 2007;539–543 (1):698–703.

139. Witzleb WC, Ziegler J, Krummenauer F, Neumeister V, Guenther KP. Exposure to chromium, cobalt and molybdenum from metal-on-metal total hip replacement and hip resurfacing arthroplasty. *Acta Orthopaed.* 2006;77(5):697–705.

140. Cobb AG, Schmalzreid TP. The clinical significance of metal ion release from cobalt-chromium metal-on-metal hip joint arthroplasty. *Proc Instit Mech Eng.* 2006;220(2):385–398.

141. Schaffer AW, Pilger A, Engelhardt C, Zweymueller K, Ruediger HW. Increased blood cobalt and chromium after total hip replacement. *J Toxicol.* 1999;37(7):839–844.

142. Koster R, Vieluf D, Kiehn M, et al. Nickel and molybdenum contact allergies in patients with coronary in-stent restenosis. *Lancet.* 2000;356(9245):1895–1897.

143. Hallab N, Merritt K, Jacobs JJ. Metal sensitivity in patients with orthopaedic implants. *J Bone Joint Surg.* 2001;83-A(3):428–436.

144. Hallab NJ, Mikecz K, Jacobs JJ. A triple assay technique for the evaluation of metal-induced, delayed-type hypersensitivity responses in patients with or receiving total joint arthroplasty. *J Biomed Mater Res.* 2000;53(5):480–489.

145. Hallab NJ, Mikecz K, Vermes C, Skipor A, Jacobs JJ. Orthopaedic implant related metal toxicity in terms of human lymphocyte reactivity to metal-protein complexes produced from cobalt-base and titanium-base implant alloy degradation. *Mole Cell Biochem.* 2001;222(1–2):127–136.

146. Merritt K, Rodrigo JJ. Immune response to synthetic materials. Sensitization of patients receiving orthopaedic implants. *Clin Orthop Relat Res.* 1996(326):71–79.

147. Jensen CS, Lisby S, Baadsgaard O, Byrialsen K,

Menne T. Release of nickel ions from stainless steel alloys used in dental braces and their patch test reactivity in nickel-sensitive individuals. *Contact dermatitis.* 2003;48(6):300–304.

148. Hillen U, Haude M, Erbel R, Goos M. Evaluation of metal allergies in patients with coronary stents. *Contact Dermatitis.* 2002;47(6): 353–356.

149. von Blomberg-van der Flier M, van der Burg CK, Pos O, et al. In vitro studies in nickel allergy: diagnostic value of a dual parameter analysis. *J Invest Dermatol.* 1987;88(4):362–368.

150. Thyssen JP, Linneberg A, Menne T, Johansen JD. The epidemiology of contact allergy in the general population—prevalence and main findings. *Contact Dermatitis.* 2007;57(5):287–299.

151. Marks JG Jr., Belsito DV, DeLeo VA, et al. North American Contact Dermatitis Group patch-test results, 1998 to 2000. *Am J Contact Dermatol.* 2003;14(2):59–62.

152. Cohen DE. Contact dermatitis: a quarter century perspective. *J Am Acad Dermatol.* 2004;51(1, suppl):S60–S63.

153. Rietschel RL, Fowler JF, Warshaw EM, et al. Detection of nickel sensitivity has increased in North American patch-test patients. *Dermatitis.* 2008;19(1):16–19.

154. Burian M, Neumann T, Weber M, et al. Nickel release, a possible indicator for the duration of antiplatelet treatment, from a nickel cardiac device in vivo: a study in patients with atrial septal defects implanted with an AMPLATZER occluder. *Int J Clin Pharmacol Ther.* 2006;44(3):107–112.

155. Dasika UK, Kanter KR, Vincent R. Nickel allergy to the percutaneous patent foramen ovale occluder and subsequent systemic nickel allergy. *J Thorac Cardiovasc Surg.* 2003;126(6):2112.

156. Ries MW, Kampmann C, Rupprecht HJ, Hintereder G, Hafner G, Meyer J. Nickel release after implantation of the AMPLATZER occluder. *Am Heart J.* 2003;145(4):737–741.

157. Singh HR, Turner DR, Forbes TJ. Nickel allergy and the amplatzer septal occluder. *J Invasive Cardiol.* 2004;16(11):681–682.

158. Anselmino M, Ribezzo M, Orzan F. Nickel allergy, how deep? *Acta Cardiol.* 2009;64(1): 104–106.

159. Reddy BT, Patel JB, Powell DL, Michaels AD. Interatrial shunt closure devices in patients with nickel allergy. *Cathet Cardiovasc Intervent.* 2009;74(4):647–651.

160. Serruys PW, Ormiston JA, Onuma Y, et al. A bioabsorbable everolimus-eluting coronary stent system (ABSORB): 2-year outcomes and results from multiple imaging methods. *Lancet.* 2009;373(9667):897–910.

161. Ramcharitar S, Serruys PW. Fully biodegradable coronary stents : progress to date. *Am J Cardiovasc Drugs.* 2008;8(5):305–314.

162. Ormiston JA, Serruys PW, Regar E, et al. A bioabsorbable everolimus-eluting coronary stent system for patients with single de-novo coronary artery lesions (ABSORB): a prospective open-label trial. *Lancet.* 2008;371(9616):899–907.

163. Waksman R. Biodegradable stents: they do their job and disappear. *J Invasive Cardiol.* 2006;18(2):70–74.

164. Sigler M, Jux C. Biocompatibility of septal defect closure devices. *Heart (Br Card Soc).* 2006.

165. van der Giessen WJ, Lincoff AM, Schwartz RS, et al. Marked inflammatory sequelae to implantation of biodegradable and nonbiodegradable polymers in porcine coronary arteries. *Circulation.* 1996;94(7):1690–1697.

166. Hooper KA, Macon ND, Kohn J. Comparative histological evaluation of new tyrosine-derived polymers and poly (L-lactic acid) as a function of polymer degradation. *J Biomed Mater Res.* 1998;41(3):443–454.

167. Kulkarni RK, Pani KC, Neuman C, Leonard F. Polylactic acid for surgical implants. *Arch Surg.* 1966;93(5):839–843.

168. Ratner BD, Hoffman AS, Schoen FJ, Lemons JE. *An Introduction to Materials in Medicine.* 2nd ed. Elsevier Academic Press; 2004.

169. Verbal communication, James Anderson, MD, PhD, Case Western Reserve University, Cleveland, Ohio.

170. Verbal communication, James Anderson, MD, PhD, Case Western Reserve University, Cleveland, Ohio.

171. Tamai H, Igaki K, Kyo E, et al. Initial and 6-month results of biodegradable poly-l-lactic acid coronary stents in humans. *Circulation.* 2000;102(4):399–404.

172. Lincoff AM, Furst JG, Ellis SG, Tuch RJ, Topol EJ. Sustained local delivery of dexamethasone by a novel intravascular eluting stent to prevent restenosis in the porcine coronary injury model. *J Am Coll Cardiol.* 1997;29(4):808–816.

173. Yamawaki T, Shimokawa H, Kozai T, et al. Intramural delivery of a specific tyrosine kinase inhibitor with biodegradable stent suppresses the restenotic changes of the coronary artery in pigs in vivo. *J Am Coll Cardiol.* 1998;32(3):780–786.

174. Bunger CM, Grabow N, Kroger C, et al. Iliac anastomotic stenting with a sirolimus-eluting biodegradable poly-L-lactide stent: a preliminary study after 6 weeks. *J Endovasc Ther.* 2006;13(5):630–639.

175. Vogt F, Stein A, Rettemeier G, et al. Long-term assessment of a novel biodegradable paclitaxel-eluting coronary polylactide stent. *Eur Heart J.* 2004;25(15):1330–1340.

176. Jain JP, Modi S, Domb AJ, Kumar N. Role of polyanhydrides as localized drug carriers. *J Control Release.* 2005;103(3):541–563.

177. Attawia MA, Uhrich KE, Botchwey E, Fan M, Langer R, Laurencin CT. Cytotoxicity testing of poly(anhydride-co-imides) for orthopedic applications. *J Biomed Mater Res.* 1995;29(10):1233–1240.

178. Laurencin C, Domb A, Morris C, et al. Poly(anhydride) administration in high doses in vivo: studies of biocompatibility and toxicology. *J Biomed Mater Res.* 1990;24(11):1463–1481.

179. Middleton JC, Tipton AJ. Synthetic biodegradable polymers as medical devices. *Med Plast Biomater Mag.* 1998.

180. Whitaker-Brothers K, Uhrich K. Investigation into the erosion mechanism of salicylate-based poly(anhydride-esters). *J Biomed Mater Res A.* 2006;76(3):470–479.

181. Williams SF, Martin DP, Horowitz DM, Peoples OP. PHA applications: addressing the price performance issue: I. Tissue engineering. *Int J Biol Macromol.* 1999;25(1–3):111–121.

182. Martin DP, Williams SF. Medical applications of poly-4-hydroxybutyrate: a strong flexible absorbable biomaterial. *Biochem Eng J.* 2003;16:97–105.

183. Ferrara SD, Zotti S, Tedeschi L, et al. Pharmacokinetics of gamma hydroxybutyric acid in alcohol dependent patients after single and repeated oral doses. *Br J Clin Pharmacol.* 1992;34(3):231–235.

184. Bunger CM, Grabow N, Sternberg K, et al. A biodegradable stent based on poly(L-lactide) and poly(4-hydroxybutyrate) for peripheral vascular application: preliminary experience in the pig. *J Endovasc Ther.* 2007;14(5):725–733.

185. Grabow N, Bunger CM, Schultze C, et al. A biodegradable slotted tube stent based on poly(L-lactide) and poly(4-hydroxybutyrate) for rapid balloon-expansion. *Ann Biomed Eng.* 2007;35(12):2031–2038.

186. Hoerstrup SP, Sodian R, Daebritz S, et al. Functional living trileaflet heart valves grown in vitro. *Circulation.* 2000;102(19, Suppl 3):III44–III49.

187. Sales VL, Mettler BA, Engelmayr GC, et al. Endothelial progenitor cells as a sole source for ex vivo seeding of tissue-engineered heart valves. *Tissue Eng Part A.* 2010; 16(1): 257–67.

188. Bourke SL, Kohn J. Polymers derived from the amino acid L-tyrosine: polycarbonates, polyacrylates and copolymers with poly(ethylene glycol). *Adv Drug Deliver Rev.* 2003;55(4):447–466.

189. Silver FH, Marks M, Kato YP, Li C, Pulapura S, Kohn J. Tissue compatibility of tyrosine-derived polycarbonates and polyaminocarbonates: an initial evaluation. *J Long-Term Effects Med Implants.* 1992;1(4):329–346.

190. Ertel SI, Kohn J. Evaluation of a series of tyrosine-derived polycarbonates as degradable biomaterials. *J Biomed Mater Res.* 1994;28(8):919–930.

191. Ertel SI, Kohn J, Zimmerman MC, Parsons JR. Evaluation of poly(DTH carbonate), a tyrosine-derived degradable polymer, for orthopedic applications. *J Biomed Mater Res.* 1995;29(11):1337–1348.

192. Kohn J, Zeltinger J. Degradable, drug-eluting stents: a new frontier for the treatment of coronary artery disease. *Expert Rev Med Dev.* 2005;2(6):667–671.

193. Macario DK, Entersz I, Bolikal D, Kohn J, Nackman GB. Iodine inhibits antiadhesive effect of PEG: implications for tissue engineering. *J Biomed Mater Res B Appl Biomater.* 2008;86(1):237–244.

194. Personal communication January 2010, REVA

Medical, Inc. (San Diego, California).

195. Choueka J, Charvet JL, Koval KJ, et al. Canine bone response to tyrosine-derived polycarbonates and poly(L-lactic acid). *J Biomed Mater Res.* 1996;31(1):35–41.

196. Burma O, Ustunsoy H, Davutoglu V, Celkan MA, Kazaz H, Pektok E. Initial clinical experience with a novel biodegradable ring in patients with functional tricuspid insufficiency: Kalangos Biodegradable Tricuspid Ring. *Thorac Cardiovasc Surg.* 2007;55(5):284–287.

197. Cikirikcioglu M, Pektok E, Myers PO, Christenson JT, Kalangos A. Pediatric mitral valve repair with the novel annuloplasty ring: Kalangos-Bioring. *Asian Cardiovasc Thorac Ann.* 2008;16(6):515–516.

198. Christenson JT, Kalangos A. Use of a biodegradable annuloplasty ring for mitral valve repair in children. *Asian Cardiovasc Thorac Ann.* 2009;17 (1):11–12.

199. Kalangos A, Christenson JT, Beghetti M, Cikirikcioglu M, Kamentsidis D, Aggoun Y. Mitral valve repair for rheumatic valve disease in children: midterm results and impact of the use of a biodegradable mitral ring. *Ann Thorac Surg.* 2008;86(1):161–168, discussion 168–169.

200. Ray JA, Doddi N, Regula D, Williams JA, Melveger A. Polydioxanone (PDS), a novel monofilament synthetic absorbable suture. *Surg Gynecol Obstet.* 1981;153(4):497–507.

201. Staiger MP, Pietak AM, Huadmai J, Dias G. Magnesium and its alloys as orthopedic biomaterials: a review. *Biomaterials.* 2006;27(9):1728–1734.

202. Peuster M, Wohlsein P, Brugmann M, et al. A novel approach to temporary stenting: degradable cardiovascular stents produced from corrodible metal-results 6–18 months after implantation into New Zealand white rabbits. *Heart (Br Card Soc).* 2001;86(5):563–569.

203. Waksman R, Pakala R, Baffour R, Seabron R, Hellinga D, Tio FO. Short-term effects of biocorrodible iron stents in porcine coronary arteries. *J Intervent Cardiol.* 2008;21(1):15–20.

204. Gray-Munro JE, Seguin C, Strong M. Influence of surface modification on the in vitro corrosion rate of magnesium alloy AZ31. *J Biomed Mater Res A.* 2009;91(1):221–230.

205. Di Mario C, Griffiths H, Goktekin O, et al. Drug-eluting bioabsorbable magnesium stent. *J Intervent Cardiol.* 2004;17(6):391–395.

206. Waksman R, Pakala R, Kuchulakanti PK, et al. Safety and efficacy of bioabsorbable magnesium alloy stents in porcine coronary arteries. *Cathet Cardiovasc Intervent.* 2006;68(4):607–617, discussion 618–609.

207. Mani G, Feldman MD, Patel D, Agrawal CM. Coronary stents: a materials perspective. *Biomaterials.* 2007;28(9):1689–1710.

208. Erbel R, Di Mario C, Bartunek J, et al. Temporary scaffolding of coronary arteries with bioabsorbable magnesium stents: a prospective, non-randomised multicentre trial. *Lancet.* 2007;369(9576):1869–1875.

209. Zartner P, Buettner M, Singer H, Sigler M. First biodegradable metal stent in a child with congenital heart disease: evaluation of macro and histopathology. *Cathet Cardiovasc Intervent.* 2007;69(3):443–446.

210. Sukavaneshvar S, Rosa GM, Solen KA. Enhancement of stent-induced thromboembolism by residual stenoses: contribution of hemodynamics. *Ann Biomed Eng.* 2000;28(2):182–193.

211. Jux C, Bertram H, Wohlsein P, Bruegmann M, Paul T. Interventional atrial septal defect closure using a totally bioresorbable occluder matrix: development and preclinical evaluation of the BioSTAR device. *J Am Coll Cardiol.* 2006;48(1):161–169.

212. Mathisen SR, Wu HD, Sauvage LR, Usui Y, Walker MW. An experimental study of eight current arterial prostheses. *J Vasc Surg.* 1986; 4(1):33–41.

213. Nunn DB, Freeman MH, Hudgins PC. Postoperative alterations in size of Dacron aortic grafts: an ultrasonic evaluation. *Ann Surg.* 1979;189(6):741–745.

214. Kreutzer J, Ryan CA, Gauvreau K, Van Praagh R, Anderson JM, Jenkins KJ. Healing response to the Clamshell device for closure of intracardiac defects in humans. *Cathet Cardiovasc Intervent.* 2001;54(1):101–111.

215. Sigler M, Jux C, Ewert P. Histopathological

workup of an AMPLATZER atrial septal defect occluder after surgical removal. *Pediatr Cardiol.* 2006;27(6):775–776.

216. Eagleton MJ, Ouriel K, Shortell C, Green RM. Femoral-infrapopliteal bypass with prosthetic grafts. *Surgery.* 1999;126(4):759–764, discussion 764–755.

217. Chiesa R, Melissano G, Castellano R, Frigerio S. Extensible expanded polytetrafluoroethylene vascular grafts for aortoiliac and aortofemoral reconstruction. *Cardiovasc Surg (London, England).* 2000;8(7):538–544.

218. Zahn EM, Wilson N, Cutright W, Latson LA. Development and testing of the HELEX septal occluder, a new expanded polytetrafluoroethylene atrial septal defect occlusion system. *Circulation.* 2001;104(6):711–716.

219. Hawe A, Rastelli GC. Late deterioration of intracardiac Ivalon sponge patches. *J Thorac Cardiovasc Surg.* 1969;58(1):87–91.

220. Bolton-Maggs PH, Motson RW. Late presentation of polyvinyl alcohol sponge (Ivalon) aortic graft failure. *Thorax.* 1979;34(4):561–562.

221. Porstmann W, Wierny L, Warnke H, Gerstberger G, Romaniuk PA. Catheter closure of patent ductus arteriosus. 62 cases treated without thoracotomy. *Radiol Clin North Am.* 1971;9(2).203–218.

222. Wierny L, Plass R, Porstmann W. Transluminal closure of patent ductus arteriosus: long-term results of 208 cases treated without thoracotomy. *Cardiovasc Intervent Radiol.* 1986;9(5–6):279–285.

223. Stokes K, Cobian K. Polyether polyurethanes for implantable pacemaker leads. *Biomaterials.* 1982;3(4):225–231.

224. Stokes K, Coury A, Urbanski P. Autooxidative degradation of implanted polyether polyurethane devices. *J Biomater Appl.* 1987;1(4):411–448.

225. Stokes K, Urbanski P, Upton J. The in vivo autooxidation of polyether polyurethane by metal ions. *J Biomater Sci.* 1990;1(3):207–230.

226. Chawla AS, Blais P, Hinberg I, Johnson D. Degradation of explanted polyurethane cardiac pacing leads and of polyurethane. *Biomater Artif Cells Artif Organs.* 1988;16(4):785–800.

227. Marchant RE, Miller KM, Anderson JM. In vivo biocompatibility studies. V. In vivo leukocyte interactions with Biomer. *J Biomed Mater Res.* 1984;18(9):1169–1190.

228. Zhao QH, McNally AK, Rubin KR, et al. Human plasma alpha 2-macroglobulin promotes in vitro oxidative stress cracking of Pellethane 2363-80A: in vivo and in vitro correlations. *J Biomed Mater Res.* 1993;27(3):379–388.

229. Benoit FM. Degradation of polyurethane foams used in the Meme breast implant. *J Biomed Mater Res.* 1993;27(10):1341–1348.

230. Sideris EB. Advances in transcatheter patch occlusion of heart defects. *J Intervent Cardiol.* 2003;16(5):419–424.

231. Sideris EB, Kaneva A, Sideris SE, Moulopoulos SD. Transcatheter atrial septal defect occlusion in piglets by balloon detachable devices. *Cathet Cardiovasc Intervent.* 2000;51(4):529–534.

232. Ciccone WJ 2nd, Motz C, Bentley C, Tasto JP. Bioabsorbable implants in orthopaedics: new developments and clinical applications. *J Am Acad Orthop Surg.* 2001;9(5):280–288.

233. Pans A, Desaive C. Use of an absorbable polyglactin mesh for the prevention of incisional hernias. *Acta Chir Belg.* 1995;95(6):265–268.

234. Buchsbaum HJ, Christopherson W, Lifshitz S, Bernstein S. Vicryl mesh in pelvic floor reconstruction. *Arch Surg.* 1985;120(12):1389–1391.

235. Abraham GA, Murray J, Billiar K, Sullivan SJ. Evaluation of the porcine intestinal collagen layer as a biomaterial. *J Biomed Mater Res.* 2000;51(3):442–452.

236. Badylak SF. Xenogeneic extracellular matrix as a scaffold for tissue reconstruction. *Transplant Immunol.* 2004;12(3–4):367–377.

237. Badylak SF, Tullius R, Kokini K, et al. The use of xenogeneic small intestinal submucosa as a biomaterial for Achilles tendon repair in a dog model. *J Biomed Mater Res.* 1995;29(8):977–985.

238. Huynh T, Abraham G, Murray J, Brockbank K, Hagen PO, Sullivan S. Remodeling of an acellular collagen graft into a physiologically responsive neovessel. *Nat Biotechnol.* 1999;17(11):1083–1086.

239. Rosen M, Roselli EE, Faber C, Ratliff NB, Pon-

sky JL, Smedira NG. Small intestinal submucosa intracardiac patch: an experimental study. *Surg Innov.* 2005;12(3):227–231.

240. Zhang Z, Wang Z, Liu S, Kodama M. Pore size, tissue ingrowth, and endothelialization of small-diameter microporous polyurethane vascular prostheses. *Biomaterials.* 2004;25(1):177–187.

241. Tsuchida H, Wilson SE, Ishimaru S. Healing mechanisms of high-porosity PTFE grafts: significance of transmural structure. *J Surg Res.* 1997;71(2):187–195.

242. Jux C, Bertram H, Wohlsein P, et al. Experimental ASD closure using autologous cell-seeded interventional closure devices. *Cardiovasc Res.* 2002;53(1):181–191.

243. Ramires PA, Mirenghi L, Romano AR, Palumbo F, Nicolardi G. Plasma-treated PET surfaces improve the biocompatibility of human endothelial cells. *J Biomed Mater Res.* 2000;51(3):535–539.

244. Sipehia R, Liszkowski M, Lu A. In vivo evaluation of ammonia plasma modified ePTFE grafts for small diameter blood vessels replacement. A preliminary report. *J Cardiovasc Surg.* 2001;42(4):537–542.

245. Chen M, Zamora PO, Som P, Pena LA, Osaki S. Cell attachment and biocompatibility of polytetrafluoroethylene (PTFE) treated with glow-discharge plasma of mixed ammonia and oxygen. *J Biomater Sci.* 2003;14(9):917–935.

246. Jarrell BE, Williams SK, Rose D, Garibaldi D, Talbot C, Kapelan B. Optimization of human endothelial cell attachment to vascular graft polymers. *J Biomech Eng.* 1991;113(2):120–122.

247. Wigod MD, Klitzman B. Quantification of in vitro endothelial cell adhesion to vascular graft material. *J Biomed Mater Res.* 1993;27(8):1057–1062.

248. Jansson K, Bengtsson L, Haegerstrand A. Time-course for in vitro development of basement membrane, gap junctions, and repair by adult endothelial cells seeded on precoated ePTFE. *Eur J Vasc Endovasc Surg.* 1998;16(4): 334–341.

249. Walluscheck KP, Steinhoff G, Kelm S, Haverich A. Improved endothelial cell attachment on ePTFE vascular grafts pretreated with synthetic RGD-containing peptides. *Eur J Vasc Endovasc Surg.* 1996;12(3):321–330.

250. Alvarez-Barreto JF, Shreve MC, Deangelis PL, Sikavitsas VI. Preparation of a functionally flexible, three-dimensional, biomimetic poly(L-lactic acid) scaffold with improved cell adhesion. *Tissue Eng.* 2007;13(6):1205–1217.

251. Avci-Adali M, Paul A, Ziemer G, Wendel HP. New strategies for in vivo tissue engineering by mimicry of homing factors for self-endothelialisation of blood contacting materials. *Biomaterials.* 2008;29(29):3936–3945.

252. Hara H, Virmani R, Ladich E, et al. Patent foramen ovale: standards for a preclinical model of prevalence, structure, and histopathologic comparability to human hearts. *Cathet Cardiovasc Intervent.* 2007;69(2):266–273.

253. Han YM, Gu X, Titus JL, et al. New self-expanding patent foramen ovale occlusion device. *Cathet Cardiovasc Intervent.* 1999;47(3):370–376.

254. Hara H, Jones TK, Ladich ER, et al. Patent foramen ovale closure by radiofrequency thermal coaptation: first experience in the porcine model and healing mechanisms over time. *Circulation.* 2007;116(6):648–653.

255. Kreutzer J, Ryan CA, Wright JA Jr, et al. Acute animal studies of the STARFlex system: a new self-centering CardioSEAL septal occluder. *Cathet Cardiovasc Intervent.* 2000;49(2):225–233.

256. Jux C, Bertram H, Wohlsein P, et al. Experimental preseeding of the STARFlex atrial septal occluder device with autologous cells. *J Intervent Cardiol.* 2001;14(3):309–312.

257. Kuhn MA, Latson LA, Cheatham JP, et al. Biological response to Bard Clamshell Septal Occluders in the canine heart. *Circulation.* 1996;93(7):1459–1463.

258. Courtman DW, Errett BF, Wilson GJ. The role of crosslinking in modification of the immune response elicited against xenogenic vascular acellular matrices. *J Biomed Mater Res.* 2001;55(4):576–586.

259. Huang LL, Sung HW, Tsai CC, Huang DM. Biocompatibility study of a biological tissue fixed with a naturally occurring crosslinking reagent. *J Biomed Mater Res.* 1998;42(4):568–576.

260. Roe SC, Milthorpe BK, True K, Rogers GJ,

Schindhelm K. The effect of gamma irradiation on a xenograft tendon bioprosthesis. *Clin Mater.* 1992;9(3–4):149–154.

261. Smith CW, Young IS, Kearney JN. Mechanical properties of tendons: changes with sterilization and preservation. *J Biomech Eng.* 1996;118(1):56–61.

262. Bechtold JE, Eastlund DT, Butts MK, Lagerborg DF, Kyle RF. The effects of freeze-drying and ethylene oxide sterilization on the mechanical properties of human patellar tendon. *Am J Sports Med.* 1994;22(4):562–566.

26

The AMPLATZER Devices for ASDs and PFOs

Trong-Phi Lê and Horst Sievert

The AMPLATZER Septal Occluder

Transcatheter devices to close structural heart defects including atrial septal defects (ASDs) have provided a widespread alternative to surgery. One of the most popular devices for occlusion of ASDs is the AMPLATZER Septal Occluder (AGA Medical Corporation, Plymouth, Minnesota). It is a self-centering device that consists of two circular retaining discs made of Nitinol wire mesh and linked together by a short connecting waist. The retaining discs are positioned on the opposite sides of the defect and the waist serves to center the device in the defect while occluding it. The entire device is a unique and complex "weave" of 0.004" to 0.008" fine Nitinol wires, which forms two circular flat discs joined to each other at the center by a smaller and slightly thicker circular waist (Fig 26.1). Both of the discs and the waist

have a separate single thin layer of polyester fabric sewn within their circumference (Fig 26.2). The polyester patches prevent flow through the device, enhance thrombosis within the device, and promote closure of the defect.

The device is available in multiple sizes with the diameter of the central waist representing the nominal size of the AMPLATZER Septal Occluder. The connecting waist is 4-mm long, corresponding to the thickness of the atrial septum. The waist is the principal occluding and retaining portion of the device, which is designed to completely fill and actually stretch into the rims of the atrial defect. The left atrial disc is slightly larger than the right atrial disc because of the higher left atrial pressure. It is 12 to 14 mm larger in diameter than the central waist, which provides a 6- to 7-mm circumferential rim around the waist on the left side of the defect. The right atrial disc is 8 to 10 mm

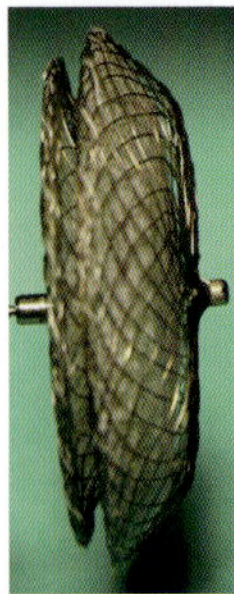

Fig 26.1–The AMPLATZER ASD Occluder connected with the delivery cable at the right atrial disc. The left atrial disc is slightly larger than the right atrial disc. The central waist is 3 mm long.

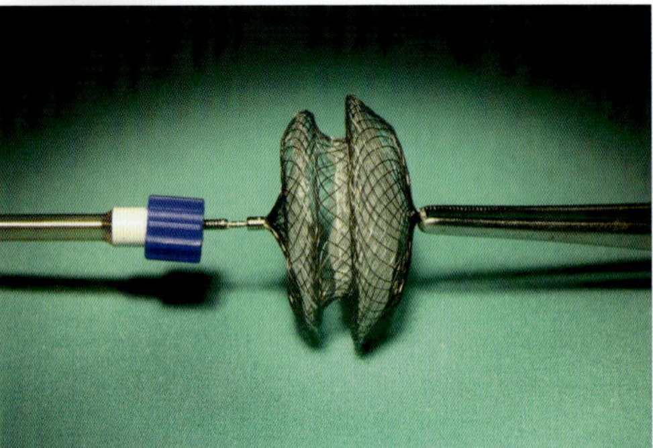

Fig 26.2—The ASD device is slightly stretched. Both the left atrial and the right atrial discs and the waist have a thin layer of polyester fabric.

larger in diameter than the central waist. It extends 4 to 5 mm radially around the connecting waist. The AMPLATZER Septal Occluders are available in sizes from 4 to 40 mm [the 40-mm size is only available outside the United States]. The devices between the 4 and 20 mm increase in size in 1-mm increments, and the devices between 20 and 40 mm are available in 2-mm increments increases.

There is a small metal pin at the center of the left atrial disc (Fig 26.3) that holds together the

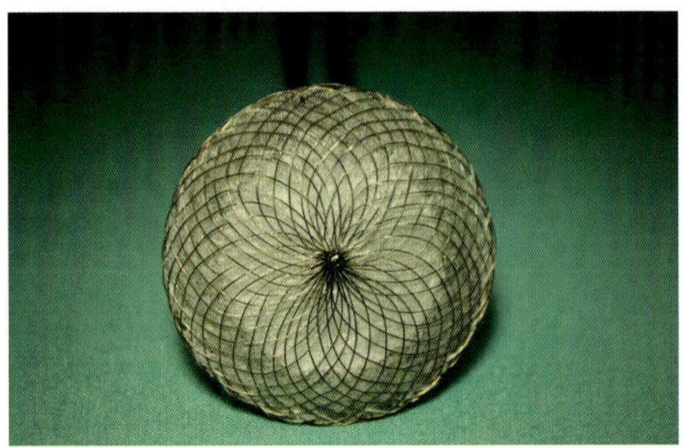

Fig 26.3—The pin at the center of the left atrial disc holds the Nitinol wires of the weave.

Nitinol wires of the weave. For the attachment to the delivery cable, there is an attach/release screw-in sleeve in a small metal strut recessed into the center of the right atrial disc (Fig 26.4). A microscrew at the end of the delivery cable attaches within the sleeve on the device.

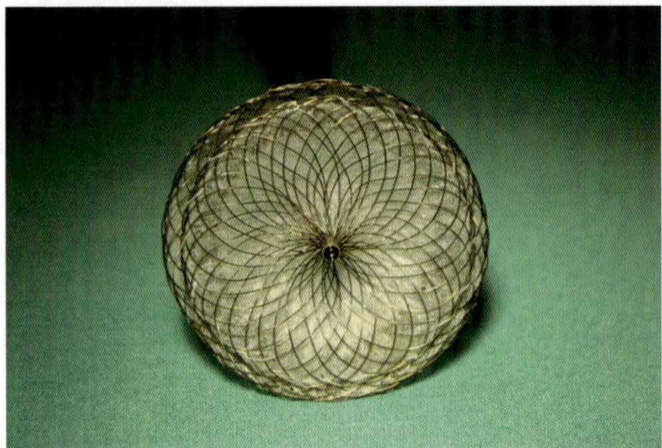

Fig 26.4—The right atrial disc of the device. There is a screw nut at the center of the disc for the attachment to the delivery cable.

The AMPLATZER Septal Occluders are delivered through long sheaths (Fig 26.5) that are manufactured by AGA. The AGA delivery sheaths are available in multiple French sizes. The smallest devices pass through a 6F delivery sheath whereas very large devices require up to a 12F sheath.

The delivery cable is passed through the Teflon loader (Fig 26.6 A), which is part of the AGA delivery sheath package. The delivery cable is attached by turning the septal occluder in a clockwise direction while the cable is fixed in position. The device is screwed onto the cable until it stops turning. Then it is recommended to back off the device in a counterclockwise direction for 1/4 or 1/8 turn to prevent too-tight attachment. The device is soaked in a flush solution and, while keeping the device under the surface of fluid and under continuous flushing, the delivery cable with the attached device is pulled into the loader. The device is stretched into a long thin strand by the traction in opposite direction to be withdrawn into the loader (Fig 26.6 B–E).

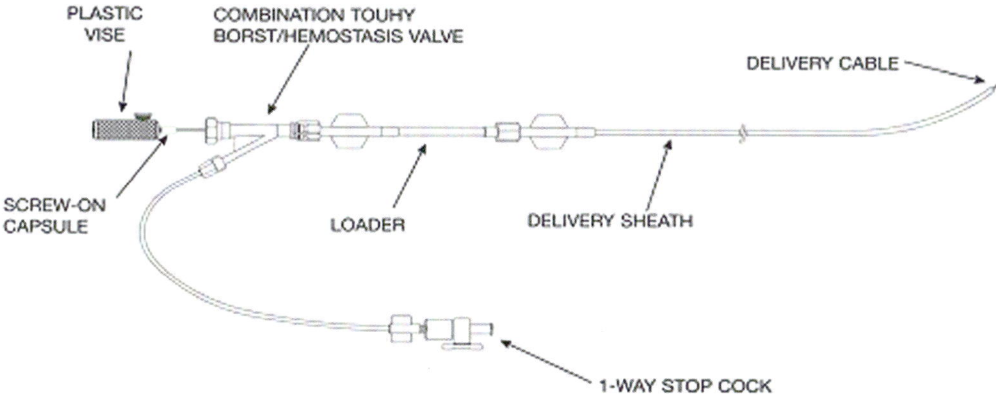

Fig 26.5—The AGA delivery system consists of the loader, the delivery cable, and the long sheath. (Courtesy of AGA Medical Corporation. Used with permission.)

Fig 26.6—A: The delivery cable is advanced through the Teflon loader. There is a microscrew on the end of the cable for the attachment with the device. B–E: The delivery cable with the attached device is pulled into the loader.

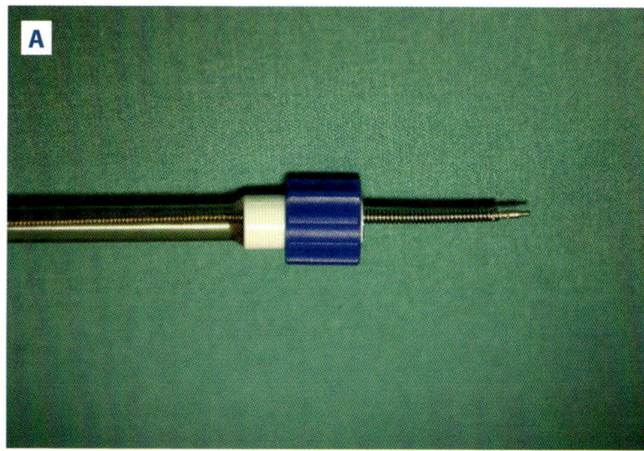
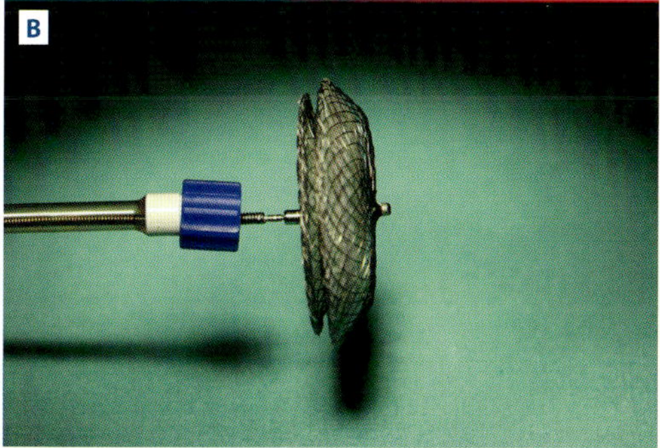
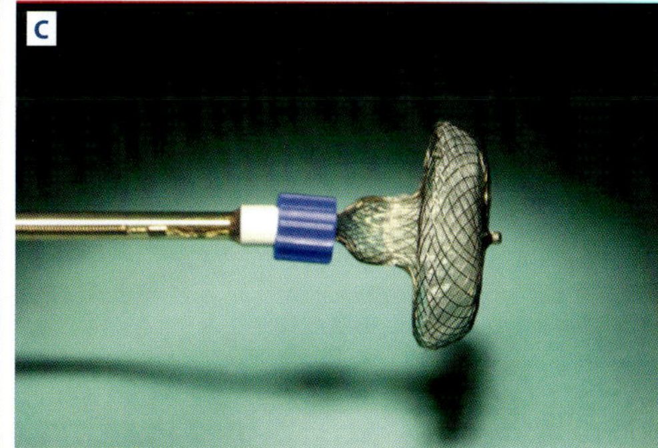
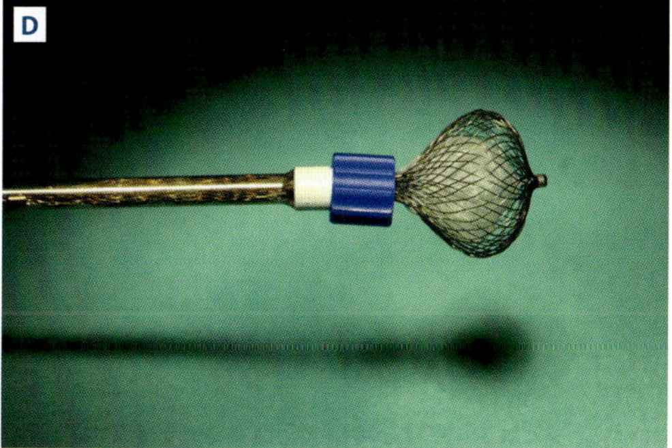
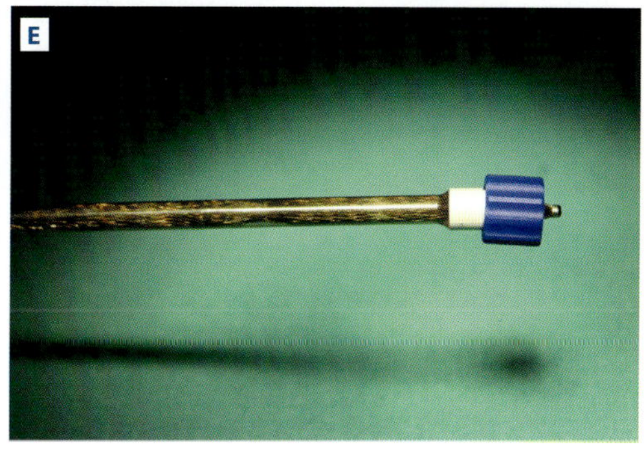

While continuing the flush on the loader with the enclosed device, it is introduced to the proximal end of the prepositioned long delivery sheath. The delivery cable is then advanced into and through the loader. By doing so the septal occluder is advanced straight into the sheath. As soon as the device has reached the end of the sheath, it is ready to be reconfigured outside the sheath to be positioned into the defect. Once the device is correctly placed into the defect, it is released by rotating the delivery cable counterclockwise.

The AMPLATZER device is also available in a configuration with a small central waist for use in patients with multiperforated aneurysm of the interatrial septum.

The AMPLATZER Multi-Fenestrated Septal Occluder—"Cribriform" (Fig 26.7) is designed for use in multiple atrial septal defects. It is placed exactly like the AMPLATZER Septal Occluder, but has a narrow waist to place it through one of the central holes in the septal wall, with the discs covering the surrounding holes. The left and right atrial disc of the AMP-LATZER Cribriform Septal Occluders are equal in size. This device is available in sizes 18, 25, 30, and 35 mm.

The AMPLATZER PFO Occluder

The AMPLATZER PFO devices (Fig 26.8) are designed specifically for the anatomy of the patent foramen ovale (PFO). They are manufactured using the same material and with a similar weave to the AMPLATZER ASD devices. The connecting waist of the PFO device, however, is very narrow and flexible. The waist is 3 mm long, and attached slightly eccentrically to the two discs. The right atrial disc is slightly larger than the left atrial disc due to the often higher pressure in the right atrium and the predominantly right-to-left shunting of these defects. The AMPLATZER PFO devices presently are available with a 35-, a 25-, or an 18-mm right atrial disc. These have corresponding left atrial discs of 25, 18, or 18 mm, respectively.

The AMPLATZER PFO devices have the same capability as the AMPLATZER ASD devices of being withdrawn easily back into the delivery sheath at any time before the purposeful release of the device from the delivery cable.

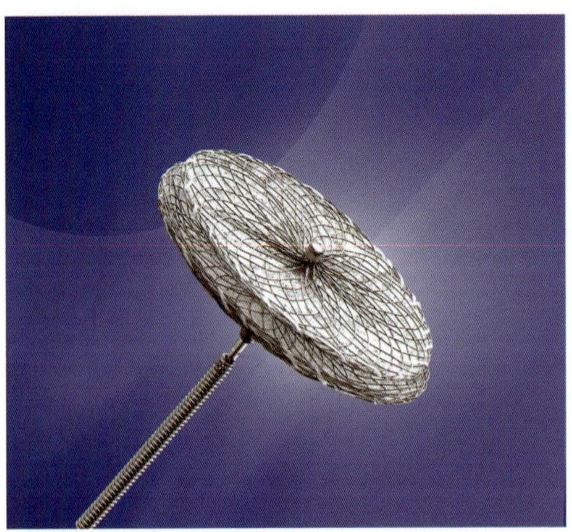

Fig 26.7—The AMPLATZER Multi-Fenestrated "Cribriform" Septal Occluder is designed for use in multiple atrial septal defects. (Courtesy of AGA Medical Corporation. Used with permission.)

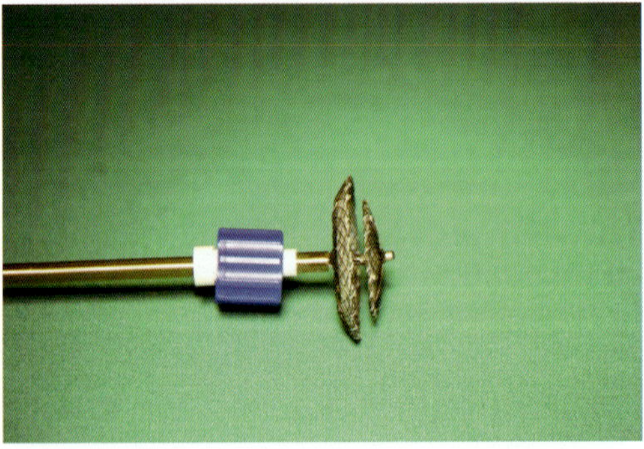

Fig 26.8—The AMPLATZER PFO Occluder. The right atrial disc is larger than the left atrial disc.

27

The GORE HELEX Septal Occluder

Ted Feldman

Introduction

For over three decades there has been a great deal of development to create the ideal device for atrial septal closure.[1-3] This device would be simple to both implant and easy to retrieve, have 100% complete closure rate, maintain a low profile on the atrial septum, have no potential for erosion or migration, and be composed of materials with proven long-term biocompatibility and mechanical integrity. An effort to design such an occlusion system began in 1995 and led to the basic features of the HELEX device.

The HELEX is composed of an implantable occluder and a catheter delivery system. The occluder is composed of expanded polytetrafluoroethylene (ePTFE) material with hydrophilic coating (Figs 27.1 and 27.2), supported by a nickel-titanium (Nitinol) super-elastic wire frame (Fig 27.3). When deployed, the occluder has double disc shape that bridges the septal defect (Fig 27.4). The delivery system consists of three components: a delivery catheter, a control catheter, and a mandrel. The control catheter has a retrieval cord to reposition and retrieve the occluder. The HELEX covers the defect and adjacent tissue with the ePTFE material supported by the wire frame. After deployment, it remains in position across the defect utilizing tension created by the wire frame and the blood pressure that pushes the ePTFE patch against the atrial septum. The ePTFE material is microporous and will become attached to the atrial septum by cellular penetration through the membrane micropores. Over time, the process of tissue attachment to the ePTFE patch will maintain the occluder in position and create a permanent defect closure. The HELEX is available in the 15, 20, 25, 30, and 35 mm diameter configurations (Fig 27.5).

Transcatheter Closure of ASDs and PFOs: A Comprehensive Assessment. © 2010 Ziyad M. Hijazi, Ted Feldman, Mustafa H. Abdullah Al-Qbandi, and Horst Sievert, editors. Cardiotext Publishing, ISBN: 978-0-9790164-9-3.

- Locking Loop
- Right Atrial Eyelet
- Retrieval Cord
- Gray Control Catheter

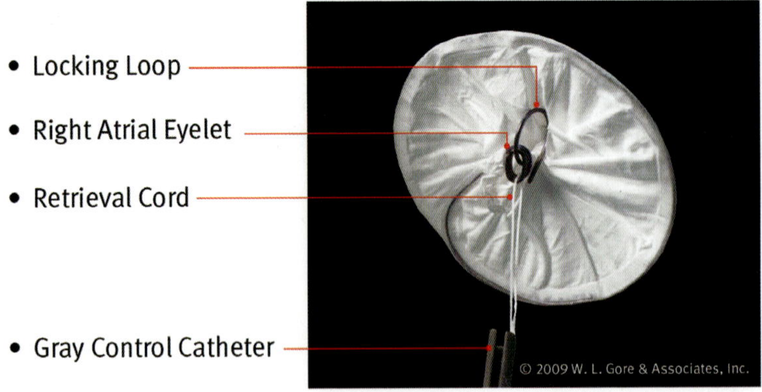

Fig 27.1—Right atrial view of the HELEX. The structural features of the device are described in detail in the text.

- ePTFE
- Central Eyelet
- Nitinol Frame
- Right Atrial Eyelet
- Green Delivery Catheter

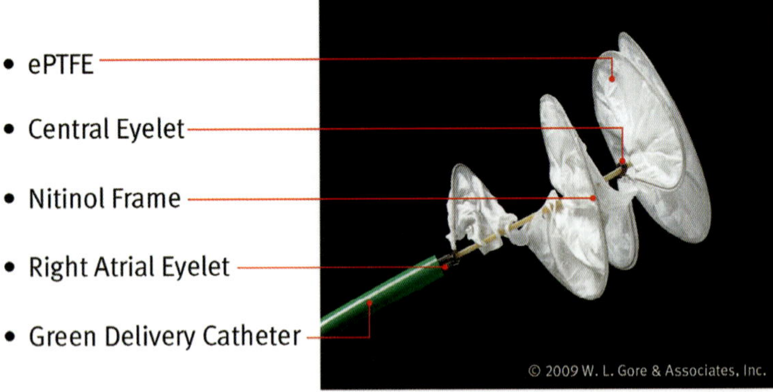

Fig 27.2—The partially undeployed HELEX device. The text details the function of each of the components of the system.

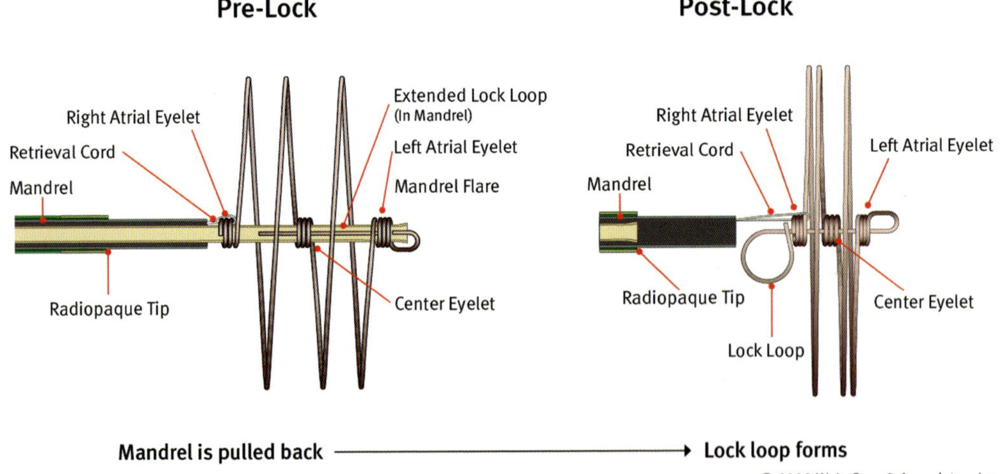

Fig 27.3—The wire frame of the HELEX device is shown in the partially opened and fully closed positions. The ePTFE membrane is strung along the entire length of the wire frame.

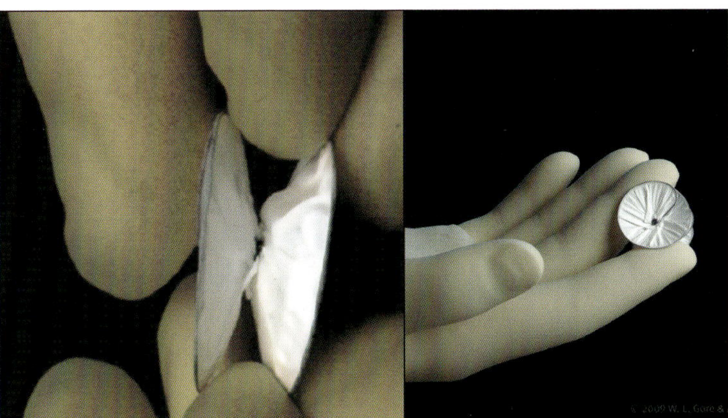

Fig 27.4—The device is shown as it would appear splayed over the atrial septum on the left panel, and from a right atrial view in the right-hand panel.

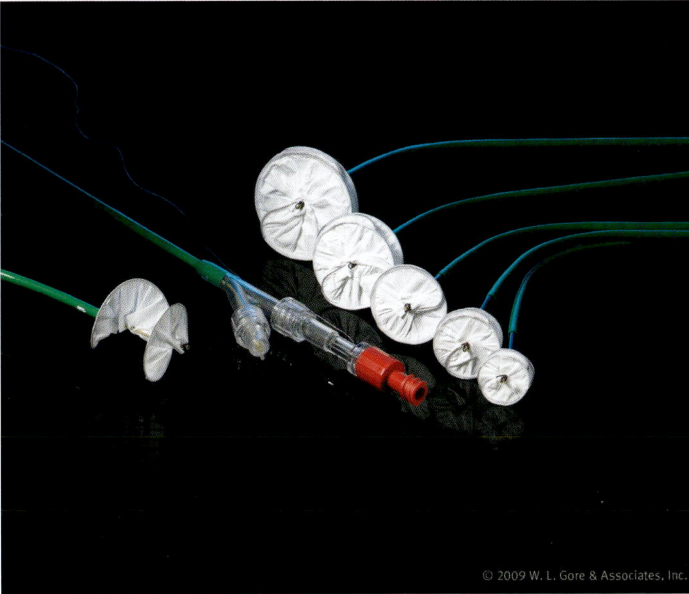

Fig 27.5—The device is available in diameters from 15 to 35 mm, in 5-mm increments. This figure illustrates the back end of the system with the red safety lock, the retrieval cord, and the tan mandrel and flushing ports of the green catheter system.

Materials

PTFE is a commonly used material for a wide range of medical devices. Polytetrafluoroethylene resin is obtained by the polymerization of tetrafluoroethylene and the subsequent coagulation of the dispersion polymer. The basic molecule of PTFE consists of a carbon atom–carbon atom bond with attached fluorine atoms such that the resultant molecule, when polymerized, forms chains of repeating units with molecular weights in the range of 400,000 to 10,000,000.

PTFE is acceptably inert and has excellent thermal and chemical stability, good nonstick properties, and excellent resistance to degradation under severe conditions. The carbon-fluorine bond is one of the strongest bonds known among organic compounds. The highly electronegative fluorine atoms form a protective sheath over the chain of carbon atoms that shields the carbon chain from the effects of most chemicals and is responsible for the chemical inertness and stability of the polymer. PTFE also has excellent thermal stability and can be used at temperatures up to 250°C.

Healing Response

The human tissue response to implantation of HELEX has been characterized in animal models (Fig 27.6).[4–5] Immediately after exposure to blood, platelets and fibrin protein deposit on the surface of the membrane to initiate the initial tissue response (Fig 27.7). As time passes, the fibrous coagulum on the device becomes organized into fibrous connective tissue (Fig 27.8). This can be seen within 3 months. Mature collagen fibrils eventually penetrate the interstices of the ePTFE. The ePTFE membrane provides a matrix for controlled tissue in-growth. Progressive neointimal proliferation extends from the disc margin toward the central portion over the course of several months. The initial coverage with fibrous connective tissue is eventually followed by coverage with true endothelial cells (Fig 27.9). After about a year, there is complete endothelialization of the device, and healing with minimal inflammation and a low risk for thrombus formation (Fig 27.10).

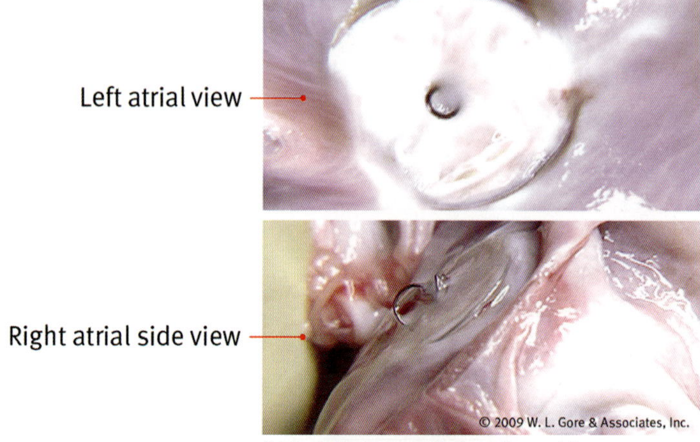

Retrieval after three months in canine model

Fig 27.6—Healing response in a canine model after 3 months shown from both sides of the septum.

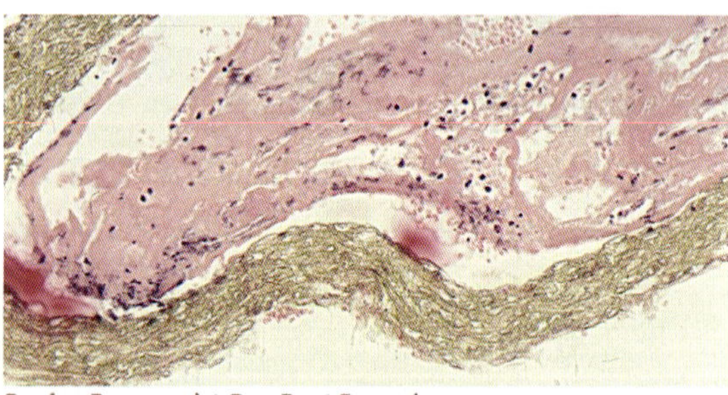

Device Removed 1 Day Post Procedure

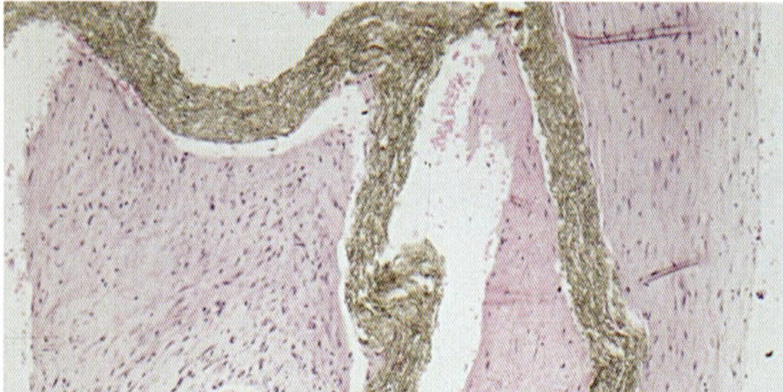

Device Removed 90 Days Post Procedure

Fig 27.7—Human tissue healing response in a device removed 1-day postprocedure in the upper panel and 90-days postprocedure in the lower panel.

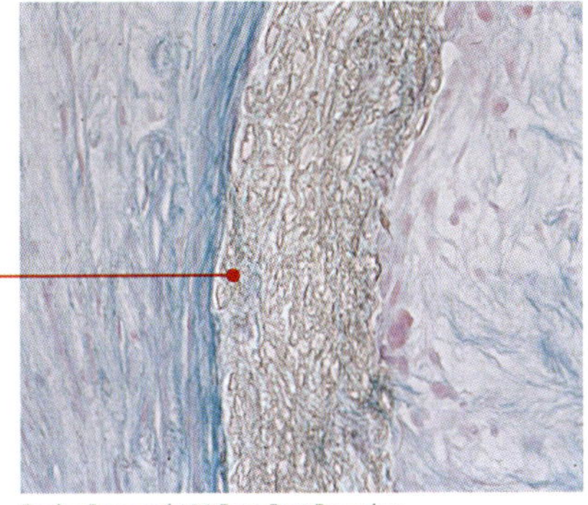

Mature collagen (blue-green) fibrils penetrate the inerstices of the ePTFE

Device Removed 139 Days Post Procedure

© 2009 W. L. Gore & Associates, Inc.

Fig 27.8—Human tissue healing response in a device removed 139-days postprocedure.

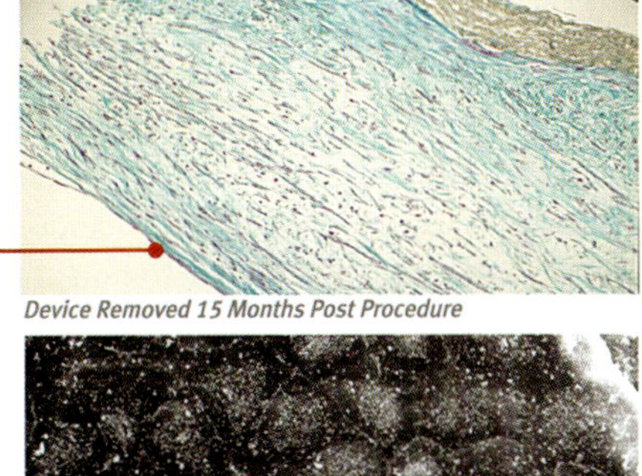

Tissue response to ePTFE characterized by endothelialization of the device

Device Removed 15 Months Post Procedure

Device Removed 8 Months Post Procedure

© 2009 W. L. Gore & Associates, Inc.

Fig 27.9—Tissue response characterized by endothelial formation shown 15 months postprocedure (upper panel), and in a scanning electron micrograph at 8 months (lower panel). The typical cobblestone appearance of normal endothelial cellular tissue can be seen in the lower panel.

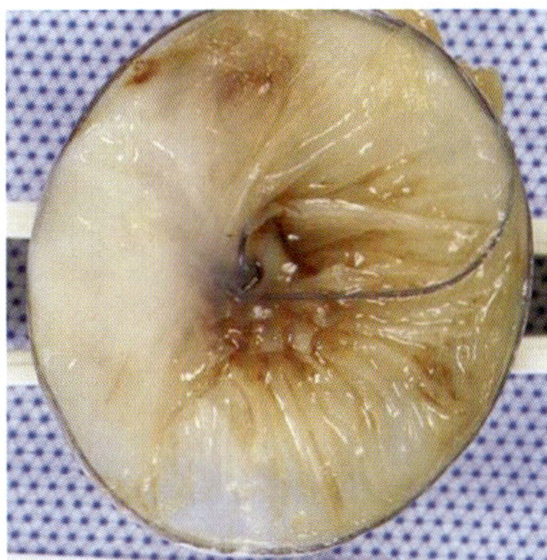

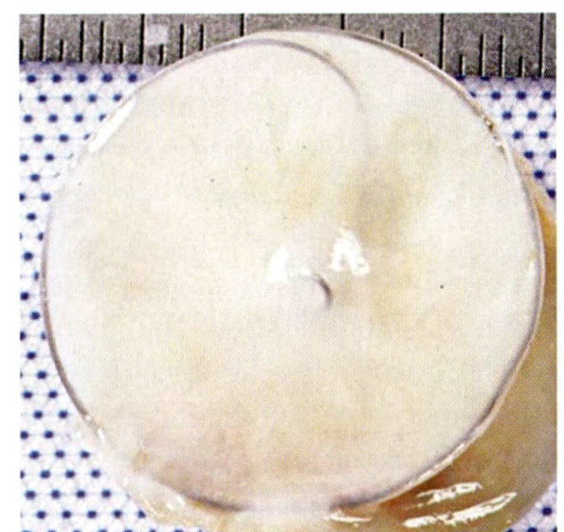

Devices Removed 8 Months (Left) and 15 Months Post Procedure (Right)

© 2009 W. L. Gore & Associates, Inc.

Fig 27.10—Tissue response after removal of the device at 8 months and 15 months. Hemosiderin is seen on the device in the left panel, and fibrotic tissue smoothly covers the device on the right.

Trial Results

Three US clinical studies were conducted to evaluate the HELEX for use in ostium secundum atrial septal defect (ASD) closure using a precursor to the current delivery system and the current occluder. The device was evaluated in a feasibility study,[6] a pivotal study,[7] and a continued access study. The pivotal study compared the device to surgical closure of ostium secundum ASDs in a nonrandomized fashion. The continued access study included 113 subjects treated with the device, with 77 subjects completing the 12-month follow-up evaluation at the time of reporting. An independent Data Safety Monitoring Board reviewed all reported adverse events to determine device/procedure relationship and event severity. There was one postoperative death in the surgical control treatment arm of the pivotal study from complications related to postpericardiotomy syndrome on Day 10 postsurgery. No deaths have been reported in the device subjects in the feasibility, pivotal, or continued access studies.

Feasibility study

Two sites participated with enrollment of 63 subjects.[6] The median age was 11 years (range: 6 months–65 years) and 65% of the subjects were female. The median estimated defect size was 12 mm (range: 4.5–20 mm). In subjects with a delivery attempt (n=59), the median stretched defect size was 18 mm (range: 6–26 mm). The HELEX was successfully implanted in 86.4% (51/59) of subjects with a delivery attempt. No deaths, device embolizations, thrombus on the device, or erosions requiring surgery were reported during 12-month follow-up. There were no repeat procedures to the target ASD. By echocardiography core laboratory review after 12 months, it was determined that successful defect closure (complete occlusion or clinically insignificant leak) had occurred in 94.6% (35/37). Clinically significant leaks were present in two subjects (5.4%) at 12 months. Clinical success, a composite of safety (no major adverse events or repeat procedure), and efficacy (clinical closure at 12 months), was achieved in 89.5%.

Multicenter pivotal study

The pivotal study enrolled 143 subjects in the device treatment arm and 128 subjects in the surgical control arm at 14 US clinical sites.[7] This was a nonrandomized, noninferiority trial comparing safety and efficacy of the HELEX with surgical repair of atrial septal defects. The primary end point was 12-month clinical success, a composite of safety and efficacy. Clinical success was defined as a residual defect classified as either completely occluded or clinically insignificant leak as determined by echocardiography core lab, no repeat procedure to the target ASD, and no major device- or procedure-related adverse events. Additional safety end points included the proportion of subjects experiencing one or more major and minor device-related and/or procedure-related adverse events through 12 months postprocedure. Additional efficacy end points included delivery success, defined as successful deployment and accurate placement of the occluder to the target ASD, and treatment efficacy, defined as the proportion of subjects with a final residual defect assessment of clinically successful closure with completely occluded or clinically insignificant leak.

Enrolled patients had echocardiographic evidence of an ostium secundum ASD and right heart volume overload (or as indicated by a QP:QS ratio of $\geq$ 1.5:1 for the device treatment arm). Patients enrolled in the device treatment arm had a defect size of 22 mm or less as measured by balloon sizing and an adequate rim to retain the device present in $\geq$ 75% of the circumference of the defect. Exclusion criteria included concurrent cardiac defect(s) that were associated with potentially significant morbidity or mortality, systemic or inherited conditions that would significantly increase patient risk, uncontrolled arrhythmia, history of stroke, contraindication to antiplatelet therapy, pulmonary artery systolic pressure greater than half the systemic systolic arterial pressure unless the indexed pulmonary artery resistance was < 5

Woods units, significant atrial septal aneurysm, or multiple defects that would require placement of more than one device, or atrial septum > 8 mm thick.

The median age of the 143 subjects enrolled in the device treatment arm of the pivotal study was 6.5 years (range: 1.4–72.4 years) and 65.7% of the subjects were female. The median estimated ASD size was 10 mm (range: 1.3–25 mm) and in subjects with a delivery attempt (n=134), the median stretched defect size was 14 mm (range: 5–24 mm). The median age of the 128 subjects in the surgical arm of the pivotal study was 4.7 years (range: 0.6 to 70.4 years), and 63.3% of the subjects were female. The median estimated defect size was 15 mm (range: 1.5–42 mm). For patients enrolled in the device treatment arm, static measurement of the ASD was obtained with echo and a measurement was taken utilizing a sizing balloon. The balloon stretched defect size was used to determine the optimal size of the occluder. In the surgical control arm, ASD repair was performed per the investigator's standard procedure, and was achieved by suturing the defect edges or by implantation of autologous or synthetic patch materials over the defect. The HELEX was successfully implanted in 88.1% (119/135) of subjects with a delivery attempt. No deaths, device-related thrombus, perforations, or erosions requiring surgery were reported. Major adverse events were reported in 5.9% of subjects with a successful delivery through the 12-month follow-up. Clinically successful closure (complete occlusion or clinically insignificant leak), as determined by echocardiographic core laboratory review, was achieved in 98.1% of subjects evaluated at 12 months postprocedure. The primary clinical success endpoint was achieved in 91.7% of subjects evaluated.

Major adverse events were reported in 10.9% of control surgical subjects. One death resulting from complications of postpericardiotomy syndrome was reported. Clinically successful closure, as determined by echocardiographic core laboratory review, was achieved in 100% of surgical subjects evaluated at 12 months postprocedure. Clinical success was achieved in 83.7% of subjects evaluated. The HELEX was successfully implanted in 85.6% of subjects with an attempt. No deaths, device-related thrombus, perforations, or erosions requiring surgery were reported. Major adverse events were reported in 3.9% of subjects with a successful delivery who have been evaluated through 12 months. Clinically successful closure, as determined by echocardiographic core laboratory review, was achieved in 98.0% of subjects evaluated at 12 months. The primary clinical success end point was achieved in 92.6% of subjects evaluated. The clinical success outcomes satisfied the primary, non-inferiority hypothesis for the pivotal study (p<0.001, with noninferiority margin of 10%).

Continued access study

The continued access study was a prospective, single arm trial intended to evaluate design modifications based on investigator input. Prior to the continued access study, the device echo images of the early device were not ideal in that one could not properly visualize the right disc on TEE. A static shield was cast by the left disc due to the air bubbles caught in the microstructure of the fabric. The hydrophilic coating that is now on the device allows the images to be much clearer because water is now able to be drawn into the ePTFE fabric when it is prepared in water. Also, the winding direction of the occluder wire was changed. Before the continued access study, the left disc would not deploy flat whereas the right disc was as flat as a pancake. By changing the direction of the wire's wind, the left disc deploys flat. The right disc now sometimes has some splay on the superior aspect of the disc. This is preferable to having the splay on the left side.

Results are described in the GORE HELEX Septal Occluder Instructions for Use (July 2007). A total of 156 subjects were enrolled at 13 US clinical sites. The median was 5.5 years (range: 0.8–51.4 years) and 66.0% of the subjects were female. The median estimated ASD size was 10 mm (range: 1.7–20.0 mm). In subjects with a delivery attempt (n=129), the median stretched defect size was 14 mm (range: 4–22 mm). The device was successfully implanted in 85.6% of subjects. No deaths, device-related thrombus, perforations, or erosions requiring surgery were reported. Major adverse events were reported in 2.2% of subjects with a successful delivery who have been evaluated through 12 months. Clinically successful closure by echocardiographic core laboratory review, was achieved in 99.1% at 12 months postprocedure. The primary clinical success end point was achieved in 96.6% of subjects evaluated. Thus, the modifications of the device did not diminish device performance.

ASD Evaluation

When selecting occluder size consider that the device size selected for the defect should achieve at least a 2:1 ratio. The occluder diameter should be no more than 90% of the measured septal length. The septal tissue margins surrounding the defect must be of sufficient size and integrity to prevent disc prolapse through the defect and embolization. Stable placement is not likely in defects > 18 mm. Evaluate the defect and atrial chamber size by TEE or ICE with color flow Doppler measurement, confirming that there is adequate space to accommodate the selected occluder size without impinging on adjacent cardiac structures (eg, A-V valves, ostia of the pulmonary veins, coronary sinus). Determine defect size using a sizing balloon across the defect. Ensure there is an adequate rim to retain the occluder in ≥ 75% of the circumference of the defect. Device size should provide a 2:1 occluder diameter-to-defect diameter ratio.

Device Preparation

Loading of the occluder into the green delivery catheter should be done with the catheter tip submerged in a heparinized saline bath. Use a large volume (20–60 mL) syringe with heparinized saline to attach to the red retrieval cord cap and flush into the bowl or sterile tray. When the initial flushing is completed, draw back on the gray control catheter with the attached syringe until only about 3 cm of the occluder remains outside the delivery catheter and the tan mandrel appears slightly curved (Fig 27.11). At that point loosen the mandrel luer and continue to draw back on the gray control catheter hub until the entire occluder has been withdrawn into the green delivery catheter. Flush the control catheter into the bowl or sterile tray. Retain the flushing syringe attached to the red cap to prevent

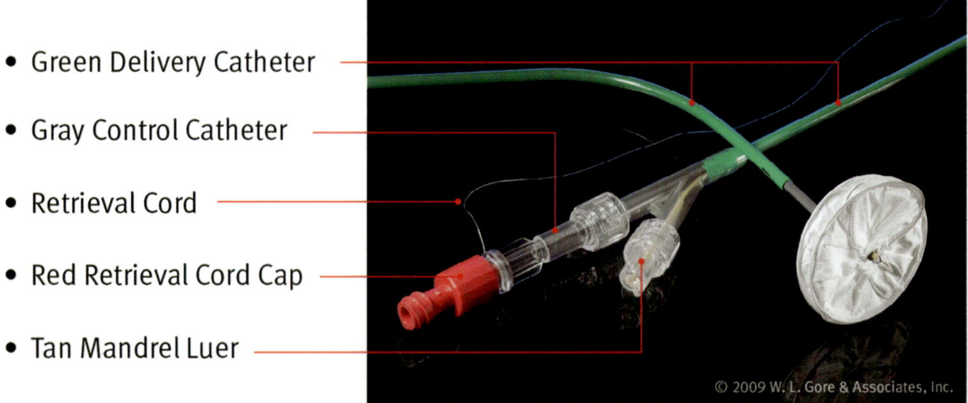

Fig 27.11—The components of the red retrieval cord cap, tan mandrel luer lock, the retrieval cord, and both the gray control catheter and green delivery catheter are seen. On careful inspection, the monorail wire port can be seen with the distal end of the green delivery catheter just before the gray control catheter exits.

air from entering into the delivery system until the catheter tip is placed inside the introducer sheath.

Device Delivery

The green delivery catheter may be used to cross an ASD directly, but the author prefers to cross the defect with a 0.035" wire and use a monorail approach to pass the delivery catheter into the left atrium. Be sure the occluder is sufficiently withdrawn into the green delivery catheter to avoid interference with the guide wire. Load the delivery catheter onto a guide wire through the guide wire port. Advance the catheter tip across the ASD until the radiopaque marker at the tip of the delivery catheter is within the left atrium and remove the wire. Use the "push-pinch-pull" method to deploy the left atrial disc. After the left atrial disc has been formed it is pulled back to gently engage the left side of the atrial septum. Deployment of the right atrial disc is counterintuitive. After the left atrial disc engages the left side of the septum, the green catheter is pulled back over the gray catheter a few centimeters until the luer lock of the tan mandrel engages the hub at its insertion point to the green catheter. At this point, the green catheter is pinned to the drape outside the venous sheath, and the gray catheter is advanced to push the wire frame of the right atrial disc toward the right atrial side of the septum. This forms the right atrial disc. When the disc is fully formed, the gray catheter can be locked to the green delivery catheter. Ultrasound can be used to interrogate the septum and evaluate the degree to which the device is opposed to the septum on both sides, and to ensure that no part of the device is caught in the tunnel, if the procedure is for a patent foramen ovale (PFO).

To summarize these steps for right atrial disc deployment again, push the gray control catheter moving the occluder into the left atrial chamber off of the septum but do not push against the atrial wall, or if chamber space is adequate, push until the tan mandrel luer stops against the Y-arm hub (approximately 2 cm). While holding the green delivery catheter to maintain position, pinch the gray control catheter, and then pull the tan mandrel back approximately 2 cm or less to form exposed segment of the occluder. Repeat the "push-pinch-pull" sequence until the center eyelet exits the green delivery catheter tip demarcated by the radiopaque marker. Once the left atrial disc is deployed, gently retract the tan mandrel to flatten the left atrial disc. Remove the flushing syringe. Verify that the red retrieval cord cap affixing the retrieval cord is securely attached to the gray control catheter. To prepare for right atrial disc deployment, hold the gray control catheter in a fixed position and gently expose a portion of the right atrial side by withdrawing the green delivery catheter until the mandrel luer stops on the Y-arm hub and tighten the mandrel luer. Deploy the right atrial disc by holding the green delivery catheter in a fixed position and pushing the gray control catheter until the control catheter luer contacts the Y-arm hub. Tighten the control catheter luer. Confirm that both left and right discs appear planar and apposed to the septum with septal tissue trapped between the discs. Up to this point it is possible to reposition the device. To do this, replace and tighten the red retrieval cord cap and tighten the mandrel luer. Reload the device into the green delivery catheter while it remains in the right or left atrium as it was initially done prior to use.

Device Release

The next steps are for lock and release of the device. Completely remove the red retrieval cord cap. The occluder can only be repositioned prior to lock release. If position and occlusion are acceptable, loosen the mandrel luer. Hold the green delivery catheter in a fixed position and release the lock by sharply pulling the tan mandrel at least 2 cm, somewhat like pulling a ripcord. At this point the occluder is still attached to the gray control catheter by the retrieval cord. If position is acceptable, remove the entire delivery system as a single unit making sure the retrieval cord moves smoothly through the control catheter hub.

Removing a Deployed Occluder with the Retrieval Cord

If the lock is released and the retrieval cord is still attached to the gray control catheter, the occluder can be removed by taking up any slack in the retrieval cord and securely reattaching the red retrieval cord cap. Position the green delivery catheter in the right atrium. Withdraw the gray control catheter while pulling the occluder into a linear form and drawing the occluder back into the green delivery catheter. Excessive force could cause the retrieval cord to break or result in occluder fracture. Withdraw 50% to 100% of the occluder into the green delivery catheter. If a portion of the locked or unlocked occluder remains outside of the delivery catheter, the control catheter and delivery catheter can be withdrawn together. If necessary, remove the introducer sheath and occluder together. Once removed, it cannot be deployed again. In the event that the occluder is malpositioned or embolized, it can be recaptured with the aid of a loop snare. A long sheath (10F or greater) positioned close to the device is ideal for recapture. A 10- or 15-mm loop snare works well. Place the loop snare around any portion of the occluder frame and pull it into the sheath using the snare. If a portion of the occluder frame cannot be retracted into the long sheath, it may be necessary to remove the occluder, loop snare, and long sheath as one unit.

Postprocedure Management

Patients should take antibiotic therapy for SBE prophylaxis. It is the author's practice to continue this for 3 to 6 months. Antiplatelet therapy with aspirin or clopidogrel, is recommended for 6 months postimplant. Aspirin is used indefinitely with clopidogrel for 1 to 6 months. The decision to continue antiplatelet therapy beyond 6 months is discretionary. In patients sensitive to antiplatelet therapy, alternative therapies, such as anticoagulants, can be used. Strenuous physical activity should be avoided for at least 2 weeks. It is recommended to follow patients with transthoracic echo the day after the procedure and then at 6 months with bubble contrast to assess residual shunt. If there is a positive study, repeat the exam at 1 year, and use TEE if there is any uncertainty. Fluoroscopy examination without contrast is recommended at 12 months postprocedure for patients with a 35-mm device with attention directed toward possible wire frame fractures. Through nonclinical testing, the HELEX has been shown to be MR safe at field strengths of 3.0 Tesla or less and a maximum whole body averaged specific absorption rate (SAR) of 3.0 w/kg for 15 minutes of MRI. Nonclinical testing has not been performed to rule out the possibility of device migration at field strengths higher than 3.0 Tesla. In this testing, the occluder produced a temperature rise $\leq 0.5°C$ at a maximum whole body averaged specific absorption rate (SAR) of 3.0 w/kg for 15 minutes of MRI. MRI quality may be compromised if the area of interest is close to the position of the device.

Predictors of Success

An analysis of factors related to successful transcatheter closure of secundum atrial septal defects using the HELEX found that the device was successfully implanted in 87% of 342 patients.[8] A major adverse event occurred in 5.8% (mostly device removal for various reasons). A significant residual leak persisted at 1 year in 2.6%. A fracture of the wire frame occurred in 8%—all were asymptomatic and only 1 required treatment. Overall composite success (no significant leak and no major adverse event) was seen in 91.5%. Patient age, body surface area, and device size had no significant influence on outcomes, except that wire frame fractures were more likely with the 35-mm device. Defect stretch diameter had the largest influence on outcomes, and implantation was possible in only 67% if the stretched diameter of the defect was > 20 mm. Device-to-defect ratio also had a significant effect on delivery success and composite success. The authors concluded that the HELEX is best suited for small to moderate ASDs with a stretched diameter < 20 mm. Although composite success was achieved in 80% of patients when a device-to-defect ratio < 1.6 was necessitated or elected, use of a device that provided a ratio > 2 resulted in 95% composite success, and is recommended when possible.

Late Assessment

Device closure of PFO in cryptogenic stroke or TIA especially in patients with atrial septal aneurysm (ASA) may result in differences in time to complete occlusion for various different closure devices. In a study of 357 patients with a history of 1 or more paradoxical embolic episodes, three different devices were used: AMPLATZER PFO (n=199), STARFlex (n=48), and HELEX occluder (n=110).[9] All patients were assigned to a postinterventional protocol with contrast-enhanced TEE at 1 and 6 months and every 6 to 12 months in case of incomplete closure. Definite closure was confirmed in at least two consecutive TEE studies. The closure time curves between the three devices were significantly different (p=0.0072). Devices of 25 mm or less had a better occlusion rate. The difference between the closure time curves of PFO and PFO+ASA concerning each device type was significant for HELEX (p=0.006) and STARFlex (p=0.030). In regard to the occlusion time for large devices, HELEX succeeded later than AMPLATZER and STARFlex (p=0.0029). Concerning the cumulative follow-up period of 1265 patient years, the recurrence/re-event rate of cerebral and peripheral thromboembolic

events was 0.7% per patient year. No relation to residual PFO shunting or to thrombus formation was seen. There were no peri-interventional technical complications. In 5 patients of the STARFlex group, thrombi were detected in the four-week TEE exams. Thus, the closure rate is dependent on occluder size and type plus the occurrence of an ASA.

Wire Frame Fracture

The HELEX is a more compliant ASD closure device than most others. It is possible that wire fracture allows the device to conform to the heart rather than forcing the heart to conform to the device. Most other closure devices have caused cardiac erosions or fistula.[12-20] To date, with worldwide use of the HELEX there has not been a single reported cardiac perforation or erosion of the aortic root or atrial free wall.

In a retrospective study of 298 subjects followed for > 12 months, 6.4% HELEX devices were found to have wire fracture (n=30 fractures). Multiple wire fractures occurred in 8 of 19 patients. Large device size was the only significant predictor of frame fracture by multivariate analysis. Fractures of the 30- and 35-mm devices accounted for 84% of fractures. All wire fracture occurred along the circumferential wire, except one in the straight portion of the locking loop. 59% of circumferential wire fractures were on the right disc. There were no clinical sequelae due to wire fracture. Due to right atrial disc mobility, the HELEX with locking loop wire fracture was percutaneously removed 6 weeks after implantation. Another report of locking loop fracture was not associated with any significant residual shunt or clinical problems and that device was left in place.

Device Comparison

A randomized trial compared procedural complications and 30-day clinical outcomes of three

PFO closure devices (AMPLATZER, HELEX, and CardioSEAL-STARFlex).[21] It examined 660 patients (361 men, 299 women, mean age 49.3 ± 1.9 years), with 220 patients per group. All patients had a history of paradoxical embolism. All PFO closures were successful technically. Exchange of devices for others was most frequently required for the HELEX occluder (7 of 220) and 2 of 220 in either of the other groups. Three device embolizations in the HELEX group were retrieved and replaced successfully. One patient with a HELEX occluder developed a transient ischemic attack and recovered without treatment. A hemopericardium in that group was punctured without affecting the device. One tamponade in the AMPLATZER group required surgical device explantation. In 8 of 660 patients in the CardioSEAL-STARFlex group, thrombi resolved after anticoagulation. Sixteen patients (11 in the CardioSEAL-STARFlex group, 3 in the AMPLATZER group, and 2 in the HELEX group) had episodes of atrial fibrillation. PFOs were closed completely in 143 of 220 patients (65%) in the AMPLATZER group, 116 of 220 patients (52.7%) in the HELEX group, and 137 of 220 patients (62.3%) in the CardioSEAL-STARFlex group at 30 days with significant differences between the HELEX and AMPLATZER occluders (p=0.0005) and the HELEX and CardioSEAL-STARFlex occluders (p=0.0003). PFO closure can be performed safely with each device. In conclusion, the HELEX occluder embolized more frequently. Device thrombus formation and paroxysmal atrial fibrillation were more common with the CardioSEAL-STARFlex occluder.

Thrombus formation has been examined in another large case series.[22] A total of 1000 consecutive patients were investigated after PFO (n=593) or ASD (n=407) closure. TEE was scheduled after 4 weeks and 6 months. Additional TEEs were performed as clinically indicated. Thrombus formation in the left atrium (n=11), right atrium (n=6), or both (n=3) was found in 5 of the 407 (1.2%) ASD patients and in 15 of the 593 (2.5%) PFO patients (p=NS). The thrombus was diagnosed in 14 of 20 patients after 4 weeks and in 6 of 20 patients later on.

The incidence was 7.1% in the Cardio-SEAL device (NMT Medical, Boston, Massachusetts); 5.7% in the StarFLEX device (NMT Medical); 6.6% in the PFO-Star device (Applied Biometrics Inc., Burnsville, Minnesota); 3.6% in the ASDOS device (Dr. Ing, Osypka Corp., Grenzach-Wyhlen, Germany); 0.8% in the HELEX device (W.L. Gore & Associates, Flagstaff, Arizona); and 0% in the AMPLATZER device (AGA Medical Corp., Golden Valley, Minnesota). The difference between the AMPLATZER device on one hand and the CardioSEAL device, the STARFlex device, and the PFO-Star device on the other hand was significant (p<0.05). A prethrombotic disorder as a possible cause of the thrombus was found in two PFO patients. Postprocedure atrial fibrillation and persistent ASA were significant predictors for thrombus formation (p<0.05). In 85% of patients with thrombus, the thrombus resolved with anticoagulation therapy with heparin or warfarin. In the remaining 15% thrombus was removed surgically. The incidence of thrombus formation on closure devices is low. The thrombus usually resolves under anticoagulation therapy.

PFO Closure

There are a number of considerations for closure of PFO.[23–26] The sizing estimation for selection of device diameter depends on use of a balloon-sizing catheter with a 2:1 size ratio remaining a rule of thumb. In addition, the balloon will demonstrate whether the PFO tunnel is rigid, compliant, or excessively long. A special consideration for PFO closure is the thickness of the bulge of the superior secundum septum. If the secundum is > 1 cm, the right atrial disc may be splayed out into the superior vena cava wall, and not apposed well to the atrial septum. Specific guidelines about size use in this setting have not been developed, and experience with PFO closure remains the only tool for device size selection and positioning.

In a multicenter study of 128 patients with PFO and cryptogenic stroke, device implantation was successful in 127 patients.[24] Device-related events during implantation or follow-up were device embolization, wire frame fracture, and retrieval cord breaks (two cases each; no sequelae). Other adverse events included atrial arrhythmia (two patients), migraine, convulsion, and transient ischemic attack (one case each). There were no recurrent strokes, deaths, perforations, or accumulations of thrombi on the device. Within a mean follow-up period of 21 ± 11 months, complete PFO closure using one device was achieved in 114 patients (90%). Five patients with a moderate-to-large residual shunt received a second device.

Among 141 patients with embolic events associated with PFO and ASA, device closure was compared with 220 patients with PFO and no septal aneurysm.[25] Device success (over 99%) and procedural complications (0.7%–3.2%) were similar in both groups. Maximal atrial septal excursion in patients with ASA + PFO decreased from 16 ± 4 mm before to 4 ± 3 mm after the intervention (p < 0.0001). At 6 months follow-up, right-to-left shunt was abolished in 85% to 86% of patients in both groups. Freedom from recurrent transient ischemic attack, stroke, and peripheral embolism at 4 years was about 95% for both groups. A residual right-to-left shunt after the intervention was the only predictor for recurrence.

Future Developments

A variety of future modifications of the HELEX system can be expected. The delivery system will be greatly simplified, with a handle and several knobs, which allows for simplified sequence of steps for delivery. In addition, several modifications of the device shape may give it more compressive force for closure of septal defects, without greatly changing its compliant, soft character. None of these enhancements have been well characterized at the time of this writing.

Also on the horizon in a randomized trial evaluating the HELEX device for prevention of recurrent stroke or TIA, the REDUCE trial. This is a prospective, randomized, multicenter, and multinational trial with up to 50 US and Nordic sites. The intended enrollment is 664 subjects with a 2 device to 1 control randomization scheme. The primary end point is freedom from recurrent ischemic stroke, imaging-confirmed TIA, or death due to stroke through 24 months postrandomization. The population will have presence of cryptogenic, ischemic stroke or transient ischemic attack with MRI or CT evidence of a presumably embolic infarction verified by a neurologist within 180 days prior to randomization. There will be a standardized antiplatelet medical therapy across treatment arms. The antiplatelet regimens for all subjects, in rank order will be aspirin alone, Aggrenox or generic equivalent (aspirin and dipyridamole), or clopidogrel for subjects with a contraindication to aspirin. Subjects will remain on antiplatelet therapy through 24 months or until an ischemic stroke or imaging-confirmed TIA. The trial is unique in that a uniform antiplatelet therapy will be used for all patients in the trial. Enrollment began in mid 2009 and may take several years.

Acknowledgment

All figures in this chapter are used with permission from W.L. GORE and Associates, Inc.

References

1. Delaney JW, Chan K-C, Rhodes JF Jr. The design and deployment of the HELEX Septal Occluder. *Congen Heart Dis.* 2006;1(5):202–209.

2. Zahn EM, Wilson N, Cutright W, Latson LA. Development and testing of the HELEX Septal Occluder, a new expanded polytetrafluoroethylene atrial septal defect occlusion system. *Circulation.* 2001;104(6):711–716.

3. Latson LA, Zahn EM, Wilson N. HELEX Septal Occluder for closure of atrial septal defects. *Curr Intervent Cardiol Rep.* 2000;2(3):268–273.

4. Zahn EM, Latson LA, Wilson N. Acute and long term follow up results with the HELEX

Septal Occluder in an animal model: Presented at the 49th Annual Scientific Session of the American College of Cardiology; March 12–15, 2000; Anaheim, Calif. *J Am Coll Cardiol.* 2000;35(2, suppl 1):498A.

5. Zahn EM, Cheatham J, Latson LA, Wilson N. Results of in vivo testing of a new Nitinol ePTFE septal occlusion device. *Cathet Cardiovasc Diagn.* 1999;47:124.

6. Mahmoud El-Sisi A, Gendi S, Dilawar M, Numan M. HELEX Septal Occluder: feasibility study of closure of atrial septal defect. *Pediatr Cardiol.* 2008;29(1):84–89.

7. Jones TK, Latson LA, Zahn E, et al; Multicenter Pivotal Study of the HELEX Septal Occluder Investigators. Results of the U.S. Multicenter Pivotal Study of the HELEX Septal Occluder for percutaneous closure of secundum atrial septal defects. *J Am Coll Cardiol.* 2007;49(22):2215–2221.

8. Latson LA, Jones TK, Jacobson J, Zahn E, Rhodes JF. Analysis of factors related to successful transcatheter closure of secundum atrial septal defects using the HELEX septal occluder. *Am Heart J.* 2006;151(5):1129:e7–e11.

9. von Bardeleben RS, Richter C, Otto J, et al. Long term follow up after percutaneous closure of PFO in 357 patients with paradoxical embolism: Difference in occlusion systems and influence of atrial septum aneurysm. *Int J Cardiol.* 2009;134(1):33–41.

10. Fagan T, Dreher D, Cutright W, Jacobson J, Latson L, for GORE HELEX Septal Occluder Working Group. Fracture of the GORE HELEX septal occluder: associated factors and clinical outcomes. *Cathet Cardiovasc Intervent.* 2009;73(7):941–948.

11. Scott PA, Wilson N, Veldtman GR. Fracture of a GORE HELEX Septal Occluder following PFO closure in a diver. *Cathet Cardiovasc Intervent.* 2009;73(6):828–831.

12. Mellert F, Preusse CJ, Haushofer M, et al. Surgical management of complications caused by transcatheter ASD closure. *Thorac Cardiovasc Surg.* 2001;49:338–342.

13. Sievert H, Babic UU, Hausdorf G, et al. Transcatheter closure of atrial septal defect and patent foramen ovale with ASDOS device (a multi-institutional European trial). *Am J Cardiol.* 1998;82:1405–1413.

14. Rao PS, Ende DJ, Wilson AD, Smith PA, Chopra PS. Follow-up results of transcatheter occlusion of atrial septal defects with buttoned device. *Can J Cardiol.* 1995;11:695–770

15. Bohm J, Bittigau K, Kohler F, Baumann G, Konertz W. Surgical removal of atrial septal defect occlusion system-devices. *Eur J Cardiothorac Surg.* 1997;12:869–872.

16. Amin Z, Hijazi ZM, Bass JL, Cheatham JP, Hellenbrand WE, Kleinman CS. Erosion of AMPLATZER septal occluder device after closure of secundum atrial septal defects: Review of registry of complications and recommendations to minimize future risk. *Cathet Cardiovasc Intervent.* 2004;63:496–502.

17. Chun DS, Turrentine MW, Moustapha A, Hoyer MH. Development of aorta-to-right atrial fistula following closure of secundum atrial septal defect using the AMPLATZER septal occluder. *Cathet Cardiovasc Intervent.* 2003;58:246–251.

18. Divekar A, Gaamangwe T, Shaikh N, Raabe M, Ducas J. Cardiac perforation after device closure of atrial septal defects with the AMPLATZER septal occluder. *J Am Coll Cardiol.* 2005;45:1213–1218.

19. Grayburn PA, Schwartz B, Anwar A, Hebeler RF Jr. Migration of an AMPLATZER septal occluder device for closure of atrial septal defect into the ascending aorta with formation of an aorta-to-right atrial fistula. *Am J Cardiol.* 2005;96:1607–1609.

20. Rickers C, Hamm C, Stern H, et al. Percutaneous closure of secundum atrial septal defect with a new self centering device ("angel wings"). *Heart* 1998;80:517–521.

21. Taaffe M, Fischer E, Baranowski A, et al. Comparison of three patent foramen ovale closure devices in a randomized trial (AMPLATZER versus CardioSEAL-STARflex versus HELEX occluder). *Am J Cardiol.* 2008;101(9):1353–1358.

22. Krumsdorf U, Ostermayer S, Billinger K, et al. Incidence and clinical course of thrombus formation on atrial septal defect and patient foramen ovale closure devices in 1,000 consecutive patients. *J Am Coll Cardiol.* 2004;43(2):302–309.

23. Ponnuthurai FA, van Gaal WJ, Burchell A, Mitchell A, Wilson N, Ormerod O. Single centre experience with GORE-HELEX Septal Occluder for closure of PFO. *Heart Lung Circ.* 2008;18(2):140–142.

24. Billinger K, Ostermayer SH, Carminati M, et al. HELEX Septal Occluder for transcatheter closure of patent foramen ovale: multicentre experience. *EuroIntervention.* 2006;1(4):465–471.

25. Wahl A, Krumsdorf U, Meier B, et al. Treatment of patent foramen ovale transcatheter treatment of atrial septal aneurysm associated with patent foramen ovale for prevention of recurrent paradoxical embolism in high-risk patients. *J Am Coll Cardiol.* 2005;45(3):377–380.

26. Sievert H, Horvath K, Zadan E, et al. Patent foramen ovale closure in patients with transient ischemia attack/stroke. *J Intervent Cardiol.* 2001;14(2):261–266.

28

The Occlutech Flex Devices for ASD and PFO Closure

Nicolas Majunke, Nina Wunderlich, and Horst Sievert

Introduction

The Occlutech Flex devices (Occlutech AB, Helsingborg, Sweden) are further developments of the initial Occlutech devices. They are technically similar to the AMPLATZER devices: double-disc devices made of a self-expanding Nitinol wire mesh, fully recapturable and repositionable before release. The devices are made of a unique braiding technology that allows a 50% reduction of meshwork material on the left atrial side in combination with a greater flexibility as compared to the AMPLATZER Occluder Device.

Unlike the AMPLATZER devices, the Occlutech devices have no hub on the left atrial side, which reduces foreign material in the left atrium and should promote quick endothelialization as well as reduce the risk for thrombosis. The new generation ASD and PFO occluder do not have any threaded hub or clamp to provide an attachment for a delivery system.

Delivery System

The amount of material implanted is reduced by utilizing a proprietary welding process to form an adaption ball called the "connector" (Fig 28.1), specifically designed for compatibility with the new delivery cable called Flex-Pusher (Figs 28.2 A–B). The new delivery system should allow significant improvements in product handling. Before release of the occluder, the system allows a tilted angle of approximately 45° without any stress or tension on the implant. Furthermore the new technology should avoid an unnoticed disconnection of the Occlutech Flex device from the Flex-Pusher.

PFO and ASD Devices

Two different PFO devices are available: A single-layered and a double-layered device. On the single-layer device (Fig 28.3) the left atrial disc is single layered, forming a very flat disc, reducing the amount of metal needed. The double-layered device is available for the so-called long-track PFO defects. This device consists of a double-layered disc on the left atrial side. The single layer PFO device is available in one size (25-mm right atrial disc/23-mm left atrial disc). The double-layer device is available in four different sizes (16/18, 23/25, 27/30, 31/35 mm).

In the Occlutech ASD device, the left atrial disc is larger than the right atrial disc. It is currently available in sizes ranging from 3 to 40 mm in 1.5-mm increments from 3 to 12 mm and 3-mm increments from 12 to 39 mm as well as a 40-mm device.

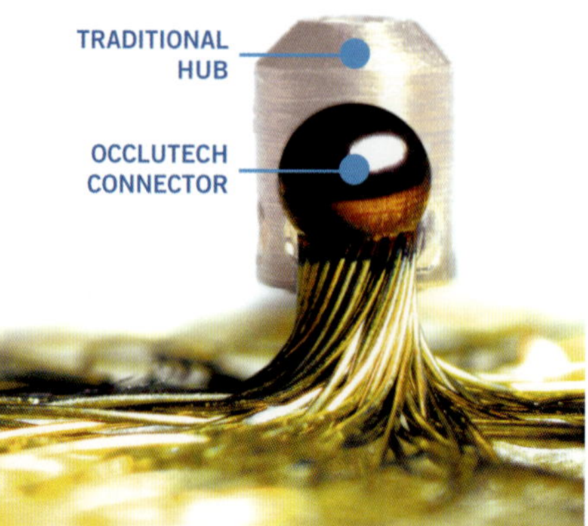

Fig 28.1—The Occlutech "connector" in comparison to the traditional right atrial hub. (Courtesy of Occlutech. Used with permission.)

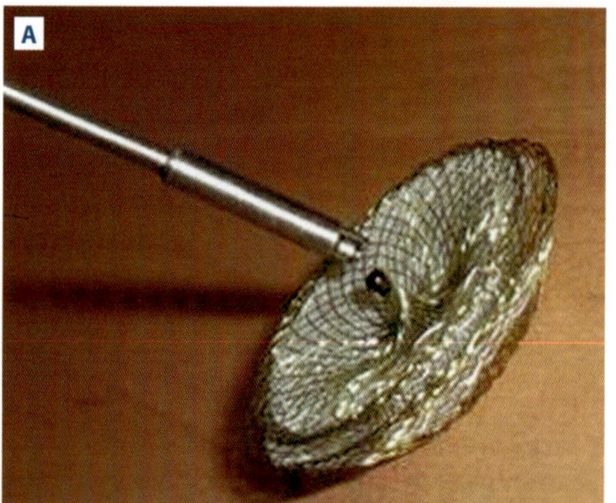

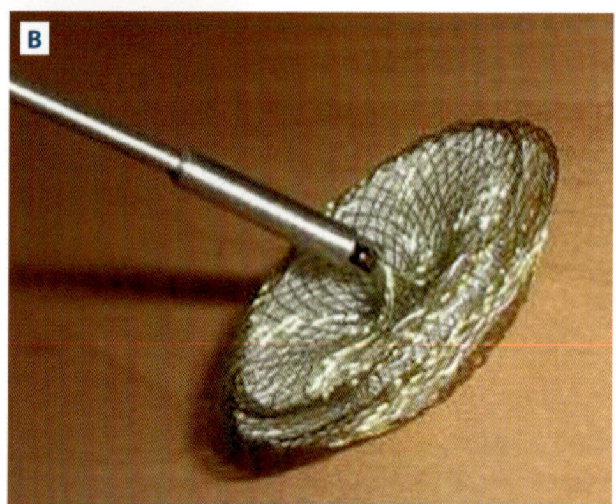

Fig 28.2 (A–B)—The Flex-Pusher delivery system. (Courtesy of Occlutech. Used with permission.)

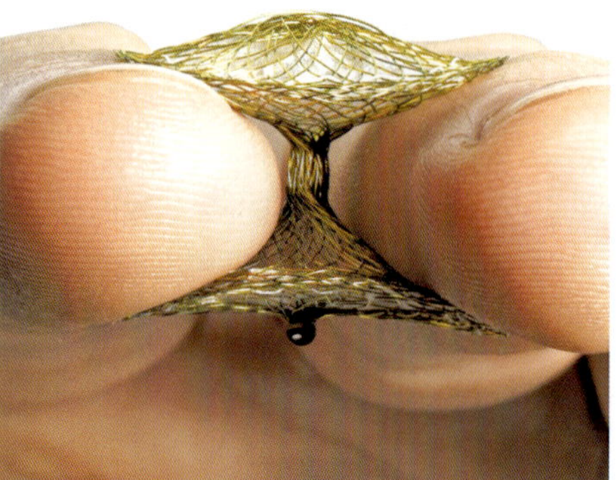

Fig 28.3—Occlutech Flex PFO Occluder. (Courtesy of Occlutech. Used with permission.)

29

Transcatheter Patch Device

Basilios E. Sideris, John D. Coulson, and Eleftherios B. Sideris

Introduction

The transcatheter patch (TP) has been used in various clinical applications since 1999. It has proven effective in occluding several cardiovascular openings including atrial septal defect (ASD), ventricular septal defect (VSD), patent ductus arteriosus (PDA), and left atrial appendage (LAA). The original TP has produced excellent acute and long-term results,[1–4] but it has proven inconvenient to use in comparison with alternative, metallic devices that can be immediately released. Since the TP was first developed, it has undergone successive improvements in regards to the time required for release. These improvements are summarized in Figure 29.1.

Initially, an accelerated-release technique was developed for the transcatheter patch using surgical adhesives.[5] This technique has been successfully used to close experimental defects in animals as well as in several clinical applications.[6,7] However, the accelerated-release technique is only effective in closing some of the aforementioned openings, and release time has varied from 45 minutes to a few hours.

In order to achieve immediate release, a new model of the TP was developed. This model incorporated features from a detachable balloon device which was used experimentally and in limited clinical cases in the late 1990s.[8,9] This device could be immediately released and showed good results with the exception of a single case in which the device embolized. The design used an occluding balloon combined with a metallic supporting disc from the right side. Attachment of the balloon to the septum or margin of an opening occurred in 6 days, it deflated within 2 months, and demonstrated gradual biodegradation and replacement by native tissue over time. The main disadvantages

Transcatheter Closure of ASDs and PFOs: A Comprehensive Assessment. © 2010 Ziyad M. Hijazi, Ted Feldman, Mustafa H. Abdullah Al-Qbandi, and Horst Sievert, editors. Cardiotext Publishing, ISBN: 978-0-9790164-9-3.

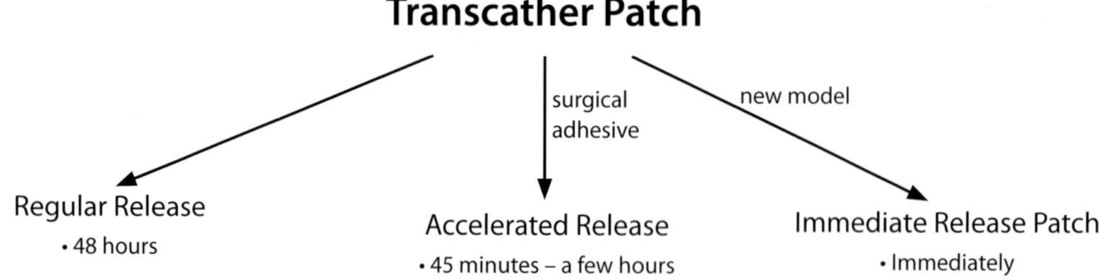

Fig 29.1—Successive improvements of the transcatheter patch.

of this device were related to the metallic supporting disc that remained on the right atrial side.

The new model of the TP, called the Immediate Release Patch (IRP) (designed by Custom Medical Devices), combines the advantages of both the original TP and the detachable balloon device. Device release is immediate and attachment to the septum, mediated by fibrin formation, takes place in approximately 48 hours. The balloon/patch becomes endothelialized in 2 to 3 weeks, and it deflates and becomes flat within 2 months. The balloon/patch later disappears, apparently undergoing biodegradation.

Devices

1. The TP device

The TP device, seen in Figs 29.2A and B, is composed of three parts: a supporting balloon catheter, a patch, and a safety thread. The patch is made from polyurethane foam and is shaped into a pouch that is placed over the tip of a balloon catheter. Depending on the size of the device, the balloon catheter contains one or two independently inflatable balloons made from latex or nylon. In cases where the double balloon catheter is used, the patch only covers the distal balloon, and the proximal balloon can be inflated for stabilization. A retrievable safety thread ensures that the patch remains on the balloon catheter prior to active release and radiopaque markers allow for device detection under fluoroscopy. Three sizes are available, and they are deliverable via 10, 12, and 13F sheaths, which are used in defects ranging from 3 to 12 mm, 13 to 20 mm, and 20 to 30 mm, respectively. The device is advanced to the relevant cardiac structure using a long sheath or over the wire using a short sheath.

2. The accelerated-release technique

The accelerated-release technique utilizes a polyethylene glycol-based surgical adhesive in conjunction with the TP.[10,11] Device delivery is carried out in the same way as with the TP by

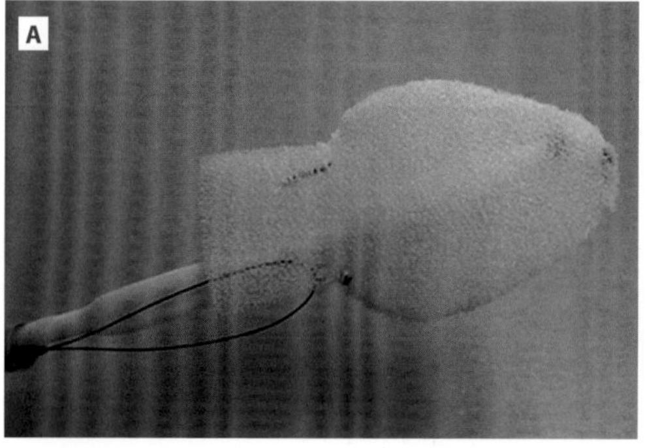

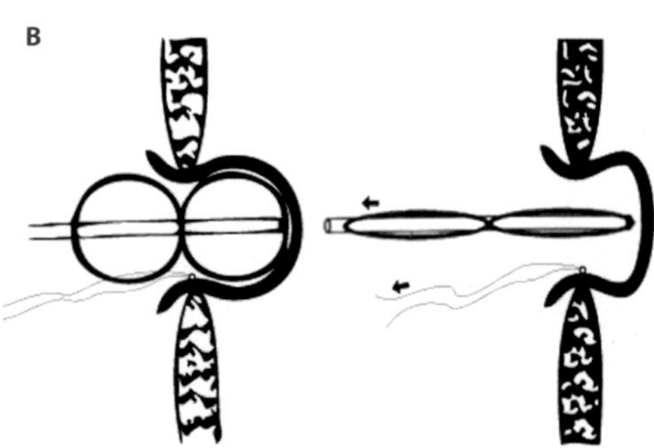

Fig 29.2—A, The transcatheter patch. B, Transcatheter patch inflation and release.

itself, except that the surgical adhesive is applied to the surface of the patch prior to implantation. The adhesive is pH sensitive and the slight alkalinity of blood causes activation. The reaction rate is slow enough to allow for correct positioning and device inflation.

3. The recently developed IRP

The recently developed IRP, seen in Figs 29.3A and B, contains the same three parts as the original TP. However, the shaft of the supporting balloon catheter is detachable, and the safety thread is bioabsorbable. The balloon catheter incorporates a detachment mechanism that allows for separation of the inflated balloon/patch from the catheter shaft after correct positioning and inflation. A removable metal stylet is kept inside the balloon catheter during implantation for support and there is only a single balloon made from latex. Three sizes are also available in this model, and they are deliverable via 9, 12, and 13F sheaths, which are used in defects ranging from 3 to 13 mm, 14 to 25 mm, and 25 to 30 mm, respectively. The safety thread is a rapidly bioabsorbable surgical suture (Vicryl) ending in a straight needle. It is used to pull the balloon/patch firmly, after it has been detached, onto the septum or margin of the opening. The safety thread is then sutured subcutaneously into the groin at the percutaneous entry point of the delivery sheath. The safety thread can also be used for device retrieval should that be necessary.

Patient selection

Patients with ASDs are initially screened by echocardiography to determine their candidacy for ASD closure. A good candidate should have an ASD of acceptable size: up to 30 mm for both the original TP and the IRP, and up to 15 mm when using the accelerated-release technique. A balloon stretched diameter of 30 mm correlates fairly well with an unstretched echocardiographic diameter of 25 mm. Therefore, the largest diameter by echocardiography should not exceed 25 mm in the transthoracic, subxiphoid four-chamber view or by transesophageal or intracardiac echocardiography. Balloon test occlusion of the ASD prior to device implantation should establish full occlusion without impairment of mitral flow or pulmonary venous return. The presence of a rim is desirable but not absolutely necessary as it is with disc devices. Therefore secundum defects with deficient rim as well as ostium primum and sinus venosus defects can be occluded provided the aforementioned criteria are met.

Exclusion criteria

Patients should be excluded when balloon test occlusion fails to fully occlude the defect or interferes with mitral flow or pulmonary venous return. Additionally, patients with associated anomalies requiring heart surgery, such as partial anomalous pulmonary vein drain-

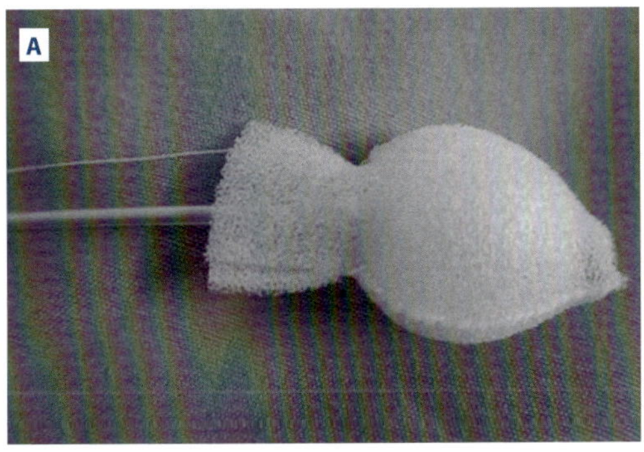
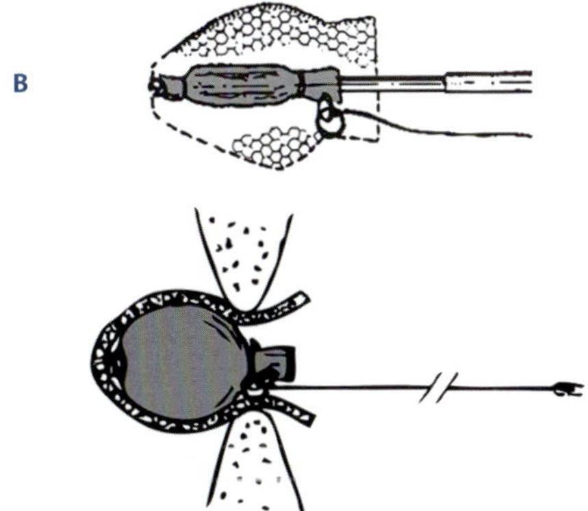

Fig 29.3—A, Immediate Release Patch. B, Immediate Release Patch introduction and defect occlusion.

age, as well as patients with severe pulmonary hypertension (PVR > 10 Wood units) should be excluded. Other exclusion criteria include IVC or pelvic vein thrombosis, sepsis, history of severe allergy to iodinated contrast, pregnancy verified by a pregnancy test completed within 7 days prior to device placement, unstable angina, decompensated left-sided heart failure, and recent myocardial infarction (less than a month). Because the procedure is carried out through a 9 to 13F sheath, patients who cannot accommodate such sheath sizes should be excluded. Patients allergic to latex should be also excluded from using TP models containing latex.

Methods

TP implantation using the accelerated-release technique

A 0.025" extra-stiff exchange wire is placed in the left upper pulmonary vein (0.021" for the small patch). The ASD is balloon sized over the wire. A 10 to 13F sheath is placed in the femoral vein and advanced to the left atrium for introduction of the TP over the wire. The dilator is removed, and the sheath is clamped to prevent air embolism. The surgical adhesive is then prepared. It is provided by the manufacturer (Baxter International, Deerfield, Illinois) in a syringe in powder form. Also provided is an additional assembly of two syringes containing acid buffer solution A and alkaline buffer solution B. The powder is diluted in solution A only. A thin film of the diluted powder is placed on the proximal half of the patch. The TP is inserted into the hemostatic valve of the long delivery sheath using a short "bypass" sheath. The external end of the exchange wire is placed through the top marker of the patch and through the central catheter lumen. All excessive adhesive is wiped away.

At this point, the short bypass sheath is pulled out of the hemostatic valve. The clamp is removed and the TP is advanced slowly over the

wire to the left atrium. After the balloon/patch is positioned in the left atrium, the balloon (distal balloon) is filled to a predetermined diameter using dilute contrast material. The balloon/patch is pulled against the atrial septum, and occlusion of the ASD is confirmed by echocardiography. Subsequently, the proximal balloon (if present) is filled to the diameter required to optimize the patch position as assessed by echocardiography and fluoroscopy. The balloon/patch should be immobilized against the septum with full occlusion of the defect and no interference with adjacent structures. The sheath and catheter are secured at the entry site in the groin using skin sutures and surgical tape. The patch is allowed to adhere to the septum for 45 minutes up to several hours.

Following the allotted time period, the patient is returned to the cardiac catheterization laboratory. The skin around the sheath entry site is reprepped using Betadine or other antiseptics. The surgical tape is removed and the skin sutures securing the sheath and the balloon catheter are removed. Deflation of the proximal balloon (if present) is carried out first. The distal balloon is test deflated to 50% diameter using echocardiography and fluoroscopy to confirm attachment of the patch to the septum and defect occlusion. If the result is satisfactory, the distal balloon is deflated and removed through the sheath followed by the sheath itself. The double nylon thread is cut and pulled out as a single strand to release the device. Pressure is applied to the groin to obtain hemostasis. A chest x-ray as well as echocardiography and fluoroscopy should be performed prior to discharge. Antibiotics (usually a cephalosporin) are given for 24 hours following the procedure with the first dose given intravenously in the catheterization laboratory.

IRP implantation

A 0.035" extra-stiff exchange wire is placed in the left upper pulmonary vein. The ASD is balloon sized over the wire. A 9 to 13F sheath is placed in the femoral vein and advanced to the left atrium for introduction of the IRP. Over-the-wire delivery of the device is optional. The dilator is removed, and the sheath is clamped to prevent air embolism. The patch is inserted into the hemostatic valve of the long delivery sheath using a short bypass sheath. At this point, the short bypass sheath is pulled out of the hemostatic valve, and the delivery sheath is well flushed. The clamp is removed and the patch is advanced slowly to the left atrium.

After the patch is positioned in the left atrium, the metal stylet is withdrawn. The balloon inside of the patch is filled to the desired diameter using dilute contrast material. Using the safety thread, the balloon/patch is pulled against the tip of the delivery sheath, and the entire complex is pulled firmly against the atrial septum. Device position is assessed using echocardiography and fluoroscopy, and occlusion of the ASD is confirmed by echocardiography. Device position and balloon volume are adjusted as necessary. With the tip of the delivery sheath held against the device, the 3F catheter is pulled out, detaching the device and sealing the balloon. The delivery sheath is withdrawn slightly, and the device is kept apposed to the septum via tension on the safety thread.

The position and stability of the device, the appropriateness of the balloon diameter, and the degree of ASD occlusion are assessed for 5 minutes before the delivery sheath is completely withdrawn. Tension is maintained on the safety thread while hemostasis is obtained. Still under considerable tension, the safety thread is then sutured subcutaneously in the catheter entry wound. A separate suture is used to close the catheter entry wound. A chest x-ray and echocardiogram should be obtained prior to discharge. Antibiotics (usually a cephalosporin) are given for 24 hours following the procedure with the first dose given intravenously in the catheterization laboratory.

Follow-up

Antibiotic prophylaxis for dental work and surgical procedures is given for 6 months if there is complete occlusion or indefinitely as long as any residual shunt persists. One baby aspirin is given daily for a month. Echocardiography is performed 1, 6, and 12 months following ASD closure. Outcomes are defined as follows:

Full occlusion: No shunt by echocardiography, angiography, or oximetry

Trivial shunt: Residual defect diameter < 2 mm by echocardiography; Qp/Qs < 1.2:1

Partial occlusion: Residual defect diameter ≥ 2 mm by echocardiography; Qp/Qs ≥ 1.2:1

Effective occlusion: Either full occlusion or trivial residual shunt.

Results

The authors analyzed 96 US and international implantation attempts, 93 of which resulted in successful occlusion. The cases included use of the original TP (n=74), the accelerated-release technique (n=9), and the IRP (n=10). Both implantation and follow-up information were recorded and the successful occlusions are summarized in Table 29.1. Both the regular and accelerated-release groups have follow-up of at least 1 year, extending up to 10 years for several patients. The mean age was 30 years (1.5–67 years) for the 48-hour release group, 33 years (8–59 years) for the accelerated-release group, and 17 years (6–48 years) for the IRP. The mean defect size was 25 mm (13–35 mm) for the TP group, 18 mm (6–25 mm) for the accelerated-release group, and 23 mm (12–26 mm) for the IRP group. The inflated balloon/patch was 1 to 2 mm larger than the defect diameter. All defects except for three were ASD secundum. Echocardiography of an ASD occlusion by the IRP can be seen in Fig 29.4. There were two occlusions of sinus venosus defects with normal pulmonary veins using the original TP, and one occlusion of ostium primum defect without mitral insufficiency using the accelerated-release technique, which is shown in Fig 29.5. Most of the patients (88%) received a large device, 10% received an intermediate device, and 2% received a small device.

Serious complications are defined as death and thromboembolic episodes including strokes and complications requiring emergency surgery (ie, perforations). No serious device-related complications occurred for any of the reported cases. In the first unsuccessful implantation attempt, there was anesthesia-related respiratory arrest 2 hours after implantation. The second unsuccessful implantation attempt was a large ASD where the inflated TP passed through after placement, initial retrieval efforts were unsuccessful due to operator error, ending in temporary pulmonary artery embolization. Successful retrieval was achieved using a snare. In the final unsuccessful occlusion attempt, the patch was not well attached in 48 hours and retrieval was performed. A second TP was subsequently implanted successfully 2 months later.

All other cases had successful device implantations. The acute full occlusion rate was 66% in the 48-hour group, 78% in the accelerated-release group, and 100% in the IRP group.

		Regular Release (n=74)		Accelerated Release (n=9)		Immediate Release Patch (n=10)	
Defect Size (mm)		13–35 (25 mean)		6–25 (18 mean)		12–26 (23 mean)	
Age (yrs)		1.5–67 (30 mean)		8–59 (33 mean)		6–48 (17 mean)	
		Immediate	Follow-up	Immediate	Follow-up	Immediate	Follow-up
Occlusion Rates (%)	Full	66	82	78	100	100	100
	Trivial	22	14	12	0	0	0
	Effective	88	96	100	100	100	100
	Partial	12	4	0	0	0	0

Table 29.1—Implantation and Follow-up Data

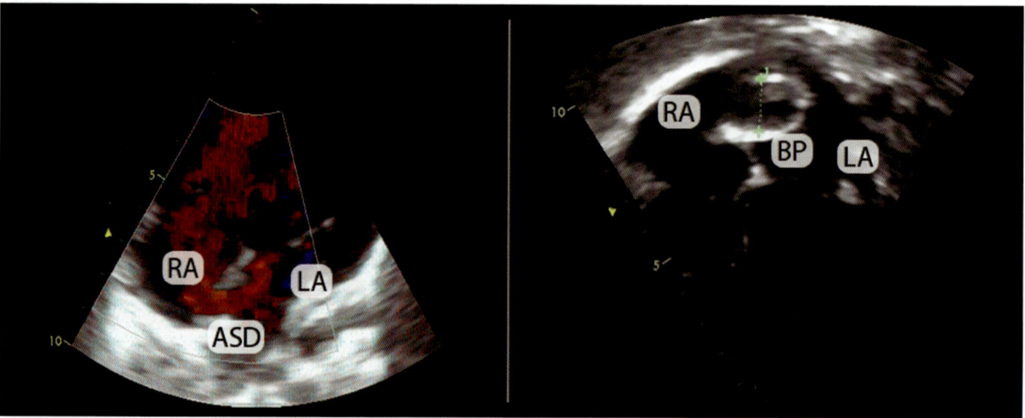

Fig 29.4—A 13-mm secundum ASD occluded by the Immediate Release Patch. Abbreviations: ASD, atrial septal defect; BP, balloon patch; LA, left atrium; RA, right atrium).

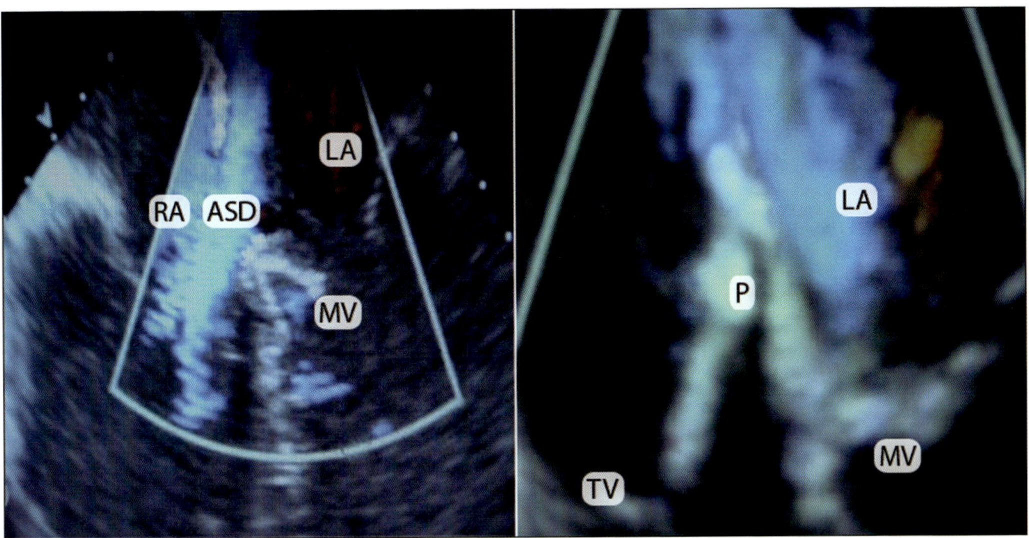

Fig 29.5—A 20-mm ostium primum ASD, occluded by the transcatheter patch using the accelerated-release technique.
Abbreviations: ASD, atrial septal defect; LA, left atrium; MV, mitral valve; P, patch; RA, right atrium; TV, tricuspid valve.

Acute effective occlusion rates (full occlusions and trivial shunts) were 82% in the 48-hour group, 100% in the accelerated-release group, and 100% in the IRP group. On latest follow-up, the full occlusion rates were 82%, 100%, and 100% for each group, respectively. In three cases from the 48-hour group in which there was partial occlusion, reintervention was carried out. Embolization of an implanted device did not occur. It is important to note that surgical retrieval or emergency surgery was not required for any case. There were a few cases in the 48-hour group in which the balloon/patch had moved from its original position at 24 hours and required readjustment with a good final result. In a few cases partial or full balloon deflation was observed before the 48-hour time period was complete. Proximal balloon deflation was inconsequential and distal balloon deflation after the first 24 hours was not crucial because the patch was already attached. No thromboembolic episodes have been reported with the device. In 4 US cases echocardiographic strands were seen on the tail of the patch upon release; the strands disappeared within a month without special treatment. They conceivably represented fibrin casts of the nylon thread.

No serious or unexpected complications were reported on follow-up in any patient with a successfully implanted device for the last 10 years. Most trivial residual shunts disappeared. Another interesting finding, presented in Fig 29.6, is the progressive disappearance of the TP under echocardiographic follow-up and the normalization of the septum (bioabsorbable device). There are several limitations in the clinical analysis and the results should be considered with caution. It is a retrospective study of an international registry of TP implantations by different investigators, in different countries, using protocols approved by different hospitals.

Patent foramen ovale occlusion

TP implantation has been used in three cases to occlude the patent foramen ovale (PFO), resulting in full occlusion. The accelerated-release technique was used for all three cases. Release of the patch was performed in 3 hours in one case (operator choice) and in 45 minutes in the other two. Although these are not enough cases to prove the safety and efficacy of the TP for PFO occlusion, favorable outcomes can be expected based on the results from ASD experience.

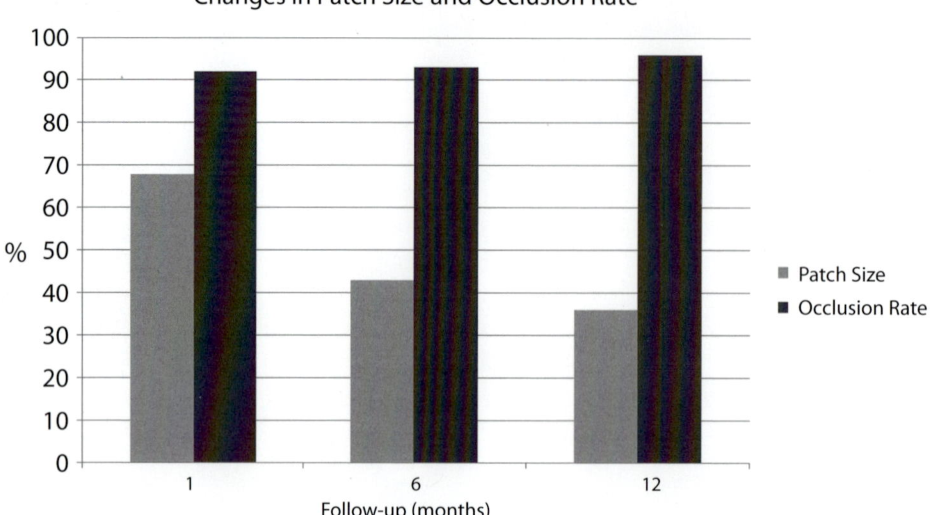

Fig 29.6—Transcatheter patch bioabsorption: Echocardiographic size of the patch (n=85), expressed as a percentage of the size on implantation, in relation to the occlusion rates.

Discussion

The transcatheter patch was developed in the late 1990s as a percutaneous occlusion device for the correction of congenital heart defects. It was first used clinically in 1999. The TP utilizes a balloon-mounted, porous polyurethane patch in conjunction with a defect bridging system for device apposition and immobilization until patch integration into adjacent tissue occurs. The device is soft, flexible, and biodegrades in situ while being replaced by native tissue. This process appears to be attributable to hydrolysis and oxidation characteristic of a foreign body reaction.[12] Histology of TP specimens removed after implantation in animals shows stimulation of macrophages and differentiation into foreign body giant cells. Aggressive tissue reaction to the TP actually appears to be advantageous by promoting device resorption.

The TP is free of metal and its associated potential complications. These include atrial perforation, aortic erosion, aortic insufficiency, mitral insufficiency, wire fracture, and heart block.[13-17] These complications are attributable to the relatively rigid nature of metal as well as to

its tendency to fatigue and break over time. Furthermore, chronic wire toxicity has been raised as a concern due to the high nickel content of commonly implanted alloys. Nickel is a known carcinogen that can cause allergy, thrombogenicity, coronary spasm, and tissue necrosis.[18]

Indeed, the TP appears to be nonthrombogenic. This characteristic is attributed to rapid incorporation of polyurethane into tissue, rapid device endothelialization, and a smooth device profile. Right-sided strands seen on echocardiography after implantation of TP may have represented fibrin casts of the safety thread within the long sheath, which was left on the right side of the heart for 48 hours. This disadvantage may have been addressed with the development of the IRP, which requires no indwelling long sheath.

The TP can be used successfully in defects with insufficient rims that are unsuitable for metallic disc devices. These defects include sinus venosus and ostium primum ASD. The TP reliably centers itself in defects, making residual shunts due to malalignment unlikely to occur and minimizing the need for repeat procedures. However, there is almost no overlapping of the defect and multiple defects and fenestrations cannot be covered as with disc devices. In addition, patients with latex allergy should be excluded from using TP models that utilize latex balloons.

In summary, experience to date suggests that the TP is comparable in safety and efficacy to available metallic disc devices. Both types of device have produced similar effective occlusion rates. Although full occlusion rates with the original TP were inferior, full occlusion rates with the newer IRP so far are excellent. An important advantage of the TP is its wider spectrum of application including defects with deficient rim and nonsecundum defects.

In 2005, the TP was approved for human implantation in the European Union (EU). The device carries the CE Mark permitting commercial distribution within the EU and many other countries outside Europe. An FDA-approved feasibility study of the 48-hour release TP model was conducted in United States centers in Cleveland and San Antonio.

References

1. Sideris E, Toumanides S, Alekyan B, et al. Transcatheter patch correction of atrial septal defects: Experimental validation and early clinical experience. *Circulation*. 2000;102(suppl 2): 588.

2. Sideris EB, Toumanides S, Macuil B, et al., Transcatheter patch occlusion of secundum atrial septal defects: early clinical experience. *Eur Heart J*. 2001;22(suppl):538.

3. Sideris EB, Macuil B, Poursanov M, Toumanides S, Moulopoulos SD. Transcatheter patch occlusion of perimembranous ventricular septal defects. *J Am Coll Cardiol*. 2003;41(6, suppl 2):473.

4. Sideris EB, Pappa PG, Sideris CE, Moulopoulos SD. Left atrial appendage and patent foramen ovale transcatheter patch occlusion in piglets: role of accelerated fibrin formation. *Cardiol Young*. 2003;13(suppl S1):60.

5. Sideris EB, Toumanides S, Sideris C, Moulopoulos SD. Accelerated transcatheter patch occlusion of heart defects: Experimental findings. *Cathet Cardiovasc Intervent*. 2004;62:93–132.

6. Calachanis M, Macuil B, Zamora R, Coulson J, Toumanides S, Sideris E. Effectiveness of transcatheter patch release with surgical adhesives in the occlusion of heart defects. *Cardiol Young*. 2007;17(suppl S1):31-014-3.

7. Sideris EB, Macuil B, Sideris VE, Moulopoulos SD. Experimental atrial septal defect occlusion using the transcatheter patch and surgical adhesive. *J Am Coll Cardiol*. 2005;4511(suppl B).

8. Sideris EB, Kaneva A, Sideris SE, Moulopoulos SD. Transcatheter atrial septal defect occlusion in piglets by balloon detachable devices. *Cathet Cardiovasc Intervent*. 2000;51(4):529–534.

9. Sideris EB, Chiang CW, Zhang JC, Wang WS. Transcatheter correction of heart defects by detachable balloon devices: A feasibility study. *J Am Coll Cardiol*. 1999; **33**(2, suppl 1):528A.

10. Hill A, Estridge TD, Maroney M, et al. Treatment of suture line bleeding with a novel synthetic surgical sealant in a canine iliac PTFE graft model. *J Biomed Mater Res*. 2001;58(3):308–312.

11. Glickman M, Gheissari A, Money S, Martin J, Ballard JL, for the CoSeal Multicenter Vascular Surgery Study Group. A polymeric sealant inhibits anastomotic suture hole bleeding more rapidly than Gelfoam/Thrombin: results of a randomized controlled trial. *Arch Surg*. 2002;137(3):326–331.

12. Coury AJ, Levy RJ, Degradation of materials in the biological environment. In: Ratner BD, Hoffman AS, Schoen FJ, Lemons JE, eds. *Biomaterials Science*. 2nd ed. Sand Diego: Academic Press. 2004:411–430.

13. Knirsch W, Dodge-Khatami A, Balmer C, et al. Aortic sinus-left atrial fistula after interventional closure of atrial septal defect. *Cathet Cardiovasc Intervent*. 2005;66(1):10–13.

14. Prieto LR, Foreman CK, Cheatham JP, Latson LA. Intermediate-term outcome of transcatheter secundum atrial septal defect closure using the Bard Clamshell Septal Umbrella. *Am J Cardiol*. 1996;78(11):1310–1312.

15. Divekar A, Gaamangwe T, Shaikh N, Raabe M, Ducas J. Cardiac perforation after device closure of atrial septal defects with the AMPLATZER septal occluder. *J Am Coll Cardiol*. 2005;45(8):1213–1218.

16. Suda K, Raboisson MJ, Piette E, Dahdah NS, Miro J. Reversible atrioventricular block associated with closure of atrial septal defects using the AMPLATZER device. *J Am Coll Cardiol.* 2004;43(9):1677–1682.

17. Rao PS, Berger F, Rey C, et al, for the International Buttoned Device Trial Group. Results of transvenous occlusion of secundum atrial septal defects with the fourth generation buttoned device: comparison with first, second and third generation devices. *J Am Coll Cardiol.* 2000;36(2):583–592.

18. Sunderman FW Jr. A review of the metabolism and toxicology of nickel. *Ann Clin Lab Sci.* 1977;7(5):377–398.

30

The CardioSEAL/STARFlex Family of Devices for Closure of Atrial-Level Defects

Paul Kramer

Introduction

In 1989, Lock and co-workers reported the first experimental use of the Clamshell device (CR Bard, Inc., Billerica, Massachusetts) to close atrial septal defects (ASDs).[1] 1990 saw the first reports of the use of this device in humans.[2,3] In 1988, Lechat et al,[4] and shortly thereafter many others,[5] reported on the strong association of cryptogenic stroke with patent foramen ovale (PFO). The identification of the relationship between PFO and multiple consequences of right-to-left shunting (e.g., stroke, transient ischemic attack, transient global amnesia, migraine, systemic thromboembolism, systemic desaturation, decompression sickness, high-altitude pulmonary edema) and the long-understood awareness of the sequelae of left-to-right and right-to-left shunting through ASDs produced a growing need for atrial defect closure. The convergence of growing clinical awareness of the pathophysiology of these sequelae and the ability to eliminate shunts with minimally invasive procedures led to the rapid growth in the number of procedures performed, the number of physicians performing them, and the number and types of catheter-based devices available for accomplishing percutaneous closure.

The Clamshell Family of Devices

The Clamshell device (Fig 30.1) consisted of two square patches of polyester fabric hand-sewn to a stainless steel skeleton resembling umbrella ribs. Each patch was secured to four ribs radiating outward from a central hub to the four patch corners. Each rib had a flexible connection with the central hub and a mid-segment coil. The central hub was intended to reside within the defect. In the case of right-to-left shunting, the right atrial umbrella was intended to cover the entrance to the pathway, while the left atrial umbrella covered the exit. The left atrial patch was rotated 45° relative to the right atrial patch, in the plane of the septum, so that the corners of the patches did not oppose one another but rather alternated around the circumference of the enveloped septum. This geometry was intended to accomplish several objectives. First, the umbrellas could be folded away from each other, enabling the Clamshell to be delivered via a reasonably sized catheter (10–12F). Secondly, it allowed the device to conform to variable anatomy through the independent and flexible mobility of each rib. As such, the device could adapt to a thick septum secundum, atrial septal aneurysm, or abutment against the anterior right atrial roof adjacent to the pulsatile aorta without imposing a rigid structure. Finally, the mid-segment rib coils enabled the corners of the patches to exert a clamping force on the septum. Alternation of this force between left and right atrial corners around the perimeter of the incorporated septum was intended to enhance securement and minimize residual shunt.

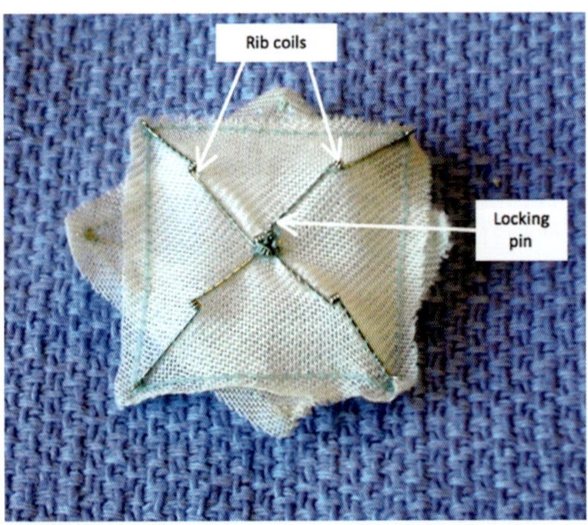

Fig 30.1—The original Clamshell device. Each umbrella consists of a square polyester patch hand-sewn to four umbrella ribs radiating to the corners from the central connecting hub. Each rib has a single mid-segment coil. (Courtesy of NMT Medical, Inc.)

As experience with the Clamshell device grew,[6] it became apparent that it suffered from some flaws, primarily rib fracture resulting from metal fatigue. Although such fracture generally did not cause clinical problems, there were some cases that caused endocardial abrasions and thrombosis. Some patients required surgical explantation. The CardioSEAL (NMT Medical, Boston, Massachusetts) (Fig 30.2) device was designed to remedy this flaw. Instead of using stainless steel, the umbrella ribs in this second-generation device were made of MP35N, a nonferrous alloy which had been used for years in pacemaker leads and been shown to be much more resistant to fatigue and fracture. In addition, the ribs were modified to incorporate two mid-segment coils in tandem, providing greater limb flexibility, device conformability, and septal clamping force. Bench testing and a subsequent large global clinical experience confirmed a dramatic reduction in rib fracture rates. The CardioSEAL became a widely adopted technology for PFO closure, but its utility in the treatment of ostium secundum ASD was limited to defects smaller than about 16 mm. This limitation resulted from the rather small caliber of the connecting hub between the two umbrellas. In contrast to the AMPLATZER Atrial Septal Occluder (AGA Medical Corporation, Golden Valley, Minnesota),[7] in which the defect is occluded by the connecting waist between the left and right atrial discs that serve to retain the waist within the defect, the CardioSEAL exerts its occlusive effect by virtue of the coverage provided by the left and right atrial umbrellas held in proximity to each other by the connecting hub. Inasmuch as this hub is much smaller in diameter than typical septal defects, it can ultimately rest in a final position anywhere within the area of the defect. This noncentering characteristic of the device necessitates that the umbrella size be more than twice the dimension of the defect to ensure adequate coverage despite eccentric hub positioning.

To overcome the limitations resulting from the non–self-centering behavior of Cardio-SEAL, the STARFlex (NMT Medical, Boston,

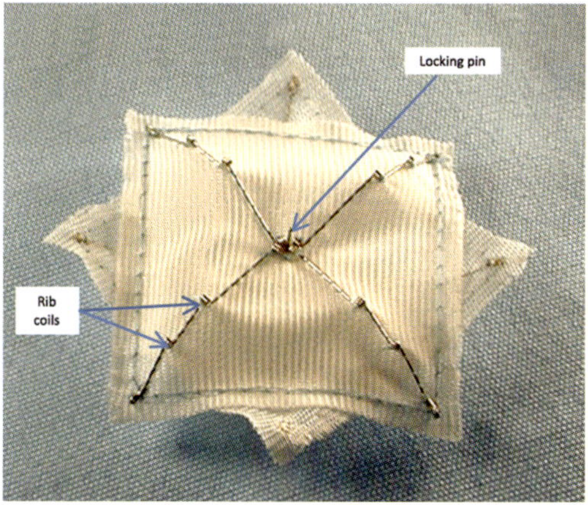

Fig 30.2—CardioSEAL device. Each square polyester patch is rotated 45° relative to its opposite. The points of the squares extend across the plane between the patches, reflecting the clamping force of the device on the septum. (Courtesy of NMT Medical, Inc.)

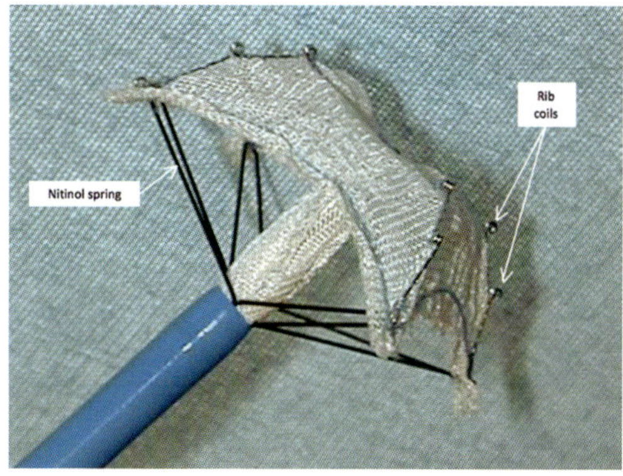

Fig 30.3—Capture of the perimeter of the right atrial umbrella of a STARFlex device. (Courtesy of NMT Medical, Inc.)

Massachusetts) device was created by adding a fine Nitinol wire coil spring that connects in sequence the corner of one patch with the adjacent corner of the opposing patch, then back to next corner of the first patch, and so on, around the entire device (Fig 30.3). There is no slack in this spring, such that when the device is deployed in a defect, whether PFO or ASD, the wire is stretched somewhat toward the central hub by the rim of the defect. This force has two major effects. First, it increases the septal clamping force of the device (Fig 30.4), which has been demonstrated to result in higher defect sealing rates. Second, the outward-pushing spring cage at the level of the defect rim serves to center the connecting hub of the device. This characteristic permits closure of larger defects with smaller devices and expands the size range of ASDs that can be treated.[8–10]

Although the safety and effectiveness of atrial level defect closure with Clamshell, CardioSEAL, and STARFlex, as well as a variety of other devices, has been demonstrated

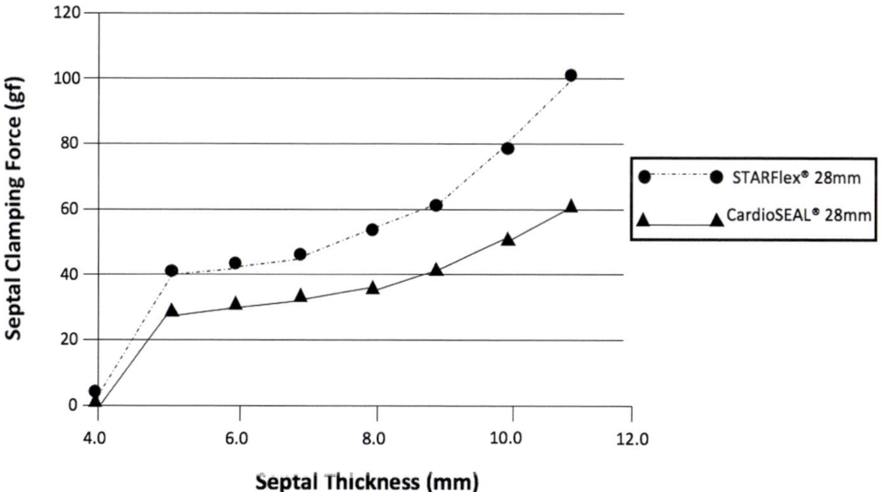

Fig 30.4—Comparative septal clamping force of STARFlex and CardioSEAL. (Courtesy of NMT Medical, Inc.)

through a large global experience, some of the consequences of the implantation of such devices are less than ideal. Chief among these is that the left atrium becomes virtually inaccessible via transseptal puncture. As technology and skills evolve to enable percutaneous left atrial appendage exclusion in patients with atrial fibrillation, mitral valve intervention (for regurgitation and stenosis), left-sided accessory pathway mapping and ablation, and antegrade access to the left ventricle and the aortic valve, the need for safe and reliable access to the left heart via transseptal puncture is certain to grow. Given the often young ages of patients who undergo percutaneous closure of atrial level defects, retaining the ability to access the left heart later in life seems desirable. The Bio-STAR (NMT Medical, Inc., Boston, Massachusetts) device is a modification of the STARFlex which features the use of a heparin-bonded, chemically modified collagen membrane[11,12] (Organogenesis, Canton, Massachusetts) in place of the polyester square patches used in the earlier devices (Fig 30.5). The bound heparin has been incorporated to address the infrequent but potentially serious development of thrombus formation on the device. In contrast to the patch, the membrane is bioabsorbable

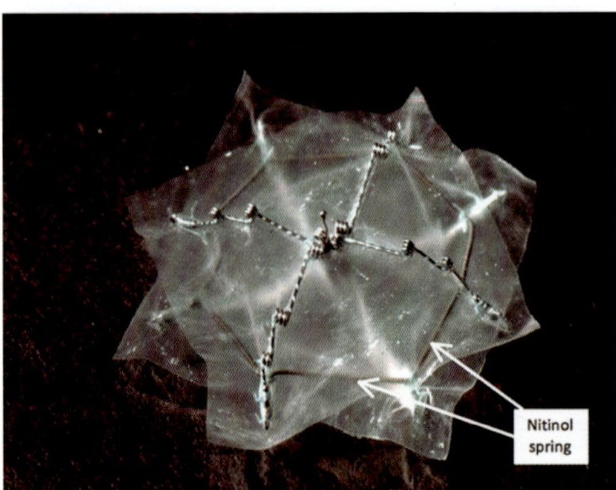

Fig 30.5—The BioSTAR. Similar in design to the STARFlex. The square patches are made of modified, heparin-bonded collagen. Each rib has two mid-segment coils. The Nitinol springs can be seen between the two bioabsorbable membranes. (Courtesy of NMT Medical, Inc.)

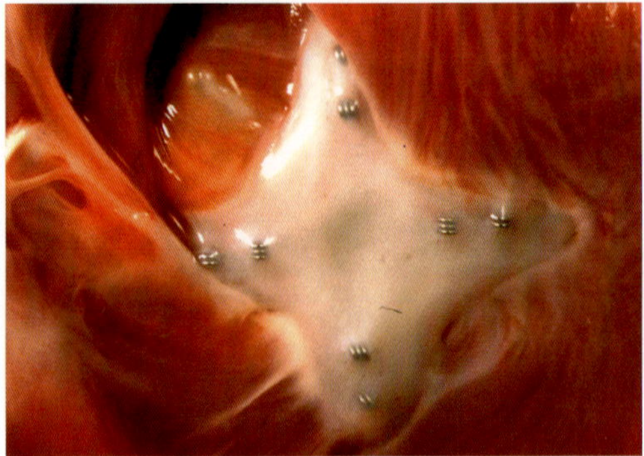

Fig 30.6—An atrial septum from the left, 6 months after BioSTAR implantation. The collagen patch has partially resorbed, and the MP35N rib coils are easily seen. (Photo courtesy of Dr. Christian Jux, University of Goettingen/Germany and Dr. Peter Wohlsein, Institute of Pathology, School of Veterinary Medicine, Hannover, Germany.)

such that, about 2 years following implantation, the membrane has been fully reabsorbed, and the atrial septum is capable of being punctured by a transseptal needle. The double-umbrella metal skeleton persists (Fig 30.6). In addition to protecting later access to the left atrium for any of a variety of procedures, the membrane behaves differently than the polyester patch at the time of implantation. Once the denatured collagen is fully hydrated, it is a more conformable material than its polyester predecessor and tends to lie flat against the septum. More intimate apposition to the septum may result in more complete early sealing and faster incorporation into the septum, although this has not been formally demonstrated.

Finally, in an attempt to leave the patient with no permanent intracardiac foreign material, the BioTREK device has been designed to be entirely bioabsorbable. The covering discs and the supporting ribs are constructed out of poly-4-hydroxybutyrate (Tepha, Lexington, Massachusetts) (Figs 30.7 and 30.8). Over time, not only do the patches resorb, but the support ribs and connecting hub eventually disappear, leaving behind only the fibrous septum previously encapsulated by the device. At the time of this writing, this device is in preclinical testing.

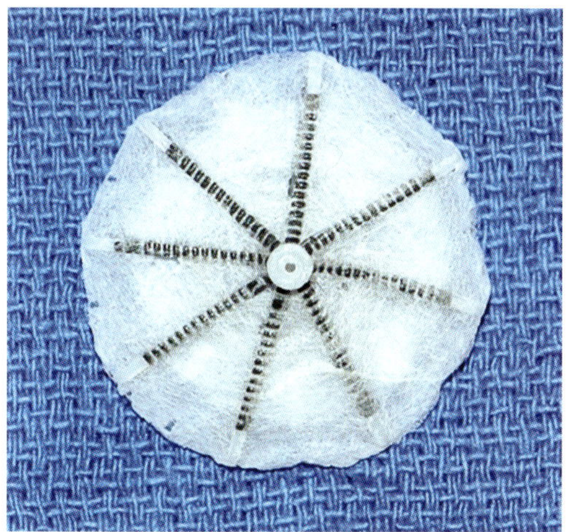

Fig 30.7—The BioTREK device. The circular patches and eight ribs are entirely bioabsorbable. (Courtesy of NMT Medical, Inc.)

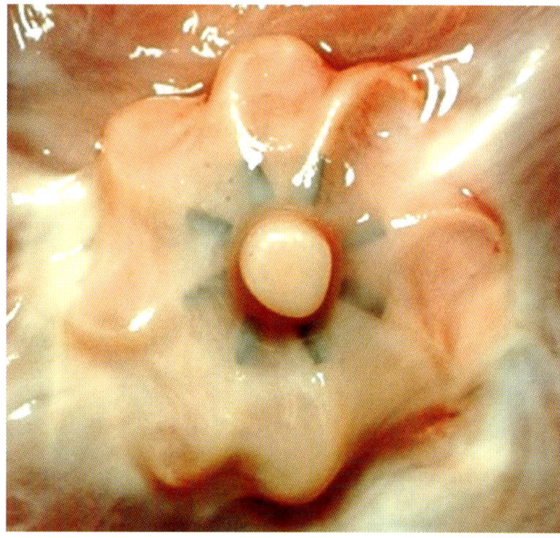

Fig 30.8—Left atrial side of a BioTREK device implanted in an ovine model 6 months earlier. Note full encapsulation of the device and partial membrane resorption around the perimeter. (Courtesy of NMT Medical, Inc.)

Technique of Defect Closure

Finding and crossing the defect

The technique for crossing atrial level defects is pretty much the same, regardless of which device is used for closure. A range of techniques has been developed, and no one method has been universally adopted. I recommend using a 6 or 7F multipurpose catheter connected to a pressure manifold and generally without the use of a guide wire. Under fluoroscopic guidance the catheter is advanced to the superior end of the inferior vena cava. It is then rotated to the 3-o'clock position, pointing straight to the patient's left. If intracardiac echocardiography (ICE) is being used, it can provide useful information about where to anticipate the location of the defect (distance from the ICE catheter tip, superior-inferior level, anterior-posterior position). Starting from below the predicted position of the defect, the catheter is simultaneously advanced superiorly while being rotated posteriorly (toward 6 o'clock). Generally, this enables transseptal passage of the catheter within one or two attempts. Advancement into the left atrium is confirmed by the fluoroscopic appearance of the catheter superimposed on the left upper

cardiac silhouette, by the ultrasound image of the catheter traversing the septum, and, in the case of PFO or restrictive ASD, the depiction of a characteristically different left atrial pressure waveform. In the case of ASD with significant right heart enlargement, the heart is rotated posteriorly. In this case, the defect is oriented closer to the 6-o'clock position than to the more typical 4 o'clock. In patients with enlarged right atria, the terminal segment of the multipurpose catheter may not be long enough to reach the septum, even though the orientation of the catheter might be correct. In this instance, the terminal segment basically needs to be made longer. This is readily accomplished by advancing a straight guide wire through the catheter, thereby functionally extending the terminal segment. The septum is then gently explored with the catheter/wire system until the defect is crossed. Finally, and least commonly, there are times when a PFO enabling a large right-to-left shunt is resistant to localization and crossing with the catheter. This most often occurs when a small PFO coexists with a large atrial septal aneurysm and when there is a long defect tunnel with an irregular interior surface or small exit portal into the left atrium. Failure to cross might lead the operator to believe no defect exists. In such a situation, a small, gentle hand injection of x-ray contrast from the tip of the catheter can be useful in confirming the presence or absence of an atrial level defect. If present, gentle manipulation of the catheter or attempting to use a hydrophilic straight or angled guide wire is almost always sufficient to cross the septum.

Once the multipurpose catheter has crossed into the left atrium, an intravenous anticoagulant is administered. The catheter is then advanced into a left pulmonary vein. An exchange wire of ≥ 180 cm is then advanced into the vein, and the catheter is removed. A stiffer wire body and shorter flexible distal end can be useful in effecting exchanges for delivery sheaths and especially for stabilizing the position of the sizing balloon, particularly in patients with large ASDs. In these patients, the torrential left-to-right shunt easily dislodges the balloon into the right atrium during the time it takes to fully inflate the balloon if a less substantial wire is used.

Defect characterization

Although it is possible to implant a variety of atrial level defect closure devices with a minimum number of steps in < 10 minutes, the purpose of closure is to eliminate, to the degree possible, the shunt through the defect. Hence, spending a few extra minutes to ensure safe and effective device deployment and shunt elimination seems reasonable. Invasive echocardiography, whether transesophageal (TEE) or intracardiac (ICE), is helpful on multiple levels. It can be used to confirm the presence of a right-to-left shunt at baseline by the use of agitated saline contrast injection, either from the femoral vein or from an upper extremity intravenous access. If such a shunt is confirmed but the septum cannot be crossed, administration of agitated contrast in the right ventricle and/ or the main or right or left pulmonary arteries can confirm and localize the presence of an intrapulmonary shunt, most often an arteriovenous fistula. Careful attention to the initial opacification of the left atrium indicates that contrast enters the chamber from a posterior, rather than a transseptal, direction. Rarely, an atrial level defect can coexist with such an intrapulmonary shunt, a phenomenon that is readily demonstrated during contrast echocardiography after closure device deployment.

Color-flow Doppler is used to demonstrate left-to-right shunting at baseline, elimination of such shunting after ASD closure, and occasionally the presence of an additional ASD. It can also demonstrate the presence of a fenestration coexistent with a PFO. It is important to exclude partial anomalous pulmonary venous return. This variant is a contraindication to percutaneous ASD closure. Although it may be recognized during preliminary ultrasound assessment, the possibility of its coexistence with the septal defect is worth considering during the catheterization procedure. When a multipurpose catheter passes from the right atrium, through an atrial defect, and into a right-sided pulmonary vein, it is impossible to distinguish the A-P fluoroscopic appearance of this catheter pathway from the alternative of passing from the right atrium (RA) into a right upper pulmonary vein directly or via the right side of the RA-SVC junction. Invasive echocardiography can demonstrate whether the catheter is traversing the septum or bypassing it. In addition, injection of agitated saline contrast from the tip of the catheter directly into the pulmonary vein can demonstrate whether it is the RA or the left atrium (LA) that is opacified first.

Other relevant findings from ultrasound performed during the closure procedure include identification of a Eustachian valve or a Chiari network, both of which may increase the risk of paradoxical embolism and interfere with proper deployment of the right atrial side of any closure device. An implanting physician aware of these anomalies can exercise extra care in ensuring full release and apposition of the right side of the device against the septum. An unusual but important ultrasound finding is the presence of a markedly thickened septum secundum, usually attributed to lipomatous atrial septal hypertrophy, in patients with PFO. This septal variant results in a greater dimension requiring coverage at the superior aspect of the fossa ovalis along the inferior rim of the septum secundum. Failure to recognize this anatomic variant could result in selecting a device size or type that does not adequately address the dimensional requirements for complete and secure device closure. The umbrella-rib construction of the CardioSEAL family of devices is uniquely suited to this anatomy by enabling the portion of the right atrial umbrella covering the septum secundum to apply a clamping force and at the same time to conform to the anatomy as a result of flexion at the rib coils. The selected device should be oversized by one size when the septum secundum exceeds 10 mm in thickness.

Although not essential for PFO closure, inflating a sizing balloon within the defect can be very helpful. In general, the size of Cardio-SEAL or earlier generations of double umbrella devices, is selected to be approximately twice the diameter of the constricted waist of the sizing balloon inflated at a low pressure. This ratio is particularly important for earlier-generation devices due to their non–self-centering characteristics. With these devices, especially in the case of ASD, the connecting hub can be very eccentrically positioned at the edge of the defect. For STARFlex and its bioabsorbable successors, due to the centering effect of the Nitinol springs, a device-to-defect size ratio of 1.5 to 2.0:1 is appropriate. Balloon sizing is mandatory in selecting the device size for ASD closure, because the gently stretched diameter can easily be > 50% greater than the diameter measured by ultrasound.

In patients with PFO, balloon sizing can indicate two problems that can interfere with successful defect closure. Not infrequently, PFO is associated with the presence of one or more fenestrations in the septum primum. When crossing the septum with a multipurpose catheter as described previously, when a fenestration exists, it tends to be anterior and inferior to the PFO itself. As a result, inasmuch as the catheter is advanced superiorly and rotated posteriorly simultaneously to cross the PFO, the first defect encountered by the tip of the catheter is the fenestration. Clues to detecting this level of

transseptal passage include: (1) the echocardiographic depiction of the catheter or exchange wire crossing the septum through the body of the septum primum rather than at the superior limbus of the fossa ovalis, and (2) the finding of a quite small stretched defect diameter ($\leq$ 5 mm) upon inflation of the sizing balloon. Either finding should alert the implanting physician that it is a fenestration that is being assessed. In addition, the finding of a persistent right-to-left shunt after deployment indicates failure to eliminate the shunt with the initial device.

Balloon characterization (not sizing per se) enables the identification of the occasional PFO associated with a long, irreducible tunnel (Fig 30.9). When the balloon is inflated at a low pressure, rather than a discrete constricting waist being imposed upon the balloon by the inferior edge of the septum secundum and the superior edge of the septum primum, two waists appear, one at the entrance to the tunnel on the right atrial side, and one at the exit from the tunnel of the left atrial side. The balloon takes on the appearance of a dog bone. Often, a bit more inflation pressure will reduce the tunnel so that a single waist is formed, but occasionally the double-waist configuration persists. In this situation, given the fixed length of the connecting hub of the double-umbrella, helical, and double-disc devices, failure to recognize this variant would result in the full deployment of one side of the device but entrapment of the other side within the tunnel, setting the stage for incomplete defect closure and/or device embolization. Two options for successful device closure in this situation include using a device with a variable connector length, such as Premere (St. Jude Medical, St. Paul, Minnesota), or avoiding the tunnel altogether by using the transseptal puncture implantation technique. In this approach, invasive ultrasound is used to position the transseptal puncture high in the fossa ovalis, at the level of the superior limbus. Once puncture has been accomplished in this location, the delivery sheath is advanced over an exchange wire, and the closure device is deployed as in a conventional procedure. In this instance, however, the left atrial umbrella does not act to cover the outlet from the tunnel. Rather, it serves to clamp the long flap of the septum primum overlapping the septum secundum onto the secundum, anchored by the right atrial umbrella, which also serves to cover the entrance to the tunnel.

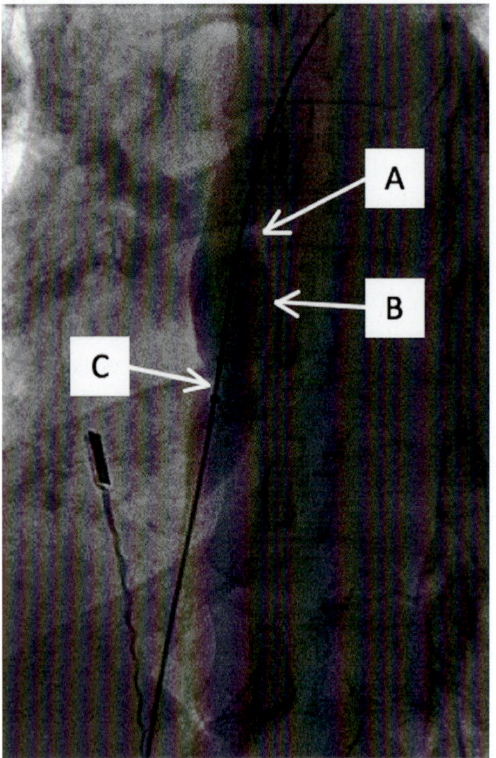

Fig 30.9—An example of the irreducible tunnel variant of PFO. The balloon takes on a characteristic "dog bone" appearance. The central portion of the balloon is inflated within the tunnel (B). A is a constraint imposed by the nondisplaced superior rim of the septum primum. C indicates the position of the lower edge of the septum secundum.

Device Deployment

Once the defect has been crossed, sized, and characterized, a transseptal delivery sheath is advanced into the left atrium over the exchange wire. The wire and dilator are withdrawn from the sheath. It is essential to recognize that the removal of the wire and dilator create a volume within the sheath. If there is no impediment to retrograde filling of the sheath with blood during dilator withdrawal, the sheath becomes blood-filled, usually with a small amount of air trapped within the external hub. At times, however, there is obstruction to backfilling with blood, and the evacuated volume of the sheath can be occupied by air aspirated via the outer end of the dilator. Recognizing this possibility is essential to preventing air embolism. The first step to undertake after removing the dilator and wire is to attach an empty syringe to the side port of the sheath, turn the stopcock, and apply negative pressure, all the while keeping the hub elevated and the side port emerging from the superior side of the hub. This orientation ensures that air will rise to the highest point, namely, the hub and the side port connection, and can be safely removed by aspiration. If there is not free aspiration, the tip of the delivery sheath may be up against the wall of the left atrium or a pulmonary vein. Gentle repositioning of the tip of the sheath will enable evacuation of the sheath contents into the aspirating syringe. Once there is oxygenated blood return into the aspirating syringe, a few forceful taps of the hub during continued aspiration will serve to evacuate any remaining air trapped within the hub. The entire delivery sheath is then flushed with heparinized saline. Some operators, as a matter of routine, will first withdraw the dilator to just within the distal end of the sheath and then remove the wire. Air is then aspirated from the wire lumen. A saline-filled syringe is connected to the distal end of the dilator, and the dilator is withdrawn slowly while injecting saline at a rate sufficient to fill the sheath as the dilator is withdrawn.

All double-umbrella devices manufactured by NMT Medical have a common method for preparation and deployment. The delivery catheters for STARFlex and later generations of devices outside of the United States are pre-attached to the closure devices and require a minor modification of the releasing step. The system currently available in the United States is similar to the original Clamshell system in that the implanting physician attaches the device to the delivery catheter. All devices have a short locking pin extending rightward from the right side of the connecting hub, perpendicularly to the plane between the umbrellas. At the terminus of the pin is a small ball (see Fig 30.1). The delivery catheter is a three-layer coaxial system of outer sheath, inner cable, and innermost locking pin and wire (Fig 30.10). During system preparation, the Tuohy-Borst adapter at

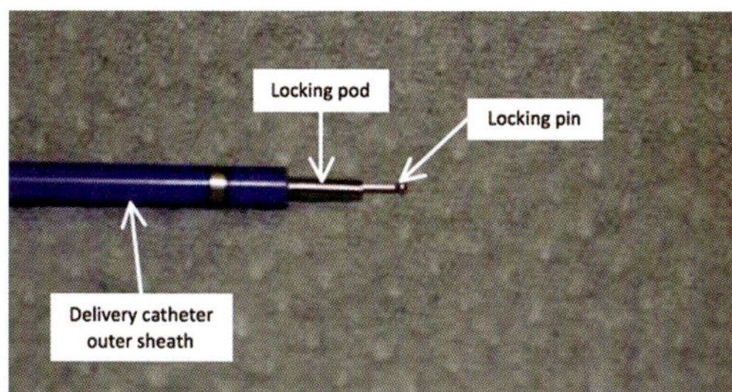

Fig 30.10—US delivery catheter. The three elements are coaxial and consist of the outer sheath, the delivery cable (retracted in this example into the outer sheath) with the locking pod at the distal end, and the locking pin. (Courtesy of NMT Medical, Inc.)

the outside end of the catheter is loosened, the locking nut securing the delivery cable to the outer sheath is loosened, the delivery cable is extended a few centimeters from the surrounding sheath, and the locking pin is extended 2 to 3 mm beyond the end of its housing, the locking pod (Fig 30.11). The Tuohy-Borst adapter is forcefully flushed during tightening of the adapter and until a bead of water emerges from the locking pod to evacuate air from the system. Once delivery catheter preparation has been completed, the closure device is attached. The locking pin of the device and the extended pin from the delivery catheter resemble each other in that both terminate in a small ball. Each ball is larger than the radius of the locking pod (Fig 30.12). The device is secured to the catheter by overlapping the pins in a parallel orientation

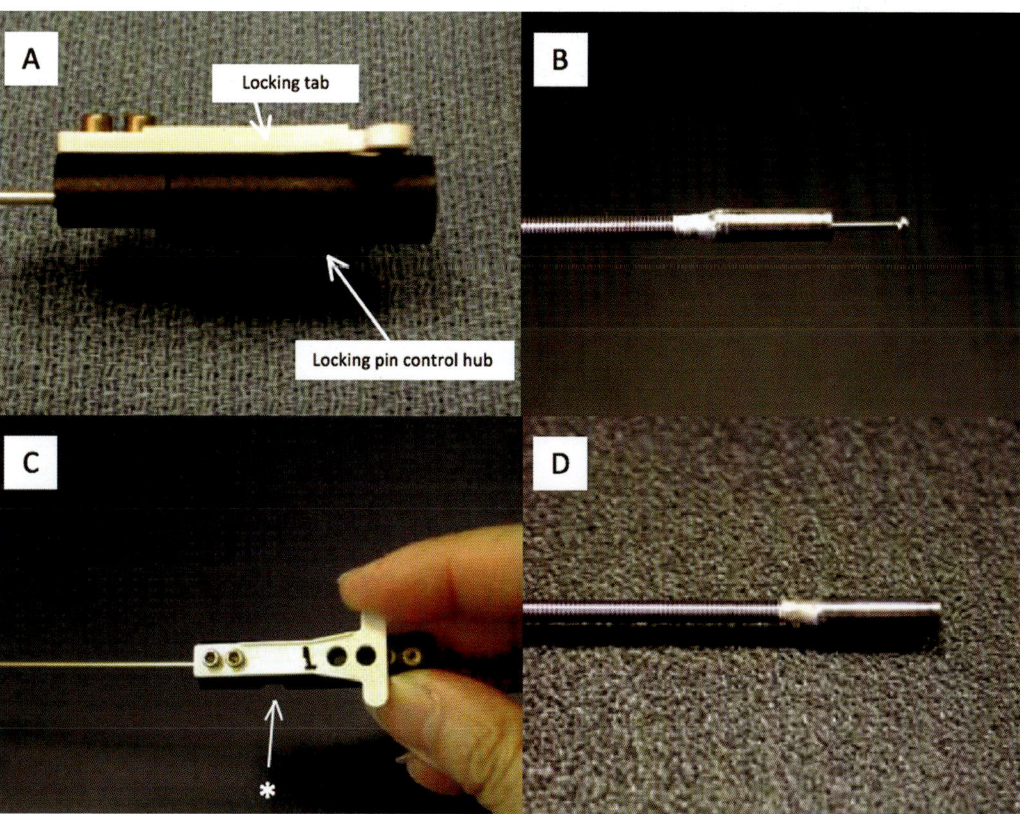

Fig 30.11—The locking mechanism of the US delivery catheter. A, The locking pin control hub is fully advanced and locked by the locking tab, and the locking pin is seen fully extended from the locking pod (B). C, The control hub has been fully retracted and locked by the locking tab, creating a gap (*) between the control hub and the rest of the handle. D, The catheter locking pin is fully retracted into the locking pod. (Courtesy of NMT Medical, Inc.)

and withdrawing the overlapped segments into the locking pod (Fig 30.13). Once inside the pod, the balls at the ends of the pins are unable to travel past each other because their combined dimension exceeds the pod diameter. The easiest method for securement is to cross the two pins at an angle of 60° to 90° (as if crossing swords), then align the pins while maintaining contact and overlap, then retract and lock the

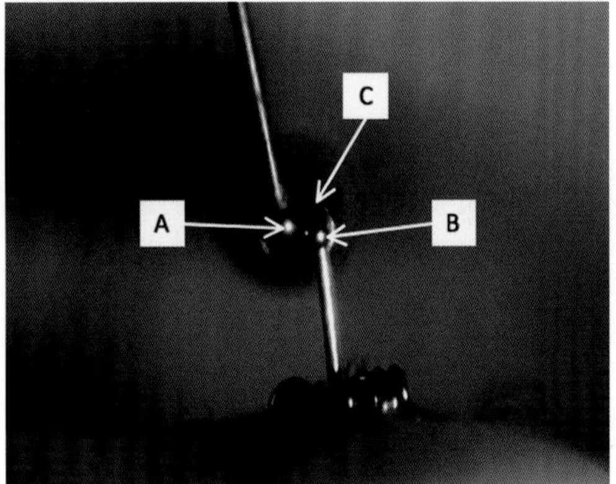

Fig 30.12—Locking mechanism of the US delivery catheter. The combined diameters of the locking pin ball of the delivery catheter (A) and of the closure device (B) exceed the diameter of the locking pod (C), preventing B from sliding over A and resultant device detachment when the locking pin is retracted into the pod. (Courtesy of NMT Medical, Inc.)

catheter's locking pin in the locking pod while keeping the closure device perpendicular to and in contact with the pod. The locking tab is then engaged (Fig 30.11).

Outside of the United States, the RT delivery catheter is preattached to the STARFlex device, and delivery catheter preparation consists of flushing the system using the syringe fitted into the deployment handle. At the time of this writing, the BioSTAR device is not preattached. Figure 30.14 shows the locking mechanism of the RT delivery catheter. The photograph depicts the relationship of the opened locking jaws to the locking pin of the BioSTAR. This mechanism enables relatively free pivoting of the attached device (Fig 30.15), minimizing distortion of the in situ device prior to release. The control handle (Fig 30.16) houses the syringe, which is used for flushing the delivery catheter. The release knob is connected to the distal locking pin and is secured in position by the locking button. This locking button must be deliberately depressed to advance the release knob, minimizing the risk of inadvertent device detachment.

After the delivery catheter has been purged of air and connected to the closure device, the next step is to collapse the device for advance-

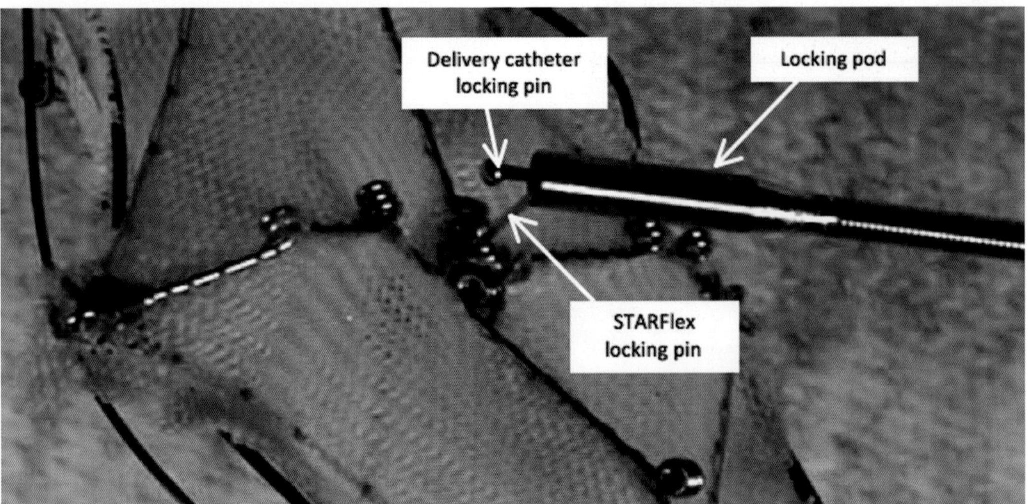

Fig 30.13—Close-up of the relationship of the closure device to the US delivery catheter just before retraction of the locking pin into the locking pod. In this case, the operator has inserted the pin of the STARFlex directly into the pod. (Courtesy of NMT Medical, Inc.)

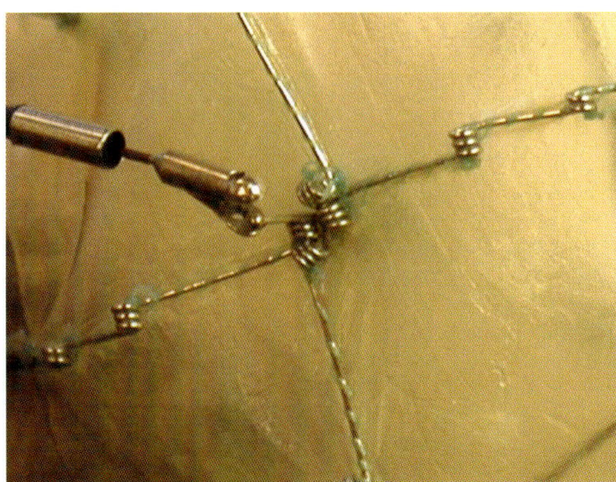

Fig 30.14—Close-up view of opened locking mechanism of the OUS RT delivery catheter poised over the ball of the BioSTAR locking pin. When locked, this mechanism permits relatively free pivoting of the engaged device, minimizing the distortion of the orientation of the device while attached. (Courtesy of NMT Medical, Inc.)

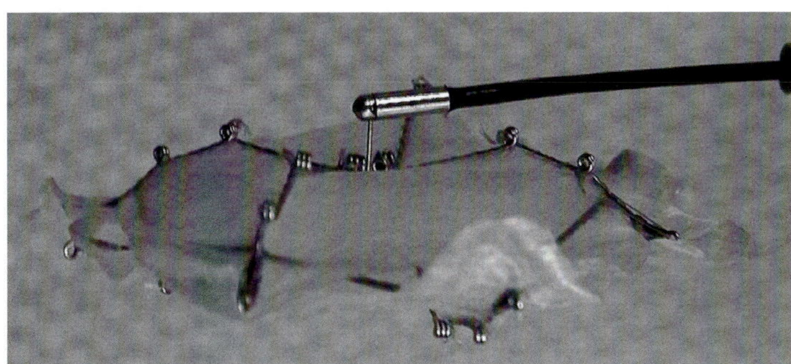

Fig 30.15—The OUS RT delivery catheter with the BioSTAR secured. Note the 90° angle to the catheter achievable by free pivoting. (Courtesy of NMT Medical, Inc.)

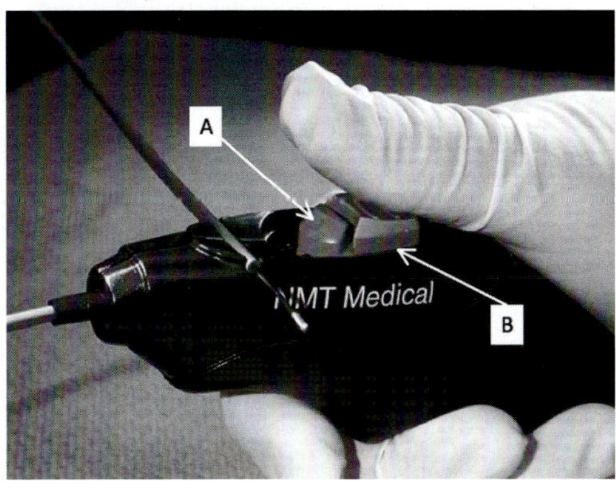

Fig 30.16—Control handle of the RT delivery catheter used outside of the United States. A, Release knob locking button. B, Release knob, which opens the securement jaws when advanced. The locking button must be forcibly depressed to permit advancement of the release knob. (Courtesy of NMT Medical, Inc.)

ment into the delivery sheath. Collapsing and loading the device is essentially the same for the United States and the RT delivery catheters. The left atrial umbrella has a suture that runs from the four corners to a small plastic button. Between the button and the umbrella is a loading tube connected to a funnel. Pulling the button away from the device pulls the four corners of the left atrial umbrella away from the right umbrella and toward each other, forming a collapsed parachute (Fig 30.17). The collapsed left atrial umbrella is pulled by the button into the funnel (Fig 30.18) and further into the loading tube (Fig 30.19). As the left atrial umbrella enters this tube, the funnel acts to fold and collapse the right atrial umbrella away from the left one, and the entire closure device is drawn into the tube. Once this has been accomplished, the suture connecting the device to the button is cut, and the suture is withdrawn and discarded, as is the protective housing around the delivery tube. A Tuohy-Borst adapter mounted on the body of the delivery catheter is then connected to the funnel. A large saline-filled syringe is

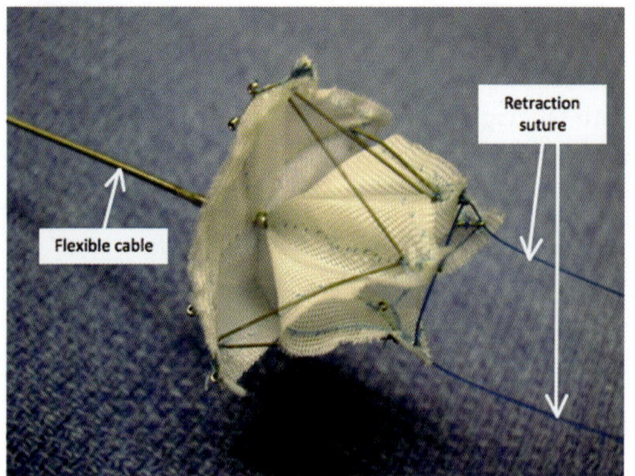

Fig 30.17—The right atrial umbrella of a STARFlex device has been partially collapsed by tension on the retraction suture. In this example, the device is attached to a US delivery catheter. (Courtesy of NMT Medical, Inc.)

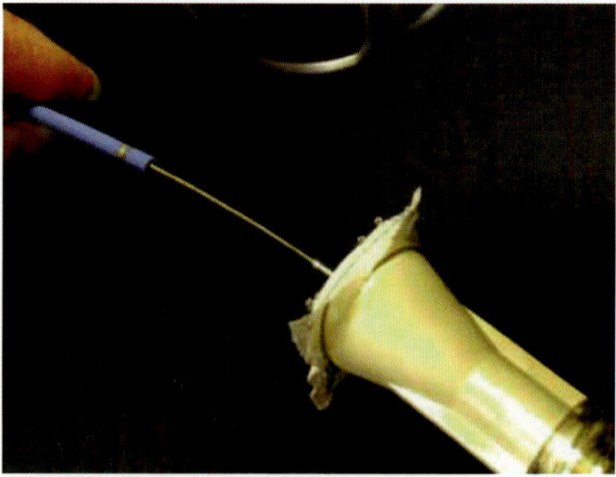

Fig 30.18—Loading the CardioSEAL device into the funnel. The left atrial umbrella has been collapsed by tension on the loading suture. (Courtesy of NMT Medical, Inc.)

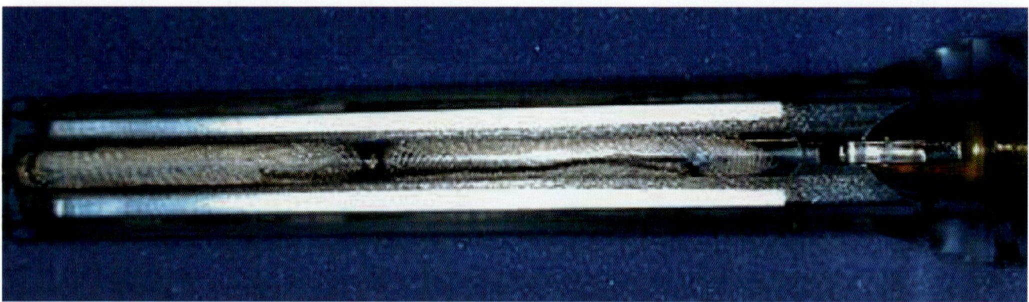

Fig 30.19—The STARFlex device has been fully loaded into the loading tube. (Courtesy of NMT Medical, Inc.)

connected to the adapter, which will allow air-less introduction of the loading tube and closure device through the hemostatic valve and into the delivery sheath without damaging the device. At this time, the outer portion of the delivery catheter is advanced to within about 10 mm of the ends of the right atrial umbrella in order to stiffen the delivery apparatus. This is accomplished by loosening the locking nut at the rear of the delivery catheter and the hemostatic valve on the adapter connected to the funnel, then gently pulling on the delivery cable within the delivery sheath, which has the effect of advancing the outer catheter over the cable. Ensure that the locking pin lock does not become disengaged during these steps and that the locking tab remains fully engaged and flat against the outside hub of the delivery catheter.

Once the outer catheter has been positioned to within 10 mm of the device, the rear locking nut is securely tightened. This step is not necessary when using the OUS RT delivery catheter.

Flushing the loaded implant within the loading tube is begun with the adapter's hemostatic valve open, and then the adapter's valve is tightened to redirect flush solution through the loading tube. The tube is advanced through the hemostatic valve of the introducer sheath while injecting flush through the tube to prevent introducing air into the sheath. The delivery catheter is then advanced 20 to 30 cm. During this step, the closure device is pushed from the loading tube and is thereafter constrained by the delivery sheath. The loading tube is then withdrawn from the delivery sheath. The delivery catheter is further advanced until, on fluoroscopy, the closure device appears at the lower level of the cardiac shadow. Next, if using the US delivery catheter, the lock nut affixing the delivery cable to the delivery sheath is loosened, and the cable is pushed inward, advancing the closure device to the distal end of the delivery sheath. The locking nut is retightened. At this stage, the more flexible delivery cable has been exposed, and the three coaxial components of the delivery catheter are secured to each other.

The left atrial umbrella is deployed as follows. First, the invasive echo image should be optimized to depict the sheath crossing the septum and, in the case of PFO, the adjacent primum and secundum components. The delivery sheath is withdrawn to the level of the connecting hub, being careful not to simultaneously permit retraction of the device itself. This is best accomplished by ensuring that the device doesn't move relative to nearby bony landmarks and generally requires a gentle pushing counterforce on the delivery catheter to overcome the frictional drag imposed by withdrawing the delivery sheath. Fluoroscopy should depict full opening of the left umbrella. However, occasionally the umbrella is constrained within a pulmonary vein, and gentle retraction of the delivery sheath and catheter together, preventing movement of one relative to the other, serves to pull the umbrella into the left atrial chamber, allowing full opening. The open umbrella is vividly depicted on invasive echocardiography. At this time, one or both hands are used to simultaneously, and without relative movement of one versus the other, withdraw the delivery sheath and catheter. In doing so, the tip of the sheath remains at the level of the connecting hub, and the right atrial umbrella remains within the sheath. Continued traction is applied until, on ultrasound, the left umbrella fully contacts the septum. At this time, the fluoroscopic image shows that with slight additional traction, the ends of the umbrella ribs don't move although the central hub elements do. If a freeze frame was retained from an image acquired at the time of balloon inflation, this can be usefully compared with the fluoroscopic image. As with any

device, excessive retraction force can pull the left atrial side of the device through the defect into the right atrium. This is of greater concern in the case of ASD, where the device is functionally replacing missing tissue, and in small PFO, where the length of the umbrella ribs is short.

Once the left atrial umbrella has "landed," the delivery sheath is withdrawn while the delivery catheter is stabilized. Ensuring that the configuration of the left umbrella doesn't change during this process and that the device doesn't move relative to adjacent bony structures facilitates the release of the right atrial umbrella without malpositioning the left. Once both umbrellas are deployed, all tension on the system should be released. Echocardiography is used to assure that each umbrella is correctly positioned on its side of the septum and that, in the case of PFO, the superior portions of the umbrellas enfold the inferior aspect of the septum secundum. Once appropriate deployment is confirmed, the device is released, allowing it to assume its unrestrained, in situ position. In the United States, this is accomplished by lifting the locking tab, thereby freeing the securement hub at the outside end of the catheter and advancing it fully inward. This serves to advance the delivery catheter locking pin out of the locking pod, releasing its attachment to the locking pin of the closure device, after which the delivery catheter is removed. Outside of the United States, the locking mechanism clamped onto the ball at the end of the device locking pin is opened by depressing the locking button with the thumb and then sliding the release button forward. Either spontaneously or after a few cardiac cycles, the delivery system can be seen to separate from the closure device. Occasionally, gentle advancing, withdrawing, and torquing of the delivery catheter and/or sheath is required to release the device.

Following successful device deployment, invasive echocardiography probes/catheters are removed, agitated saline echocardiography is performed to assure elimination or near-elimination of the shunt, the introducer and delivery sheaths are withdrawn, and hemostasis is achieved.

Troubleshooting and Avoiding Complications

It is important to recognize and address complications promptly and effectively, but, as always, the best strategy is to avoid, to the degree possible, any complications in the first place. Using invasive echocardiography, characterizing the defect with balloon inflation, meticulous attention to keeping the delivery system free of air and thrombus, and not taking irreversible steps during deployment until it is clearly safe to do so can serve not only to implant the closure device but to eliminate the consequent shunt and to avoid complications. Pretreatment of patients with a combination of aspirin and a thienopyridine for at least four days prior to implantation is recommended to avoid excessive early platelet adhesion to the device. Aspirin is continued for at least 6 months, perhaps indefinitely, and the thienopyridine is usually stopped after 3 months. Antibiotic prophylaxis is recommended for 6 months. As with any catheterization procedure, the leading risk of percutaneous atrial level defect closure is bleeding at the femoral vein access site(s). This risk is minimized by using a modest dose of anticoagulant, performing the closure procedure expeditiously, and ensuring hemostasis at the conclusion. Lingering excessively with apparatus in the vascular space, especially in the left atrium, may increase the likelihood of thrombus formation on the delivery system. Advance preparation of the delivery sheath, delivery catheter, sizing balloon, exchange wire, and closure device, to the degree possible, minimizes the time during which such thrombosis can occur and lessens the need to administer supplemental anticoagulation during the procedure. Hemostasis can be achieved by manual compression, application of any of a variety of compression devices, and/or the use of the "figure-of-eight" mattress suture. Protamine should not be administered to reverse heparin anticoagulation, as this might be associated with an increased risk of device thrombosis. Because of the sizes of the introducer and delivery sheaths used, a period of strict bed rest of 6 to 8 hours is advisable. Valsalva strain should be avoided for several days.

The need to remove an NMT Medical double umbrella device is rare and avoidable. Adhering to basic "rules of the road" essentially eliminates the need to remove these devices. These rules include, first, ensuring that the closure device is securely attached to the delivery catheter. Whether premounted or attached by the operator, a gentle tug on the device while attached confirms securement. Make sure that the locking mechanism at the outside end of the delivery catheter is fully engaged. These simple steps require only a few seconds and can help avoid inadvertent detachment within the delivery sheath. Second, attempting to deploy these devices in long, irreducible tunnels can result in the full opening of either the left or the right umbrella but constrained opening of the opposite one within the tunnel. While uncommon, releasing the device from the delivery catheter in these circumstances sets the stage for device embolization and its potentially catastrophic consequences. It takes < 1 minute to identify this anatomic variant with balloon characterization, and the procedure is then modified to implant the device using the transseptal puncture technique (see page 389).

Deployment of both umbrellas in the left atrium is best avoided by using invasive echocardiography to ensure full retraction of the left atrial umbrella against the septum before the right atrial umbrella is released by further sheath withdrawal. In addition to the use of ultrasound, it is strongly recommended that a single operator perform the actions of left atrial umbrella retraction against the septum, delivery catheter stabilization, and delivery sheath withdrawal to release the right atrial umbrella. This strategy serves to eliminate the possibility that a momentary lack of communication and coordination between two operators can produce an undesirable and potentially catastrophic result. Similarly, care should be exercised to avoid deployment of both umbrellas in the right atrium. More likely to occur during attempted ASD closure because of the relative tissue deficit in comparison with PFO, excessive traction on the left atrial umbrella can result in prolapsing one or more umbrella rib ends across the septum and into the right atrium. The device should be thoroughly scanned by ultrasound during the time that the LA umbrella is being retracted against the septum and before the sheath is retracted to release the RA umbrella to ensure that such prolapse has not occurred. Following release of the RA umbrella, relax any tension that has been applied to the system. Use ultrasound to ensure that the two umbrellas are entirely situated on their appropriate sides of the septum, and then release the device from the delivery catheter without undue delay. Prolonged attachment to the delivery system after full and appropriate deployment increases the opportunity for misadventure and shifting of the device position. Scrupulous adherence to these rules will minimize the likelihood that device retrieval and/or repositioning will be necessary.

In the event that retrieval or repositioning is necessary, the technique depends upon the nature of the event. If the left atrial umbrella is malpositioned or is deemed too small for the defect, it is a simple and straightforward procedure to reconstrain it within the delivery sheath, as long as the right atrial umbrella has not yet been uncovered. Making sure that the locking mechanism has not been inadvertently released, if the LA umbrella is on the left side of the septum, advance the delivery sheath and catheter as a unit into the body of the LA, and then withdraw the delivery catheter back into the sheath within the LA chamber. The umbrella should easily collapse away from the hub (as during the initial introduction into the loading tube) and slide into the sheath. If part of the LA umbrella has prolapsed into the RA, it is best to pull the device all the way into the RA and then recapture the LA umbrella as previously explained. Once the closure device has been fully reconstrained within the delivery sheath, the sheath/catheter/device needs to be removed from the femoral vein, unless the angulated delivery sheath can be advance easily back through the defect and into the left atrium

(much more likely with ASD). The device cannot reliably be withdrawn through the hemostatic valve in the hub of the delivery sheath when using the loading device included with the US delivery system. The femoral vein then needs to be reentered and device delivery needs to resume from the beginning of the process. Outside of the United States, the loader (called Qwik Load) can be readvanced into the sheath hub, and the collapsed implant can be removed from the sheath, basically reversing the initial steps of the procedure. As such, the sheath position can be maintained.

If the RA umbrella is deployed before the need to retrieve or reposition the device is recognized, retrieval is more difficult, highlighting the need to ascertain optimal LA umbrella positioning before unmasking of the RA side. In the unlikely event that both umbrellas are deployed within the LA, the device can be easily pulled through an ASD to the RA, first ensuring that the locking mechanism is securely engaged. If the defect is a PFO, attempts should be made to retract the device through the defect, but this may not be possible. If that is the case, an attempt to at least partially reconstrain the device within the tip of the delivery sheath should be made. In attempting to reconstrain the RA umbrella, regardless of the chamber in which it is being attempted, it is important to be aware that, unlike the case of recapturing the LA umbrella, the coils of the RA umbrella face the delivery sheath. As such, they may engage the lip of the sheath and prevent retraction into it. Magnified fluoroscopy can help the operator to manipulate the sheath and the delivery catheter to coaxially align the two and thereby facilitate passage of the coils into the sheath. It is important to understand that in doing so, the RA umbrella is being collapsed in a direction opposite from that during initial device preparation, and the umbrella may not fully reenter the delivery sheath. Nevertheless, by partially collapsing the device, its profile is reduced, and pulling it back through the defect into the RA is facilitated. It is important to maintain a moderate degree of retraction force on the delivery catheter during this maneuver. Once the device is completely within the right atrium, the entire system is withdrawn to the femoral vein entry site. An attempt can then be made to forcefully withdraw the system in its entirety from the vein, but this can be quite difficult and can result in inadvertent device detachment. For this reason, an assistant should apply gentle compression over the vein above the level of the device to prevent embolism to the right heart and beyond. Cutting down on the vein may be necessary to extract the device. For the less experienced operator, given the complexity of these maneuvers, it is recommended that a 14F sheath be preloaded to the back end of the transseptal delivery sheath. In the event that device retrieval becomes necessary and it cannot be fully reconstrained within the transseptal delivery sheath, the 14F sheath is advanced over the delivery sheath and into the femoral vein. Using the same traction technique described earlier to partially reconstrain the fully uncovered device, the entire delivery system is withdrawn into the 14F sheath. The large size of this sheath generally accepts the profile of the device, enabling atraumatic removal from the femoral vein.

Summary

The Clamshell family of devices has been in evolution for over 20 years. The development of improved materials, mechanical characteristics, and operator skills, along with the growing awareness of the wide variety of potential consequences of right-to-left as well as of left-to-right shunts, has produced a rapidly growing, global interest in definitive, minimally invasive methods for shunt elimination. PFO was first reported as a regular finding in young patients with cryptogenic stroke only 22 years ago. The first large, multicenter, randomized trial of PFO closure as compared with antithrombotic therapy has been completed and will be analyzed and reported this year (2010). The latest generations of these devices are simple, safe, and effective for the percutaneous closure of almost all PFOs and of most ostium secundum ASDs $\leq$ 18 mm in diameter. The active septal clamping force of these devices distinguishes them from all others and may be particularly desirable in patients with certain anatomic variants, such as lipomatous atrial septal hypertrophy. The bioabsorbable versions of these devices possess the attractive feature of enabling transseptal access to the left atrium for future potential therapies, such as mitral valve repair, left atrial appendage exclusion, and antegrade access to the left ventricle and aortic valve.

Acknowledgments

The author wishes to thank Carol Devellian and NMT Medical, Inc., for their assistance in providing the figures (except 30.6 and 30.9) used in this chapter.

References

1. Lock JE, Rome JJ, Davis R, et al. Transcatheter closure of atrial defects. Experimental studies. *Circulation.* 1989;79(5):1091–1099.
2. Rome JJ, Keane JF, Perry SB, et al. Double-umbrella closure of atrial septal defects. Initial clinical applications. *Circulation.* 1990;82(3): 751–758.
3. Bridges ND, Newburger JW, Mayer JR. Transcatheter closure of the secundum ASD in pediatric patients. *Am J Cardiol.* 1990;66:522.
4. Lechat P, Mas J-L, Lacault G, et al. Prevalence of patent foramen ovale in patients with stroke. *N Engl J Med.* 1988;318:1148–1152.
5. Webster MW, Chancellor AM, Smith HJ, et al. Patent foramen ovale in young stroke patients. *Lancet.* 1988;2:11–12.
6. Prieto LR, Foreman CK, Cheatham JP, et al. Intermediate-term outcome of transcatheter secundum atrial septal defect closure using the Bard Clamshell Septal Umbrella. *Am J Cardiol.* 1996;78(11):1310–1312.
7. Masura J, Gavora P, Formanek A, Hijazi ZM. Transcatheter closure of atrial septal defects using the new self-centering AMPLATZER septal occluder. Initial human experience. *Cathet Cardiovasc Diagn.* 1997;42:388–393.

8. Hausdorf G, Kaulitz R, Paul T, et al. Transcatheter closure of atrial septal defect with a new flexible, self-centering device (the STARFlex Occluder). *Am J Cardiol.* 1999;84(9):1113–1116, A1110.

9. Nugent AW, Britt A, Gauvreau A, et al. Device closure rates of simple atrial septal defects optimized by the STARFlex device. *J Am Coll Cardiol.* 2006;48(3):538–544.

10. Law MA, Josey J, Justino H, et al. Long-term follow-up of the STARFlex device for closure of secundum atrial septal defect. *Cathet Cardiovasc Onterv.* 2009;73(2):190–195.

11. Jux C, Wohlsein P, Bruegmann M, et al. A new biological matrix for septal occlusion. *J Interv Cardiol.* 2003;16(2):149–152.

12. Jux C, Bertram H, Wohlsein P, et al. Interventional atrial septal defect closure using a totally bioresorbable occluder matrix. Development and preclinical evaluation of the BioSTAR device. *J Am Coll Cardiol.* 2006;48(1):161–169.

31

Bioabsorbable Devices:
The BioSTAR and BioTREK for ASDs and PFOs

Ryan Ko and Michael J. Mullen

Introduction

BioSTAR and BioTREK are both devices developed by NMT Medical (Boston, Massachusetts) for the closure of atrial septal defect (ASD) and patent foramen ovale (PFO). Both technologies are unique in that they utilize bioabsorbable materials to optimize the biological response to ASD and PFO closure and reduce the burden of prosthetic material that remains in the heart once closure has occurred. With increasing numbers of devices being placed in clinical practice, often in a young patient population, the benefits of this approach are both intuitive as well as of practical benefit. Achieving this represents somewhat of a challenge in choosing materials with appropriate characteristics that preserve structural integrity while allowing absorption in a controlled and predictable fashion. This chapter describes the devices, the characteristics of the materials used, and the techniques for their deployment and use in patients with ASD and PFO.

BioSTAR

The design of the BioSTAR device is predicated on previous successful umbrella closure devices developed by NMT Medical. Using an identical MP35N frame to the CardioSEAL and STARFlex devices, in the BioSTAR, the polyester fabric scaffold is replaced with a bioabsorbable tissue engineered porcine intestinal collagen layer (ICL) scaffold (Organogenesis, Canton, Massachusetts). The two square umbrellas each supported by four arms are offset by 45° such that when viewed en face the device has the appearance of an eight-point star (Fig 31.1). Torsion

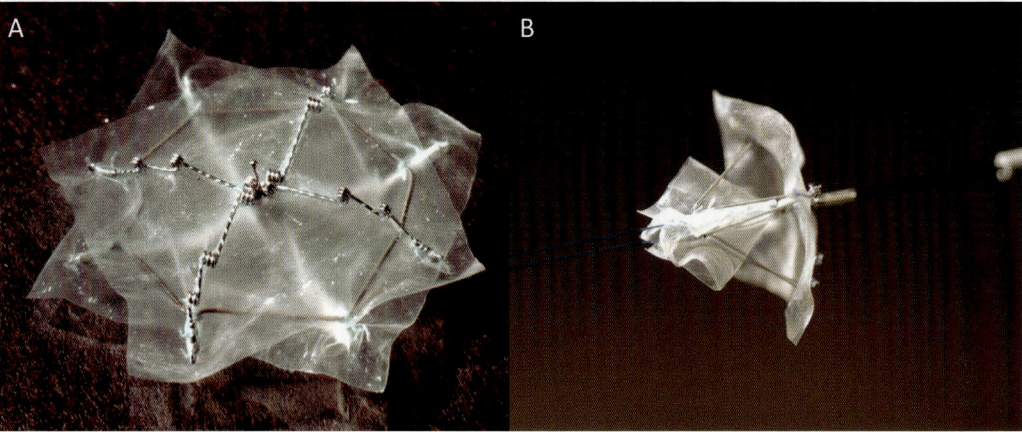

Fig 31.1—The BioSTAR septal closure device. A, The double umbrella design resembles an 8-point star when view en face. Note the torsion springs along the length of the arms. B, The right atrial umbrella attached to the Rapid Transport Delivery Catheter. The left atrial umbrella is everted before loading into the delivery sheath. (Courtesy of NMT Medical, Inc.)

springs are incorporated along its length, which facilitate both flexibility and conformation to variable anatomy and give the device a degree of clamping force to facilitate closure. Each spring arm has a platinum marker at its distal tip to enhance fluoroscopic visibility. The device retains the self-centering Nitinol springs of the STARFlex device, which facilitates its use in larger PFO and ASDs. The BioSTAR is available in three sizes: 23, 28, and 33 mm, based upon diagonal length.

The collagen used in the BioSTAR is derived from the tunica submucosa of the porcine small intestine. Cells and noncellular debris (e.g., DNA, glycosaminoglycans, lipids) are removed during cleaning utilizing a number of proprietary processes, such that a layer of virtually pure Type I collagen is produced. Structural integrity is ensured by crosslinking a number of layers of collagen. Finally, the whole device is coated with a heparin benzalkonium chloride complex (HBAC), which in animal experiments reduced protein deposition early after implant.

Implant Technique

The BioSTAR device is implanted by a similar technique to that used for previous genera-tions of NMT devices. Following puncture of a femoral vein, the PFO is crossed from the right atrium and a guide wire placed in the left upper pulmonary vein. Sizing of the PFO can be by transesophageal echo, angiography, or balloon distension. An appropriate device size is between 1.5× and 2× the diameter of the defect, although other factors such as the thickness of the secundum septum, the length of the PFO tunnel, and whether the primum septum is aneurysmal also may be factors in choosing the correct device size.

The device is supplied with the collagen in a desiccated state and therefore requires reconstitution in heparinized saline, for approximately 5 minutes, prior to loading and deployment. It is important to handle the device carefully during loading to avoid disturbing the heparin coating on the device. The device is connected to the delivery system by means of a pin that projects from the center of the right atrial umbrella. This is secured to the delivery catheter by means of small jaws similar to a bioptome at the distal tip of the catheter. This arrangement allows the device to swivel freely while still attached, which results in a more comfortable alignment with the atrial septum after deployment. The device is supplied with a nylon suture through the distal arms of the left atrial umbrella. This allows eversion of the left atrial disc and loading into the delivery system. Once loaded, care must be taken to fully irrigate and deair the device and delivery system. The device is then transferred to an 11F transseptal sheath, which has been positioned with its distal tip within the left atrium. The device is advanced to the left atrium using fluoroscopic guidance.

Device deployment and positioning can be fluoroscopically guided alone or in conjunction with transesophageal or intracardiac echocardiographic imaging (Fig 31.2). We have found that the best angle for device deployment is with the image intensifier at LAO 50°. The initial step is to deploy the left atrial umbrella by slow retraction of the transseptal sheath while the device position is kept stationary. Once the sheath reaches the midpoint of the device the umbrella will open spontaneously. The device and sheath are then withdrawn until the left atrial umbrella engages with the atrial septum.

This can be seen fluoroscopically by gentle lifting of the arms and confirmed by echocardiography. The right atrial umbrella can then be deployed by again retracting the sheath while maintaining the device position within the atrial septum. Before releasing the device, its position should be checked by echo and/or angiography, which can be performed through the transseptal sheath. The device can then be released by opening the jaws using the controls on the delivery catheter. Care should be taken to ensure the jaws have become detached before the delivery system is withdrawn.

The BioSTAR device is ideal for many types of PFO, the majority of which can be closed using the smallest 23-mm device. In patients with particularly long tunnels, as is common with other umbrella type devices, the BioSTAR device may remain partially deployed within the tunnel resulting in poor apposition to the atrial

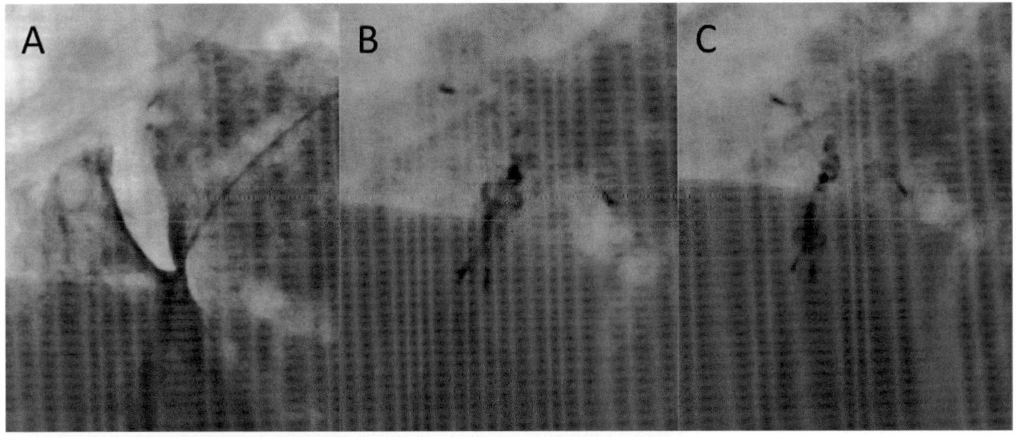

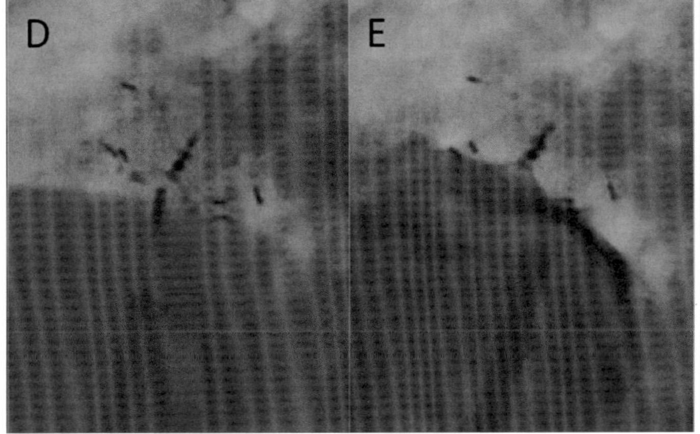

Fig 31.2—Implantation of BioSTAR septal closure device. A, Predeployment angiogram of LAO 50° projection to delineate the PFO anatomy. B, Deployment of the left atrial umbrella by retracting the transeptal sheath to the midpoint. C, After the left atrial umbrella is engaged onto the atrial septum, the sheath is further retracted to expose the right atrial umbrella. D, Successful deployment of both umbrellas on the atrial septum. Note the device is still attached to the delivery catheter. E, Post-deployment angiogram after release of the device.

septum and the potential for residual leaks. This may be overcome by modification of the tunnel[1] or by performing a transseptal puncture at the level of the tip of the secundum septum and placing the device through this.

BioSTAR has also been used to close ASDs up to 20 mm in diameter. The deployment procedure is the same as for PFO except that care should be taken to only withdraw the center of the device as far as the atrial septum prior to deploying the right atrial umbrella, so as to avoid inadvertent deployment of a left atrial arm within the right atrium. This is best achieved using echocardiographic guidance.

Retrieval
of the BioSTAR

In the case of malposition, if only the left atrial umbrella has been deployed it can be carefully withdrawn into the delivery sheath and redeployed. Once the right atrial umbrella has been deployed, the device can be withdrawn but cannot be reused. In this case, both umbrellas are inverted in the same direction and withdrawn into the sheath. It is important to ensure that all four torsion springs at the center of the device are adequately captured within the sheath before gently withdrawing the device up to the level of the next set of torsion springs. The device is then withdrawn via the backup 14F sheath on the 11F long transseptal sheath.

Preclinical Data

In preclinical studies conducted in sheep, the ICL matrix undergoes rapid endothelialization with a complete layer of endothelium by 30 days.[2,3] Subsequent ingress of host cells initiates a process of remodeling and absorption of ICL occurs by phagocytosis and enzymatic digestion. In the sheep model, complete resorption

of the porcine collagen and replacement with native tissue occurred over a period of up to 2 years. This contrasts with the healing response seen in synthetic devices, which is characterized by a chronic low-grade inflammatory response.[4]

Clinical Data

The safety and efficacy of the BioSTAR has been reported in one multicenter study,[5] a number of small single center studies,[6–8] and a long-term registry is currently being undertaken. In the BioSTAR Evaluation Study (BEST),[5] 58 unselected patients underwent PFO or ASD closure using the BioSTAR device. Procedure success was achieved in 98% of patients. High rates of closure were noted at 30 days (92%) and 6 months (96%), assessed by contrast transthoracic echocardiography. This reflects not only the excellent conformation of the device to native anatomy but also the impermeable nature of the ICL layer. High rates of acute closure have been reported, especially when the smaller 23-mm device is used, and it is important not to oversize as the device may not conform as well. The efficacy of BioSTAR has also been reported in patients with an ASD.[8] Complete closure was reported in all eight patients. The efficacy of BioSTAR in pediatric patients with an ASD is currently being investigated in the BASIC study.

Adverse events are rare following BioSTAR implantation. Atrial arrhythmia has been reported in up to 10% of patients although these are usually transient and settle spontaneously. The presence of an atrial septal aneurysm may be an important factor in the generation of these arrhythmias. Arm fractures have not been reported to date. Although long-term data is awaited, the overall efficacy and safety record of the device appears excellent. Importantly, the advantage of a bioabsorbable implant is highlighted by the finding that it facilitates transseptal puncture at a lower force and to a greater extent than other synthetic implants.

BioTREK

The BioTREK device is the latest technology being developed by NMT Medical. The rationale for the device is similar to that of BioSTAR, recognizing the need to leave as little permanent synthetic material in the heart as possible. The BioTREK is an entirely bioabsorbable device manufactured from a synthetic polymer poly-4-hydroxybutyrate (P4HB). The configuration of the BioTREK device is similar to other double umbrella PFO and ASD devices with two conformable discs connected by a fixed length

mal experiments using a variety of different device configurations and bioactive coatings are currently underway and the first human trials will follow.

Conclusion

With increasing indications for PFO closure in an ever-younger population, there is a growing requirement for devices to be safe and effective but have little impact on

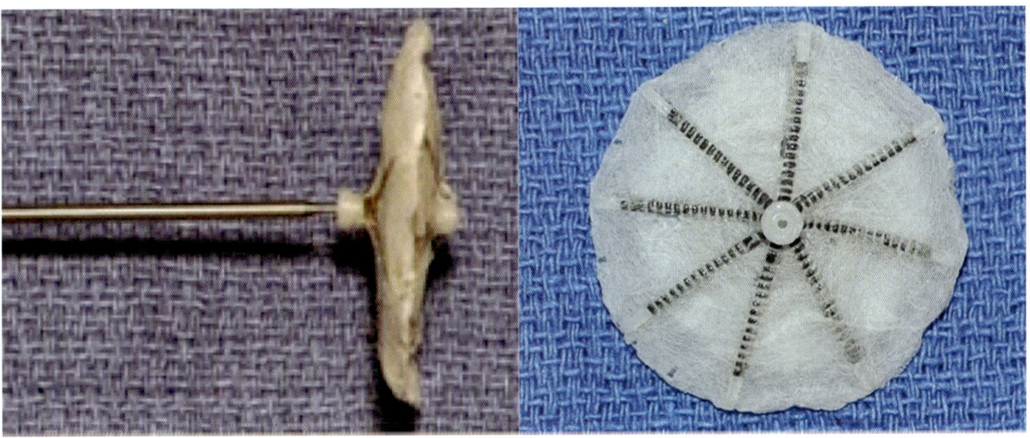

Fig 31.3—Two views of the BioTREK septal closure device. It is an entirely bioabsorbable device made from poly-4-hydroxy-butyrate (P4HB). (Courtesy of NMT Medical Inc.)

central pin (Fig 31.3). The device is designed to be both radiopaque and echogenic and easily retrievable and repositionable.

P4HB is an ideal polymer for structural heart devices, synthesized by a process of fermentation using recombinant DNA technology (Tepha, Lexington, Massachusetts). It is more flexible and associated with less inflammatory response than other commonly used bioabsorbable polymers. It degrades by a combination of bulk hydrolysis and surface erosion to a naturally occurring metabolite 4HB. This results in a gradual loss of polymer while maintaining the structural integrity of the device until this process is advanced at which point the device should be fully endothelialized (Fig 31.4). Ani-

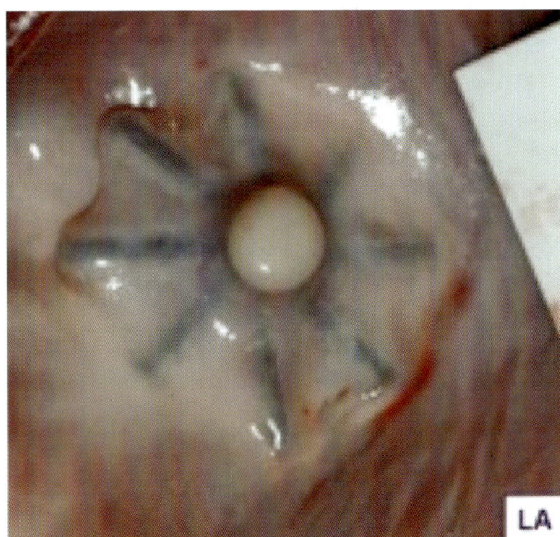

Fig 31.4—View from the left atrium of an animal model showing complete endothelialization of the BioTREK septal closure device. (Courtesy of NMT Medical Inc.)

the long-term health of the heart. BioSTAR and BioTREK represent the first bioabsorbable devices developed for the treatment of structural heart disease in humans. The safety and efficacy of BioSTAR has been shown and future research will determine whether such benefits can be extended to the completely absorbable BioTREK technology.

References

1. Spence MS, Khan AA, Mullen MJ. Balloon assessment of patent foramen ovale morphology and the modification of tunnels using a balloon detunnelisation technique. *Cathet Cardiovasc Interv.* 2008;71(2):222–228.

2. Jux C, Wohlsein P, Bruegmann M, et al. A new biological matrix for septal occlusion. *J Intervent Cardiol.* 2003;16(2):149–152.

3. Jux C, Bertram H, Wohlsein P, et al. Interventional atrial septal defect closure using a totally bioresorbable occluder matrix: development and preclinical evaluation of the BioSTAR device. *J Am Coll Cardiol.* 2006;48(1):161–169.

4. Sigler M, Jux C. Biocompatibility of septal defect closure devices. *Heart.* 2007;93(4):444–449.

5. Mullen MJ, Hildick-Smith D, De Giovanni JV, et al. BioSTAR Evaluation STudy (BEST): a prospective, multicenter, phase I clinical trial to evaluate the feasibility, efficacy, and safety of the BioSTAR bioabsorbable septal repair implant for the closure of atrial-level shunts. *Circulation.* 2006;114(18):1962–1967.

6. Ussia GP, Cammalleri V, Mule M, et al. Percutaneous closure of patent foramen ovale with a bioabsorbable occluder device: single-centre experience. *Cathet Cardiovasc Interv.* 2009;74(4):607–614.

7. Van den Branden BJ, Post MC, Jaarsma W, et al. New bioabsorbable septal repair implant for percutaneous closure of a patent foramen ovale: short-term results of a single-centre experience. *Cathet Cardiovasc Interv.* 2009;74(2):286–290.

8. Hoehn R, Hesse C, Ince H, et al. First experience with the BioSTAR-device for various applications in pediatric patients with congenital heart disease. *Cathet Cardiovasc Interv.* 2010;75(1):72–77.

32

Cardia Devices

Daniel R. Turner and Thomas J. Forbes

Introduction

Cardia, Inc. (Eagan, Minnesota) was formed in 1997 as a device manufacturer committed to developing and improving transcatheter septal occluder technology. Since then, Cardia has developed several generations of septal occluders designed for closure of patent foramen ovale (PFO) and secundum atrial septal defect (ASD). Device improvement has specifically addressed the complex and varied interatrial septal anatomy and the need for a closure device that adapts to these anatomic variations. To date, over 12,000 successful septal closures have been performed throughout the world using Cardia devices, primarily outside of the United States.

Device Description

Generation I

The PFO-Star was the first septal occluder developed by Cardia (Fig 32.1). The device had a double-umbrella, four-arm frame made from two crossing wire struts of solid Nitinol with titanium end caps. The right and left atrial umbrellas or sails were made from 2-mm-thick square pieces of Ivalon/polyvinyl alcohol (PVA) foam. The end caps provided an area for suturing the PVA to the frame and "softened" the tips of the strut wires. A 2-mm center post separated the sails. Animal and human data were collected. After encountering non-clinically significant fractures of the solid Nitinol struts (17%), residual shunts (9%), and device thrombus (2.5%), Generation II modifications were made.

Transcatheter Closure of ASDs and PFOs: A Comprehensive Assessment. © 2010 Ziyad M. Hijazi, Ted Feldman, Mustafa H. Abdullah Al-Qbandi, and Horst Sievert, editors. Cardiotext Publishing, ISBN: 978-0-9790164-9-3.

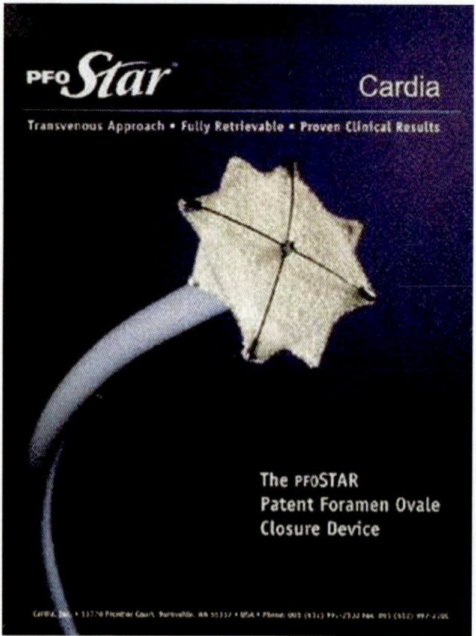

Fig 32.1—PFO-Star device. (Courtesy of Cardia, Inc.)

Generation II

The frame of the Generation II Cardia Star device was strengthened by using seven strands of Nitinol in each strut wire. This increased the fatigue life of the struts while the spring rate of the device was maintained. The center post separating the left and right atrial sails was available in both 3- and 5-mm lengths to accommodate a longer PFO tunnel and/or thicker septum secundum. Further strut wire and sail improvements resulted in the Generation III device.

Generation III

The strut wires of the Cardia PFO device were further enhanced by using 19 strands of Nitinol, improving the fatigue life and spring rate of the frame. An additional strut was added (six arms per side), making the device sails hexagonal instead of square (Fig 32.2). The PVA foam was reinforced, decreasing device bulk and increasing durability. The PVA sail material was placed on the outside of the left atrial arms of the device, decreasing the possibility of clot formation on the left-sided frame.

A tuft of PVA was added to the center post for enhanced closure of the PFO tunnel. Center post lengths of 3 and 5 mm remained available. The Generation IV device was made due to persistent residual shunt in patients after using the 5-mm center post devices.

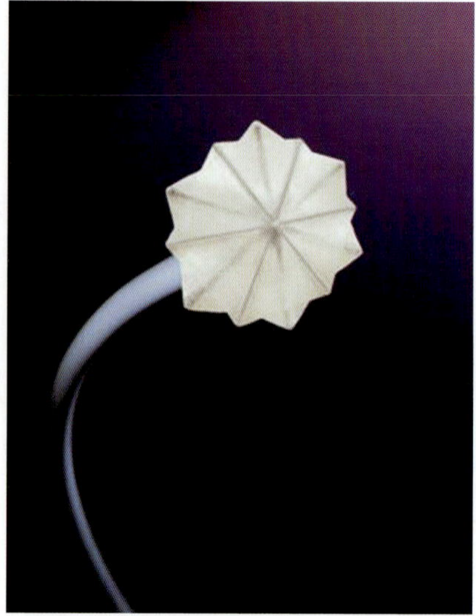

Fig 32.2—Cardia PFO device. (Courtesy of Cardia, Inc.)

Generation IV

The INTRASEPT was the first PFO device with articulating sails (Fig 32.3).

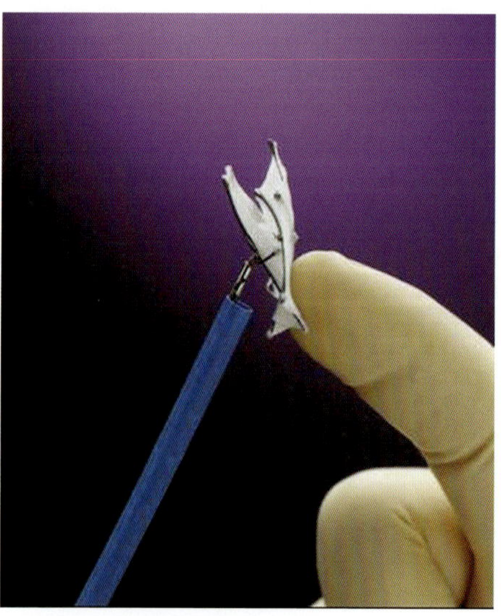

Fig 32.3—INTRASEPT device. (Courtesy of Cardia, Inc.)

A titanium, multijointed center post permitted each sail to move independently from the other in three dimensions, resulting in optimal device adaptation to septal anatomy and the least amount of stress on the device and surrounding structures. The device conformed to the septum immediately after delivery, allowing for increased confidence in device position before release. The INTRASEPT was available in 20-, 25-, 30-, and 35-mm sizes (the length of the strut wires), each with a 3-mm center post only. The INTRASEPT was a common device used for transcatheter closure of PFO outside the United States.[1]

Although the INTRASEPT device was used to close small secundum ASDs, lack of a centering mechanism made closure of medium or large defects difficult. For this reason, a varied diameter centering ring or "honeycomb" of PVA was added at the center of the device, creating the first actual Cardia ASD device called the Cardia Septal Occluder (Fig 32.4).

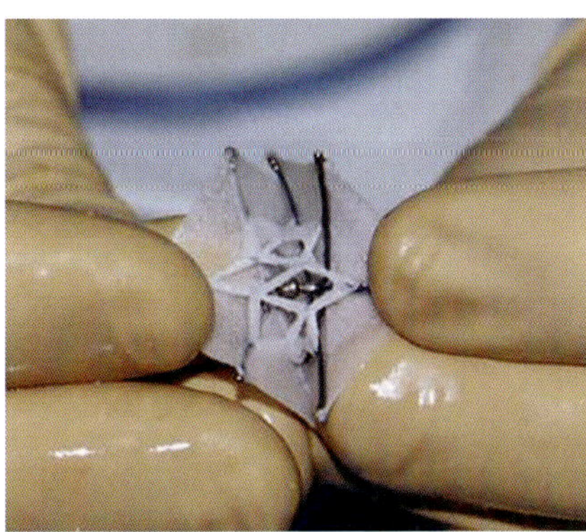

Fig 32.4—The Cardia ASD device, a modification of the INTRASEPT device with a PVA centering mechanism. (Courtesy of Colette Squire, RN, Dominican Republic.)

The centering ring allowed device stability within larger defects. Although initial results were positive, improvements in the centering mechanism were necessary.[2-4] Both the INTRASEPT and Cardia Septal Occluder evolved into the currently available ATRIASEPT.

Generation V

The ATRIASEPT generation of devices is available for closure of secundum ASD (ATRIASEPT I/II-ASD) and PFO (ATRIASEPT I/II-PFO). The ATRIASEPT I devices shared all of the INTRASEPT's characteristics, but had enhanced centering/sail articulation and easier device loading and retrieving features. The frame was 13-stranded Nitinol (Fig 32.5).

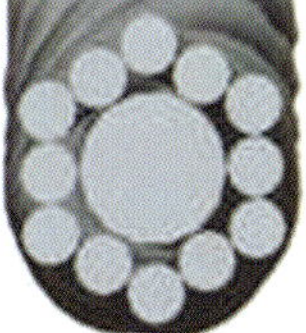

Fig 32.5—Cross-sectional view, ATRIASEPT Nitinol frame. (Courtesy of Cardia, Inc.)

The ability of each PVA sail to articulate independently of the other was preserved. For the first time, loading the right atrial side did not require manual insertion of the tips of the struts into the loader (Fig 32.6).

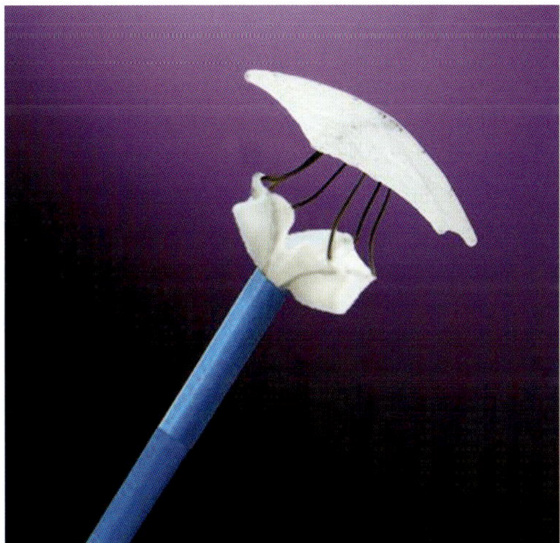

Fig 32.6—ATRIASEPT I-ASD showing loading/retrieval of right atrial sail within delivery sheath. (Courtesy of Cardia, Inc.)

The device can be delivered and retrieved multiple times in vivo without withdrawing and reloading the device, enhancing device safety.

In the ATRIASEPT I-ASD, a centering ring was made by the unique attachment of the left-sided struts to the tips of the right atrial arms (Fig 32.7).

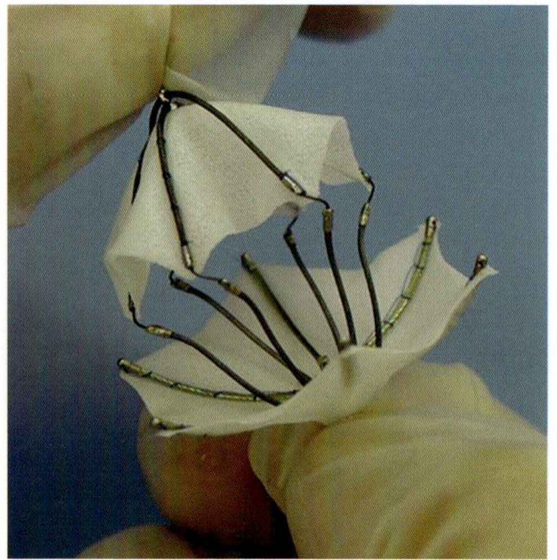

Fig 32.7—ATRIASEPT I-ASD centering mechanism. (Courtesy of Cardia, Inc.)

ATRIASEPT I-ASD device sizes were available in diameters from 6 to 32 mm (in 2-mm increments). The labeled size of the device represented the centering ring diameter and was chosen to closely match the balloon-stretched diameter of the ASD. The total diameter (arm length) of the device was 14 mm greater than the centering ring/labeled diameter. For example, if a 20-mm ATRIASEPT-ASD was used for a 20-mm stretched diameter ASD, the total device diameter was 34 mm. Devices were delivered through 10F (8–12 mm), 11F (14–18 mm), 12F (20–24 mm), and 13F (26–32 mm) long delivery sheaths such as Mullins or Hausdorf (Cook Inc., Bloomington, Indiana). The larger delivery sheaths were used without difficulty in children < 15 kg.[5]

The ATRIASEPT I-PFO was similar to the ASD version, but the left- and right-sided arms were attached so that no centering ring was formed. While there was no center post, each sail articulated independently and conformation to the septal anatomy was superb. ATRIASEPT I-PFO devices were available in 20-, 25-, 30-, and 35-mm sizes (total arm length).

Devices were delivered through 10F (20–25 mm), 11F (30–mm), and 12F (35–mm) long delivery sheaths.

Although initial ATRIASEPT I-ASD results were encouraging[5–7] one center reported two cases of asymptomatic perforation of the aortic sinus by a left atrial arm.[8] Realizing that device design could be enhanced, the ATRIASEPT II was made.

The ATRIASEPT II-ASD and -PFO devices were released in late 2008 and have all the characteristics listed previously with the addition of an enhanced left atrial sail. The wire orientation is improved, making the sail round and eliminating wire tips and end caps (Fig 32.8).

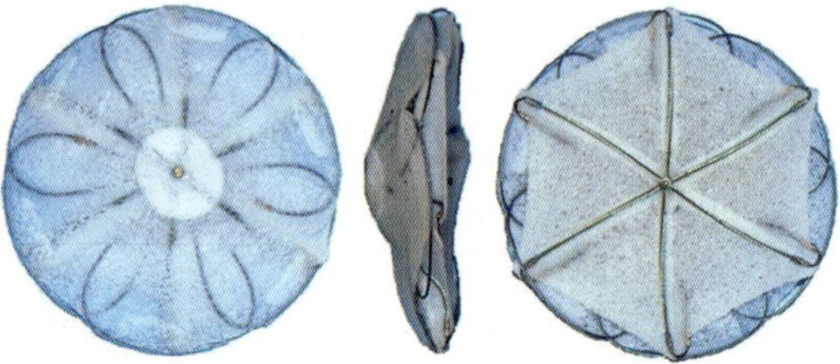

Fig 32.8—ATRIASEPT II-ASD with a round left atrial sail (left) and hexagonal right atrial sail (right). (Courtesy of Cardia, Inc.)

Sail articulation is superb in both the ASD and PFO versions (Fig 32.9).

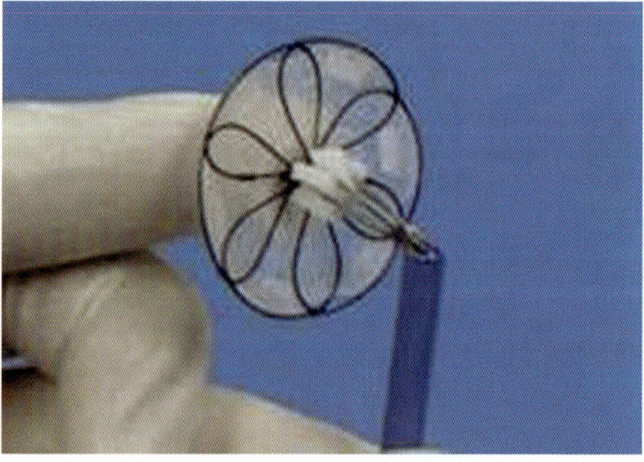

Fig 32.9—ATRIASEPT II-PFO showing the round left sail with 90° articulation from the right sail that remains in the delivery sheath. (Courtesy of Cardia, Inc.)

The round shape of the left sail distributes the left-sided forces evenly around the circumference of the sail. This force distribution reduces the potential for perforation. The right side of the device remains hexagonal with titanium end caps.

Sheath and device sizes are identical to the ATRIASEPT I version. The ATRIASEPT II-ASD and ATRIASEPT II-PFO are currently the only Cardia devices available for use outside of the United States. Use of Cardia devices for transcatheter PFO closure approximates 25% to 30% of the global marketplace. The first early study of the ATRIASEPT II-ASD device is in progress.

Generation VI

The ULTRASEPT is the latest Cardia septal occluder, incorporating all of the previous features with additional safety and performance improvements. The right atrial struts and end caps have been replaced with a rounded wire sail similar to the left sail (Fig 32.10). There are no pointed ends whatsoever, enhancing the safety profile of the device. Device fatigue resistance and sail tension is optimal. The device will be available soon for human trial.

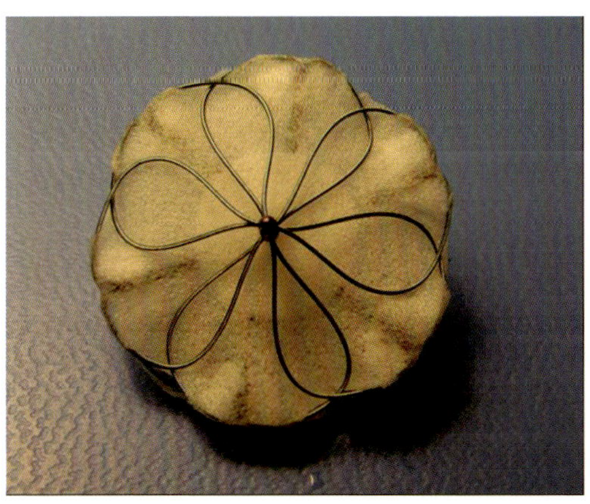

Fig 32.10—ULTRASEPT device, round right atrial sail. (Courtesy of Cardia, Inc.)

Device Loading and Retrieval

All Cardia devices are loaded and delivered using a specially made bioptome to grasp the rounded right atrial center post (Figs 32.11 and 32.12). The bioptome jaws have a hole at the tip in order to close firmly around the center post. The bioptome has a locking mechanism on the handle to prevent premature release of the device.

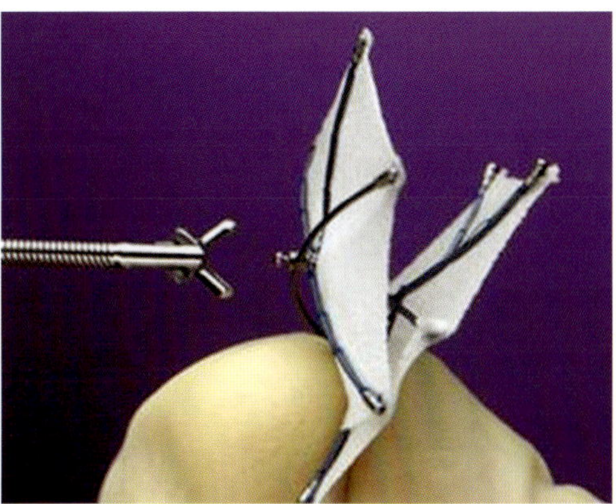

Fig 32.12—Bioptome and device prior to loading. (Courtesy of Cardia, Inc.)

After advancing the bioptome through any standard 12 to 13F short sheath (loading sheath) and the fluted loading assist tube (tube) packaged with the device, the bioptome is opened and the ball of the right atrial center pin is grasped. The bioptome locking mechanism is activated. The remaining loading sequence is completed under water to limit air entry into the tube or loading sheath.

For the INTRASEPT, the right-sided arms of the device were manually inverted and pulled into the tube and loading sheath. For the ATRIASEPT I/II and ULTRASEPT, manual insertion of the right-sided arms into the

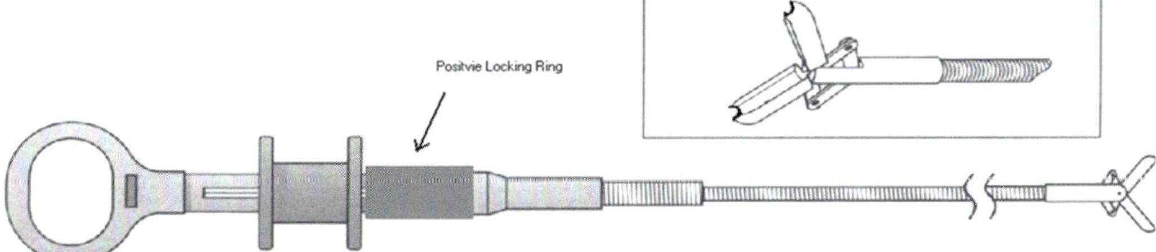

Fig 32.11—Modified bioptome for device loading and delivery. (Courtesy of Cardia, Inc.)

tube is not required. After grasping the device with the bioptome, the device is pulled into the tube and loading sheath in one smooth movement. Once within the loading sheath, copious flushing with heparinized saline is performed to remove any air trapped within the device or sheath.

After device delivery and prior to release, all Cardia devices may be pulled back into the delivery sheath and removed from the body. This maneuver is similar to loading the device. With the INTRASEPT, the right atrial arms become inverted, requiring the device to be removed from the body and properly reloaded (with manual inversion of the right atrial arms) before redelivery. With the ATRIASEPT I/II and ULTRASEPT, the device may be pulled back into the delivery sheath and then redelivered without removal from the body. Multiple redeliveries are possible.

Retrieval after complete release of the device is simple. The rounded, right-sided center post may be grasped by a gooseneck snare or even the delivery bioptome for withdrawal into the delivery sheath. In fact, any of the wire portions of the device may be snared or similarly grasped with a retrieval device and pulled into the delivery sheath due to the flexibility of the Nitinol.

Animal Data

Animal implant testing was done using Generation I devices implanted in an ovine PFO model. Macroscopic postmortem testing showed satisfactory device endothelialization with a thin, but complete covering of the PVA foam sails at 29 days postimplant. After 53 days the entire implant was completely covered with fibromuscular tissue (Fig 32.13), and at 131 days the fibromuscular ingrowth was complete with growth of tissue into the PVA foam (Figs 32.14 and 32.15).

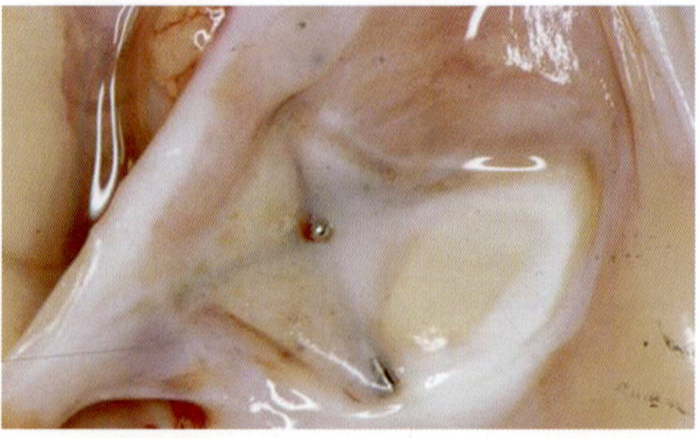

Fig 32.13—Device endothelialization, PFO-Star, 53 days. (Courtesy of Cardia, Inc.)

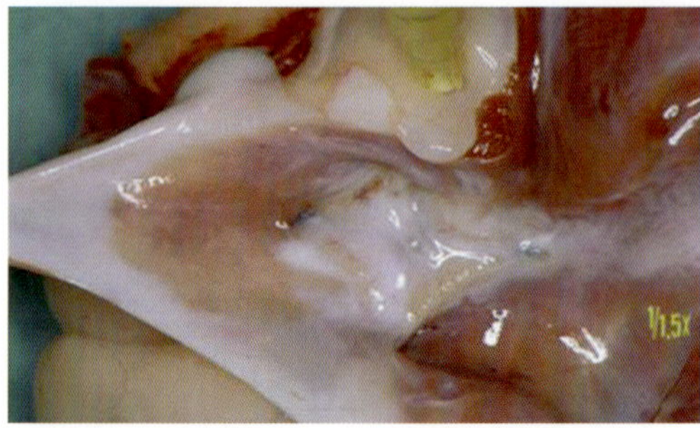

Fig 32.14—Device endothelialization, PFO-Star, 131 days. (Courtesy of Cardia, Inc.)

A histological analysis showed no inflammation or foreign body reaction to the device.[1]

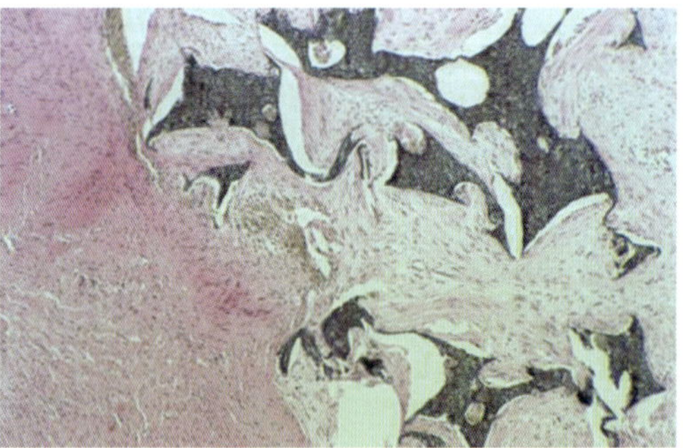

Fig 32.15—Photomicrograph, device endothelialization, showing tissue growth into the PVA foam sail. Darker blue areas represent PVA. (Courtesy of Cardia, Inc.)

Device Selection

Device size selection for closure of PFO using the ATRIASEPT I/II-PFO is largely based upon the preference of the operator and less so on experimental data. Some feel that a smaller device is optimal using the "less is more" philosophy. Others like the security of a larger diameter device for greater overlap of septal tissue, especially in longer tunnel defects or those with atrial septal aneurysm.

For secundum ASD, device choice is more straightforward. After static balloon sizing using the stop-flow method, a device with similar centering ring diameter (± 1–2 mm) is chosen. In the first ATRIASEPT study, the median centering ring–defect stretched diameter ratio was 1.08 (range 0.86–2). The median device arm length–defect stretched diameter ratio was 1.88 (range 1.62–3.75).[5] Overall, slightly smaller devices may be satisfactory as more experience with the ATRIASEPT is gathered. A slightly larger device may be chosen if rim deficiency is present or a slightly smaller device may be necessary for closure of a larger defect in a smaller patient.

Procedural/ Technical Considerations

Patent foramen ovale

Patients meet the criteria for transcatheter closure of PFO according to the operator. This could include patients with single or recurrent cerebrovascular accident or transient ischemic attack, severe migraine headaches, ortho-deoxia-platypnea syndrome, sleep apnea, or commercial scuba divers. Most procedures are done with moderate sedation or occasionally with general anesthesia. Primarily intracardiac or occasionally transesophageal echocardiography (TEE) is used for additional imaging. Heparin is administered to achieve an activated clotting time of ≥ 300 seconds. A right heart hemodynamic catheterization is recom-

mended, especially if there is the possibility of pulmonary hypertension. The PFO is crossed antegrade using an end-hole catheter placed in the left upper pulmonary vein. Balloon sizing is done at the discretion of the operator. A Mullins sheath is advanced over a wire to the right atrium. Removing the dilator and flushing the long sheath in the right atrium is recommended before advancing it to the left atrium to reduce the risk of air embolus. A smaller PFO tunnel may not allow this. The device is loaded into the loading sheath as described previously. While continually flushing the loading sheath, the sheath is pushed through the Mullins sheath hemostasis valve until it stops. The device is then advanced to the tip of the delivery sheath. The left atrial sail is delivered by withdrawal of the delivery sheath. The sheath and device are pulled back together until the left atrial sail contacts the atrial septum. The device lays flat on the septum due to the articulating properties of each sail. A small amount of flexing of the left-sided arms is seen. While maintaining slight tension on the bioptome to keep the left sail on the septum, further withdrawal of the delivery sheath delivers the right atrial sail. Assessment with echocardiography or angiography is performed prior to release. To release the device, the bioptome is first actively squeezed to keep the jaws closed. The locking mechanism is unscrewed. Under fluoroscopy, the bioptome is released to open the jaws and the device is released. An anticoagulation and/or antiplatelet regimen is recommended for at least 6 months after the procedure.

Secundum atrial septal defect

The criteria for recommending transcatheter closure of secundum ASD usually includes a large-enough left-to-right shunt to cause right atrial and right ventricular enlargement. Adequate tissue rims surrounding the defect are preferred, although successful closure with deficient anterior-superior rim is usually possible. In children or patients with complex anatomy or larger defects, procedures are usually done with general anesthesia and TEE. Moderate sedation and intracardiac echocardiography are used in most adults and simpler cases. Heparin is administered as described earlier. A right heart hemodynamic catheterization is recommended. Defect balloon sizing is recommended using the stop-flow technique. The delivery sheath is positioned as with PFO closure. The left atrial sail is delivered by withdrawal of the delivery sheath in the left atrium. The sheath and device are pulled back together until the left atrial sail approaches the atrial septum. In small to moderate size defects, the device lays flat on the surrounding septum due to the articulating properties of the sail. A small amount of flexing of the left-sided arms may be seen. Further withdrawal of the delivery sheath delivers the right atrial sail. Assessment with echocardiography or angiography is performed prior to release (Fig 32.16). Release is as described previously. Antiplatelet therapy is recommended for 6 months.

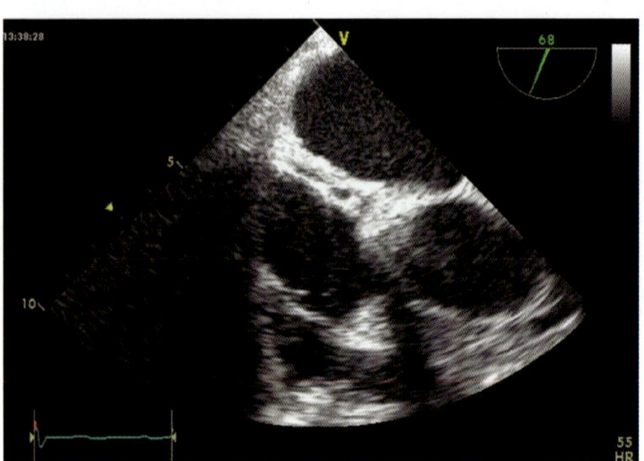

Fig 32.16—TEE of ATRIASEPT I device after release. (Courtesy of Cardia, Inc.)

For deficient anterior-superior rim, the left sail may be opened some distance from the atrial septum when initiating delivery of the right sail. This technique, along with the articulation of the sails, allows the centering mechanism to help orient the device parallel to the septum during delivery. Recapturing and redelivery of the device is simple and safe and may be done multiple times.

Clinical Results

Patent foramen ovale

Transcatheter closure of PFO seems to be a safe and effective treatment for the prevention of recurrent cerebrovascular accident. Literature review including all available devices from 1992 to 2003 showed a stroke recurrence rate of 1.9% to 4.2% and a residual shunt rate of 6.3% at 12 months.[9] Clinical data using the INTRASEPT device was reported in 189 patients, 50% with atrial septal aneurysm. Device placement was achieved in all patients. Transient ST segment elevation occurred in two patients and misplacement of the device occurred in one patient due to incorrect initial loading of the device. During follow-up of 0.5 to 3.3 years, a recurrent stroke rate of 1.4% per year was found. Residual shunt rate was 10.7% at 6 months. There were no device thrombi, wire fractures, or perforations.[1] Additionally, prospective data reported from the United States Cardia stroke trial in 90 patients showed a recurrent stroke rate of 1.1%.[10] Unfortunately, the trial was ended prematurely due to recruitment difficulties.

Cardia PFO devices have also been used successfully for the management of obstructive sleep apnea,[11] scuba divers with decompression illness,[12] and may play a role in the future management of migraine headaches.[13,14]

Secundum atrial septal defect

The use of a modified, self-centering INTRASEPT was successful for closing ASD.[2-4] Several additional studies investigated the use of both ATRIASEPT I- and II-ASD.

Turner et al[5] used the ATRIASEPT I-ASD in 58 patients with a median age of 25.7 years and a median defect size of 16.6 mm (range 8–26 mm). Immediate results showed that all patients had successful device delivery. A small residual shunt was present in 6/58 (10%), mitral regurgitation in 1/58 (2%) in a 13-kg child, 1/58 (2%) required device retrieval with placement of a larger device, and 1/58 (2%) developed a small pericardial effusion that did not require drainage. At median follow-up of up to 12 months, all had stable device position and sinus rhythm. Residual shunt resolved in 5, leaving only 1/58 (2%) with small, insignificant residual shunt. The pericardial effusion and mitral regurgitation resolved spontaneously at 1 and 3 months, respectively.

More recently, Steiger et al[8] reported the early European multicenter experience using the ATRIASEPT I-ASD in 76 patients with a mean age of 37 years (range 1–75 years). The mean defect size was 15 mm (range 5–30 mm) and there was deficient anterior-superior (aortic) rim in 7 patients. There was one each (1.5%) device embolization with retrieval, transient and clinically insignificant pericardial effusion, and increased tricuspid regurgitation. At 6-month follow-up in 64 of these patients, complete closure was noted in 90%. No other complications were encountered. The authors' conclusion was that the ATRIASEPT I-ASD was safe and effective and that further large studies are required to confirm these favorable early results.

The rare complication of cardiac perforation has been reported after the use of almost every ASD device. Brown et al[7] reported two cases of perforation of the aortic sinus 1 year after use of the ATRIASEPT I-ASD device. A 20-mm device was used in a 14-year-old patient. Due to a second, separate ASD, she was taken back to the catheterization lab for reinvestigation. The preprocedure TEE and subsequent fluoroscopy and angiography showed protrusion of a left atrial strut through the atrial limbus and into the noncoronary aortic sinus. The perforating device arm clearly moved out of synchrony with the others during real-time imaging. A 9.5-year-old patient with a 16-mm ATRIASEPT I-ASD similarly had the abnormality discovered at 1 year during a routine follow-up transthoracic echocardiogram. Transesophageal imaging confirmed the perforation, which was identical to the previous case. The first patient had surgical removal and repair due to the second ASD and the other patient is being managed medically.

Each of these ATRIASEPT I-ASD devices was of the original, dual-sided hexagonal design.

In addition, each had a thin, circumferential wire through the tips of the left atrial struts to decrease device prolapse during delivery (a modification used for a short time before the development of ATRIASEPT II-ASD). The circumferential left-sided wire was broken in each of these patients, possibly freeing the left atrial arm to then cause penetration into the aorta. The rigidity and memory of the 19-stranded Nitinol were thought to be additional possible etiologic factors. As a result, the ATRIASEPT II was developed, with a new, round left sail and elimination of the wire tips and end caps. The round shape distributes the left-sided forces evenly around the circumference of the left atrial sail. This new shape and force distribution reduces the potential for perforation. In the ATRIASEPT II devices, the right side of the device remains hexagonal with titanium end caps. The ULTRASEPT further decreases potential perforation by making the right sail round as well.

Conclusions

In just over a decade, the Cardia family of devices has evolved and improved significantly in response to clinical data and the desire for continued quality improvement. Preliminary results using the ATRIASEPT I-PFO and ASD devices are encouraging and we await ATRIASEPT II data. As the ULTRASEPT becomes available, further PFO and ASD investigation will be required. Additional animal study and a multicenter United States FDA-approved trial are planned. The ULTRASEPT may become one of the common devices used to close PFO and secundum ASD in the future.

References

1. Schraeder R. The Cardia-INTRASEPT PFO closure device. In: Brecker S, ed. *Percutaneous Device Closure of the Atrial Septum*. London: Informa Healthcare; 2006;151–162.

2. Turner DR, Chessa M, Zurkurnai Y, et al. Initial experience with the Cardia Septal Occluder: A

new device for transcatheter closure of secundum atrial septal defect. *Cathet Cardiovasc Interv.* 2007;69:S90–S91.

3.   Goy JJ, Stauffer JC, Yusoff Z, et al. Percutaneous closure of atrial septal defect type ostium secundum using the new INTRASEPT Occluder: Initial experience. *Cathet Cardiovasc Interv.* 2006;67:265–267.

4.   Chessa M, Butera G, Carminati M. Preliminary experiences closing secundum atrial septal defect using the modified Cardia INTRASEPT PFO device. *J Invasive Cardiol.* 2007;19:142–144.

5.   Turner DR, Sabiniewicz R, Chessa M, et al. Initial experience with the ATRIASEPT: A new device for transcatheter closure of secundum atrial septal defect. *Cathet Cardiovasc Interv.* 2007;70:S8.

6.   Chessa M, Turner DR, Sabiniewicz R, et al. Initial experience with the ATRIASEPT: A new device for transcatheter closure of secundum atrial septal defect. *J Cardiovasc Med.* 2007;8:S38.

7.   Steiger V, Chessa M, Aubry P, Juliard J-M, Schraeder R, Berger A, Goy J-J. Closure of ostium secundum atrial septal defect with the ATRIASEPT occluder. Early European experience. *Cathet Cardiovasc Interv.* 2009 (in press, published online 17 Dec 09).

8.   Brown S, Gewillig M. Perforation of the aortic sinus after closure of atrial septal defects with the ATRIASEPT occluder. *Cathet Cardiovasc Interv.* 2009;74:289–301.

9.   Schraeder R. Indication and techniques of transcatheter closure of patent foramen ovale. *J Intervent Cardiol.* 2003;16:543–551.

10. Savage MP, Fischman DL, Jasti B, Mooney M, Greenbaum A, Turner DR. Transcatheter closure of patent foramen ovale to prevent recurrent stroke: Initial experience with the Cardia PFO closure device. *J Am Coll Cardiol.* 2002;39:352A.

11. Agnoletti G, Iserin L, Lafont A, Sidi D, Desnos M. Obstructive sleep apnea and patent foramen ovale: Successful treatment of symptoms by percutaneous foramen ovale closure. *J Intervent Cardiol.* 2005;18:393–395.

12. Chessa M, Clai F, Vigna C, et al. Patent foramen ovale in scuba divers. A report of two cases and a brief review of the literature. *Ital Heart J.* 2005;6:73–76.

13. Post MC, Thijs V, Herroelen L, Budts W. Closure of patent foramen ovale is associated with a decrease in prevalence of migraine. *Neurology.* 2004;62:1439–1440.

14. Schwerzmann M, Wiher S, Nedeltchev K, et al. Percutaneous closure of patent foramen ovale reduces the frequency of migraine attacks. *Neurology.* 2004;62:1399–1401.

33

The Solysafe Septal Occluder
for the Closure of ASDs and PFOs

Peter Ewert

Introduction

The Solysafe Septal Occluder (Swissimplant AG, Solothurn, Switzerland) is a relatively new device for transcatheter closure of atrial septal defects (ASDs) and patent foramen ovale (PFOs) (Fig 33.1). Its name pays tribute to the inventor of the basic principle of the occluder, Dr. Laszlo Solymar, assistant professor of pediatric cardiology in Gothenburg, Sweden. The occluder consists of a self-centering device with two foldable polyester patches attached to eight metal wires made of Phynox, a cobalt-based alloy that has been used in surgical implants for many years (Fig 33.2A). Two wire holders keep the wires fixed at the proximal (right atrial) and distal (left atrial) end of the device. As a consequence of this arrangement, the occluder has two stable configurations: The first position is

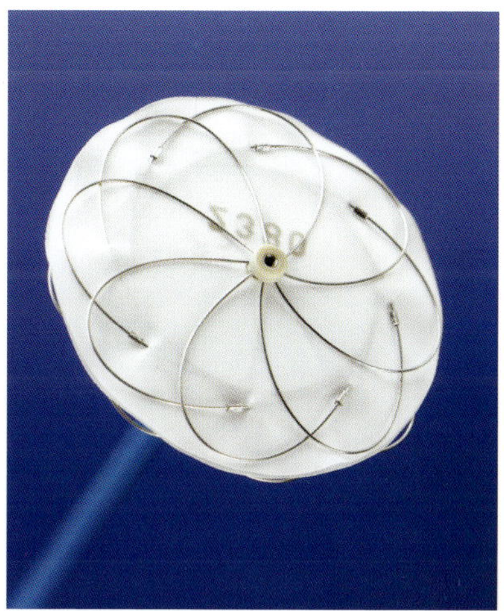

Fig 33.1—The Solysafe Septal Occluder configured. Two polyester patches are fixed on eight wires of Phynox that are fixed at the ends on two wire holders. (Courtesy of SwissImplant AG.)

Transcatheter Closure of ASDs and PFOs: A Comprehensive Assessment. © 2010 Ziyad M. Hijazi, Ted Feldman, Mustafa H. Abdullah Al-Qbandi, and Horst Sievert, editors. Cardiotext Publishing, ISBN: 978-0-9790164-9-3.

with the wires stretched in parallel position in its mid portion and stabilized by their course through the polyester patches. The device can be forced into a second stable position by approaching the wire holders to each other, so that the wires themselves rear up and twist, ending up in a very flat, flowerlike shape (Fig 33.2B–D). It is noteworthy that the course of the wires through the patches enables the device to self-center in defects of a considerable variety of diameters whereas the maximal diameter is given by the distance the wires are fixed to in the patches. For practical purposes, this distance is used to name the different occluder sizes, namely, in a 15-mm device the fixation points of the eight wires in the patches form a circle of 15 mm in diameter, and accordingly in the larger devices. However, as indicated, the device can be placed into considerably smaller defects without bulging. Just by more torque of the left and right atrial portions to each other, the course of the wires in the center of the device tightens. Despite the relatively stable second configuration, it is additionally secured by

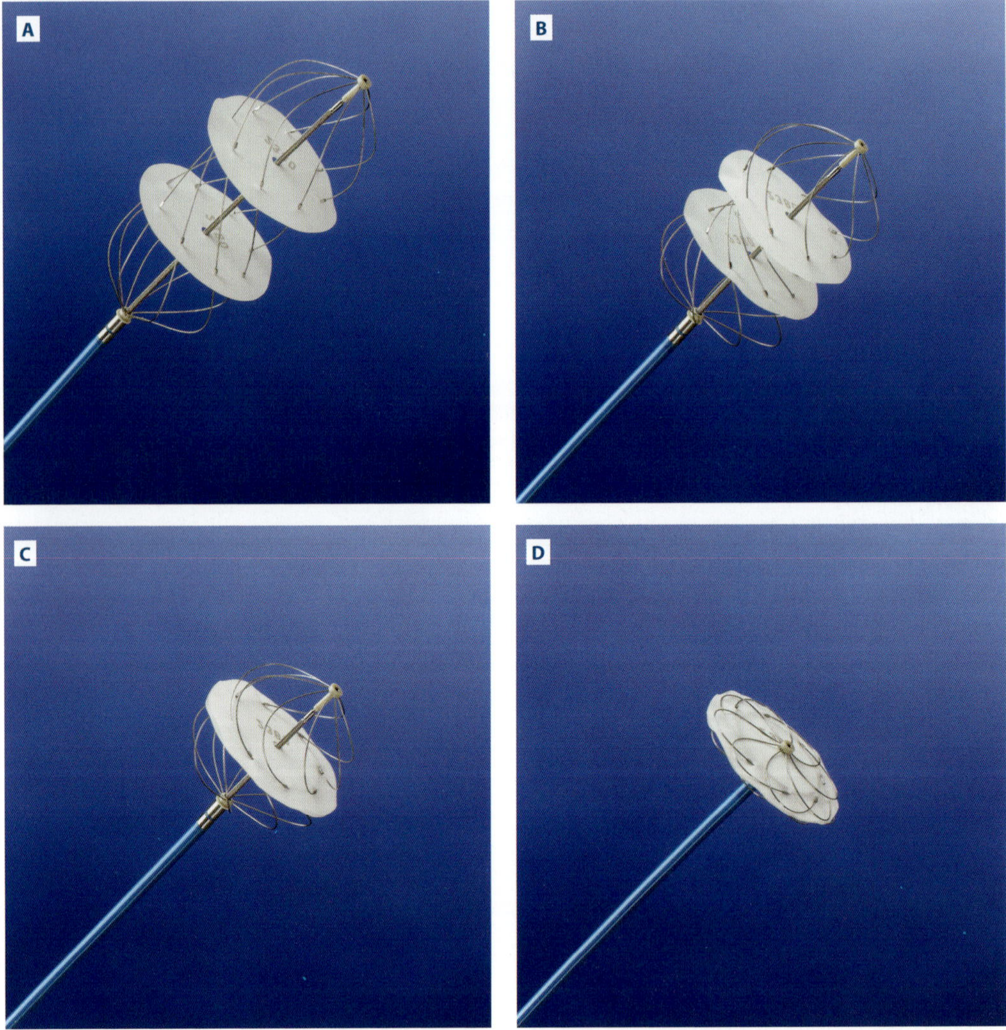

Fig 33.2A–D—The Solysafe Septal Occluder. The occluder is stretched by two coaxial position controls and can be easily configured to a flat double disc device by approximating both ends. (Courtesy of Swissimplant AG.)

a locking mechanism, which is fixed, when the two wire holders are pressed against each other, so that they are connected by a clicking mechanism. The device can be reopened by pulling the wire holders apart, which reverses the clicking mechanism.

The device is mounted on a delivery catheter to implant it into the atrial septum. It consists of two coaxial catheters, called position controls. The outer catheter, the proximal position control, is a 7F catheter with a screw thread at its distal tip, taking the corresponding thread on the proximal wire holder of the device. Inside the catheter, the thin distal position control can be advanced through the center line of the device to the distal wire holder. Here a counterclockwise thread ensures the fixation of the distal end of the occluder. Changes in configuration can be performed by pushing the distal position control (stretching the device) or pulling it (flatten the device). Devices with patch diameters of 15, 20, 25, 30, and 35 mm are available (Table 33.1). A specially designed PFO-Occluder is developed but still not commercially available.

Patient and Device Selection

The Solysafe Septal Occluder is designed for the closure of secundum ASD and is suitable for the closure of PFO. It has been successfully used in patients of all ages, however, due to a minimal sheath size of 10F it seems advisable not to use it in children < 10 kg body weight. Due to its self-centering capabilities, it is possible to close even large ASDs up to 30 mm. Also defects with absent rim behind the aortic root have been successfully closed with this device. In contrast to its very flat design, the device tends to align only partially to the septum in narrow PFOs, especially if combined with long tunnel formations. On the other hand, large PFO, especially with aneurysms, can be closed very elegantly, because the device flattens and, due to its variable self-centering capabilities, it adapts favorably to the width of the PFO and simultaneously stabilizes the septum.

Because of the unique self-centering capabilities, sizing is not as meticulously necessary

Solysafe Septal Occluder	Defect size (stretched)	Ø Patch (X)	Length distal end to distal Patch (Ldp)	Introduction Sheath (20–63 cm)	Solysafe Peel Away	Solysafe Position Controls
Type 15 (Ref 010.0001)	4–12 mm	25 mm	25 mm	10 F	10 F	7 F / 80 cm
Type 20 (Ref 010.0002)	13–17 mm	27 mm	25 mm	10 F	10 F	7 F / 80 cm
Type 25 (Ref 010.0003)	18–22 mm	32 mm	30 mm	10 F	10 F	7 F / 80 cm
Type 30 (Ref 010.0004)	23–26 mm	39 mm	40 mm	14 F	12 F	7 F / 80 cm
Type 35 (Ref 010.0005)	27–30 mm	44 mm	45 mm	14 F	12 F	7 F / 80 cm

Table 33.1—Device selection for Solysafe septal occluders.

as with other devices. In general, the nominal diameter of the device should exceed the defect diameter by at least 3 mm (Table 33.1). However, oversizing is relatively forgiving and does not result in excessive bulging. This is the reason why devices in 5-mm increments are sufficient to cover the full range of defects from just a few to 30 mm in diameter. Thus, a balloon sizing in clear-cut cases may be unnecessary.

Implantation

For implantation, the device is fixed with the wire holders onto the two coaxial control catheters. The inner catheter is screwed in a counterclockwise direction onto the distal wire holder;

the outer one in regular, clockwise direction onto the proximal wire holder. By pushing the inner catheter and pulling the outer catheter, the device can be straightened and introduced through a 10F or a 14F (for the 30 and 35 devices) short sheath into the femoral vein over a stiff 0.018" guide wire already placed in the left atrium or a left pulmonary vein. Over the wire, the device can be advanced without the assistance of a long sheath into the defect until the patches of the device are located on each side of the defect (Fig 33.3A). Then, the two wire holders at the end of the stretched device are moved toward each other by pulling the inner and pushing the outer control catheter until the wires snap into the second stable position, forming the flat flowerlike disc on each side of the septum (Fig 33.3B–D). Simultaneously, the wires stretch the patches over the defect while

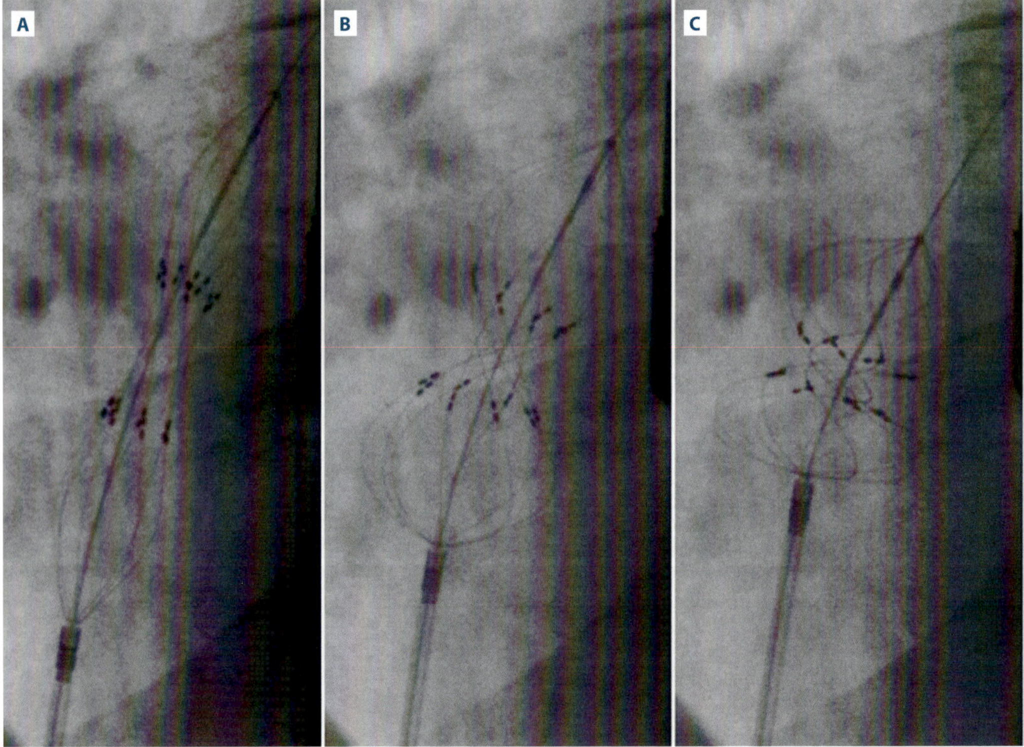

Fig 33.3—Configuration of the Solysafe Septal Occluder under fluoroscopy (45° LAO, 15° cranial tilt). A, Stretched device placed in the defect. B–D, Configuration by pulling the distal and pushing the proximal position control. E, Device after release of the position controls. The 0.018" guide wire crossing the device is still in place. If desired, the device can be explanted by reversing steps A–D. If not, the wire is pulled out to finish the implantation.

figure continues on following page

the wires between the patches form a stentlike section to center the device (Fig 33.3A). By further pulling the distal and pushing the outer control catheter, the clicking mechanism locks the wire holders to each other.

Next, the control catheters are unscrewed and pulled back while the guide wire remains in place (Fig 33.3E). The device aligns itself with the septum, and closure and stable positions are confirmed by echocardiography and/or fluoroscopy. At this point, if desired, all maneuvers can be reversed. The device is fully reattachable and can be unclicked, straightened, and removed. Otherwise, if placement is satisfactory, the thin guide wire is removed as the last step in definitive implantation. The fully deployed occluder shows a very flat configuration (Fig 33.4).

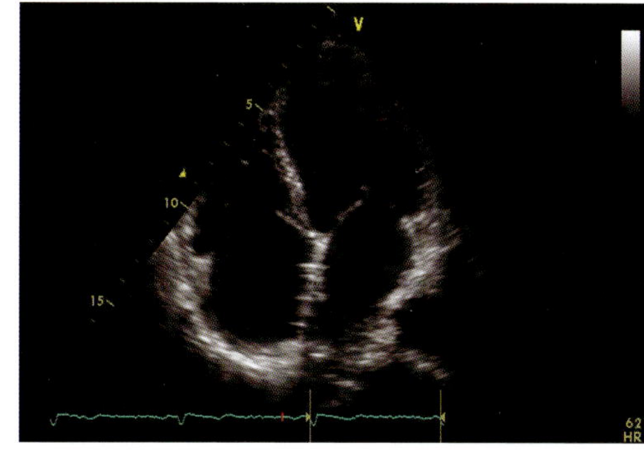

Fig 33.4—The Solysafe Septal Occluder fully implanted in a four-chamber view of transthoracic echocardiography. The occluder demonstrates its flat design and the excellent alignment to the atrial septum.

Fig 33.3 (cont.)

Results

Reports have been published on two studies with 44 and 32 patients,[1,2] respectively. Interestingly, closure rates were 100% after 6 months in both studies. However, defects with absent rim behind the aorta were treated with reserve.[3] This is mainly due to the lack of experience, which is only slowly increasing in the presence of other well-established devices. Nevertheless, treatment of defects with absent superior anterior rim (retroaortic) is possible, especially if an implantation technique is used with the guide wire placed in the left inferior pulmonary vein to stabilize the stretched device prior to configuration directly behind the aortic root. The total number of implanted occluders worldwide is about 1400.

Discussion

Several devices for the closure of interatrial communications (ASD and PFO) are currently available, and each has its possible advantages and disadvantages. The purpose of the Solysafe Septal Occluder was to create a device with explicit self-centering capabilities but with the possibility of adaptation to different defect sizes, so that a few occluder sizes would be sufficient to close a broad spectrum of defects. With the five occluder sizes of 15, 20, 25, 30, and 35 mm, defects with stretched diameters of up to 30 mm can be closed.

One of the most interesting differences of the Solysafe Septal Occluder in comparison to all other devices for interatrial defect closure on the market is the configuration mechanism: The conventional method is to configure first the left and then the right atrial component of the different devices. Especially in larger defects, this bears the problem that the occluder may slip through the defect before the device is properly configured.[4] In the Solysafe device left and right discs configure simultaneously, so that no pull on the system is necessary. On the other hand, it is even possible to configure the right disc first and develop the left disc by pushing the system against the atrial septum. The possibilities of this mechanism are certainly not completely discovered yet, and new techniques for implantation may develop in the future. The configuration of the device over the wire in the left lower pulmonary vein is only one example.

All currently available devices for ASD and PFO closure have to be advanced into the defect through a guiding catheter or a long sheath. Although different strategies to avoid air embolism are recommended, this remains a possible serious adverse event. The fact that the Solysafe Septal Occluder does not require a sheath in the left atrium, but is advanced through the inferior caval vein over the wire without the use of any sheath or guiding catheter makes air embolism to the left atrium very unlikely.

Conclusion

The Solysafe Septal Occluder in its present form is a safe, self-centering device for transcatheter closure of large PFOs and small to large ASDs in adults and children. With the five sizes of the device, defects with a stretched diameter of up to 30 mm can be effectively closed with very high occlusion rates.

References

1. Ewert P, Soderberg B, Dahnert I, et al. ASD and PFO closure with the Solysafe septal occluder—results of a prospective multicenter pilot study. *Cathet Cardiovasc Interv.* 2008;71:398–402.

2. Kretschmar O, Sglimbea A, Daehnert I, Riede FT, Weiss M, Knirsch W. Interventional closure of atrial septal defects with the Solysafe Septal Occluder—Preliminary results in children. *Int J Cardiol.* 2009;13:13.

3. Divekar A, Gaamangwe T, Shaikh N, Raabe M, Ducas J. Cardiac perforation after device closure of atrial septal defects with the AMPLATZER septal occluder. *J Am Coll Cardiol.* 2005;45:1213–1218.

4. Knirsch W, Dodge-Khatami A, Valsangiacomo-Buechel E, Weiss M, Berger F. Challenges encountered during closure of atrial septal defects. *Pediatr Cardiol.* 2005;26:147–153.

34

The pfm Device for ASD Closure

Miguel Granja and Franz Freudenthal

Introduction

Dr. Franz Freudenthal has developed a new generation of closure devices for pfm Medical AG. They are the PFO-R (Fig 34.1A), the PDA-R (Fig 34.1B), and the ASD-R devices (Fig 34.1C). They are all constructed in Nitinol wire mesh, woven with a single wire, without welding or hubs, and they acquire their final form by a reverse configuration of the distal side.

Animal experience with these devices has been done by implantation in 15 pigs, and it was possible to prove that complete endothelization had been achieved at the third week (Fig 34.2A and 2B), without significant inflammatory response (Fig 34.2C).

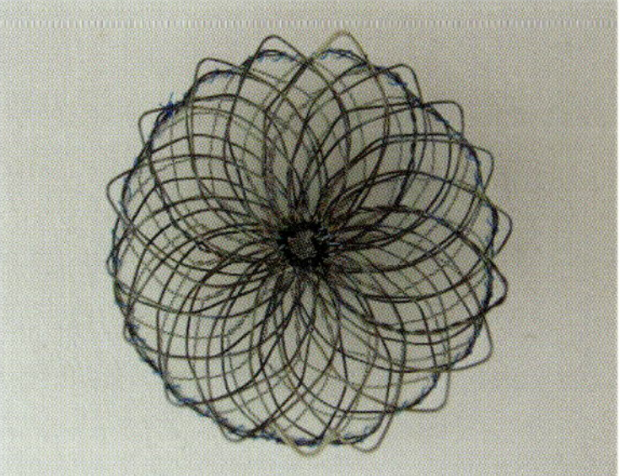

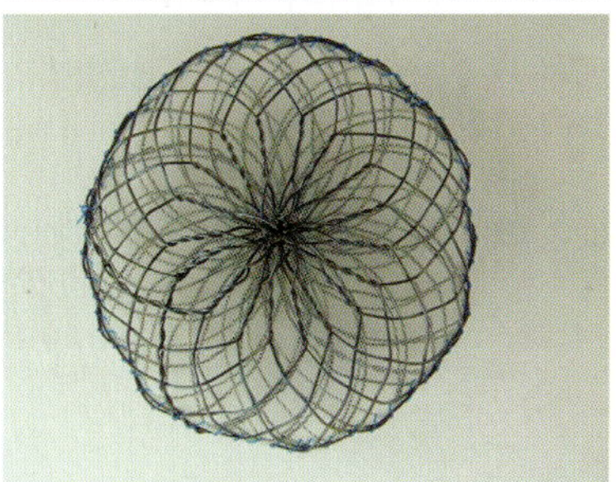

Fig. 34.1A—PFO-R device by pfm Medical, left atrial view (above) and right atrial view (below).

Transcatheter Closure of ASDs and PFOs: A Comprehensive Assessment. © 2010 Ziyad M. Hijazi, Ted Feldman, Mustafa H. Abdullah Al-Qbandi, and Horst Sievert, editors. Cardiotext Publishing, ISBN: 978-0-9790164-9-3.

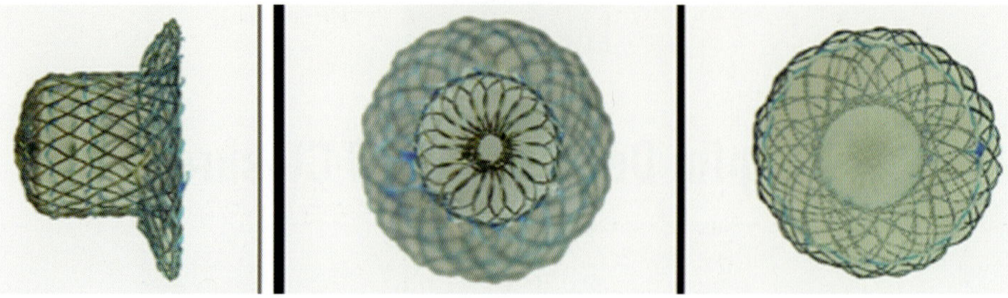

Fig. 34.1B—Three views of the PDA-R device by pfm Medical.

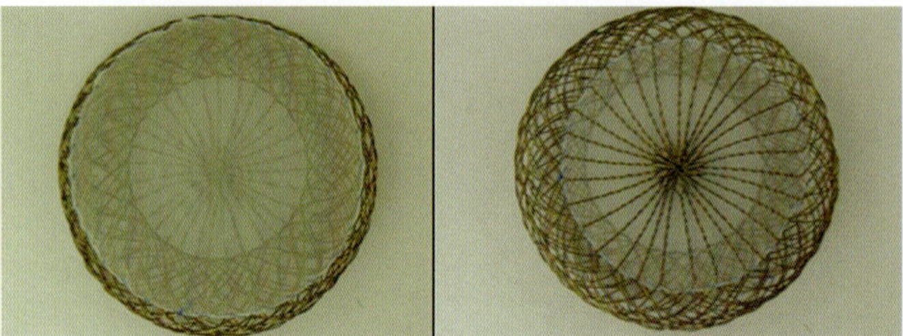

Fig. 34.1C—PFO-R device by pfm Medical, left atrial view (left) and right atrial view (right).

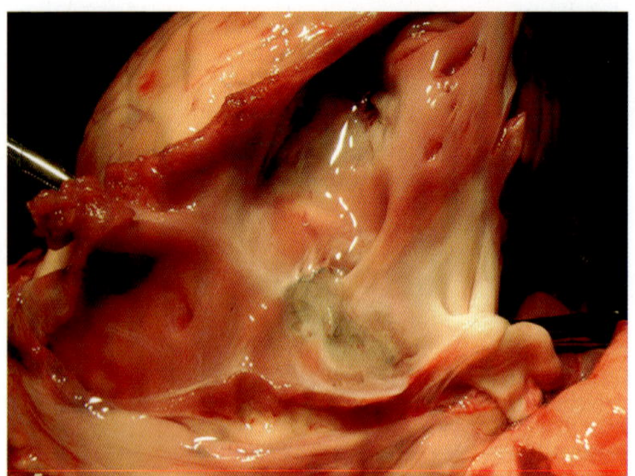

Fig. 34.2A—Macroscoptic view of device in an animal on day 74.

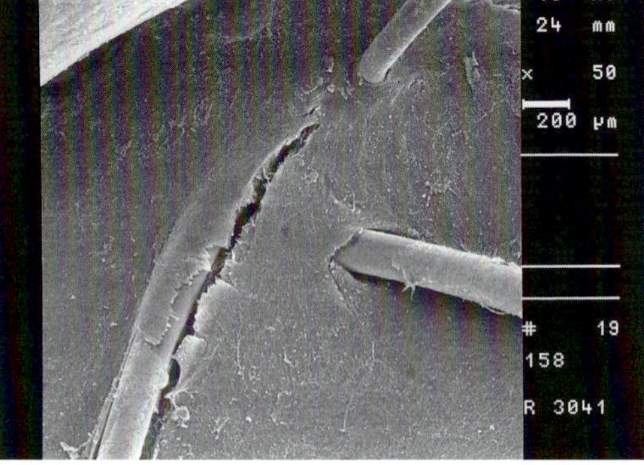

Fig. 34.2C—Microscoptic view of device in an animal on day 24.

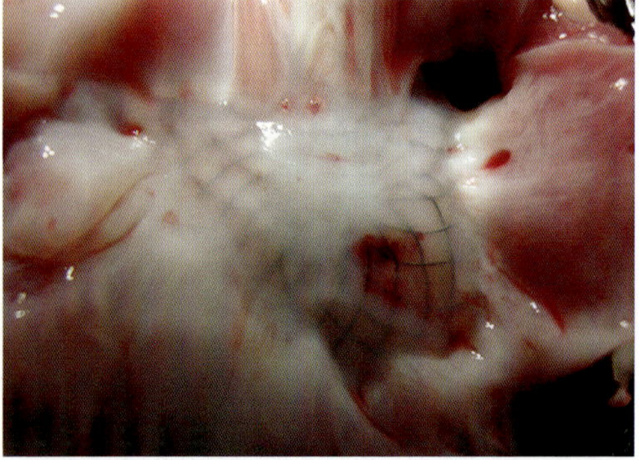

Fig. 34.2B—Another macroscoptic view of device in an animal on day 74.

Device Features

The pfm ASD-R is a double disc device constructed from Nitinol wire, tightly woven in a single piece without welding or hubs in either of its sides and this could be of potential benefit to reduce the chance of clot formation on the surface of discs. Its final double disc configuration with a self-centering waist is achieved by the reverse configuration of the distal (left atrial side) disc. The left atrial side is completely covered by

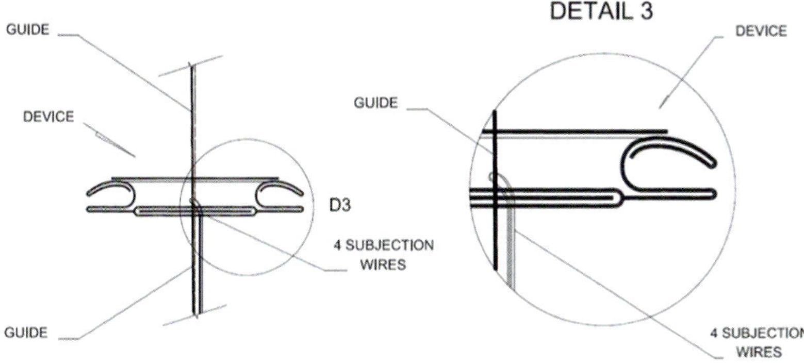

Fig. 34.3—Delivery system diagram for ASD-R..

polyester fabric sutured to the borders, minimizing contact between the metal and blood in this side in comparison with other devices. This could also be of benefit, reducing the chance of clot formation on the left atrial disc.

The delivery system is very flexible and consists of a wire with a very thin movable core that goes through the device and is attached to the right atrial side by a loop as it is described in detail in Fig 34.3. The delivery system proximal to the device is covered by a blue catheter that allows good drainage of air in the system and is also good for heparinization of the wire, an important component in avoiding clot formation (Fig 34.4).

The device is fully retrievable and repositionable prior to its release, and the implantation technique is very similar to that of other commonly used devices. Therefore, the learning curve is very short for operators familiar with ASD device closure techniques.

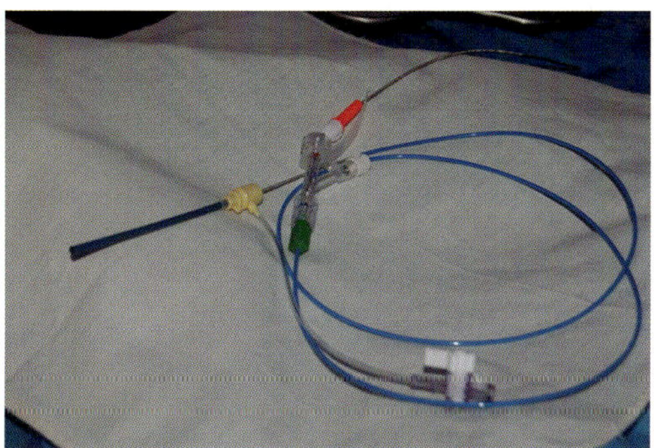

Fig. 34.4—Delivery system.

Preparation

Step-by-step preparation of the device to be implanted can be seen in Figs 34.5 and 34.6. The first step is loading the device into the loader (Fig 34.5A–L). The second step is carefully flushing the delivery system and loader, then loading the device into delivery sheath.

Implantation

The implantation procedure begins with the selection of the size of the device to be implanted. Under transesophageal/intracardiac echocardiographic guidance, catheterization is performed routinely and balloon sizing of the defect is done using the ¨stop flow¨ technique. A device is selected similar in size to the measured diameter of the balloon. Then, the device is loaded in the sheath and advanced until the left atrial (reverse) disc is configured. The left atrial (LA) disc borders are so soft that it can be delivered (if necessary) into a pulmonary vein and then retrieved to be configured in the reverse manner. Then, the left atrial disc is brought close to the septum where the sheath is retracted to deploy the waist and the right atrial disc.

To assess device position and stability, a gentle pull and push similar to the "Minnesota wiggle" is performed under fluoroscopy and echocardiography. Once good device position is confirmed, the device is detached.

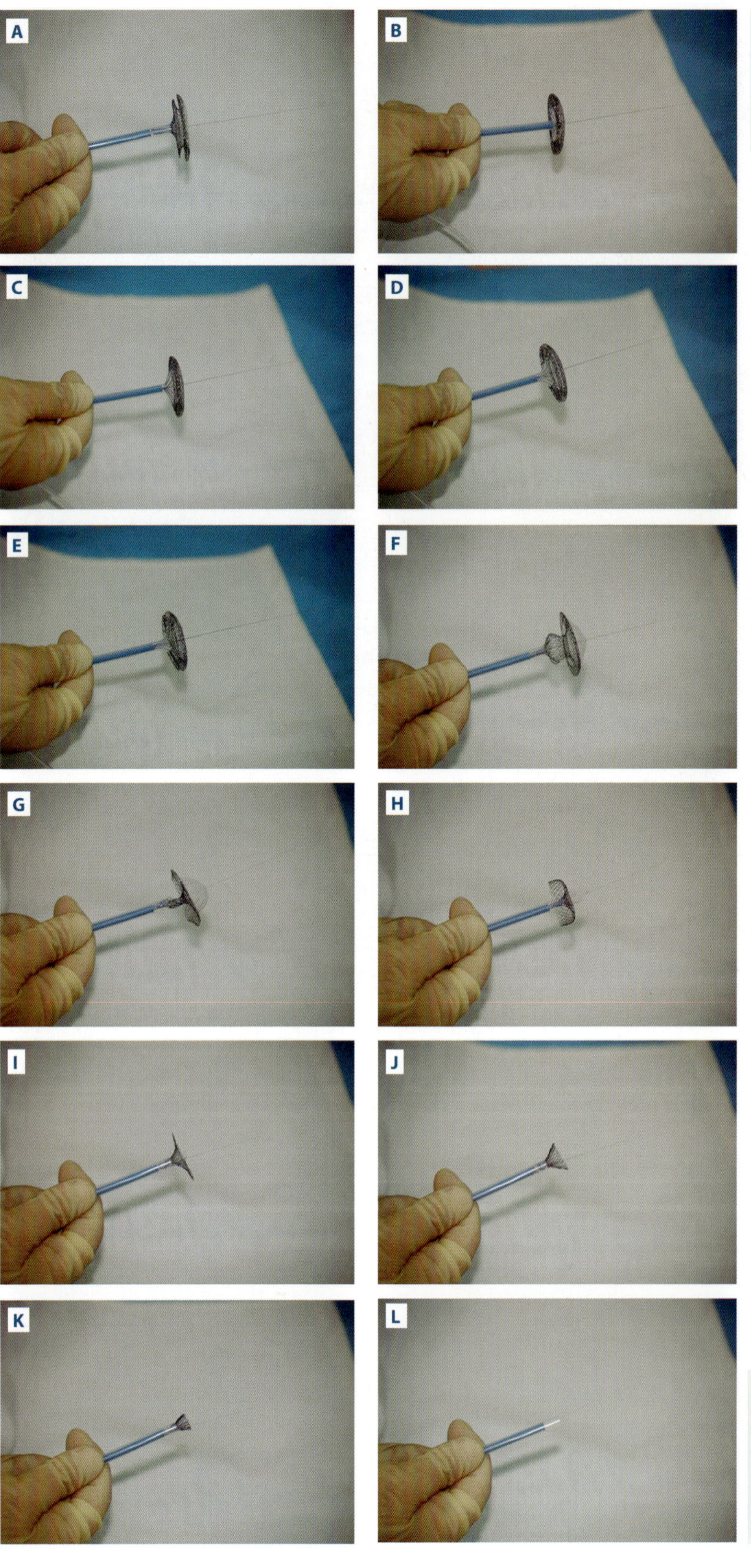

Fig. 34.5A–L— The first step is loading the device into the loader.

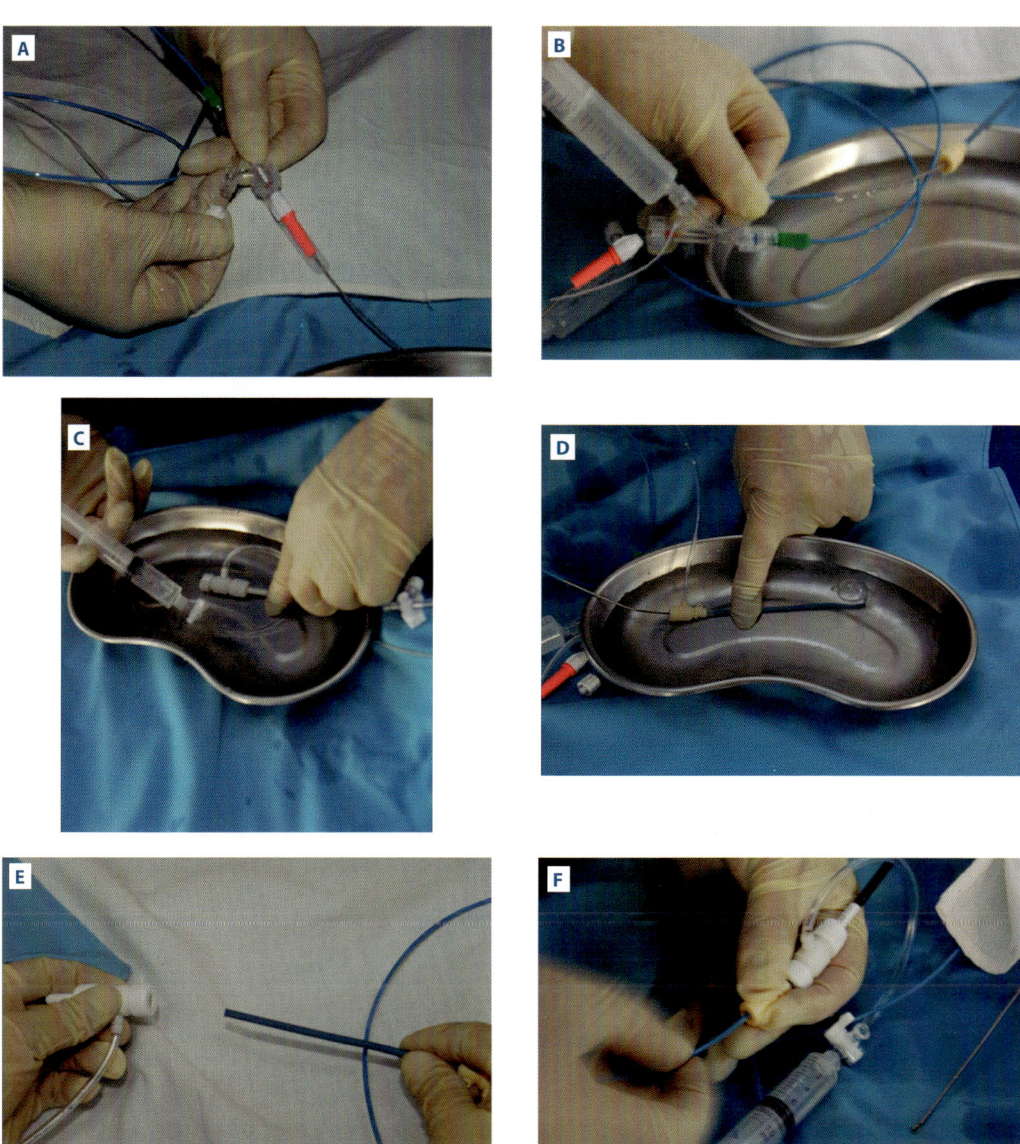

Fig. 34.6A–F—The second step is carefully flushing the delivery system and loader, then loading the device into delivery sheath.

Detachment Procedure

The detachment procedure begins by releasing the locking mechanism on the back of the delivery system (Fig 34.7), and then pulling the wire (Fig 34.8). On fluoroscopy it can be seen how the very thin distal part of the core wire is retrieved, until the device is very softly detached. The flexibility of the whole system can be seen in movie #8. The process can be seen in detail in the brief movies on the website for this book at www.cardiotext publishing.com/sites/transcatheter-closure.

After release, it is easy to recapture and

retrieve the device in vitro; however, it has not been done yet in human cases. The device could be retrieved using a lasso or a biopsy forceps technique.

The initial clinical experience has been started in Bolivia, where the Health Regulatory Authority has approved the device. Between 2007 and 2009 and under the direction of Dr. Alexandra Heath and Dr. Franz Freudenthal, 23 patients have been treated with excellent results and no significant complications (Table 34.1).

These initial results were very encouraging and have been the basis for the next step.

In 2010, the Regulatory Authority in Argentina (AMMAT), will approve an extensive clinical experience phase II protocol in which 100 patients will be involved in at least four centers.

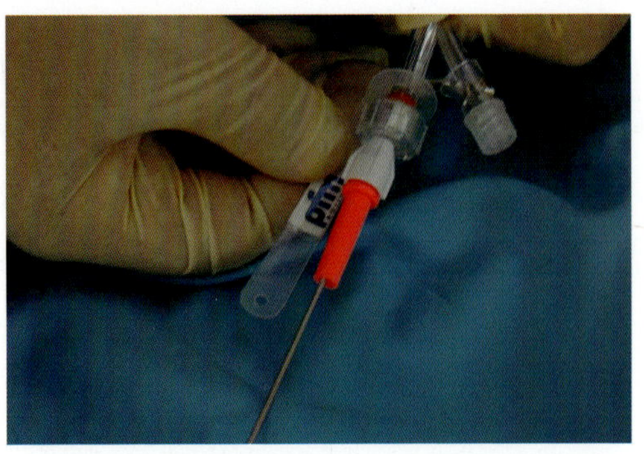

Fig. 34.7—Releasing the locking mechanism on the back of the delivery system during the detachment procedure.

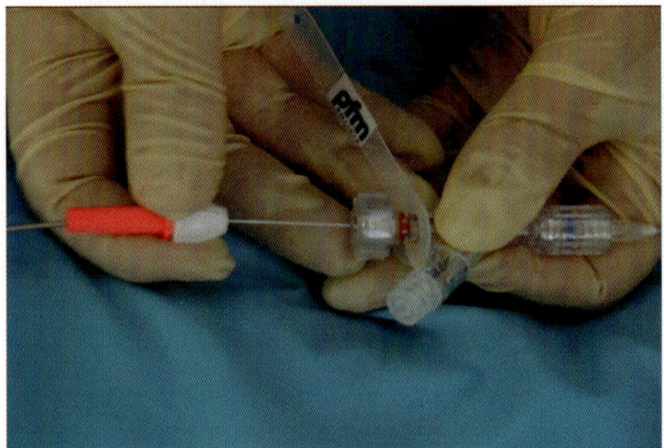

Fig. 34.8—Pulling the wire during the detachment procedure.

Nº	Patient	Birth date	Age (yrs)	Weight (kg)	ASD diameter*	QP/QS	Device size	Date of intervention	Device	Date of last control	Dx post control
1	A	2/19/1988	19	68	16	1.9	19	5/15/2007	ASD-R	6/11/2008	ASD closed. NO residual shunt, mild PAH
2	B	12/6/2004	12	44.5	16	2.4	14	9/28/2007	ASD-R	10/30/2008	ASD closed. No residual shunt normal PAP
3	C	3/10/1987	20	57.7	10	1.8	3	10/23/2007	PFO	11/17/2008	ASD closed. No residual shunt normal PAP
4	D	3/7/1983	21	51	13	1.7	19	11/8/2007	ASD-R	11/10/2007	ASD closed. No residual shunt normal PAP
5	E	6/18/2002	5	17	14	2.4	13	3/4/2008	ASD-R	3/5/2009	
6	F	6/10/1962	45	67	16	1.7	17	3/4/2008	ASD-R	6/13/2008	ASD closed. No residual shunt normal PAP

Table 34.1—Experimental trial results in Boliva during 2007–2009. *Stop flow balloon sizing.

table continues on following page

Nº	Patient	Birth date	Age (yrs)	Weight (kg)	ASD diameter*	QP/QS	Device size	Date of intervention	Device	Date of last control	Dx post control
7	G	5/11/1967	41	55	21	1.8	24	5/13/2008	ASD-R	6/6/2008	ASD closed. No residual shunt normal PAP
8	H	7/14/1998	9	39	21	2.2	20	6/3/2008	ASD-R	6/6/2008	ASD closed. No residual shunt .MILD PAH
9	I	8/7/1993	14	52.6	18	1.9	17	7/29/2008	ASD-R	11/7/2008	ASDclosed. No residual shunt normal PAP
10	J	6/26/1991	17	63	15		21	8/28/2008	ASD-R	3/5/2009	No control registered
11	K	5/26/1955	53	46	19	2.3	21	10/31/2008	ASD-R	3/20/2009	ASD closed. NO residualshunt, mild PAH
12	L	12/1/2002	5	22	7	1.5	26	11/9/2008	PFO		No control registered
13	M	1/16/1998	10	32	6	1.3	10	11/9/2008	ASD-R	5/19/2009	No control registered
14	N	6/16/1997	11	37	16	1.8	17	11/9/2008	ASD-R	12/12/2008	No control registered
15	O	6/16/1997	11	37	21	1.8	17	12/9/2008	ASD-R	12/12/2008	ASD closed. No residual shunt normal PAP
16	P	4/13/1971	37	51	17	1,9/1	20	1/15/2009	ASD-R	1/19/2009	ASD closed. No residual shunt normal PAP
17	Q	7/14/1991	17	58	15		17	1/20/2009	ASD-R	5/4/2009	ASD closed. No residual shunt normal PAP
18	R	10/13/1995	13	47	17	1,7/1	20	1/24/2009	ASD-R	1/29/2009	ASD closed. NO residualshunt, mild PAH
19	S	4/5/2002	6	43.4	14	1.6	16	2/5/2009	ASD-R	2/9/2009	ASD closed. No residual shunt normal PAP
20	T	9/12/1999	5	15.5	17	2.3	16	8/11/2009	ASD-R	9/4/2009	ASD closed. No residual shunt normal PAP
21	U	4/23/1989	20	49	17.9	2,4/1	21	8/18/2009	ASD-R	10/9/2009	ASD closed. NO residualshunt, mild PAH
22	V	5/28/1982	27	73	20	1,2/1	20	11/12/2009	ASD-R		
23	W	1/4/2006	3	15.7		1,8/1		12/1/2009	ASD-R		

Table 34.1 (cont.) Blank spaces represent incomplete data at time of publication.

35

The Coherex FlatStent

Olaf Franzen and Stephan Baldus

Introduction

In the 20 years since 1989, when James Lock and colleagues performed the first transcatheter closure in a patient with presumed paradoxical embolism and a patent foramen ovale (PFO),[1] various types of PFO closure devices have been developed. Most of these are derivations of that first device used in Boston. Although there are differences in the materials used—varying from Nitinol mesh to Dacron fabric, polytetrafluoroethylene (PTFE), or intestinal collagen—most of them are single or double disc umbrella-type devices that block flow through the PFO by the application of patches to the septum proper. Typical examples of such devices are the STARFlex Umbrella (NMT Medical, Inc.)[1] and the AMPLATZER PFO Occluder (AGA Medical Corporation, Golden Valley, Minnesota).[2] High closure rates in excess of 90% have

been reported with "patch devices."[3] However, the material left behind in the heart can cause problems such as erosion or perforation, particularly if it is rigid as in metal frames or meshwork.[4] Material exposed to the blood can cause thrombus formation.[5] Consequently, some clinicians include "minimal material left behind" as one of the attributes of the "ideal" PFO closure device.

Intuitively, devices that treat only the PFO tunnel without placing large patches on the interatrial septum do meet the postulation of leaving little material behind. One such approach uses mechanical suturing with a catheter system; this device has been used in a feasibility trial, with complete closure achieved at 3 months in only 1 of 11 patients.[6] Attempts have been made to leave no material at all behind by closing the PFO with radiofrequency current. Although this approach was demonstrated to be feasible and safe in 144 patients, the closure rate of 55% at 6 months did not meet expectations.[7] Recently, CE mark approval was granted to a device that closes the PFO via placement of a stentlike device inside the tunnel. This device, the Coherex FlatStent EF PFO Closure System,[8] is reviewed here.

nel length by incorporating small micro-tines along the framework. The tines engage tunnel tissue and work to further stabilize the implant in the tunnel. Thus, anchors, center-section lateral force, and micro-tines work in combination to engage the tunnel and hold the device in place.

Description of the Coherex FlatStent EF PFO Closure System

The Coherex FlatStent EF PFO Closure System (Coherex Medical, Inc., Salt Lake City, Utah) is a Nitinol-based lattice framework, onto which medical-grade polyurethane foam is attached (Fig 35.1). Along the framework, at specified points, tantalum markers are placed to aid in visualization. The system is available in two sizes, 13 and 19 mm. The size designation indicates the width of the center portion of the FlatStent, that is, the part of the implant that lies within the PFO tunnel. The left atrial anchors, which are intended to engage the PFO tunnel on the left side of the septum, extend 4 mm beyond the designated FlatStent size. Thus, a 19-mm FlatStent has a 27-mm overall anchor span. Similarly, the right atrial anchors, which engage the right atrial side of the PFO tunnel, extend 3 mm outside the center section. However, these anchors are designed to engage the tunnel proper independent of tun-

Description of the Coherex FlatStent Delivery Catheter

The implant arrives preattached to the delivery system. The delivery system is a multilumen catheter of rapid-exchange (monorail) design with a 12F holding pod (Fig 35.2) at its distal end, into which the implant is collapsed for delivery to the PFO. The control handle at the proximal end (Fig 35.3) consists of a stationary handle with a deployment slide on it. The stationary handle is in functional continuity with the outer catheter, whereas the deployment slide is connected to an inner deployment system with tethers at its distal end. These tethers are connected to the implant; two are connected to the outer aspects of the right atrial anchor, and the third tether is connected to the center of the right atrial anchor (Fig 35.4). Advancing the deployment slide on the handle collapses the implant into the distal holding pod of the outer catheter, while retraction deploys the device. The implant can be released from the delivery

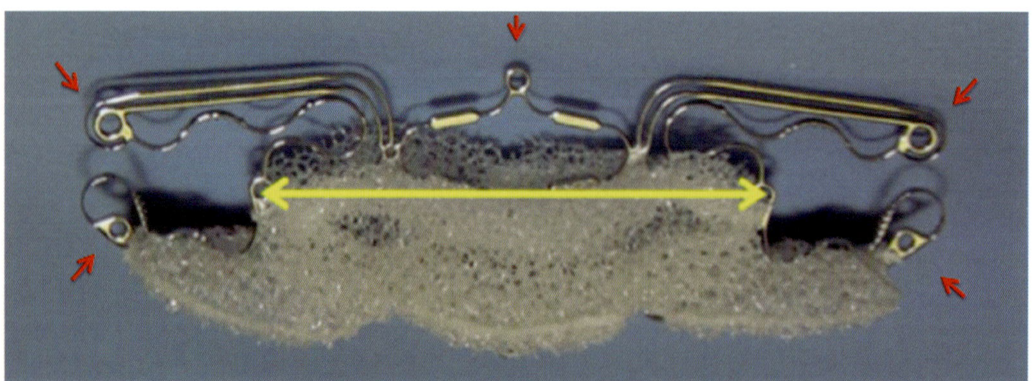

Fig 35.1—The FlatStent device. Red arrows indicate radiopaque markers. (Courtesy of Coherex. Used with permission. Modified by the authors.)

catheter through activation of a release knob located at the end of the handle.

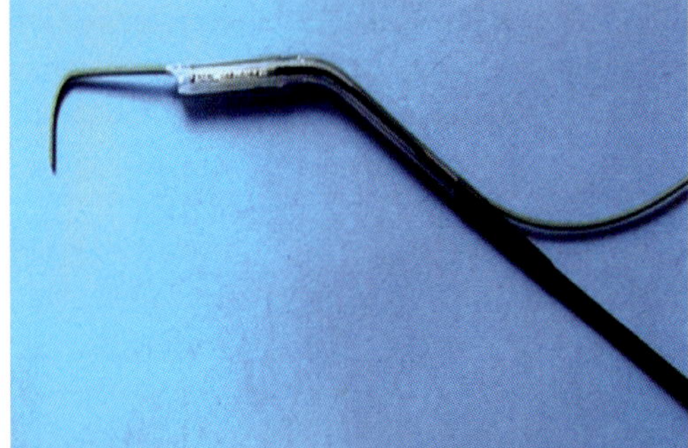

Fig 35.2—Distal end of the delivery catheter with the device collapsed in the holding pod, demonstrating the monorail design of catheter. (Courtesy of Coherex. Used with permission.)

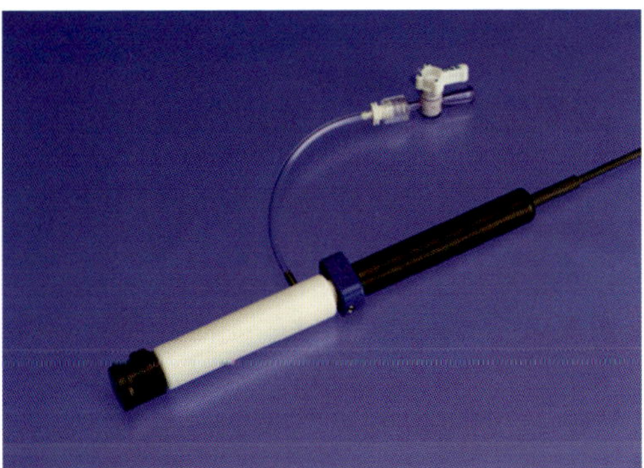

Fig 35.3—Control handle of the delivery system with the stationary handle, the blue sliding handle, and the black release knob at the end of the catheter. (Courtesy of Coherex. Used with permission.)

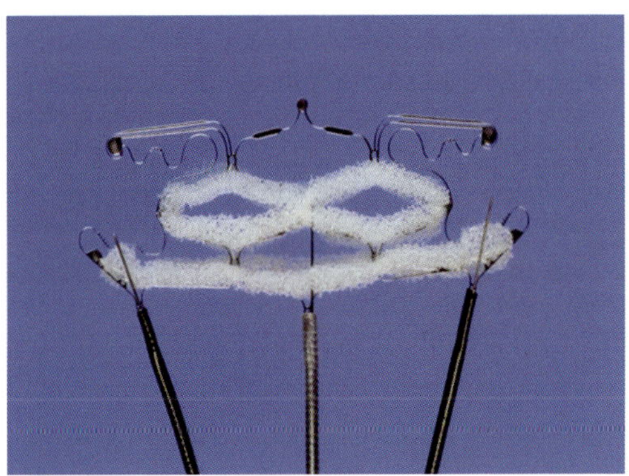

Fig 35.4—Three tethers are connected to the device on three points. (Courtesy of Coherex. Used with permission.)

Working Principle of the Device in Relation to PFO Morphology

A PFO can be described as a flat, open tunnel between the septum primum and septum secundum which have failed to fuse postpartum and therefore overlap like theater curtains. In context with the Coherex FlatStent device, the length of the overlap in which the septum primum lies parallel on the septum secundum is defined as the functional tunnel length (Fig 35.5). It is important to note that with this definition of functional tunnel length the septum primum needs to lie parallel on the septum secundum during all phases of the heart cycle. A region of overlap between the septa, in which the septum primum temporally shifts away from the septum secundum and forms an almost perpendicular appearance, does not contribute to the functional tunnel length (Fig 35.6). The diameter between the lateral borders

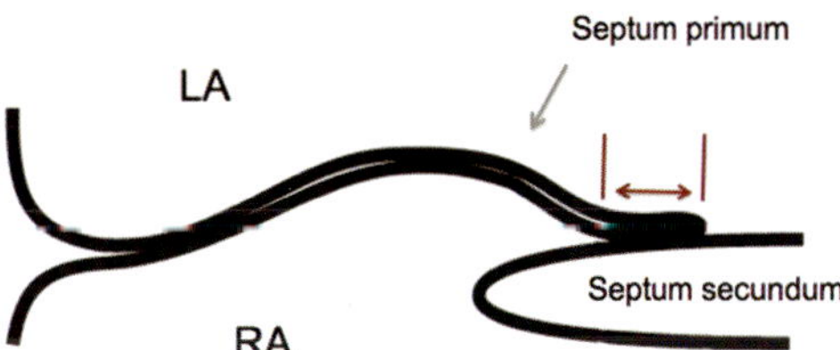

Fig 35.5—Sketch of PFO amenable to treatment with the FlatStent device. Functional tunnel length is indicated by red arrow between the red marker lines. (Courtesy of Coherex. Used with permission. Modified by the authors.)

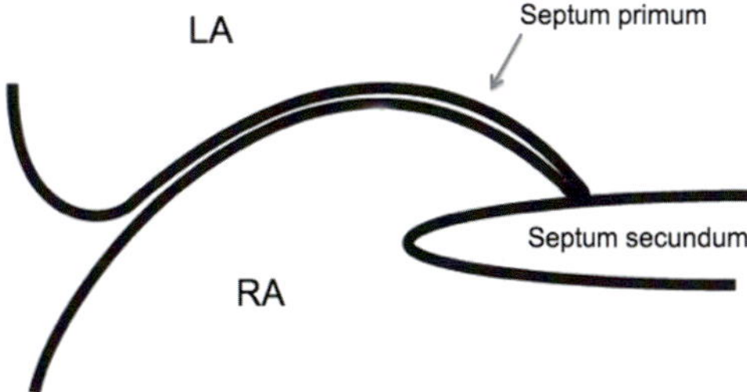

Fig 35.6—Sketch of PFO unfavorable to treatment with the FlatStent device. Septum primum lifts completely from septum secundum (no functional tunnel length). (Courtesy of Coherex. Used with permission. Modified by the authors.)

of the tunnel is defined as the tunnel width. The apices of the PFO tunnel are where the septa eventually join the lateral aspects of the tunnel on both the right and left atrial sides. The working principle underlying the design of the FlatStent is to engage the apices of the tunnel and gently stretch the tunnel along its width, thereby drawing septum secundum and septum primum in close apposition to each other (Fig 35.7). A polymer matrix on the implant helps to fill the tunnel and once endothelialized causes septum secundum and septum primum to fuse.

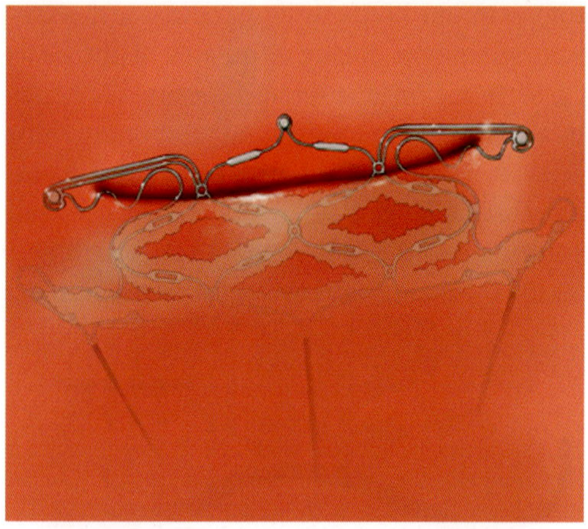

Fig 35.7—Left atrial anchors of the device engaged at the apices of the PFO tunnel. (Courtesy of Coherex. Used with permission.)

Deployment of the FlatStent EF

A 12F sheath is placed in the right femoral vein and the PFO is crossed using a 0.038" or 0.035" standard or stiff wire in concert with a 5 or 6F diagnostic catheter or with the catheter alone. Once the PFO is crossed, a wire is placed in one of the pulmonary veins to provide a stable rail for the sizing balloon and the delivery system. Following balloon sizing of the PFO, a FlatStent EF of appropriate size is selected. The implant is collapsed into the delivery catheter, flushed of air, and inserted over the wire. The implant is advanced such that the tip of the delivery system is in the left atrium.

Deployment of the implant is achieved as follows. By partially pulling back the deployment slide and holding the stationary handle stable, the left atrial anchors and center section of the implant are advanced out of the delivery catheter. The delivery catheter, and thereby the implant, is then retracted toward the septum until the left atrial anchors engage the septum primum. The remainder of the implant is revealed by full retraction of the deployment slide along the stationary handle. After confirming the correct and stable implant position, the guide wire is retracted into the inferior vena cava. The implant can be released from the delivery catheter by activating the release knob located at the end of the stationary handle. As long as it is not released, the implant may be recollapsed within the delivery catheter, redeployed, or retrieved.

Preprocedural, Intraprocedural, and Postprocedural Imaging

The FlatStent EF is readily visible on both fluoroscopy (Fig 35.8) and echocardiography (Fig

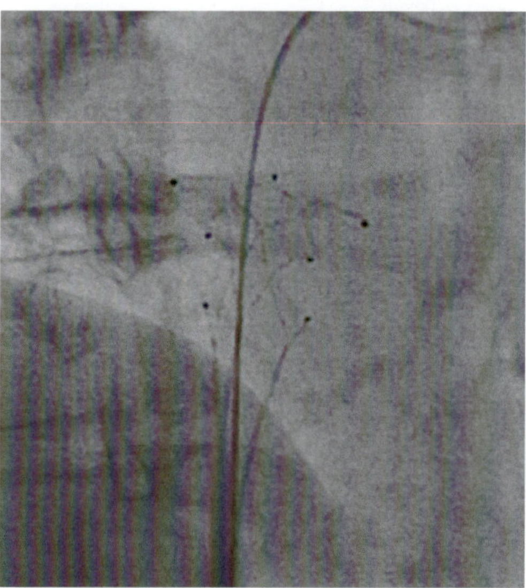

Fig 35.8—Fluoroscopic 30° right anterior oblique view of the Flatstent still attached to the tethers of the delivery catheter.

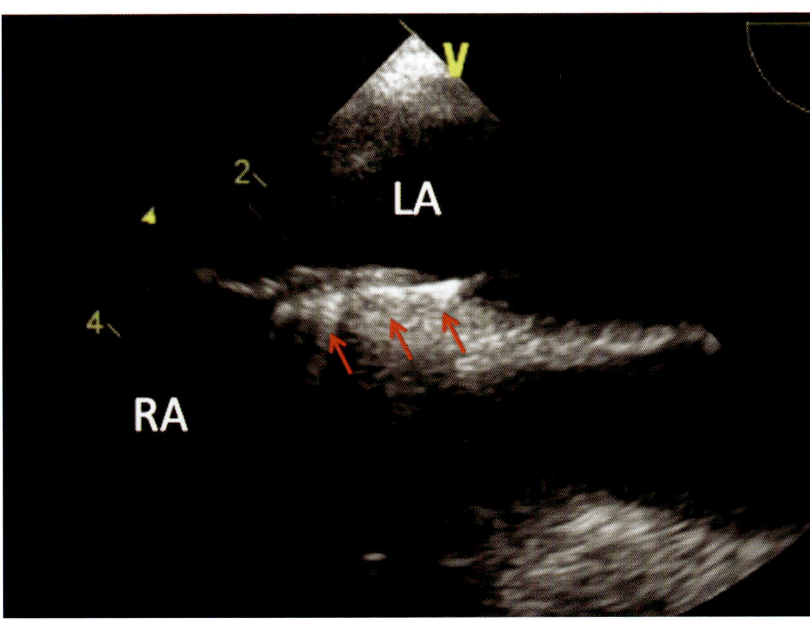

Fig 35.9—TEE "bicaval view" showing correct position of the device after release (arrows) between septum primum and septum secundum. Abbreviations: LA, Left atrium; RA, right atrium.

35.9). Both imaging modalities have their specific advantages in regard to the procedure. A major advantage of echocardiography is that it can directly characterize septal tissue in detail. With fluoroscopy, the septal anatomy can be only indirectly visualized by contrast injection. On the other hand, a metal device with a flat architecture may present a problem for two-dimensional echocardiographic visualization as is can be challenging to find an imaging plane in which the expansions of the device can be properly determined.

Preprocedural Echocardiographic Evaluation

For the exact preprocedural evaluation of the interatrial septum and the PFO, transesophageal echocardiography (TEE) or intracardiac echocardiography (ICE) is mandatory. The morphology of the PFO tunnel must be carefully evaluated because the variety of tunnel morphologies is large. Important TEE imaging planes to characterize PFO morphology prior to FlatStent implantation are the 45° mid-esophageal view ("aortic valve short-axis view") and the 70° to 90° midesophageal view ("bicaval view"). The main question preprocedural echocardiography needs to answer is whether the specific PFO morphology is suitable for FlatStent implantation. Given the design of the device, there are logical aspects for defining suitable tunnel morphology: In the area of the overlap of septum primum and secundum there should be at least 4 mm of functional tunnel (i.e., 4 mm along which the septum primum is parallel to the septum secundum during all phases of the cardiac cycle). The gap between the septa in this functional tunnel should not exceed 8 mm. Unfavorable or unsuitable tunnel morphologies are: (1) too small an overlap of septum secundum and septum primum (< 4 mm) that may not allow stable and anatomically correct device position; and (2) too large a gap between septum primum and secundum (> 8 mm) because it may increase the risk of a residual shunt (the size of this gap is best determined in the bicaval view).

Currently, there is no reliable echocardiographic method to determine the tunnel width. Therefore, the correct size of the device must be determined periprocedurally by balloon sizing or contrast injection. Attention must also be given to fenestrations of the interatrial septum because an in-tunnel device will not cover those.

Periprocedural imaging

Exact image guidance to position the implant in the functional tunnel is crucial for a successful procedure. But the use of echocardiographic guidance may be difficult. Aside from the principal reasons mentioned previously, this is primarily because—given the flat design of the implant—the wire and the implant echoes may merge, making it difficult to distinguish between the two. However, the combination with fluoroscopy allows detailed monitoring of the deployment process.

To achieve fluoroscopic contrast images, a long sheath on the guide wire with the tip directly placed before the right atrial inlet of the PFO tunnel can be used. In standard (50°) left anterior oblique and ~30° right anterior oblique views, contrast injection is performed through the sheath to profile the septum secundum, septum primum, and PFO tunnel (Fig 35.10). The same views are used to perform balloon sizing

of the PFO. In concert with the echocardiographic examination, these images determine tunnel morphology, including tunnel length and tunnel width, as well as the extent of septal mobility. Based on this information, device size is selected. For a tunnel width between 4 and 8 mm, the 13-mm FlatStent is recommended; for a tunnel width > 8 mm, the 19-mm device is recommended.

For deployment of the implant, the ~30° right anterior oblique view is used, placing the device in an "en face" view parallel to the septal plane. In this view the different stages of device deployment can be readily monitored with fluoroscopy. If necessary, the implant is rotated clockwise or counterclockwise to improve alignment with the septal plane. When the left atrial anchors begin to engage the apices of the PFO tunnel, they will bend slightly so that the rest of the implant can be deployed in the PFO tunnel under fluoroscopic visualization. The correct device position in the PFO is verified in the 50° left anterior oblique view by another contrast injection (Fig 35.11). This injection also tests for complete closure of the PFO.

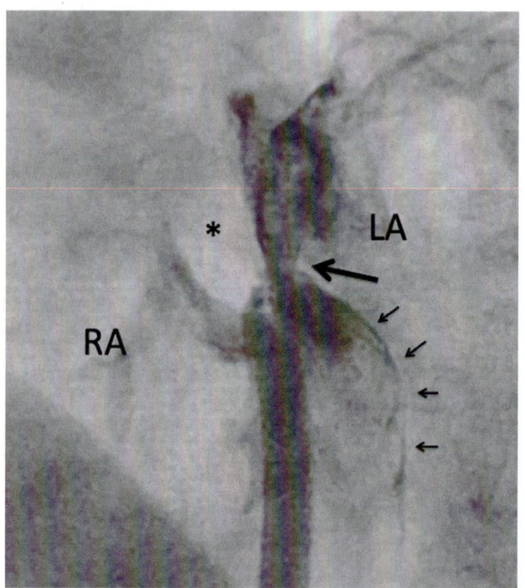

Fig 35.10—Fluoroscopic 50° left anterior oblique view with contrast injection into the PFO tunnel, asterisk (*) indicating septum secundum, small arrows indicating septum primum, large arrow indicating PFO tunnel. Abbreviations: LA, Left atrium; RA, right atrium.

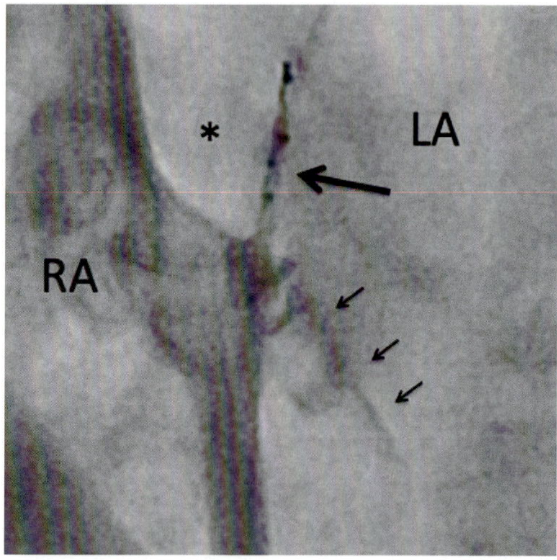

Fig 35.11—Fluoroscopic 50° left anterior oblique view with contrast injection prior to release of the device, demonstrating correct position and complete PFO closure, asterisk (*) indicating septum secundum, small arrows indicating septum primum, large arrow indicating Flatstent implant within PFO tunnel. Abbreviations: LA, Left atrium; RA, right atrium.

Correct orientation of the implant in the tunnel or misalignment that holds the tunnel open and prevents complete closure can also be assessed by TEE. Carefully pushing and pulling the device under fluoroscopy will demonstrate a bowing of the tethers and a bowing of the left atrial anchors, retrospectively. After release of the implant, both fluoroscopy and echocardiography (see Fig 35.9) can correctly determine device position and complete closure.

Follow-up echocardiography

Detection of a residual shunt, assessment of device position, and exclusion of complications are the purposes of follow-up echocardiography examinations. Device position can be readily determined by TEE even though there is not much solid-body material in the septum. In unclear situations during follow-up, an x-ray examination of the chest can exclude device embolization.

Postprocedural Care

Patients receive acetylsalicylic acid for 3 months and clopidogrel for 1 month after device implantation.

Preliminary Clinical Results with the Coherex FlatStent EF PFO Closure System

The results from the CE mark trial for the Flat-Stent have been reported in abstract form; the final results of the trial await completion of long-term follow-up. Based on abstract presentations at major interventional cardiology meetings, some early observations can be reported and preliminary conclusions made.[9-14]

First, although the FlatStent EF has been reported as easy to use, there is a need to better understand tunnel morphology. The FlatStent performs best with tunnel lengths of 4 mm or longer.

Second, acute and short-term follow-up results have demonstrated clinically effective closure rates on the order of 94% (15 of 16 patients with complete closure after 180 days[9]).

Third, device embolization in the learning phase with this implant has occurred in 3 of 49 patients[9]; in all cases the device was implanted in a tunnel length < 4 mm. All three devices were retrieved by catheter. Use of the push-pull test may reduce the risk of embolization by providing ample proof of device stability prior to release. There have been no reports of thrombus, perforation, erosion, air embolus, or transient or persistent arrhythmia.

Summary and Conclusions

The Coherex FlatStent EF PFO Closure Device is a self-expanding device with only a small amount of foreign material implanted. It is placed in the PFO tunnel such that only a small amount of material is exposed to the blood in the left and right atria. The device is fully repositionable and retrievable and can be implanted via 12F venous access. Patients selected for treatment with this device should have an overlap of at least 4 mm of the septum primum and secundum. Exact positioning of the device is important. Device implantation can be guided by fluoroscopy and echocardiography. Initial preliminary clinical follow-up data have been reported orally, demonstrating high closure rates and a low risk profile. Embolization was an issue in the early learning phase with this device.[9-14] Published follow-up is pending.

The concept of "leaving less material behind"—and only in the PFO tunnel—instead of "patching" the atrial septum is appealing; particularly, since more and more interventions emerge that require access to the left atrium. Furthermore, some complications of percutaneous PFO closure are related to the size and material of the closure devices.[4] Therefore, less material could also mean fewer complications. On the other hand, earlier devices utilizing the concept of minimal or no material could not demonstrate the same high closure rates of established patch devices.[1-3,6,7] High closure rates with minimal or no complications must be the dictum of all new PFO devices. Initial preliminary data of the FlatStent are encouraging, also in regard to closure rates.[9-14] After further confirmation of these data it seems worthwhile to strengthen the efforts to prove the potential advantages of the system.

Acknowledgments

The authors wish to thank Coherex Medical, Inc., (in particular, Mr. Rudy Davis) for photography, illustrations, and technical descriptions of the device.

References

1. Bridges ND, Hellenbrand W, Latson L, Filiano J, Newburger JW, Lock JE. Transcatheter closure of patent foramen ovale after presumed paradoxical embolism. *Circulation.* 1992;86:1902–1908.

2. Han YM, Gu X, Titus JL, et al. New self-expanding patent foramen ovale occlusion device. *Cathet Cardiovasc Intervent.* 1999;47:370–376.

3. Spies C, Reissmann U, Timmermanns I, Schräder R. Comparison of contemporary devices used for transcatheter patent foramen ovale closure. *J Invasive Cardiol.* 2008;20:442–447.

4. Amin Z, Hijazi ZM, Bass JL, Cheatham JP, Hellenbrand WE, Kleinman CS. Erosion of AMPLATZER septal occluder device after closure of secundum atrial septal defects: review of registry of complications and recommendations to minimize future risk. *Cathet Cardiovasc Intervent.* 2004;63:496–502.

5. Krumsdorf U, Ostermayer S, Billinger K, et al. Incidence and clinical course of thrombus formation on atrial septal defect and patient foramen ovale closure devices in 1,000 consecutive

patients. *J Am Coll Cardiol.* 2004;43:302–309.

6. Majunke N, Baranowski A, Zimmermann W, et al. A suture is not always the ideal solution: problems encountered in developing a suture-based PFO closure technique. *Cathet Cardiovasc Intervent.* 2009;73:376–382.

7. Sievert H, Ruygrok P, Salkeld M, et al. Transcatheter closure of patent foramen ovale with radiofrequency: acute and intermediate term results in 144 patients. *Cathet Cardiovasc Intervent.* 2009;73:368–373.

8. Reiffenstein I, Majunke N, Wunderlich N, Carter P, Jones R, Siever H. Percutaneous closure of patent foramen ovale with a novel FlatStent. *Expert Rev Med Devices.* 2008;5:419–425.

9. Sievert H, Wunderlich N, Grube E, et al. Interim results of a multi-center study to evaluate the safety and efficacy of the Coherex FlatStent EF PFO Closure System. Oral presentation. 32nd Annual Scientific Sessions of the Society for Cardiac Angiography and Interventions; May 6–9, 2009; Las Vegas, Nev.

10. Jones R. The Coherex FlatStent: Closure inside the PFO. Oral presentation. EuroPCR09; May 19–22, 2009; Barcelona, Spain,

11. Muller D. The Coherex FlatStent EF: New device, short learning curve. Oral presentation. Transcatheter Cardiovascular Therapeutics 2009; September 21–25, 2009; San Francisco, Calif.

12. Ruygrok P. The Coherex FlatStent EF: A case based review. Oral presentation. Transcatheter Cardiovascular Therapeutics 2009; September 21–25, 2009; San Francisco, Calif.

13. Sievert H. The Coherex FlatStent EF PFO Closure System: Lessons learned from the clinical experience. Oral presentation. Transcatheter Cardiovascular Therapeutics 2009; September 21–25, 2009; San Francisco, Calif.

14. Ruygrok P. The Coherex FlatStent EF: Results from the CE trial. Oral presentation. Transcatheter Cardiovascular Therapeutics 2009; September 21–25, 2009; San Francisco, Calif.

36

The St. Jude Medical Premere Device for PFO Closure

Jennifer Franke, Stefan Bertog, and Horst Sievert

Introduction

The Premere PFO Closure System from St. Jude Medical, Inc., is specifically designed for PFO closure (Fig 36.1). It is known that the individual variation of the PFO tunnel morphology depends highly on the length of its tunnel, the configuration of the right and left atrial openings and the thickness of the interatrial septum itself. To suit the individual needs of these PFO and septal characteristics without causing tissue distortion, the Premere device features two cross-shaped nitinol anchors. The right-sided anchor is positioned between two membranes of knitted polyester. The left-sided nitinol anchor is uncovered. As shown in Figure 36.2, a flexible polyester braided tether connects the two nitinol anchors of the device and allows the left and right anchor arms to

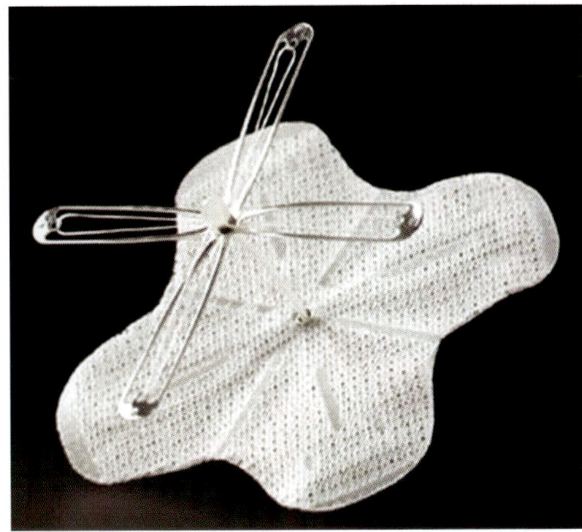

Figure 36.1—The Premere PFO Closure System. (Courtesy of St. Jude Medical, Inc.)

conform independently to different variations in septal thickness without any distortion of

---

the atrial anatomy. One end of the tether is linked to the left-sided anchor, and the other end is connected to the external side of the delivery system. The right-sided anchor is connected to the delivery guide-wire. Once the right-sided anchor is released, the distance between the two anchors can be adjusted according to the unique anatomy of a patient's PFO. Thereafter, the position of the right-sided anchor is locked. The final position is shown in Figures 36.3–36.5. More important features of the Premere device are the open architecture and low profile of the left anchor arm. The low amount of nitinol used for the nitinol cross-shaped anchor architecture allows high flexibility and rapid endothelialization. Furthermore, this specific design may minimize the risk of thrombus formation on the device and reduce the potential for atrial tissue erosion. The device is available in diameters of 20 and 25 mm, whereas a 30 mm device is currently under development. The Premere PFO Closure System has CE mark.

Trial Studies

The safety and efficacy of the Premere device has been demonstrated in several prospective studies. To date, the largest published study is the CLOSEUP trial.[1] Sixty-seven patients with cryptogenic stroke or transient ischemic attack and PFO were enrolled to receive the Premere device. It was successfully implanted in all patients with no major complications. At a follow-up at 6 months with contrast echocardiography, the closure rate was 86%. Importantly, there were no recurrent cerebral ischemic events. Likewise, a closure rate of 94% was reported in 104 patients with cryptogenic stroke, transient ischemic attack or peripheral embolism.[2] There were no major complications except device embolization to the pulmonary artery in one patient with successful percutaneous retrieval. Once again, at 12 months follow-up, there were no recurrent embolic events. Finally, excellent closure rates have been reported in several smaller studies.[3–5]

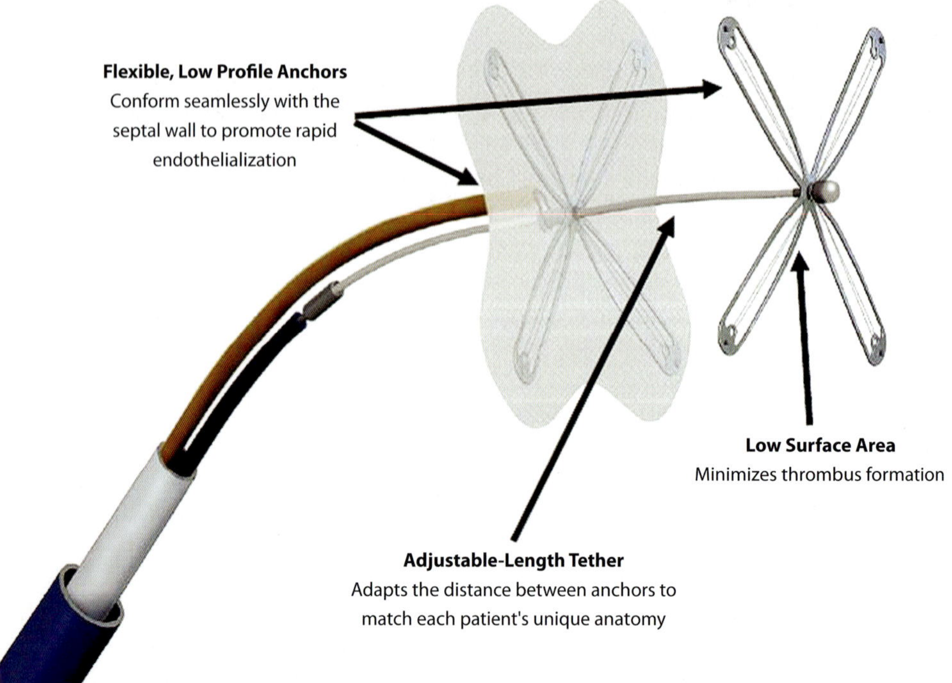

Figure 36.2—Implant Assembly of the Premere PFO Closure System. (Courtesy of St. Jude Medical, Inc.)

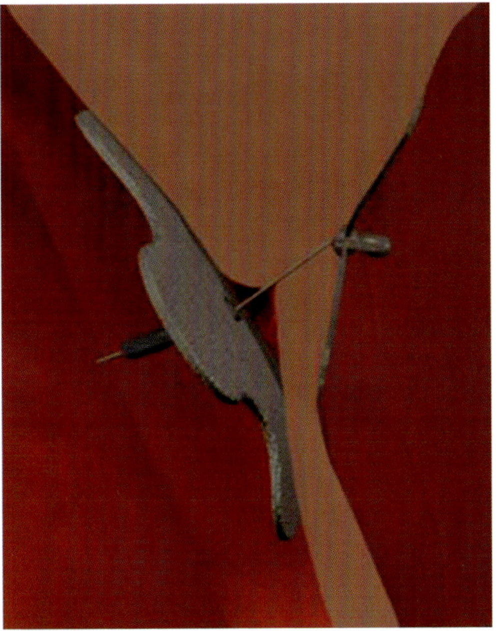

Figure 36.3—Scheme of Final Position of the Premere PFO Closure System after Release. (Courtesy of St. Jude Medical, Inc.)

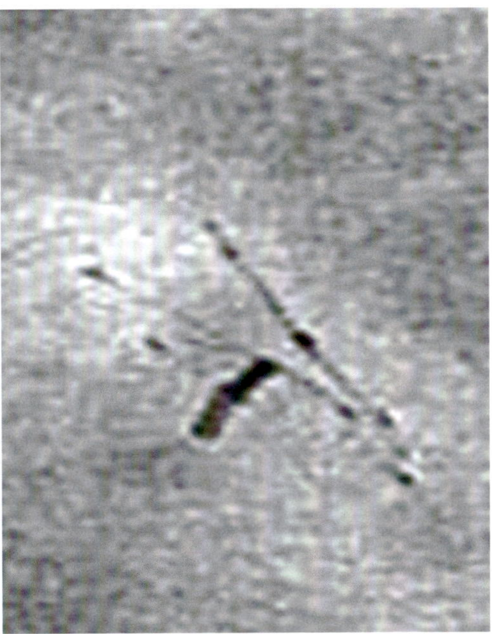

Figure 36.4—Final Position of the Premere PFO Closure System as seen in Fluoroscopy. (Courtesy of St. Jude Medical, Inc.)

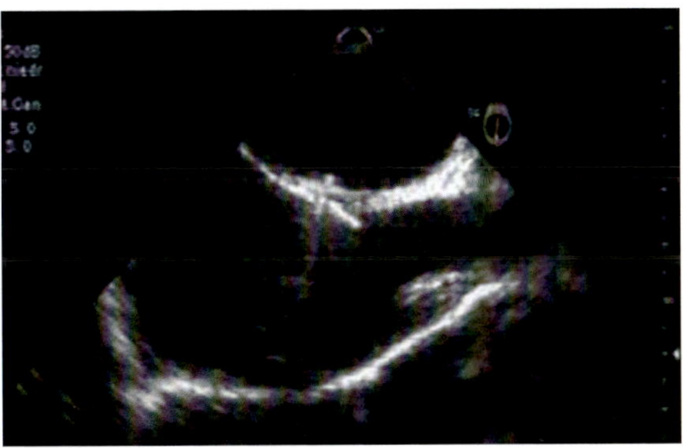

Figure 36.5—Final Position of the Premere PFO Closure System as seen in TEE. (Courtesy of St. Jude Medical, Inc.)

References

1. Büscheck F, Sievert H, Kieber F, et al. Patent foramen ovale using the Premere device: the results of the CLOSEUP trial. *J Interv Cardiol.* 2006;19(4):328–33.

2. Nobel D, Weilenmann O, Kretschmar F, et al. Interventional PFO-closure using the Premere device: A triple-centre experience. In *European Society of Cardiology Scientific Meeting.* 2008: Munich, Germany.

3. Rigatelli G, Cardaioli P, Braggion G, et al. Resolution of migraine by transcatheter patent foramen ovale closure with Premere Occlusion System in a preliminary series of patients with previous cerebral ischemia. *Catheter Cardiovasc Interv.* 2007; 70(3):429–33.

4. Rigatelli G, Dell'Avvocata F, Ronco F, et al. Patent oval foramen transcatheter closure: results of a strategy based on tailoring the device to the specific patient's anatomy. *Cardiol Young.* 2010; 20(2):144–49.

5. Reyes, RM, Galeote G, Moreno R, et al. Percutaneous PFO closure using the Premere device occluder: initial experience. *Rev Port Cardiol.* 2009; 28(11):1225–30.

Boxes are indicated by b, figures by f ,
and tables by t following the page number.